PHARMACOKINETIC BASIS FOR DRUG TREATMENT

Pharmacokinetic Basis for Drug Treatment

Editors

Leslie Z. Benet, Ph.D.

Professor and Chairman
Department of Pharmacy
School of Pharmacy
University of California, San Francisco
San Francisco, California

Neil Massoud, M.S., Pharm.D.

Postdoctoral Fellow
Division of Clinical Pharmacology
Departments of Medicine and Pharmacy
University of California, San Francisco
San Francisco, California

John G. Gambertoglio, Pharm.D.

Associate Clinical Professor
Division of Clinical Pharmacy
School of Pharmacy
University of California, San Francisco
San Francisco, California

Raven Press ■ New York

Raven Press, 1140 Avenue of the Americas, New York, New York 10036

Made in the United States of America

Library of Congress Cataloging in Publication Data
Main entry under title;

Pharmacokinetic basis for drug treatment.

Includes bibliographical references and index.
1. Pharmacokinetics. 2.Chemotherapy. I. Benet,
Leslie Z. II. Massoud, Neil. III. Gambertoglio,
John G. [DNLM: 1. Drug therapy. 2. Pharmacology,
Clinical. QV 38 P532]
RM301.5.P46   1983   615.7   83-9512
ISBN 0-89004-874-6

Preface

In 1973, Mitenko and Ogilvie attempted to develop a logical theophylline dosage regimen based on the drug's established pharmacokinetics and pharmacodynamics. Although the temporary acceptance of the recommendations by the general medical community represented a great step forward for clinical pharmacokinetics as a science, the acceptance proved to be premature and reverberations are still being felt today. The problem was that their recommendations were appropriate only for nonacutely ill asthmatics. An enormous variability in the true patient population was soon found, and patients were often seriously overdosed or underdosed. In time, subpopulations with distinct physiologically altered pharmacokinetics were identified, and an entirely new set of recommendations presently exists for theophylline dosage among these populations.

At any point in the history of health care, our knowledge was considered to be quite extensive; however, in perspective, the knowledge of yesterday seems to have been very limited, just as today's knowledge can be expected to seem one day as such. It is apparent that a great void exists and, as a result, there continues to be a need to expand and accumulate knowledge and information. In this expansion, clinical pharmacokinetics has evolved as a new science in health care. As such, it often has given answers that were ambiguous or, as with the initial theophylline dosage guidelines, highly questionable. For this reason, in the development of this science, one must always question ideas and constantly challenge assumptions made in the process of developing this field. Fundamental in applying basic scientific and mathematical concepts to patient care is an appreciation of the physiologic constraints placed on these concepts and an appreciation of how disease and/or physiologic changes can further affect these constraints.

This book covers pharmacokinetics in all the common diseases, as well as drug clearance, and altered plasma protein binding. It provides values for patients with specific diseases, along with normal values obtained from volunteers. It is comprehensive, with chapters discussing aspects of pharmacokinetics in regard to the care of pediatric and geriatric patients, the effects of smoking and pregnancy, and the placental transfer of drugs.

To date, this is the only book to provide the pharmacokinetic concepts and relevant parameters necessary to design more tailored dosage regimens for specific patient populations. This book will be of interest to pharmacists, pharmacologists, and prescribing physicians.

Acknowledgments

The editors wish to acknowledge the following individuals: Dr. G. O. Barbezat of the University of Otago, New Zealand; Dr. Jorden L. Cohen of the University of Southern California; Dr. Gedy Gudauskas at the Cancer Control Agency of British Columbia; Dr. Martha Harkey at the French Hospital Medical Center, San Francisco; Dr. John H. Holbrook of the University of Utah; and Dr. Beatrice Krauer at the Hospital Cantonal, Geneva. The editors also acknowledge their colleagues at the University of California, San Francisco: Drs. Donald Alexander, Nicholas H. G. Holford, Robert H. Levin, Diane Dan-Shya Tang-Lui, Michael E. Winter, and Robert A. Upton. All of the above individuals provided critical evaluations of specific chapters in this text.

Contents

Contributors

Stuart L. Beal, Ph.D.
Associate Professor of Biostatistics
Department of Laboratory Medicine
and Departments of Pharmacy
and Medicine
Division of Clinical Pharmacology
University of California, San
Francisco
San Francisco, California 94143

Leslie Z. Benet, Ph.D.
Professor and Chairman,
Department of Pharmacy
School of Pharmacy
University of California, San
Francisco
San Francisco, California 94143

Neal L. Benowitz, M.D.
Associate Professor of Medicine,
Clinical Pharmacology Unit,
Medical Service
San Francisco General Hospital
Medical Center
and
Department of Medicine
University of California,
San Francisco
San Francisco, California 94143

Robert A. Branch, M.D.,
M.R.C.P.
Associate Professor, Departments
of Medicine and Pharmacology
School of Medicine
Vanderbilt University
Nashville, Tennessee 37232

D. Craig Brater, M.D.
Associate Professor of
Pharmacology and Internal
Medicine
The University of Texas Health
Science Center at Dallas
Department of Pharmacology
5323 Harry Hines Boulevard
Dallas, Texas 75235

Polavat Chennavasin, M.D.
Assistant Professor of
Pharmacology and Internal
Medicine
The University of Texas Health
Science Center at Dallas
Department of Pharmacology
5323 Harry Hines Boulevard
Dallas, Texas 75235

Robert M. Elenbaas,
Pharm.D.
Associate Professor, Schools of
Pharmacy and Medicine
University of Missouri
Kansas City, Missouri 64108

John G. Gambertoglio,
Pharm.D.
Associate Clinical Professor,
Division of Clinical Pharmacy
School of Pharmacy
University of California,
San Francisco
San Francisco, California 94143

Thomas P. Green, M.D.
Assistant Professor, Division of
Clinical Pharmacology
Departments of Pediatrics and
Pharmacology
University of Minnesota
Minneapolis, Minnesota 55455

Erna Halberg, Ph.D.
Research Associate, Chronobiology
Laboratories
Department of Laboratory Medicine
and Pathology
University of Minnesota
Minneapolis, Minnesota 55455

Franz Halberg, M.D.
*Professor of Laboratory Medicine
and Director, Chronobiology
Laboratories
Department of Laboratory Medicine
and Pathology
University of Minnesota
Minneapolis, Minnesota 55455*

William J. Jusko, Ph.D.
*Professor of Pharmaceutics,
Director, Division of Clinical
Pharmacy Sciences
Department of Pharmaceutics
School of Pharmacy
State University of New York
at Buffalo
Amherst, New York 14260*

Lawrence J. Lesko, Ph.D.
*Associate Professor, Clinical
Pharmacokinetics Laboratory
School of Pharmacy
University of Maryland
610 West Lombard Street
Baltimore, Maryland 21201*

**Neil Massoud, M.S.,
Pharm.D.**
*Postdoctoral Fellow, Division of
Clinical Pharmacology
Schools of Medicine and Pharmacy
University of California, San
Francisco
San Francisco, California 94143*

**Bernard L. Mirkin, Ph.D.,
M.D.**
*Director, Division of Clinical
Pharmacology
Departments of Pediatrics and
Pharmacology
University of Minnesota
Minneapolis, Minnesota 55455*

William A. Parker, Pharm.D.
*Associate Professor, College of
Pharmacy
Dalhousie University
Halifax, Nova Scotia, Canada B3H 3J5*

Carl C. Peck, M.D.
*Associate Professor of Medicine,
Chief of the Division of Clinical
Pharmacology
Departments of Medicine and
Pharmacology
Uniformed Services
University of the Health Sciences
Bethesda, Maryland 20014*

C. E. Pippenger, Ph.D.
*Department of Biochemistry
Cleveland Clinic Foundation
Cleveland, Ohio 44106*

**Susan M. Pond, M.B., B.S.,
M.D.**
*Assistant Professor of Medicine,
Medical Service and Division of
Clinical Pharmacology
San Francisco General Hospital
Medical Center
and
Department of Medicine
University of California,
San Francisco
San Francisco, California 94110*

**Douglas E. Rollins, M.D.,
Ph.D.**
*Acting Director, Division of
Clinical Pharmacology
Departments of Medicine and
Pharmacology
University of Utah School of
Medicine
Salt Lake City, Utah 84132*

Robert A. Roth, Jr., Ph.D.
*Associate Professor of
Pharmacology and Toxicology,
Department of Pharmacology
and Toxicology
Michigan State University
East Lansing, Michigan 48824*

Ronald J. Sawchuk, Ph.D.
*Associate Professor of
Pharmaceutics, Department of
Pharmaceutics
College of Pharmacy
University of Minnesota
Minneapolis, Minnesota 55455*

Lewis B. Sheiner, M.D.
Professor, Departments of
Laboratory Medicine and
Medicine
School of Medicine
University of California,
San Francisco
San Francisco, California 94143

Thomas N. Tozer, Ph.D.
Professor of Pharmacy and
Pharmaceutical Chemistry,
Department of Pharmacy
School of Pharmacy
University of California,
San Francisco
San Francisco, California 94143

Peter G. Welling, Ph.D.
Professor of Pharmaceutics, School
of Pharmacy
University of Wisconsin, Madison
Madison, Wisconsin 53706

Grant R. Wilkinson, Ph.D.
Professor of Pharmacology,
Department of Pharmacology
School of Medicine
Vanderbilt University
Nashville, Tennessee 37232

Roger L. Williams, M.D.
Assistant Professor of Medicine and
Pharmacy
Departments of Medicine and Pharmacy
University of California,
San Francisco
San Francisco, California 94143

Pharmacokinetic Basis for Drug Treatment,
edited by L. Z. Benet et al., Raven Press,
New York © 1984

Chapter 1

Pharmacokinetics

Leslie Z. Benet and *Neil Massoud

*Department of Pharmacy and *Division of Clinical Pharmacology, Schools of Pharmacy
and Medicine, University of California, San Francisco, California 94143*

Drug treatment, or therapeutics, has historically been associated with pharmacodynamics, the study of "what the drug does to the body." It has long been recognized that disease states may modify the relationship between drug dosing and both drug efficacy and drug toxicity. More recently, it has become obvious that disease states may modify pharmacokinetics and/or pharmacodynamics, and that it is impossible to isolate the particular effect of a disease on these two processes without investigating the time course of a drug and its metabolites in the patient. The aim of this volume is to provide a comprehensive review and critical compilation of the information available concerning the effects of disease states on pharmacokinetics, that is, the information which describes "what the body does to the drug." This information may then serve to provide a rational basis for the initial adjustment of drug treatment in a particular patient. Neither the title of this volume, nor the encyclopedic compilation of clinical pharmacokinetic information provided should be interpreted as implying that the effects of disease on pharmacodynamics are unimportant. However, at this point in time, few studies have addressed the separation of the effect of disease on pharmacokinetics and pharmacodynamics. When available, the information is provided in the chapters which follow.

When a clinician prescribes a drug, and a patient takes it, their fundamental concern is with the beneficial effect of the agent on the patient's disease. However, as illustrated in Fig. 1, several processes are interposed between administration of the dose, the resulting plasma or blood concentration, and the appearance of the drug's therapeutic effect. Physiological processes determine how rapidly, at what concentration, and for how long the drug will appear at the target organ. Three steps shown in Fig. 1—bioavailability, distribution, and clearance (loss)—represent three major pharmacokinetic variables (1). In most cases, the drug will be administered to the body via the most convenient site that meets the requirements for speed and completeness of availability. The pattern of the concentration/time curve measurable in the blood is a function of the bioavailability, distribution, and loss factors. The various chapters in this book will address how each of the pharmacokinetic factors may be modified in disease (see Fig. 1).

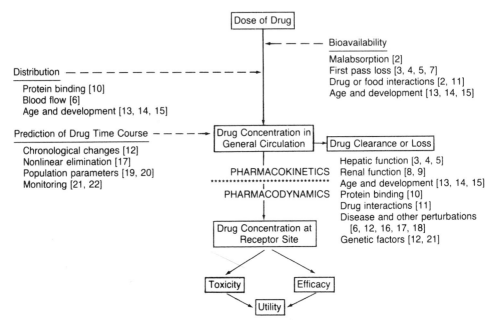

FIG. 1. Schematic interrelationship of pharmacokinetics and pharmacodynamics *(above and below starred line)* in the dose–utility paradigm. Numbers in brackets refer to chapters in this volume where pharmacokinetic concepts are discussed.

Pharmacokinetics is the mathematical relationship that exists between the dose of a drug and the concentration of the drug in a readily accessible site in the body (e.g., plasma or blood). Pharmacodynamics extends this relationship to the correlation between measured concentrations of drug and the pharmacologic effect. This mathematical relationship has been documented for many drugs (2,3) (see Appendixes A–C), although for some drugs, no direct or simple relationship has been found between pharmacologic effect and plasma or blood concentrations. In most cases, the concentration of drug in the general circulation will be related to the concentrations of drug at its site(s) of action (Fig. 1). The drug at the site of action may then elicit a number of pharmacologic effects. These pharmacologic effects can include the desired clinical effect or one or more toxic effects, and in some cases there may be effects unrelated to either the desired effect or toxicity of the drug. The clinician must balance the toxic potential of a particular dose of a drug with its efficacy in determining the utility of the drug.

Pharmacokinetics and pharmacodynamics play roles in the dose–efficacy scheme by describing the quantitative relationship between drug efficacy and dose by means of measurements of drug concentrations in various biological fluids. The importance of pharmacokinetics in patient care rests on the improvement in drug efficacy that can be attained when measurements of drug concentrations in the general circulation are combined with traditional methods of predicting drug dosages (see Chapters 21 and 22). With knowledge of the pharmacokinetic profile of a particular medication and the relationship between efficacy and drug concentration measurements, the

clinician can take into account the various pathological and physiological features that make a particular patient different from the normal individual in responding to a dose of the drug. This will be especially important for a drug with a narrow therapeutic index (e.g., digoxin) where there is only a small difference between the concentration producing therapeutic benefit and the concentration that will produce toxic manifestations. Application of the principles presented in this and subsequent chapters will be of further value in cases where the response is inadequate, where target concentrations may not have been achieved, or in an overdose situation.

PHARMACOKINETIC PARAMETERS

The various pathological and physiological variables that dictate dosage adjustment in individual patients do so by modifying specific pharmacokinetic parameters. The two basic independent parameters are clearance, a measure of the body's ability to eliminate drug, and volume of distribution, a measure of the apparent space in the body available to contain the drug.

CLEARANCE

Clearance is the most important concept to be considered in defining a rational drug dosage regimen. In most cases the clinician would like to maintain steady state drug concentrations within a known therapeutic range (see Appendixes A–C). The steady state will be achieved when the rate of drug elimination equals the rate of input:

$$\text{Dosing rate} = CL \cdot C_{ss} \qquad (1)$$

Thus, if the desired steady state concentration (plasma or blood) is known, the clearance value in that patient will dictate the dosing rate.

Drug clearance principles are similar to the clearance concepts in renal physiology, in which creatinine clearance is defined as the rate of elimination of the creatinine in the urine relative to the plasma creatinine concentration (see Chapter 8). At the simplest level, clearance of a drug is the rate of elimination by all routes relative to the concentration of drug in any biologic fluid:

$$CL = \text{rate of elimination}/C \qquad (2)$$

It is important to remember that clearance does not indicate how much drug is being removed but rather the volume of blood or plasma which would be completely cleared of drug if it were present. Clearance can thus be expressed as a volume per unit of time.

Clearance *(CL)* is usually further defined as blood clearance *(CL_b)*, plasma clearance *(CL_p)*, or clearance based on unbound or free drug concentration *(CL_u)*, depending on the concentration measured *(C_b, C_p, or C_u)*.

In Appendix B, the plasma clearance for ampicillin is reported as 270 ml/min, with 90% of the drug excreted in the urine unchanged. In other words, the kidney is able to completely remove this drug at a rate of approximately 240 ml of plasma

per minute. Because clearance is usually assumed to remain constant in a stable patient, the rate of ampicillin elimination will depend on the concentration of drug in the plasma, as described by Eq. 2. Propranolol is cleared at a rate of 800 ml/ min, almost exclusively by the liver. In this case, the liver is able to remove the drug from 800 ml of plasma per minute. For the drugs listed in Appendix B, one of the highest plasma clearance values is for imipramine, 1,400 ml/min, a value often exceeding plasma flow to the liver, the dominant organ of elimination for this drug. However, because this drug apparently partitions readily into red blood cells (C_{rbc}/C_p = 2.7), the amount of drug delivered to the excretory organ is considerably higher than plasma flow indicates. The relationship between plasma and blood clearance at steady state is given by:

$$\frac{CL_p}{CL_b} = \frac{C_b}{C_p} = 1 + H \left(\frac{C_{rbc}}{C_p} - 1\right) \tag{3}$$

One may solve for imipramine clearance in blood by substituting the red blood cell to plasma concentration ratio and the average value for the hematocrit (H = 0.45). Then, imipramine clearance, when measured in terms of blood concentration (800 ml/min) is in the physiologic range of blood flow measurements. Thus, like the volume of distribution (to be explained later in this chapter), the plasma clearance may assume proportions that are not "physiologic." A drug with an extremely low plasma concentration that is concentrated in the red blood cells (e.g., mecamylamine) can show a plasma clearance of tens of liters per minute. However, if blood concentration is used to define clearance, the maximum clearance possible is equal to the sum of blood flow to the various organs of elimination (Table 1) (4). For a drug eliminated solely by the liver, blood clearance is therefore limited by the flow of blood to that organ, approximately 1,500 ml/min.

It is important to note the additive character of clearance. Elimination of drug may occur as a result of processes occurring in the kidney, the liver, and other organs. Dividing the rate of elimination at each organ by a concentration of drug (e.g., plasma concentration) will yield the respective clearance at that organ. Added together, these separate clearances will equal total systemic clearance:

$$CL_{renal} + CL_{hepatic} + CL_{other} = CL_{systemic} \tag{4}$$

The example provided in Eq. 4 indicates that the drug is eliminated by liver (see Chapters 3 and 4), kidney (Chapters 8 and 9), and other tissues and that these routes of elimination are additive except for drugs additionally removed by the lung (see Chapter 7). Other routes of elimination could include saliva (Chapter 21), sweat, partition into the gut (see Chapter 2), and additional sites of metabolism such as hydrolysis in blood or muscle.

The two major sites of drug elimination are the kidney and liver. Clearance of drug detected unchanged in the urine is represented by renal clearance. Within the liver, drug elimination occurs via biotransformation of unchanged drug to one or more metabolites (see Chapters 3, 4, 21) and/or excretion of unchanged drug into the bile (see Chapter 5). For most drugs, clearance is constant over the plasma or blood concentration range encountered in clinical settings (linear): that is, elimi-

TABLE 1. *Volumes and blood supplies of different body regions for a standard man[a,b]*

Tissue	Vol. (liters)	Blood flow (ml/min)	Blood flow (ml/100 ml tissue × min)	Vol. of blood in equilibrium with tissue (ml)
Adrenals	0.02	100	500	62
Kidneys	0.3	1,240	410	765
Thyroid	0.02	80	400	49
Gray matter	0.75	600	80	371
Heart	0.3	240	80	148
Other small glands and organs	0.16	80	50	50
Liver plus portal system	3.9	1,580	41	976
White matter	0.75	160	21	100
Red marrow	1.4	120	9	74
Muscle	30.0	300/600/1,500	1/2/5	185/370/925
Skin				
Nutritive	3.0	30/60/150	1/2/5	18/37/92
Shunt		1,620/1,290/300	54/43/10	
Nonfat subcutaneous	4.8	70	1.5	43
Fatty marrow	2.2	60	2.7	37
Fat	10.0	200	2.0	123
Bone cortex	6.4	0	0	0
Arterial blood	1.4	—	—	—
Venous blood	4.0	—	—	—
Lung parenchymal Tissue	0.6	—	—	—
Air in lungs	2.5 + half tidal volume	—	—	1,400[c] 999/795/185[d]
Total	70.0[e]	6,480		5,400

[a]Data compiled by Dedrick and Bischoff (5), from mean estimates of Mapleson (6).
[b]Standard man = 70-kg body weight, 1.73 m^2 surface area, 30–39 years old.
[c]Arterial blood.
[d]Skin-shunt venous blood.
[e]Excluding the air in the lung.

nation is not saturable, and the rate of drug elimination is directly proportional to concentration (Eq. 2). For drugs that exhibit saturable or dose-dependent elimination (nonlinear), clearance will vary depending on the concentration of drug that is achieved (see Chapters 17 and 21). Dosage adjustments with such drugs are more complex.

A further definition of clearance is useful in understanding the effects of physiologic and pathologic variables on drug elimination, particularly with respect to an individual organ. The rate of elimination of a drug by an individual organ can be defined in terms of the blood flow entering and exiting from the organ and the concentration of drug in the blood. The rate of presentation of drug to the organ is the product of blood flow and entering drug concentration ($Q \cdot C_A$), and the rate of exit of drug from the organ is the product of blood flow and exiting drug concentration ($Q \cdot C_V$) (Fig. 2). The difference between these rates at steady state is the rate of drug elimination.

Mass balance across liver

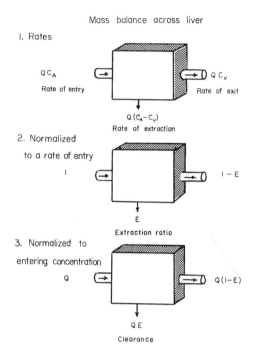

I. Rates

$Q\,C_A$
Rate of entry

$Q\,C_V$
Rate of exit

$Q\,(C_A - C_V)$
Rate of extraction

2. Normalized
to a rate of entry

1

$1 - E$

E

Extraction ratio

3. Normalized to
entering concentration

Q

$Q\,(1-E)$

$Q\,E$
Clearance

FIG. 2. The principles of mass balance can be used to illustrate the extraction of a drug in the liver. **1:** The difference between the rates in and out of the organ is the *rate of extraction*. **2:** Normalizing the rates to the rate of entry provides a measure of the fraction extracted, the *extraction ratio*. **3:** Normalizing the rates to the entering drug concentration gives the volume of entering blood from which the drug appears to be extracted, the *clearance*. (From Tozer, ref. 7, with permission.)

$$\text{Rate of elimination} = Q \cdot C_A - Q \cdot C_V \qquad (5)$$

(At steady state the amount of drug reaching the systemic circulation will equal the amount being eliminated.) Dividing Eq. 5 by concentration of drug entering the organ of elimination (C_A), an expression for organ clearance of drug is obtained:

$$CL_{\text{organ}} = \frac{Q \cdot C_A - Q \cdot C_V}{C_A} \qquad (6a)$$

$$= Q\,\frac{C_A - C_V}{C_A} = Q \cdot E \qquad (6b)$$

As shown in Eq. 6b, the expression $(C_A - C_V)/C_A$ can be referred to as the extraction ratio of the drug (E).

The concepts developed in Eqs. 6a and 6b have important implications for drugs that are eliminated by the liver. Consider a drug that is efficiently removed from the blood by hepatic processes. In this instance, the concentration of drug in the blood leaving the liver will be low, the extraction ratio will approach unity, and the clearance of the blood will become limited by hepatic blood flow. Drugs highly extracted by the liver (Table 2) (see Chapters 3 and 4) are restricted in their rate of elimination not by intrahepatic processes but by the rate at which they can be transported in the blood to hepatic sites of elimination. The concepts embodied in Eqs. 5 and 6 can be derived from consideration of mass balance of a drug across an eliminating organ at steady state. However, simple expressions for clearance,

TABLE 2. *Selected drugs with high (>0.5) and low (<0.3) hepatic extraction ratios*[a]

Low	High
Acetaminophen	Aldosterone
Amobarbital	Alprenolol
Antipyrine	Arabinosyl cytosine
Azapropazone	Bromosulfophthalein
Chloramphenicol	Chlormethiazole
Chlordiazepoxide	Desipramine
Chlorpromazine	Hydrocortisone
Clindamycin	Imipramine
Dapsone	Indocyanine green
Diazepam	Isoproterenol
Digitoxin	Labetalol
Ethchlorvynol	Lidocaine
Griseofulvin	Lorcainide
Hexobarbital	Meperidine
Isoniazid	Metoprolol
Lincomycin	Metyrapone
Lorazepam	Morphine
Minocycline	Nitroglycerin
Oxazepam	Nortriptyline
Phenobarbital	Pentazocine
Phenytoin	Phenacetin
Phenylbutazone	Phenylephrine
Prednisolone	Propranolol
Probenecid	Propoxyphene
Quinidine	Salicylamide
Salicylic acid	Verapamil
Sulfadimethoxine	
Theophylline	
Thiopental	
Tolbutamide	
Warfarin	

[a]These drugs primarily undergo hepatic elimination. For more specific information, see Chapters 3 and 4. Adapted from Benet and Sheiner (2) and Tozer (7,8).

blood flow, and extraction cannot account for the full complexity of hepatic or renal drug elimination. For example, these equations do not account for drug protein binding to blood and tissue components, nor do they permit an estimation of the intrinsic ability of the liver or kidney to eliminate a drug in the absence of limitations imposed by blood flow (see Chapters 10 and 11, and 3, 4, 8, and 9, respectively). To extend the relationships of Eq. 6 to include expressions for protein binding and intrinsic clearance, it is necessary to formulate a model to describe organ elimination of drugs. The most straightforward and most commonly employed model relating the extraction ratio to physiologic parameters is the so-called venous equilibration or well-stirred model (9,10) which assumes that the unbound drug concentration leaving the organ is equal to the unbound concentration inside the organ (Fig. 2) and that the intrinsic ability to metabolize or clear drug (CL^u_{int}) is equal to the rate of elimination divided by the unbound concentration in the organ. The clearance (with respect to blood concentration) for the eliminating organ then becomes

$$CL = Q \; \frac{fu_b \cdot CL^u_{int}}{Q + fu_b \cdot CL^u_{int}} \qquad (7)$$

where fu_b is the unbound fraction of drug in blood and Q is the blood flow. This model indicates that when the capability of the eliminating organ to metabolize the drug is large in comparison with the rate of drug presentation to the organ $(fu_bCL^u_{int} >> Q)$, the clearance will approximate the organ blood flow:

$$CL = Q \qquad (8)$$

that is, drug elimination is blood flow rate limited and the compound is called a high extraction ratio drug. This is further explained in Chapters 3 and 4, for drugs predominantly eliminated by the hepatic process. Table 2 provides a listing of high hepatic extraction ratio drugs.

In contrast, when the metabolic capability is small in comparison to the rate of drug presentation $(Q >> fu_bCL^u_{int})$, the clearance will be proportional to the unbound fraction of drug in blood and the intrinsic clearance, that is,

$$CL = fu_bCL^u_{int} \qquad (9)$$

The drug is then called a low extraction ratio drug. A listing of low hepatic extraction ratio drugs is provided in Table 2. When the capability for elimination is of the same order of magnitude as the blood flow, clearance would be dependent upon the blood flow as well as the intrinsic clearance and plasma protein binding (Eq. 7). An appreciation of Eq. 7 allows the investigator to understand a number of experimental results, heretofore unclear. For example, enzyme induction or hepatic disease may change the rate of drug metabolism in an isolated hepatic microsomal enzyme system but no change in clearance is found in the whole animal. For a high extraction ratio drug, clearance is blood flow rate limited (Eq. 8) and changes in CL^u_{int} due to enzyme induction or liver disease should have no effect on clearance. Similarly, for high extraction ratio drugs, changes in protein binding due to disease or competitive binding should have no effect on clearance (Eq. 8). In contrast, changes in intrinsic clearance and protein binding will affect the clearance of low extraction ratio drugs, but blood flow should have little affect on clearance (Eq. 9).

Pharmacokinetic changes in renal disease may also be explained in terms of clearance concepts. However, the complications which relate to filtration, active secretion, and reabsorption must also be considered. Renal clearance can theoretically be described by the following equation:

$$CL_{renal} = (CL_{RF} + CL_{RS}) (1 - FR) \qquad (10)$$

where CL_{RF} is renal filtration clearance, CL_{RS} is the net renal secretion clearance, and FR is the fraction of drug filtered and secreted that is reabsorbed. The rate of filtration depends on the volume of fluid that is filtered in the glomerulus and the unbound concentration of drug in plasma because proteins and drugs bound to proteins are not filtered. The volume filtered is usually estimated by inulin or creatinine clearance. The renal filtration is therefore usually expressed as:

$$CL_{RF} = fu_b \cdot CL_{cr}$$

where CL_{cr} is the creatinine clearance.

The secretion of drug in the kidney will depend on the relative binding of drug to the active transport carriers in relation to the binding to plasma proteins, the degree of saturation of these carriers, transfer of the drug across the tubular membrane, and the rate of delivery of the drug to the secretory site. A model that combines these factors can be set up in a manner similar to Eq. 7, where CL_{RS} may be defined in terms of kidney blood flow, fu_b and the intrinsic clearance of the kidney to transport unbound drug across the tubular membrane. The influences of changes in protein binding, blood flow, and number of functioning nephrons are analogous to the examples given earlier for hepatic elimination. For comments concerning the adjustments of dosage regimens in renal failure, see Chapters 8 and 9.

Volume

The second fundamental kinetic parameter useful in discussing processes of drug disposition is volume *(V)*. The volume of distribution *(V)* relates the amount of drug in the body to the concentration of drug *(C)* in the blood or plasma, depending upon the fluid measured. This volume does not necessarily refer to identifiable physiologic volume but merely to the fluid volume which would be required to account for all the drug in the body:

$$V = \text{amount of drug in body}/C \tag{11}$$

The plasma volume of a normal 70-kg man is 3 liters, blood volume is about 5.5 liters, extracellular fluid outside the plasma is 12 liters, and total body water is approximately 42 liters. However, many drugs exhibit volumes of distribution far in excess of these known fluid volumes as shown in Table 3. For example, if 500 µg of digoxin were in the body of a young healthy 70-kg male, a plasma concentration of approximately 0.7 ng/ml would be expected. Dividing the amount of drug in the body by the plasma concentration yields a volume of distribution for digoxin of about 700 liters, approximately 10 times greater than the total body volume of a 70-kg man. This serves to emphasize that the volume of distribution does not represent a real volume but rather must be considered as the size of the pool of body fluids that would be required if the drug were equally distributed throughout all portions of the body. In fact, digoxin, which is relatively hydrophobic, distributes into muscle and adipose tissue, leaving a very small amount of drug in the plasma. As might be expected, volume of distribution can change as a function of the patient's age (see Chapters 14 and 15), gender, disease (Chapters 6 and 9), and body composition (Appendix D). For example, the same 500 µg of digoxin in a middle-aged congestive heart failure patient might yield a 1-ng/ml concentration corresponding to a 500-liter volume of distribution.

The volume of distribution may vary widely depending on the pK_a of the drug (Table 4), the degree of plasma protein binding (see Chapter 10), the partition coefficient of the drug in the fatty tissues, differences in regional blood flow, as

TABLE 3. Mean volumes of distribution for selected drugs (liters/kg)[a]

V	Drug
0.05	Spironolactone
0.06	Heparin
0.08	Clofibrate (CPIB)
	Dicloxacillin
	Insulin
	Phenylbutazone[b]
0.10	Furosemide
	Warfarin[b]
0.14	Aspirin
	Cefazolin
	Cefoxitin
	Cephapirin
	Cromoglycate
	Ibuprofen
	Probenecid
	Tolbutamide
	Valproic acid
0.16	Cefamandole
	Fusidic acid
	Glipizide
	Piroxicam
	Sulfafurazole
	Sulfinpyrazone
0.18	Carbenicillin
	Chlorpropamide
0.20	Amikacin
	Bumetanide
	Chlorothiazide
	Diazoxide
	Sisomicin
	Sulfamethoxazole
0.23	Aminosalicylic acid
	Cephalexin
	Gentamicin
	Ticarcillin
0.25	Cefuroxime
	Cephalothin
	Cephradine
	Kanamycin
	Streptomycin
	Tobramycin
0.30	Benzylpenicillin
	Chlordiazepoxide
	Glibenclamide
	Ampicillin
0.35	Bacampicillin
	Cloxacillin
	Methyldopa
	Nalidixic acid
	Nitroglycerin
	Sulfadiazine
	Sulfametazine
0.40	Amoxicillin
	Propicillin
	Bleomycin
	5-Fluorouracil
	Hetacillin
	Methotrexate

V	Drug
	Oxacillin
	Minocycline
0.45	Vancomycin
0.50	Cyclophosphamide
	Digitoxin
	Lincomycin
	Prednisolone
	Theophylline
0.55	Ethanol
	Flucytosine
0.60	Isoniazid
	Magabe
	Phenazone
	Prazosin
	Primidone
	Sulfadimidine
0.65	Alphaxalone
	Clindamycin
	Insulin (regular)
	Oxazepam
	Phenytoin
0.70	Atenolol
	Sotalol
	Erythromycin
	Ethosuximide
	Griseofulvin
	Metronidazole
	Phenoxymethylpenicillin
0.80	Amylbarbital
	Disopyramide
	Hydrochlorothiazide
	Lithium
	Phenobarbital
	Rolitetracycline
0.90	Midazolam
	Pyridostigmine
1.0	Acetaminophen
	Bupivacaine
	Chloramphenicol
	Hexobarbital
	Indomethacin
	Lidocaine[b]
	Meclastine
	Methacycline
	Nafcillin
	Prednisone
1.2	Acebutolol
	Carbamazepine
	Chlortetracycline
	Diazepam[b]
	Lorazepam
	Mepivacaine
	N-acetylprocainamide
1.5	Doxycycline
	Ethambutol
	Hydralazine
	Oxytetracycline
	Phenacetin

V	Drug
	Rifampicin
	Tetracycline
1.6	Tocainide
	Viloxazine
	Metolazone
	Timolol
2.0	Cimetidine
	Clonidine
	Isosorbide
	Nadolol
	Etidocaine
	Pindolol
	Procainamide
	Trimethoprim
2.3	Colchicine
	Flunitrazepam
	Nitrazepam
2.8	Glutethimide
	Quinidine
3.0	Alprenolol
	Amphotericin B
	Atropine
	Chlorthalidone
	Clonazepam
	Minoxidil
	Morphine
	Naloxone
	Pentazocine
3.5	Bromocriptine
	Diphenhydramine
4.0	Metoprolol
	Propranolol
	Verapamil
4.5	Meperidine
5.0	Amiloride
6.0	Amantadine
	Methaqualone
6.5	Hydroflumethiazide
	Nomifensine
	Pizotifen
	Lorcainide
7.0	Bethanidine
8.0	Amitriptyline
10	Digoxin
14	Fenfluramine
	Imipramine
20	Chlorpromazine
	Doxepin
	Maprotiline
	Miconazole
	Nortriptyline[b]
	Ouabain
	Perphenazine
	Protriptyline
	Thioridazine
25	Haloperidol
35	Desipramine
40	Mianserin

[a]Where there may have been a conflict, data were preferentially selected from Benet and Sheiner (2). For additional data, see Appendixes A and B.

[b]There may be considerable differences between individuals in the V for certain drugs, as shown by the following examples (the ratio of the upper value to lower value is given in parentheses): diazepam, 0.18–1.30 (7.22); phenylbutazone, 0.04–0.15 (3.75); lidocaine, 0.58–1.91 (3.29).

well as the degree of binding to other tissues within the body. For example, plasma volumes of distribution ranging from 0.06 liter/kg (heparin) to 35 liters/kg (desipramine) are represented in Table 3 (and Appendix B). The latter has been reported to exhibit an apparent volume of distribution approaching 2,500 liters (35 liters/ kg × 70-kg person = 2,500 liters), implying extensive uptake into one or more organs or tissues. For a drug extensively bound (i.e., greater than 90%) to plasma proteins (albumin) but not bound to tissue components, the volume of distribution will have a lower limit of approximately 7 liters, as may be exemplified by furosemide and warfarin in Table 3. In contrast, drugs such as imipramine, nortriptyline, and propranolol have high volumes of distribution, even though over 90% of the drug in the blood is bound to plasma proteins. It would appear that these drugs either are even more extensively bound to tissue than to plasma proteins or are more highly soluble in adipose or other peripheral tissues than in blood. If plasma protein binding is more sensitive to pathological changes than tissue binding, we might expect to see a linear relation between V and fu, the unbound fraction in plasma, as has been shown for propranolol in patients with liver disease (see Chapters 4 and 10). Other sources of variation in this volume term may result from interindividual differences due to pathological factors (i.e., renal failure, see Chapter 9), environmental factors, drug interactions (see Chapter 11), as well as age (see Chapters 14 and 15). For example, the extracellular fluid volume accounts for 40% of body weight in the infant (see Chapter 14), 20% in the normal adult, 18% to 20% in the elderly (see Chapter 15), and 30% in the pregnant woman (see Chapter 13).

Several volume terms are commonly used and are derived in a number of ways. The volume of distribution defined in Eq. 11 considers the body as a single homogeneous compartment. Much useful pharmacokinetic information and data interpretation can come from this simplified model of the body which is depicted in Fig. 3. In this "one compartment" body model all drug administration occurs directly into the body (or central) compartment where drug is instantaneously distributed throughout volume V. Clearance of drug from this compartment occurs in a first order fashion as defined in Eq. 2, that is, the amount of drug eliminated per unit time depends on the amount of drug in the body compartment. Figure 3B and Eq. 12 describe the decline of plasma concentration with time for a drug injected into the body compartment.

$$C = \frac{\text{dose}}{V} e^{-kt} \qquad (12)$$

where k is the rate constant for elimination of drug from the body compartment. This rate constant is inversely related to the half-life of the drug ($k = .693/T_{1/2}$).

Let us now compare our noncompartmental definition of clearance (Eq. 2) and a model specific relation between C, V, and k (Eq. 12):

$$C = \text{rate of elimination}/CL \qquad C = \frac{\text{dose}}{V} e^{-kt}$$

TABLE 4. *Ionization constants (pK$_a$ values) of selected drugs*

Drug	pK$_a$ Values[a] Acid	Base	Drug	pK$_a$ Values[a] Acid	Base
Acebutolol		9.4	Epinephrine	10.2	8.7
Acetaminophen	9.5		Erythromycin		8.8
Acetazolamide	7.2		Ethacrynic acid	3.5	
Adrenaline	10.2	8.7	Ethambutol		9.5, 6.7
Allopurinol		9.4	Ethosuximide	9.5	
Alprenolol		9.7	Fenfluramine		9.1
Amiloride		8.7	Fenoprofen	4.5	
Aminocaproic acid		10.8	5-Fluorouracil		8.1
Amitriptyline		9.4	Fluphenazine		8.0, 3.9
Amobarbital	7.9		Furosemide	3.9	
Amoxicillin	2.7, 7.4, 9.6		Glutethimide	4.5	
Amphetamine		9.8	Guanethidine		11.4, 8.3
Amphotericin B	5.5	10.0	Haloperidol		8.7
Ampicillin	2.5	7.2	Homatropine		9.7
Apomorphine		7.2	Hydralazine		7.1
Aspirin	3.5		Hydrochlorothiazide	7.9, 9.2	
Atenolol		9.6	Hyoscine		8.1
Atropine	8.9	9.7	Ibuprofen	4.4, 5.2	
Baclofen	3.9, 9.6		Imipramine		9.5
Benzocaine		2.5	Indomethacin	4.5	
Benztropine		10.0	Indoramin		7.7
Benzylpenicillin	2.8		Isoniazid		10.8
Bupivacaine		8.1	Isoxsuprine		8.0
Buprenorphine		8.5, 10.0	Isoproterenol		8.6
Butacaine		9.0	Kanamycin		7.2
Caffeine		0.8	Levodopa	2.3	
Carbenicillin	2.6		Lidocaine		7.9
Cephalexin	5.2		Lincomycin		7.6
Cephalothin	2.5		Lysergide		7.8
Chlorambucil		8.0	Mecamylamine		11.3
Chlordiazepoxide		4.6	Mefenamic acid	4.2	
Chloroquine		8.4, 10.8	Meperidine		8.6
Chlorphentermine		9.6	Mephentermine		10.3
Chlorothiazide	6.8, 9.4		Mepivacaine		7.6
Chlorpromazine		9.3	Mepyramine		8.9
Chlorpropamide	5.0		Metaraminol		8.6
Clindamycin		7.5	Metformin		11.5, 2.8
Clonidine		8.3	Methadone		8.5
Cocaine		8.5	Methamphetamine		10.0
Codeine		8.2	Methapyrilene		8.9, 4.0
Colchicine		1.9	Methicillin	2.8	
Cromoglycate	2.0		Methotrexate	4.8	
Cyclizine		8.2	Methotrimeprazine		9.2
Dantrolene	7.5		Methoxamine		9.2
Dapsone	1.2	2.4	Methoxyphenamine		10.1
Desipramine		10.2	Methyldopa	2.2, 9.2	10.6
Dextromethorphan		8.8	Methysergide		6.6
Dextropropoxyphene		6.3	Metoprolol		9.7
Diazepam		3.3	Morphine	9.9	7.9
Dicloxacillin	2.7		Nafcillin	2.7	
Dicoumarol	5.7		Nalidixic acid	6.7	
Dihydrocodeine		8.8	Nalorphine		7.8
Diphenhydramine		9.0	Naphazoline		10.9
Diphenoxylate		7.1	Naproxen	5	
Disopyramide		9.6	Nicotine		7.9, 3.1
Dopamine	10.6	8.9	Nitrofurantoin	7.2	
Doxylamine		9.2	Norepinephrine	9.8	8.6
Droperidol		7.6	Noscapine		6.2
Emetine		8.3, 7.4	Orphenadrine		8.4
Ephedrine		9.4	Pentazocine	11.2	9.7

TABLE 4. *(continued)*

Drug	pK_a Values[a] Acid	pK_a Values[a] Base	Drug	pK_a Values[a] Acid	pK_a Values[a] Base
Phenindamine		8.2	Quinine		8.4, 4.1
Pheniramine		9.3	Salbutamol		9.3
Phenmetrazine		8.5, 8.0	Salicylamide	8.4	
Phenobarbital	7.4		Salicylic acid	3.0	
Phentermine		10.1	Strychnine		8.0, 2.3
Phenylbutazone	4.5		Sulfasoxizole	5.0	
Phenylephrine	8.8	9.8	Sulfamethoxazole	5.6	
Phenylpropanolamine		9.0	Synephrine	9.3	10.2
Phenoxymethylpenicillin	2.7		Terbutaline		10.1
Phenytoin	8.3		Tetracycline	3.3, 7.7	9.7
Physostigmine		7.9, 1.8	Theophylline	8.8	0.7
Pilocarpine		6.9, 1.4	Thioridazine		9.5
Pindolol		8.8	Thiopental	7.6	
Probenecid	3.4		Ticarcillin	2.5, 3.4	
Procainamide		9.2	Tolbutamide	5.3	
Procaine		9.0	Tolazoline		10.6
Prochlorperazine		8.1	Tranexamic acid	4.3	10.6
Promazine		9.4	Trifluoperazine		8.1
Promethazine		9.1	Trimethoprim		6.4
Propranolol		9.4	Valproic Acid	4.8	
Propylthiouracil	8.3		Viloxazine		8.13
Pseudoephedrine		9.8	Vincristine		7.4, 5.4
Pyrimethamine		7.0	Warfarin	5.0	
Quinidine		4.3, 8.5			

[a]The pK_a values are listed under the nature of the drug (i.e., acid or base). In the case where the drug's pK_a values are listed under both categories, the drug is considered amphoteric.
Adapted from Bowman and Rand (11), and from Heel and Avery (12).

Integration of these two equations over the entire time course of drug in the body (i.e., from time zero to time infinity) yields the area under the plasma or blood concentration-time curve, defined as AUC.

$$AUC = \frac{\text{amount eliminated}}{CL} \qquad\qquad AUC = \frac{\text{dose}}{V \cdot k} \qquad (13)$$

Since for an intravenous dose the amount of drug eliminated from the body will equal the dose administered to the body, it is obvious that clearance is the product of volume and the elimination rate constant for the one compartment body model depicted in Fig. 3A. If drug kinetics is adequately described by a one compartment body model, Fig. 3A, then the volume of distribution may be calculated in two different ways. The first is depicted in Fig. 3C which represents the logarithmic transformation of Fig. 3B and Eq. 12, where the y-axis intercept of the log concentration time curve is the zero time concentration of drug in the body compartment, that is, C_0 which equals the injected dose divided by V. The second method is to determine clearance from the AUC (Eq. 13) and then determine V by dividing CL by the rate constant for elimination. This latter method is more generally followed since this procedure will allow one to calculate a volume of distribution even when drug kinetics is described by more than one body compartment as depicted in Fig. 4. This multicompartment volume term is designated V_{area} and it may be calculated as follows:

$$V_{area} = \frac{CL}{\lambda_z} = \frac{F \cdot dose}{\lambda_z \, AUC} \qquad (14)$$

where λ is the terminal disposition constant determined from the log-linear portion of the plasma concentration time curve, that is, the "β" phase for the two-compartment body model depicted in Fig. 4, and F is the bioavailability of the dose administered as will be discussed in the following section. Area under the curve, AUC, can be obtained mathematically by the trapezoid rule, utilizing the time points and corresponding plasma concentrations (14). AUC in a one-compartment model (Fig. 3C) can be approximated by dividing the extrapolated intravenous C_0 by the elimination rate constant *(k)*, which is equal to 0.693 divided by the elimination half-life. For further discussion of the uses of AUC, refer to Gibaldi and Perrier (14), who have provided an excellent review.

Most of the volume of distribution values listed in the literature, as compiled in Table 3 and Appendix B, are calculated using Eq. 14 and represent V_{area}. This is an easy parameter to calculate and the volume term may be determined following intravenous and enteral routes of administration. However, another multicompartment distribution volume may be more useful, especially when determining the effect of disease states on pharmacokinetics. The volume of distribution at steady state *(Vss)* represents the volume in which a drug would appear to be distributed during steady state if the drug existed throughout that volume at the same concentration as in the measured fluid (plasma or blood). This volume can be determined by the use of areas as described by Benet and Galeazzi (15):

$$V_{ss} = (Dose^{iv}) \, (AUMC)/AUC^2 \qquad (15)$$

where AUMC is the area under the first moment of the plasma or blood concentration time curve, that is, the area under the curve of the product of time, t, and plasma or blood concentration, C, over the time span zero to infinity.

Although V_{area} is a convenient and easily calculated parameter, this volume term varies when the rate constant for drug elimination changes, even when there has been no change in the distribution space. As the rate constant for elimination decreases, V_{area} approaches V_{ss}. Since we may wish to know whether a particular disease state influences either clearance or the distribution of the drug within the body independently, it is preferable to define volume in terms of a parameter that is theoretically independent of changes in the rate of elimination. The difference between these two volume terms is illustrated in Table 5 where pharmacokinetic parameters for cefamadole in 6 normal volunteers (16) is compared with those obtained in 3 uremic patients (17). Since cefamadole is almost exclusively eliminated by the renal route, a marked difference in clearance (24-fold change) is noted between normals and uremics. However, the terminal half-life, $T_{1/2}$, and the terminal rate constant for elimination only change by a factor of 11. Note that a significant difference, more than a twofold change, is observed in V_{area}. This could be interpreted to mean that changes in renal function not only affect the elimination of cefamadole as reflected by the clearance changes, but that there is also a decrease

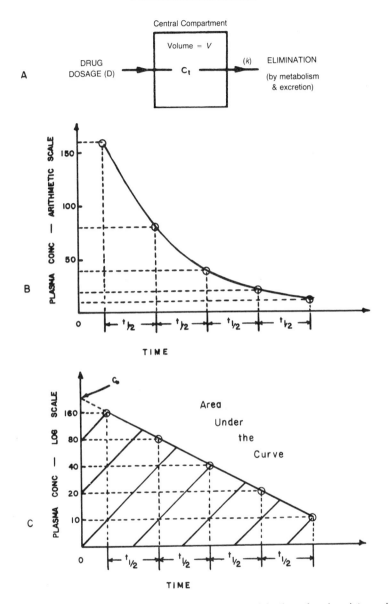

FIG. 3. Single-compartment kinetics. Rapid intravenous injection of a drug into a single-compartment model (A) gives the resulting plasma concentration/time plot on a linear scale (B). Replotting with the concentration (C_t) on a logarithmic scale gives a straight line *(C)*. This plot is easily extrapolated back to zero time to give C_0, the theoretical initial concentration. The elimination half-life of the drug is represented by $T_{1/2}$. The elimination rate constant (k) is equal to $0.693/T_{1/2}$. This latter value indicates the amount of drug eliminated from the body per unit time. The constant k is also CL/V. (From Paxton, ref. 13, with permission.)

in the distribution volume of this drug. However, when V_{ss} is compared it is obvious that no significant difference in the distribution volume between these two patient populations is noted.

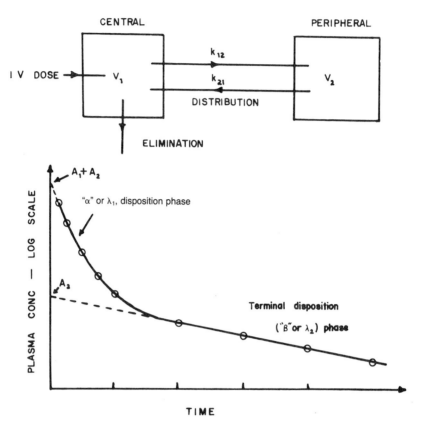

FIG. 4. Two-compartment kinetics. Rapid intravenous injection of a drug into a two-compartment model results in a semilogarithmic plasma concentration/time plot that shows two distinct linear portions. k_{12} and k_{21} are transfer rate constants between the two compartments and V_1 and V_2 are the apparent volumes of distribution of the two compartments. The terminal elimination or disposition phase is often designated as the β phase with the faster disposition phase designated the α phase. More recent pharmacokinetic terminology would designate these phases as λ_2 (or λ_z) and λ_1, respectively. (From Paxton, ref. 13, with permission.)

Half-Life

Two other pharmacokinetic terms, half-life and bioavailability, are necessary for designing appropriate drug dosage regimens. For the simplest case (and the most useful) in designing drug dosage regimens the body can be considered as one compartment. As seen in Fig. 3 half-life is the time it takes for the plasma concentration to be reduced by 50%. However, when drug concentrations in the body are described by two or more compartments (e.g., Fig. 4), then each disposition phase has a characteristic half-life. The relevance of these half-lives depends upon both pharmacokinetic and pharmacodynamic considerations as recently reviewed by Benet (18). Generally, however, the half-life is determined from plasma concentration measurements during the terminal or elimination phase.

$$T_{1/2} = \frac{0.693}{\lambda_z} \qquad \lambda_z = \frac{\ln(Cp_1/Cp_2)}{t_2 - t_1} \qquad (16)$$

TABLE 5. *Cefamandole kinetics in normals and uremics*

Parameter	Normals[a]	Uremics[b]	Significance
CL (ml/min · kg)	2.81 ± 0.98	0.115 ± 0.023	$p < 0.05$
$T_{1/2_z}$ (hr)	1.2 ± 0.2	13.0 ± 4.5	$p < 0.05$
λ_z (hr^{-1})	0.576 ± 0.096	0.0534 ± 0.0187	$p < 0.05$
V_{area} (liters/kg)	0.298 ± 0.104	0.138 ± 0.048	$p < 0.05$
V_{ss} (liters/kg)	0.161 ± 0.050	0.134 ± 0.045	ns

[a]Aziz et al., ref. 16.
[b]Gambertoglio et al., ref. 17.

Elimination of unchanged drug from the body (clearance) can only occur from the blood or plasma in direct contact with the organs of elimination, and the amount of drug in the blood or plasma at any time will depend on the volume of distribution. Thus, the time course of drug in the body will depend on both the clearance and the volume of distribution.

$$T_{1/2} \approx 0.693 \ V/CL \qquad (17)$$

Early studies of drug pharmacokinetics in disease were compromised by their reliance on drug half-life as the sole measure of alteration in drug disposition. Diseases can affect either or both of the physiologically related parameters volume and clearance; thus, the derived parameter, $T_{1/2}$, will not necessarily reflect changes in drug disposition (see Chapter 4). Although a poor indicator of drug elimination, $T_{1/2}$ does provide a good indication of the time required to reach steady state (four half-life periods to reach approximately 90% of a new steady state), the time for a drug to be removed from the body, and a means to estimate the appropriate dosing interval.

Bioavailability

Bioavailability *(F)* is defined as the fraction of the dose reaching the systemic circulation as unchanged drug following administration by any route. For a drug administered orally, bioavailability may be less than unity, for several reasons. The drug may be incompletely absorbed. It may be metabolized in the gut, the gut wall, the portal blood, or the liver prior to entry into the systemic circulation (see Fig. 5). It may undergo enterohepatic cycling with incomplete reabsorption following elimination into the bile (see Chapter 5). Biotransformation of some drugs in the liver following oral administration is an important factor in the pharmacokinetic profile, as will be discussed further. Bioavailability measures following oral drug administration are given in Appendix B as the percentage of the dose available to the systemic circulation.

ABSORPTION, BIOAVAILABILITY AND ROUTES OF ADMINISTRATION

The difference between the extent of availability, F (often designated solely as bioavailability), and the rate of availability is illustrated in Fig. 6 which depicts the concentration/time curve for a hypothetical drug formulated into three different

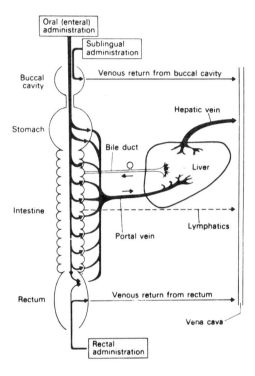

FIG. 5. Passage of drugs from the alimentary tract into the bloodstream. (From Bowman and Rand, ref. 11, with permission.)

dosage forms. Dosage forms A and B are designed so that the drug is put into the blood circulation at the same rate, but twice as fast as for dosage form C. The times at which drug concentrations reach a peak are identical for dosage forms A and B and occur earlier than the peak time for dosage form C. In general, the relative order of peak times following the administration of different dosage forms of the drug corresponds to the rates of availability of the drug from the various dosage forms. The extent of availability can be measured by using either drug concentrations in the plasma or blood, or amounts of unchanged drug in the urine. The area under the blood concentration/time curve (area under the curve, AUC) for a drug can serve as a measure of the extent of availability. In Fig. 6, the areas under curves A and C are identical and twice as great as the area under curve B. In most cases, where drug clearance is constant, the relative areas under the curves or the amount of unchanged drug excreted in the urine will quantitatively describe the relative availability of the drug from the different dosage forms. However, even in nonlinear cases, where clearance is dose dependent, the relative areas under the curves will yield a measurement of the rank order of availability from different dosage forms or from different routes of administration.

Because there is usually a target concentration for a drug in the blood (as designated in Fig. 6) that is necessary to elicit a clinical effect (i.e., effective concentrations in Appendixes A–C), both the rate and extent of input or availability can affect the clinical efficacy of a drug. In the majority of cases the duration of

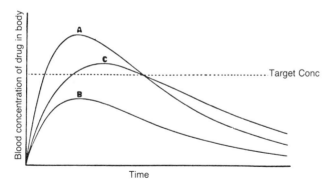

FIG. 6. Blood concentration/time curves illustrating how changes in the rate and extent of drug availability can influence both the duration of action and the efficacy of a dose of a drug. The dotted line indicates the target concentration (T_C) of the drug in the body. Case A: Drug is absorbed and is available rapidly and completely. This product produces a prompt and prolonged response. Case B: Drug is absorbed at the same rate as in case A, but is only 50% as available. There will be no response from this dose of the drug, because the T_C is not reached. Case C: Drug is absorbed at one-half the rate seen in cases A and B, but is 100% available. The product produces a delayed and less prolonged response when compared with case A. (From Benet, ref. 19, with permission.)

pharmacologic effects will be a function of the length of time the blood concentration curve is above the target concentration, and the intensity of the effect for many drugs will be a function of the height of the blood concentration curve above the target concentration (see Chapters 21 and 22).

Thus, for the three different dosage forms depicted in Fig. 6, there will be significant differences in the levels of clinical effectiveness. Dosage form B will require that twice the dose be administered to attain blood levels equivalent to those for dosage form A. Appendixes A through C contain measures of the extent of availability of selected drugs following oral dosing. No measures of the rate of availability are provided, because the fractional extent (F) is more useful than the rate of availability to estimate the amount of drug in the body. Differences in rate of availability may become important for drugs given as a single dose, such as hypnotic drugs used to induce sleep or those drugs designed specially to be released slowly (e.g., TheoDur®, Slo-Phyllin®, Contact®). Drug from dosage form A will reach the target concentration earlier than drug from dosage form C; concentrations from A will reach a higher level and remain above the minimum effective concentration for a longer period of time. In a multiple dosing regimen, dosage forms A and C will yield the same average blood concentrations, although dosage form A will show somewhat greater maximum and lower minimum concentrations.

For most drugs, rate of disposition or loss from the biological system is independent of rate of input, once the drug is absorbed. Disposition is defined as what happens to the active drug after it reaches a site in the blood circulation where drug concentration measurements can be made, referred to here as the systemic circulation. Although disposition processes may be independent of input, the inverse is not necessarily true, because disposition can markedly affect the extent of availability. Drug absorbed from the stomach and the intestine must first pass through the liver before reaching the circulation (Fig. 5). Thus, if a drug is metabolized in

the liver or excreted in bile, some of the active drug absorbed from the gastrointestinal tract will be inactivated by hepatic processes before the drug can reach the general circulation and be distributed to its sites of action. If the metabolizing or biliary excreting capacity of the liver is great, the effect on the extent of availability will be substantial. Knowing the extraction ratio *(E)* for a drug across the liver (see Fig. 2 and Eq. 6), it is possible to predict the maximum oral availability (F_{max}) for this drug if hepatic metabolism follows first order kinetic processes.

$$F_{max} = 1 - E = 1 - (CL_{hepatic}/Q_{hepatic}) \qquad (18)$$

Thus, if the hepatic blood clearance $(CL_{hepatic})$ for the drug is large relative to hepatic blood flow $(Q_{hepatic})$, the extent of availability for this drug will be low when it is given by a route that yields first-pass metabolic effects (see Fig. 5). This decrease in availability is a function of the physiologic site from which absorption takes place, and no amount of dosage-form modification can improve the availability under linear conditions. Of course, therapeutic blood levels can be reached by this route of administration if larger doses are given. Therefore, the toxicity potential and elimination kinetics of the metabolites must be thoroughly understood before a decision to administer a large oral dose is made.

Figure 7 depicts the variation in blood levels which result following intravenous (upper panels) and oral (lower panels) dosing following increases in hepatic total intrinsic clearance (CL_{int}) for a low extraction ratio drug (left panels) and a high extraction ratio drug (right panels). Note that CL_{int}, the parameter which approximately doubles for each of the drugs in Fig. 7, is the product of fraction unbound to plasma proteins (fu_b) and the intrinsic ability of the liver to clear unbound drug (CL^u_{int}) as described previously in Eq. 7. That is, the changes noted in Fig. 7 for each drug could have resulted from changes in two different pharmacokinetic characteristics or from a combination of both. For the high extraction drug (right panels) very little change in blood levels is seen following intravenous dosing since clearance is blood flow rate limited (Eq. 8), but marked differences are noted following oral dosing since the extraction ratio is close to unity (Eq. 18). It is important to realize that drugs with high extraction ratios will show marked intersubject variability in bioavailability because of variations in hepatic function or blood flow or both (e.g., see Table 1 in Chapter 4). For the drug with an extraction ratio of 0.90 that increases to 0.95 (Fig. 7, right panels), the bioavailability of the drug will be halved, from 0.10 to 0.05. These relationships can explain the marked variability in plasma or blood drug concentrations that occurs among individuals given similar doses of a highly extracted drug. Small variations in hepatic extraction between individuals will result in large differences in availability and plasma drug concentrations.

For the low extraction ratio drug (left panels) a marked change in blood levels is seen following both intravenous and oral dosing when CL_{int} is doubled. For this low extraction ratio drug, clearance varies with CL_{int} (Eq. 9). However, since blood levels change significantly following both oral and intravenous dosing, bioavailability does not vary significantly, (i.e., *F* decreases from 0.90 to 0.82). Further consideration of changes in pharmacokinetic parameters for drugs primarily eliminated by the liver may be found in Chapters 3 and 4.

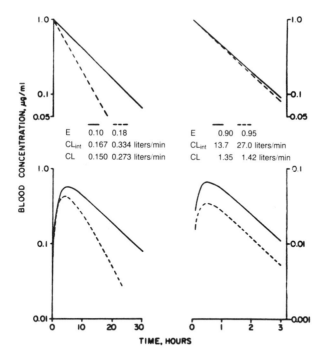

FIG. 7. The effect of increasing hepatic total intrinsic clearance (CL_{int}) on the total blood concentration/time curves after intravenous *(upper panels)* and oral *(lower panels)* administration of equal doses of two totally metabolized drugs. The left panels refer to a drug with an initial CL_{int} equivalent to an extraction ratio of 0.1 at a liver blood flow of 1.5 liter/min, and the right panels refer to one with an initial extraction ratio of 0.9. The *AUC*s after oral administration are inversely proportional to CL_{int}. (From Nies et al., ref. 21, with permission.)

The first-pass effect can be avoided to a great extent by use of sublingual tablets and by topical preparations (e.g., nitroglycerin ointment) and can be partially avoided by using rectal suppositories (see Fig. 5). The capillaries in the lower and middle sections of the rectum drain into the inferior and middle hemorrhoidal veins, which in turn drain into the inferior vena cava, thus bypassing the liver. However, suppositories tend to move upward in the rectum into a region where veins that lead to the liver predominate, such as the superior hemorrhoidal. In addition, there are extensive anastomoses between the superior and middle hemorrhoidal veins, and thus probably only about 50% of a rectal dose can be assumed to bypass the liver (20). The lungs represent a good temporary clearing site for a number of drugs, especially basic compounds by partition into lipid tissues, as well as serving a filtering function for particulate matter that may be given by intravenous injection. In essence, the lung may cause first-pass loss by excretion and possible metabolism for drugs input into the body by the nongastrointestinal routes of administration (see Chapter 7).

PHARMACOKINETICS IN DESIGNING A DOSAGE REGIMEN

Dosage regimen describes both the route and time course of drug administration and knowledge of pharmacokinetic principles is important in making such decisions.

Maintenance Dosage

In most situations, drugs are administered in a series of repetitive doses or as a continuous infusion in order to maintain a steady state plasma concentration within a given therapeutic window. Thus, calculation of the appropriate maintenance dosage is a primary goal. To maintain the chosen steady state, the rate of drug administration is adjusted so that the rate of drug input into the body equals the rate of drug loss. This relation was previously defined at steady state in Eq. 1:

$$\text{Dosing rate} = CL \cdot C_{ss} \tag{1}$$

Dosing rate is also defined as the product of the extent of availability *(F)* and the dose divided by the dosing interval (τ). If the clinician chooses the desired average plasma drug concentration and knows the clearance and availability for that drug in a particular patient, the appropriate dose per dosing interval can be calculated as follows:

$$\frac{\text{Dose}}{\tau} = \frac{CL \cdot C_{ss}}{F} \tag{1a}$$

Example: A steady state plasma level of theophylline of 15 mg/liter is desired to relieve acute bronchial asthma in a patient. If the patient is a nonsmoker and otherwise normal except for the asthmatic condition, we can use the mean clearance given in Appendix A, that is, 0.65 ml/min/kg or 2.7 liters/hr (70 kg). Because the drug is to be given as an intravenous infusion, $F = 1$.

$$
\begin{aligned}
\text{Dosing rate} &= CL \cdot C_{ss} \\
&= 2.7 \text{ liters/hr} \times 15 \text{ mg/liter} \\
&= 41 \text{ mg/hr}
\end{aligned}
$$

Therefore, in this patient the proper infusion rate will be 41 mg/hr per 70 kg body weight. However, all intravenous preparations of theophylline are available as the ethylenediamine salt (aminophylline), which contains 85% theophylline. Therefore, the infusion rate will be (41 mg/hr)/(0.85) = 48 mg/hr aminophylline. Once the clinical situation is appropriate for oral dosing, the clinician will then want to maintain levels using oral aminophylline dosing at intervals of 6, 8, or even 12 hr. When a series of multiple doses is given, the concentration term in Eq. 1 becomes the average of plasma concentrations over the dosing interval C_{avg}:

$$\frac{(S)(F) \cdot \text{Dose}}{\tau} = CL \cdot C_{avg}$$

$$\text{Dose} = 41 \text{ mg/hr} \cdot \tau/0.85 \approx 50 \text{ mg/hr}$$

In the above equation, the term *S* is added to indicate the fraction of the salt form of the drug containing the active species ($S = 0.85$ for aminophylline), the oral availability $F = 1$ (see Appendix A), and the dose rate is rounded off to a convenient number consistent with the solid dosage forms commercially available. Therefore, in this patient, oral aminophylline should be dosed as 300 mg every 6 hr, or 400 mg every 8 hr, or 600 mg every 12 hr. Note that when dosing rate is

maintained, the steady state plasma level on continuous infusion or the average plasma level following multiple dosing depends only on the primary disposition parameter clearance. The values of volume of distribution and half-life are not needed to determine the average plasma concentration for a given dosing rate, or for the reverse, determining the dosing rate for a desired plasma steady state concentration. However, the C_{ss} is determined by a number of input parameters: dose, bioavailability (F), and rate of administration (τ) in addition to clearance (CL). Any changes in these parameters will alter the C_{ss}, as shown in Table 6.

Although the foregoing equations are the most useful in reaching a given average level, it is important to realize that at different dosing intervals the plasma level/time curves will have different maximum and minimum values, even though the average level will always be 15 mg/liter. (A simulation for a hypothetical drug with a clearance of 6.67 liters/hr and a half-life of 4 hr given at a dosing rate of 500 µg/hr is depicted in Fig. 8 for four different dosing regimens.) If the clinician chooses to infuse aminophylline at a continuous rate of 48 mg/hr, then the level of 15 mg/liter will be maintained continuously. However, if an intermittent dosing schedule is chosen, as suggested, at intervals of 6, 8, or 12 hr, then the maximum and minimum levels will differ. A simplified way of calculating these maximum $[C_{ss(max)}]$ and minimum $[C_{ss(min)}]$ values is given in the following equations:

$$C_{ss(max)} = \frac{(S)(F) \cdot \text{dose}/V}{\text{fraction lost in a dosing interval}} = \frac{(S)(F) \cdot \text{dose}/V}{1 - e^{-\lambda_z \tau}} \qquad (19)$$

$$= \frac{(0.85)\,(1)\,(400 \text{ mg})\,/35 \text{ liters}}{0.50} \quad \text{or} \quad \frac{0.85\,(1)\,(600 \text{ mg})/35 \text{ liters}}{0.65}$$

$$= 20 \text{ mg/liter (dosing every 8 hr)} \quad \text{or} \quad 22.4 \text{ mg/liter (dosing every 12 hr)}$$

$$C_{ss(min)} = C_{ss(max)} \cdot \text{fraction remaining after dosing interval} \qquad (20)$$
$$C_{ss(min)} = C_{ss(max)} \cdot e^{-\lambda_z \tau}$$
$$= (20 \text{ mg/liter})\,(0.5) = 10 \text{ mg/liter (dosing every 8 hr)}$$
$$\text{or}$$
$$(22.4 \text{ mg/liter})\,(0.35) = 7.8 \text{ mg/liter (dosing every 12 hr)}$$

The calculations for Eqs. 18 and 19 were made assuming intermittent oral aminophylline doses of 400 mg every 8 hr and of 600 mg every 12 hr in a patient having a 35-liter volume of distribution, an 8-hr half-life, and an oral availability of approximately 1 (Appendix A). The denominator in Eq. 19, the fraction lost in a dosing interval, may be easily calculated when one knows the half-life. For example, with the 8-hr dosing interval, assuming a half-life of 8 hr, 50% of the dose will be lost in the first 8 hr, 75% in 16 hr, and 88% in 24 hr. Correspondingly, only 50% will remain at the end of the 8-hr dosing interval. Thus, with this dosing regimen, a maximum level of 20 ml/liter and a minimum level of 10 mg/liter will be achieved. Example calculations are also given for the 12-hr dosing interval. In this case, the fraction lost in a dosing interval is 0.65, as calculated from $\lambda_z\,(=0.693/T_{1/2})$ and τ using the expression in the denominator of Eq. 19, and the fraction

TABLE 6. *Effects of changes in pharmacokinetic parameters on steady state plasma concentrations*

Change in parameter	Possible rationale or explanation for change	Effect on C_{ss}
↑ Dose *(D)*	To improve clinical response	↑
↑ Bioavailability *(F)*	Change to a different route of administration or to a dosage form that is better absorbed	↑
↑ Total body clearance *(CL)*	Drug interaction causing an enhanced rate of drug elimination or improvement in a physiologic or pathologic condition	↓
↑ Dosing interval (τ)	To improve compliance for greater patient convenience	↓

Adapted from Mayersohn, ref. 22.

remaining is 0.35. Thus, with this dosing regimen, a maximum level of 22.4 and a minimum level of 7.8 mg/liter are calculated.

In contrast to the situation with Eq. 1 in which dosage rates and average steady state levels can be determined independent of drug distribution (using only clearance), determination of maximum and minimum steady state levels requires pharmacokinetic model assumptions. Equations 18 and 19 are derived assuming that the drug follows a one-compartment-body model (Fig. 3A) and the absorption rate is much faster than the elimination rate. Most likely, the only clinically relevant consequences of these assumptions, for the majority of drugs, will be that the calculated $C_{ss(max)}$ will be overestimated. Therefore, in choosing the appropriate dosage regimen, either the more convenient 600 mg twice a day or 400 mg three times a day, the clinician must consider the consequences which may result when plasma theophylline concentrations are less than the reported minimum effective concentration (C_{mec} = 10 mg/liter). The time during which concentrations are below the minimum effective concentration ($t_{<mec}$) may be calculated using Eq. 21 and would equal 2.4 hr for the 12-hr dosing interval example above.

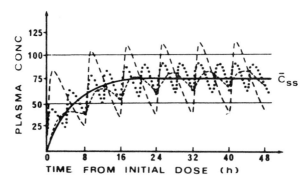

FIG. 8. Simulations of plasma concentrations achieved during four continuous administration regimens of a drug with a clearance of 6.67 liters/hr, a half-life of 4 hr, and a therapeutic range of 50 to 100 μg/liter. *Key:* 0.05 mg/hr constant intravenous infusion, *solid line*; oral dosing, 400 mg every 8 hr, *long-dashed line*; oral dosing, 200 mg every 4 hr, *dotted line*; oral dosing of sustained-release preparation, 400 mg every 8 hr, *short-dashed line*. (Adapted from Paxton, ref. 13, with permission.)

$$t_{<\text{mec}} = \frac{\ln \left[C_{\text{mec}}/C_{ss(\text{min})} \right]}{\lambda_z} \qquad (21)$$

More recently, a number of drugs have been formulated as prolonged release dosage forms, with the goal of (a) decreasing blood level fluctuations about the average concentration and (b) increasing the dosage interval. Under these conditions, the assumption that the absorption rate is much faster than the elimination rate may not hold, and Eqs. 19 and 20 will overestimate the peak and underestimate the trough concentration. Specific equations are available to predict $C_{ss(max)}$ and $C_{ss(min)}$ if the absorption rate constant or the time to peak is known (14). However, there appears to be little rationale for making such calculations. The primary relation between the dosing rate, clearance, and the desired steady state concentration (Eq. 1) is valid independent of the input rate. Therefore, for theophylline prolonged release dosage forms, a dosing rate of 41 mg/hr or approximately 500 mg every 12 hr will yield an average plasma concentration of 15 mg/liter, the same average concentration which would be obtained with a 600-mg dose of a quick releasing dosage form of aminophylline every 12 hr as detailed in the sample calculations above. However, maximum and minimum concentrations for the prolonged release dosage form should be significantly closer to C_{avg} than the values calculated above. For example, the package insert for one prolonged action theophylline product indicates an average peak-trough difference of only 4 mg/liter upon reaching steady state after multiple dosing every 12 hr.

When prolonged release dosage forms act properly, the plasma concentration profile begins to approach that observed for the continuous infusion as depicted in Fig. 8. With peak and trough variation minimized, it may be possible to select a lower average plasma concentration, thereby lowering the dosing rate, while still maintaining $C_{ss(\text{min})}$ above C_{mec}. For example, with a theophylline prolonged release dosage form it may be possible to select 12 mg/liter as the steady state concentration, thereby requiring a 32.4 mg/hr dosing rate or approximately 400 mg every 12 hr for the patient used in the sample calculations above. In any case, it should be emphasized that all of the above calculations were based on literature data for an average, nonsmoking, 70-kg patient, otherwise normal except for his asthmatic condition. However, the accuracy of these preliminary projections for the time course of theophylline concentrations must be checked by plasma theophylline concentration measurements in the patient being treated (see Chapters 21 and 22).

In the foregoing examples the fraction of drug in the body eliminated was derived from realizing that 50% of the amount remaining to be eliminated is eliminated within the time frame of each successive half-life. Thus, it takes five half-lives after the cessation of therapy for a drug to be virtually entirely (i.e., 97%) eliminated from the body. This same principle also applies to drug accumulation within the body toward a plateau that occurs with multiple dosing and constant rates of intravenous infusion (Fig. 8).

In many clinical situations, dosages are not given on exact schedules of 6, 8, or 12 hr. In such cases, the following equation may be used to determine the concentration observed:

$$C_{\text{obs}} = \frac{F}{V} \ (D_1 \cdot e^{-\lambda_z t_1} + D_2 \cdot e^{-\lambda_z t_2} + D_3 \cdot e^{-\lambda_z t_3} + \ldots) \tag{22}$$

Here, as with $C_{ss(\text{max})}$ and $C_{ss(\text{min})}$, the plasma concentration is a reflection of previous doses; however, as a result of inconsistent time intervals, we must account for each dose individually. We will not need to go back more than four half-lives, because 93% of the drug will have been eliminated from that time. Here, we again assume that the absorption rate is much faster than the elimination rate and t_1 is the elapsed time since the first dose (D_1) was given, etc.

LOADING DOSE

When the time to reach the steady state is appreciable, as it is for drugs with long half-lives, it may be desirable to administer a loading dose that promptly raises the concentration of drug in plasma to the projected steady state value. In theory, only the amount of the loading dose need be computed, not the rate of its administration; to a first approximation, this is so. The amount of drug required to achieve a given steady state concentration is the amount that will eventually be in the body when the desired steady state is reached. (For intermittent dosage schemes, the amount is that at the average concentration.) The volume of distribution *(V)* is the proportionality factor that relates that total amount of drug in the body to the plasma concentration:

$$\text{Loading dose} = C_{ss} \cdot V \tag{23}$$

For the theophylline example given earlier, the loading dose will be 525 mg (i.e., 15 mg/liter $\times$ 35 liters). For most drugs, the loading dose can be given as a single dose by the chosen route of administration. Up to this point, we have ignored the possibility that drugs follow complicated multicompartment pharmacokinetics (e.g., the distribution process as exemplified by the two-compartment model in Fig. 4). This is justified in the great majority of cases, where pharmacokinetic tools are used in developing drug dosage regimens and in elucidating or predicting the effects of physiologic and pathologic changes in the patient. However, in some cases, the distribution phase cannot be ignored, particularly when a loading dose is administered. If the rate of absorption is rapid relative to distribution (this is always true for intravenous bolus administration), the concentration of drug in plasma that results from an appropriate loading dose can initially be considerably higher than desired. This is true, since initially the drug will distribute only in the central compartment volume (V_1 in Fig. 4) and time is required before distribution occurs into the larger whole body volume of distribution. Unwanted effects may occur transiently, and these may be severe. This may be particularly important, for example, in the administration of an antiarrhythmic drug, where almost immediate toxic response is obtained when plasma concentrations exceed a particular level. Thus, whereas usually only the amount of a loading dose need be calculated, the rate of administration can sometimes be crucial, and slow administration of an intravenous drug (over minutes rather than seconds) is almost always wise. For intravenous doses

of theophylline, initial injections are recommended to be given over a 20-min period to avoid plasma levels during the distribution phase.

EFFECTS OF DISEASE STATES ON PHARMACOKINETICS

Disease states can modify a number of kinetic parameters altering steady state concentrations. The ability to predict or understand how pathologic conditions can modify drug kinetics requires an understanding of the interrelationships among the various parameters. Clearance is the most critical parameter in the design of drug dosage regimens. It is also the most easily calculated and utilized parameter. For drugs following first order kinetic processes, clearance may be calculated independent of the number of compartments in a pharmacokinetic model using area under the curve measurements. During steady state dosing clearance may be calculated from the dosing rate and the measured average concentration (Eq. 1). Clearance does not have the same ambiguities associated with volume of distribution and the various half-lives which characterize multicompartment pharmacokinetic models. However, these other parameters must be estimated if one wishes to characterize the time course of drug concentrations following intermittent doses, particularly the expected maximum and minimum steady state concentrations. Bioavailability must also be determined. If an intravenous dose of the drug is given, calculation of this parameter is straightforward. However, even when only oral doses are available, the bioavailability parameter is incorporated into the unknown estimate of clearance (see Eq.1a). Then, the relation between dosing rate and measured average concentration yields CL/F values, which may be characterized just as readily in various patient populations. In the chapters to follow, further elucidation of the effects of the various disease states and physiologic processes on drug pharmacokinetics will be provided in particular patient populations.

REFERENCES

1. Benet, L. Z. (1982): Pharmacokinetics: I, Absorption, distribution, and excretion. In: *Basic and Clinical Pharmacology*, edited by B. G. Katzung, pp. 22–33. Lange Publications, Los Altos, California.
2. Benet, L. Z., and Sheiner, L. B. (1980): Design and optimization of dosage regimens: Pharmacokinetic data. In: *Goodman and Gilman's The Pharmacological Basis of Therapeutics*, 6th Ed., edited by A. G. Gilman, L. S. Goodman, and A. Gilman, pp. 1675–1737. Macmillan, New York.
3. Evans, W. E., Schentag, J. J., and Jusko, W. J. (editors) (1980)! *Applied Pharmacokinetics: Principals of Therapeutic Drug Monitoring*. Applied Therapeutics, San Francisco.
4. Benet, L. Z. (1978): Effect of route of administration and distribution on drug action. *J. Pharmacokinet. Biopharm.*, 6:559–585.
5. Dedrick, R. L., and Bischoff, K. B. (1968): Pharmacokinetics in applications of the artificial kidney. *Chem. Eng. Prog. Sym. Ser.*, 64:32–44.
6. Mapelson, W. W. (1963): An electric analogue for uptake and exchange or inert gases and other agents. *J. Appl. Physiol.*, 18:197–204.
7. Tozer, T. N. (1981): Concepts basic to pharmacokinetics. *Pharmacol. Ther.*, 12:109–131.
8. Rowland, M., and Tozer, T. N. (1980): *Clinical Pharmacokinetics: Concepts and Applications*. Lea & Febiger, Philadelphia.
9. Rowland, M., Benet, L. Z., and Graham, G. G. (1973): Clearance concepts in pharmacokinetics. *J. Pharmacokinet. Biopharm.*, 1:123–136.
10. Wilkinson, G. R., and Shand, D. G. (1975): A physiological approach to hepatic drug clearance. *Clin. Pharmacol. Ther.*, 18:377–390.

11. Bowman, W. C., and Rand, M. J. (1980): *Textbook of Pharmacology*, 2nd Ed., pp. 40.1–40.58. Blackwell, London.

12. Heel, R. C., and Avery, G. S. (1980): Drug data information. In: *Drug Treatment*, 2nd Ed., edited by G. S. Avery, pp. 1211–1222. ADIS press, New York.

13. Paxton, J. W. (1981): Elementary pharmacokinetics in clinical practice; 3, Practical pharmacokinetic applications. *N.Z. Med. J.*, 94:381–384.

14. Gibaldi, M., and Perrier, D. (1982): Pharmacokinetics, 2nd Ed., pp. 1–43, 84–109, 445–449. Marcel Dekker, New York.

15. Benet, L. Z., and Galeazzi, R. L. (1979): Noncompartmental determination of the steady-state volume of distribution. *J. Pharm. Sci.*, 68:1071–1074.

16. Aziz, N. S., Gambertoglio, J. G., Lin, E. T., and Benet, L. Z. (1978): Pharmacokinetics of cefamandole using HPLC assay. *J. Pharmacokinet. Biopharm.*, 6:153–164.

17. Gambertoglio, J. G., Aziz, N. S., Lin, E. T., Grausz, H., Naughton, J. L., and Benet, L. Z. (1979): Cefamandole kinetics in uremic patients undergoing hemodialysis. *Clin. Pharmacol. Ther.*, 26:592–599.

18. Benet, L. Z. (1983): Pharmacokinetic parameters: Which are necessary to define a drug substance? *Eur. J. Resp. Dis. (in press)*.

19. Benet, L. Z. (1974): Input factors as determinants of drug activity: Route, dose, dosage regimen, and the drug delivery system. In: *Principles and Techniques of Human Research and Therapeutics*, edited by F. G. McMahon, Jr., pp. 9–23. Furtura Publishing, Mount Kisco, New York.

20. de Boer, A. G., Moolenaar, F., de Leede, L. G. J., and Breimer, D. D. (1982): Rectal drug administration: Clinical pharmacokinetic considerations. *Clin. Pharmacokinet.*, 7:285–311.

21. Nies, A. S., Shand, D. G., and Wilkinson, G. R. (1976): Altered hepatic blood flow and drug disposition. *Clin. Pharmacokinet.*, 1:135–155.

22. Mayersohn, M. (1980): Clinical pharmacokinetics: Applying basic principles to therapy. *Drug Ther.*, September: 79–91.

Pharmacokinetic Basis for Drug Treatment,
edited by L. Z. Benet et al., Raven Press,
New York © 1984

Chapter 2

Effects of Gastrointestinal Disease on Drug Absorption

Peter G. Welling

School of Pharmacy, University of Wisconsin, Madison, Wisconsin 53706

The great majority of systemically acting drugs are administered by the oral route, because this method is generally more convenient and less painful and often is just as efficient as parenteral dosage routes. By administering drugs orally, one uses the natural processes by which the body obtains essential nutrients.

The efficiency with which an orally administered drug is absorbed is a function of many variables. A drug product should be sufficiently water-soluble to dissolve in gastrointestinal fluids and yet be sufficiently lipophilic to diffuse across the lipoidal epithelial lining of the gastrointestinal tract into the splanchnic circulation. Acid-labile drugs must be protected from acidic gastric secretions, whereas a drug that is an irritant to the gastrointestinal mucosa must be formulated to prevent or minimize this irritation (e.g., potassium chloride tablets). The oral absorption of a drug is thus a function of its chemical nature and the type of formulation, and also various interactions between the drug, the formulation, and the components of the gastrointestinal tract. These include the following: variable pH; gastric, pancreatic, and intestinal secretions; intestinal motility; enzymic activity within the lumen and epithelium of the gastrointestinal tract and the liver; a host of other interactions involving both endogenous and exogenous components. Drugs for oral use are therefore available in a huge variety of formulations that are designed to optimize drug absorption characteristics and also to provide a dosage form that is stable, attractive, and convenient to use (1).

Drug absorption into the systemic circulation (i.e., drug bioavailability) is usually examined in healthy volunteers under carefully controlled conditions, and data arising from such studies are used by regulatory agencies and by health science practitioners to establish drug absorption characteristics and appropriate dosages.

The clinical situation in which a drug is administered may, however, be far different from that prevailing in a controlled study in healthy volunteers. The patient may receive a larger number of drugs simultaneously. These may be taken before, with, or shortly after meals and may be ingested with varying fluid volumes. The patient may also be suffering from a variety of conditions that may influence the efficiency of drug absorption.

The purpose of this chapter is to describe some conditions that can affect (and in some cases have been shown to affect) the absorption characteristics of orally administered drugs, with particular reference to gastrointestinal disease. In this respect, the discussion will be limited to those disease conditions directly involving the gastrointestinal tract. Diseases involving other organs and systems (e.g., liver disease and cardiovascular disease) affecting drug absorption are covered in Chapters 3, 4, and 6. The present discussion is limited to those drugs that are swallowed and therefore absorbed into the splanchnic circulation.

DISEASES OF THE GASTROINTESTINAL TRACT

Gastrointestinal and liver diseases are major causes of morbidity and mortality. In 1968 in the United States, digestive diseases were responsible for 9% of all deaths, 10 to 15% of hospital admissions, one-third of all major operations, and 11% of chronic illnesses, with a total estimated cost of $15 billion (2).

Many conditions involving the gastrointestinal tract are likely to cause changes in drug absorption. Whereas a considerable amount of information is available on the malabsorption of nutrients and other substances (3), little attention has been paid to the effect of gastrointestinal disease on the absorption and bioavailability of drugs.

With an organ system as complex as the gastrointestinal tract, the number of disease conditions and drug interactions, often of unpredictable intensity, that can interfere with drug absorption is almost infinite. For the purposes of this discussion, however, it is convenient to consider the various diseases and interactions under the headings listed in Table 1.

GASTROINTESTINAL MOTILITY

It is generally accepted that passive absorption is favored when a drug is in the un-ionized and more lipophilic form (4). Thus, the absorption of weak acids might be considered to be optimal in the acidic environment of the stomach, whereas absorption of bases might be favored in the relatively alkaline small intestine. However, owing to the large surface area created by the presence of microvilli in

TABLE 1. *Conditions that can influence drug absorption from the gastrointestinal tract*

1. Gastrointestinal motility
2. Diseases of the stomach
3. Gastric and intestinal surgery
4. Diseases of the small intestine
5. Diseases of the large intestine
6. Gastrointestinal infections
7. Interactions with other substances

the small intestine, this organ is the major absorption site for most drugs. Any factor that accelerates stomach emptying is therefore likely to increase the rate at which a drug is absorbed, and any factor delaying stomach emptying is likely to decrease the rate at which a drug is absorbed.

Stomach emptying is delayed by disease conditions such as atrophic gastritis, gastric carcinoma, pyloric stenosis, pancreatitis, migraine, and gastric ulcer (5). Other factors that can delay stomach emptying include the ingestion of food, alcohol, antacids, anticholinergic agents, and drugs such as propantheline (Table 2). A more comprehensive discussion of the effects of drug interactions on absorption is provided in Chapter 11. On the other hand, stomach emptying may be accelerated by such conditions as celiac disease, calcular cholecystitis, duodenal ulcer, stress, and gastroenterostomy, and also after ingestion of large fluid volumes and such drugs as reserpine and metoclopramide. The condition of achlorhydria has been claimed to increase (6) but also to delay (7) stomach emptying. However, these studies were carried out under different conditions, and the precise nature of the influence of achlorhydria on stomach emptying is uncertain (8). The absorption of orally administered lidocaine is markedly delayed in patients premedicated with atropine prior to laparoscopy, the mean peak plasma concentration of lidocaine occurring at 3 hr, as compared with 45 min in healthy volunteers (9). The absorption rate of orally administered quinidine sulfate was increased twofold to threefold in rats subjected to stress, whereas the absorption of salicylate was essentially unchanged under the same conditions (10). The increased absorption of the basic quinidine molecule was associated with more rapid stomach emptying and a decreased intestinal transit rate in stressed animals, as compared with controls.

A bizarre case of inhibited drug absorption due to delayed stomach emptying occurred in a 68-year-old woman who had ingested 66 enteric coated aspirin tablets during an 11-day period prior to hospital admission with hypertrophic pyloric stenosis. Of the 66 tablets ingested, 61 were recovered virtually intact from the stomach by gastrotomy (11).

Faster stomach emptying has been implicated in the apparently increased absorption of some therapeutic agents in patients suffering from celiac disease (12,13). However, the underlying mechanisms associated with increased drug levels in these patients are controversial and will be considered separately.

Metoclopramide accelerates stomach emptying and is used to prevent gastric reflux. It thus has the opposite effect to the antispasmodic agent propantheline, which decreases the rate of stomach emptying. Metoclopramide has been shown to increase the rate of absorption of several compounds, including aspirin (14), acetaminophen (15), levodopa (16), lithium (17), pivampicillin, and tetracycline (18). Propantheline, on the other hand, decreases the absorption rate for acetaminophen (15), levodopa (16), lithium (17), pivampicillin, and tetracycline (18). In one study, digoxin behaved differently from the foregoing compounds in that the absorption rate from tablets was decreased by metoclopramide but increased by propantheline (19). Rapid gastrointestinal transit due to metoclopramide presumably reduced the time available for tablet dissolution, while propantheline had the op-

TABLE 2. *Factors that influence the rate of gastric emptying*

Syndrome	Increased gastric emptying rate	Decreased gastric emptying rate
Physiological	Liquids; gastric distension; posture (prone or right side); energy density of food	Solids; acids; fat; increased osmotic pressure; amino acids; gastrin[a]
Pathological	? Chronic calcular cholecystitis; duodenal ulcer; atrophic gastritis, for liquids; gastroenterostomy; Zollinger-Ellison syndrome; medullary carcinoma of the thyroid; pancreatic cholera syndrome; chronic pancreatitis (with pancreatic insufficiency)	Acute abdomen; laparotomy; trauma and pain; labor of childbirth; myocardial infarction; gastric ulcer; hepatic coma; hypercalcemia; gastric volvulus; intestinal obstruction; uremia; pneumonia (severe, pneumococcal); secretin[a]; cholecystokinin[a]; glucagon[a]; diabetes mellitus; myxedema; malnutrition; migraine; raised intracranial pressure; atrophic gastritis, for solids; pyloric stenosis; heavy-metal poisoning; acute pancreatitis
Pharmacological	Metoclopramide; reserpine; anticholinesterases; sodium bicarbonate; aluminum hydroxide; magnesium hydroxide; guanethidine; dantrolene; cholinergic agents (i.e., bethanechol)	Anticholinergic drugs (atropine, propantheline, amitriptyline, nortriptyline, maprotiline, trihexyphenidyl, methylatropine nitrate); ganglion blocking drugs (hexamethonium, diphenoxylate, loperamide); narcotic analgesics (morphine, codeine, pethidine [meperidine], diamorphine, pentazocine); isoniazid; orphenadrine HCl; sodium nitrite; vincristine; vinblastine; alcohol; poldine methylsulfate; ? phenytoin; potassium chloride tablets; ? aluminum hydroxide; ? magnesium hydroxide

[a]Physiological role uncertain; question mark indicates questionable relevance.
Adapted from Nimmo (5), with permission.

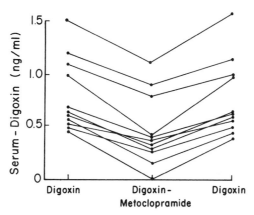

FIG. 1. Serum digoxin concentrations during treatment with digoxin and metoclopramide in 11 patients on digoxin therapy. (From Manninen et al., ref. 19, with permission.)

posite effect. The negative effect of metoclopramide on serum digoxin levels in 11 patients who received 10 mg metoclopramide three times daily for 10 days during long-term digoxin therapy is shown in Fig. 1.

The absorption of riboflavin is also increased by propantheline, but the absorption rate is delayed (20). The absorption of isoniazid is delayed by aluminum hydroxide gel (21), and it has been shown that aluminum salts and magnesium hydroxide delay the absorption of sulfadiazine sodium and quinine in rats, probably because of delayed stomach emptying or drug binding (22). Both magnesium and aluminum hydroxide retarded sodium pentobarbital absorption and delayed the onset of sleep in rats (22).

Rapid intestinal transit due to diarrhea may inhibit drug absorption. This is likely to be a problem with enteric coated and slow-release formulations, and it has been implicated in reduced absorption of sulfisoxazole and in delayed absorption of aspirin (23). Pregnancy has occurred after the use of oral contraceptives during a period of diarrhea (24).

DISEASES OF THE STOMACH

One condition of the stomach that has been studied for its effect on drug absorption is achlorhydria. This condition tends to occur in elderly patients and, apart from its uncertain effect on stomach emptying rate (8), has been considered as a possible causative factor influencing drug absorption by a direct pH effect. However, the results obtained in three separate studies are inconclusive. Achlorhydria had no effect on absorption of cephalexin, penicillin V (25), tetracycline (26), or acetaminophen (8), whereas the absorption of aspirin (measured as total salicylate) was significantly increased. Because the raised gastric pH in achlorhydria would be expected to inhibit aspirin absorption, because more of the drug is in the ionized form, it was postulated that the dissolution step may be rate-limiting in absorption,

and this would be favored in the achlorhydric patient. For further consideration of the effect of achlorhydria on absorption, see Chapters 14 and 15.

Diseases of the antrum and prepyloric area (e.g., carcinoma or peptic stricture) have profound effects on absorption, because gastric retention results. However, these have not been studied extensively.

SURGERY OF THE STOMACH AND SMALL INTESTINE

Surgical procedures involving the gastrointestinal tract might be expected to alter drug absorption, either directly through a reduction in epithelial surface area or indirectly through changes in gut motility and secretory patterns. In 10 patients who had undergone antrectomy with gastroduodenostomy and selective vagotomy, the serum levels and 6-hr urinary excretion of the acidic, basic, and neutral compounds sulfisoxazole, quinidine, and ethambutol were markedly reduced (27). The serum levels resulting from this study are shown in Fig. 2. In patients undergoing antrectomy with gastroduodenostomy without vagotomy, there were few changes in the absorption patterns of these three drugs, and it was suggested that decreased absorption after vagotomy may be associated with delayed stomach emptying. Vagotomy with pyloroplasty has been a frequently performed operation for many years, but it is now declining in popularity. This operation results in rapid gastric emptying of water-soluble substances and slower passage of solids. The form of medication (liquid or tablet) might well have a marked effect on its absorption rate.

Billroth II gastrectomy, a common surgical treatment for peptic ulcer disease, has been shown to reduce the absorption of nitrofurantoin, sulfamethoxazole, and cephalexin, but it does not influence the absorption of ampicillin or digoxin (28–33). This operation also has little effect on the absorption of tetracycline, despite the removal of essentially all acid-secreting cells (34). The unpredictable relationships between gastric surgery and drug absorption should perhaps not be unexpected, because the optimal absorption surface of the small intestine remains intact. Removal of part of the small intestine, as in intestinal shunt surgery for obesity, might be expected to have a more profound influence on drug absorption. However, this is not the case, because the small intestine is only partially bypassed. Whereas mal-

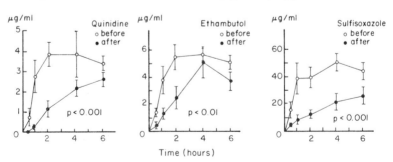

FIG. 2. Mean serum concentrations (± SE) for quinidine, ethambutol, and sulfasoxazole in 9 patients before and after antrectomy with gastroduodenostomy and selective vagotomy. (From Venho et al., ref. 27, with permission.)

absorption of nutrients and of some drugs such as norethindrone (35) and hydro-chlorothiazide (36) has been demonstrated, the absorption of antipyrine (37), propylthiouracil, and ampicillin (38) appears to be unaffected. In the case of hy-drochlorothiazide, urinary recovery of unchanged drug in postoperative patients was reduced to one-half of that observed in healthy volunteers.

Delayed gastrointestinal motility following other surgical procedures, and also after strong analgesics, may also give rise to impaired drug absorption (39). The absorption of antipyrine is reduced in cholecystectomy patients (40), the absorption of pivampicillin is reduced and variable following urological surgery (41), and the absorption of acetaminophen is reduced by meperidine and heroin (42).

DISEASES OF THE SMALL INTESTINE

The two diseases of this region in the gastrointestinal tract that have received most attention in the literature are celiac disease, or gluten-sensitive enteropathy, and Crohn's disease. These conditions have different etiologies and tend to affect different regions of the intestine. Celiac disease is an inflammatory condition of the proximal small intestine brought about by ingestion of gluten, a viscous protein contained in cereals. The condition can be controlled by a gluten-free diet, but control is lost if the diet is not maintained. Crohn's disease, on the other hand, is an inflammatory condition of largely unknown etiology that is associated primarily with the distal small intestine and proximal large bowel. This disease is a very heterogeneous condition that can also involve obstruction, bacterial overgrowth, liver disease, and gross debility. Whereas celiac disease can generally be controlled by means of a gluten-free diet, Crohn's disease is routinely treated with steroids and salicylazosulfapyridine (sulfasalazine). The efficacy of the latter is still debat-able. Patients with Crohn's disease often require surgical resection procedures.

Both of these diseases are associated with malabsorption syndromes, and their influences on drug absorption have undergone intensive study recently. The ab-normalities associated with the two conditions are summarized in Table 3. The variable effects on drug absorption that may be predicted from the data in Table 3 have been shown to occur in practice, and interpretation of the results of reported studies has been controversial. In most cases, celiac patients have been studied while on a gluten-free diet and therefore while in remission. However, these studies have given rise to somewhat unexpected results. Drugs whose absorption has been studied in patients suffering from celiac disease or Crohn's disease are summarized in Table 4. There is clearly no obvious pattern of relationships between the two diseases and the drugs that have been studied. Although, as seen in Table 3, there is significant overlap between the two diseases (reduced surface area, increased rate of gastric emptying, enzyme deficiencies of the gut wall), their influences on drug absorption often differ. Circulating levels of cephalexin are increased in celiac disease but are reduced in Crohn's disease. Conversely, circulating levels of clin-damycin are increased in Crohn's disease but are unchanged in celiac patients. The absorption of sodium fusidate is apparently increased in both conditions. Whereas

TABLE 3. *Abnormalities in celiac disease and Crohn's disease that can affect drug absorption*

Celiac disease		Crohn's disease	
Abnormality	Possible effect	Abnormality	Possible effect
Increased rate of stomach emptying	Drugs delivered more rapidly to small intestine	Reduced surface area available for absorption	Malabsorption of drugs whose major site of absorption is at the site of disease
Increased permeability of gut wall	Increased transport of passively absorbed drugs	Thickening of bowel wall	Impaired drug diffusion
Enzyme deficiencies at brush border	Impaired hydrolysis of esterified drugs to their constituents	Bowel flora changed to predominantly anaerobic population	Absorption patterns of drugs active against anaerobes would be important
Altered intestinal drug metabolism	Increased absorption of unchanged drug	Slower intestinal transit rate	Unpredictable patterns of absorption
Steatorrhea	Malabsorption of fat-soluble drugs and vitamins		
Reduced enterohepatic cycling of bile acids	Impaired absorption of drugs that require micelle formation for optimal absorption	Diarrhea due to bacterial overgrowth	Impaired absorption

Adapted from Parsons (46), with permission.

circulating levels of digoxin are reduced in celiac disease, there is no evidence of digoxin malabsorption in patients with chronic pancreatitis (45).

Of particular interest to the writer are the increased levels of propranolol in celiac disease and the even greater increase in patients with Crohn's disease. The dramatic increase in circulating propranolol levels in patients with Crohn's disease, compared with patients with celiac disease in remission and normal controls, is shown in Fig. 3 (47). The precise mechanisms causing the elevated circulating propranolol levels are not clear, nor is their clinical significance. Although it is tempting to ascribe the increased levels of propranolol to improved absorption, and an altered microclimate of hydrogen ions at the luminal surface of the intestinal epithelium might contribute to this (49), altered drug distribution may play an important, perhaps dominant, role.

Recent studies have shown that other pathological conditions such as ulcerative colitis, rheumatoid arthritis, and staphylococcal pneumonia also give rise to increased circulating levels of orally administered propranolol, and it is unlikely that all of these conditions increase propranolol absorption efficiency (50).These and other studies (51) have identified two factors, an increased erythrocyte sedimentation

TABLE 4. *Influence of celiac disease or Crohn's disease on circulating drug concentrations*[a]

Condition	Drug	Effect on drug levels	References
Celiac disease	Acetaminophen	Slightly reduced	68
	Amoxicillin	Unchanged	12,43
	Ampicillin	Unchanged	12,43
	Aspirin	Faster absorption gave increased levels during 30 min post dosing	13
	Cephalexin	Increased	44
	Clindamycin	Unchanged	12,43
	Digoxin	Reduced	45
	Erythromycin ethyl succinate	Unchanged	12,43
	Erythromycin stearate	Increased, but renal clearance is decreased	12,43
	Fusidic acid	Increased	43
	Indomethacin	Unchanged	13
	Lincomycin	Unchanged	12,43
	Pivampicillin	Slightly reduced	12,43
	Practotol	Delayed	46
	Propranolol	Increased	46,47
	Rifampicin	Unchanged	12,43
	Sodium fusidate	Increased	12,46
	Sulfamethoxazole	Increased, but renal clearance is decreased	12,43
	Trimethoprim	Unchanged	12,43
Crohn's disease	Acetaminophen	Slightly reduced	68
	Cephalexin	Reduced	44
	Clindamycin	Increased	48
	Erythromycin ethyl succinate	Unchanged	48
	Erythromycin stearate	Reduced	48
	Lincomycin	Reduced	48
	Propranolol	Marked increase	47
	Rifampicin	Unchanged	48
	Sodium fusidate	Increased	48
	Sulfamethoxazole	Marked increase	44
	Trimethoprim	Delayed	44

[a]For detailed studies, see original references.

rate and elevated levels of the acute-phase protein α_1-acid glycoprotein in plasma, that are common to all of these conditions. Propranolol and other basic drugs bind to α_1-acid glycoprotein, and Piafsky and associates (52) have demonstrated a high correlation between circulating levels of α_1-acid glycoprotein and the binding of propranolol and also of chlorpromazine. It is therefore likely that in Crohn's disease, which is associated with elevated α_1-acid glycoprotein levels, increased binding of propranolol causes a distribution shift that favors drug concentrations in plasma,

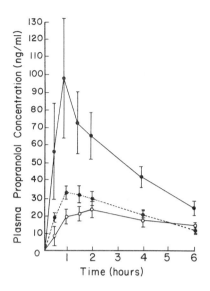

FIG. 3. Mean plasma concentrations of propranolol ($\pm$ SE) in patients with Crohn's disease (upper curve), treated patients with celiac disease (middle curve), and control subjects (lower curve) following a 40-mg oral dose. (From Schneider et al., ref. 47, with permission.)

thus giving rise to increased circulating drug concentrations that may be unrelated or only partially related to absorption changes. Support for this concept has recently been obtained in studies using an animal model (53). For further discussion concerning α_1-acid glycoprotein, see Chapter 10.

In 10 patients with symptoms of clinical malabsorption associated with intestinal villous atrophy, the absorptions of isoniazid, chloramphenicol, salicylate, and cycloserine were similar to those in healthy controls (54). Sulfafurazole absorption was delayed, whereas serum levels of quinine were elevated. However, increased levels of quinine were attributed to lower body weight and less subcutaneous fat in patients.

DISEASES OF THE LARGE INTESTINE

Because drug absorption occurs predominantly in the proximal small intestine, the effect of localized disease of the large intestine on drug absorption is unlikely to be clinically significant in most cases. However, for drugs that are absorbed throughout the gastrointestinal tract, and, in particular, for rectal dosage forms, diseases of the large bowel may be important. Typically, nonspecific or pseudomembranous colitis, diarrhea, bowel obstruction, amebic dysentery, and constipation may influence drug absorption. To the writer's knowledge, however, there have been no reports of substantially altered drug absorption under these conditions.

GASTROINTESTINAL INFECTIONS

The gastrointestinal tract is susceptible to a wide variety of infections and infestations, and any influence these may have on drug absorption will depend on the condition and on the drugs that are being used to treat it. Many such conditions

cause diarrhea, which can give rise to drug and nutrient malabsorption. Among these are shigellosis (bacillary dysentery), *Salmonella* gastroenteritis, cholera, staphylococcal food poisoning, and infestations by worms or protozoa (e.g., *Giardia lamblia*).

The absorption of ampicillin and nalidixic acid is reduced by diarrhea (55), but the extent of reduction in the absorption of these compounds depends on the severity of the condition. In infants and children with shigellosis, circulating levels of both compounds were markedly reduced in "poor absorbers" but not in "good absorbers." The poor absorbers tended to be younger, with lower body weight and with more severe diarrhea, than the good absorbers.

The activity of sulfasalazine in the treatment of Crohn's disease or ulcerative colitis is partially dependent on the bacterial microflora in the large bowel. Although some of the drug is absorbed intact, the majority is cleaved at the azo linkage by bacteria to release the active moiety 5-aminosalicylate (56). Sulfasalazine is ineffective in patients with Crohn's disease who have had a relapse following colonic resection, but it is effective in patients with intact colons (57). Its lack of effect in the former group is presumably due to loss of colonic bacteria with resection.

INTERACTIONS WITH OTHER SUBSTANCES

Orally administered drugs and drug formulations are subjected to a variety of interactions with other substances that can influence their absorption. For further discussion, see Chapter 11. Patients with gastrointestinal diseases may be on a number of medications, on special or restricted diets, or on controlled fluid intake. All of these factors can give rise to interactions, both direct and indirect, affecting drug absorption. Some indirect interactions concerning such agents as metoclopramide and propantheline were discussed earlier in this section (1,58,59) and will be reviewed in Chapter 11. Reduced absorption of tetracyclines and other compounds due to interactions with antacids is well documented (61). Similarly, absorption of many drugs, including digitoxin (62), thiazide diuretics (63), triiodothyronine (64), and warfarin (65), is impaired by cholestyramine, which may be used in cases of biliary obstruction or hyperlipoproteinemia.

The influence of food and specific dietary components on drug absorption has been studied extensively during recent years. However, as with gastrointestinal disease, the result of food-drug interactions on drug absorption is a function of a number of different processes and is difficult to predict (66,67). A brief summary of such studies is provided in Table 5 (2,58,60,66,74,77,78).

The physiological and physicochemical interactions associated with ingested food and varying fluid volumes that may affect drug absorption are described in Table 6. As indicated in Table 5, these have variously been shown to increase, delay, and reduce the absorption of different drugs from the gastrointestinal tract (66,67). The inhibitory effect that ingested food has on the absorption of erythromycin stearate is indicated in Fig. 4, and the apparent increases in circulating levels of the β-receptor antagonists propranolol and metoprolol due to food are illustrated in Fig. 5.

TABLE 5. *Drugs whose absorption is reduced, delayed, not affected, or increased by food[a]*

Group I: reduced	Group II: delayed	Group III: not affected	Group IV: increased
Amoxicillin	Acetaminophen	Acetaminophen	Alafosfin
Ampicillin	Alclofenac	Some penicillins	Carbamazepine
Antipyrine	Amoxicillin	Some sulfonamides	Chlorothiazide
Aspirin	Aspirin	Bendroflumethiazide	Diazepam
Erythromycin base	Bumetanide	Cephradine	Dicoumarol
Ethyl alcohol	Cefaclor	Chlorpropamide	Diftalone
Fluorouracil	Cephradine	Diazepam	Erythromycin ethyl
Hydrochlorothiazide	Cephalexin	Digoxin	succinate
Isoniazid	Cimetidine	Doxycycline	Erythromycin stearate
Ketoconazole	Cinoxacin	Erythromycin estolate	Griseofulvin
Levodopa	Diflunisal	Erythromycin ethyl	Hydralazine
Penicillin V	Digoxin	carbonate	Labetalol
Phenethicillin	Erythromycin	Glibenclamide	Lithium
Phenacetin	Furosemide	Glipizide	8-Methoxsalen
Pivampicillin	Indoprofen	Indoprofen	Metoprolol
Propantheline	Nitrofurantoin	Melperone	Nitrofurantoin
Rifampicin	Potassium ion	Metronidazole	Phenytoin
Sotalol	Sulfadiazine	Minocycline	Propoxyphene
Tetracycline	Sulfisoxazole	Oxazepam	Propranolol
Theophylline	Theophylline	Prednisone	Riboflavin
Trazodone	Valproic acid	Propylthiouracil	Spironolactone
Captopril[b]		Spiramycin	Hetacillin[c]
Doxycycline[b]		Sulfonylureas	
Erythromycin[b]		Theophylline	
		Tolbutamide	

[a]Data compiled from several sources (1,58,59,60,66,74,77,78). Some drugs, e.g., erythromycin, are listed in more than one category, reflecting variable results from different studies.
[b]Slightly reduced.
[c]Slightly increased.

Unlike the situation with ingested food, the influence of fluid volume on drug absorption is more predictable. Gastric distension is the only known natural stimulus to stomach emptying, and drugs that are ingested with a large fluid volume will tend to be emptied from the stomach into the optimum absorption area of the proximal small intestine at a faster rate than those ingested with a smaller fluid volume. This, together with improved dissolution characteristics, gives rise in the vast majority of cases to improved and more reproducible drug absorption. Four examples of increased circulating drug levels resulting from large accompanying fluid volumes are shown in Fig. 6. It has been shown also that the nutritive density (kcal/ml) may determine the rate of stomach emptying (ml/min) and that this supersedes consideration of volume alone (75).

TABLE 6. *Physiological and physicochemical interactions due to ingested food and fluid that can influence drug interactions*

Physiological function	Effect of food on physiological function	Possible effect on drug absorption
Stomach emptying rate	Decreased rate with solid meals, fats, high temperature, acids, solutions or high osmolarity; increased rate with large fluid volumes	Absorption generally delayed, may be reduced with unstable compounds, may be increased due to drug dissolution in stomach; absorption increased with large fluid volumes
Intestinal motility	Increased	Faster dissolution and decreased diffusional path promotes absorption; shorter transit time may inhibit absorption
Splanchnic blood flow	Generally increased, but may be decreased by ingestion of glucose	Absorption increased with faster blood flow; variable effects on first-pass metabolism, depending on drug characteristics
Bile secretion	Increased	Absorption may be increased due to faster dissolution or decreased due to complexation
Acid secretion	Increased	Increased absorption of basic drugs provided they are acid-stable; decreased absorption of acid-labile compounds
Enzyme secretion	Increased	Increased or decreased absorption depending on drug characteristics
Active absorption process	Increased	Active drug absorption reduced by competitive inhibition

Physicochemical interactions		Possible effect on drug absorption
Fluid volume		Absorption rate may decrease with large fluid volumes due to reduced concentration gradient, but absorption efficiency may be increased due to faster dissolution, osmotic effect, and exposure of drug molecules to greater GI surface area
Food and food components		Absorption decreased due to chelation, absorption, adsorption, physical blockade, but may be increased due to increased solubility with some diets; variable effects due to pH changes

From Toothaker and Welling (66), with permission.

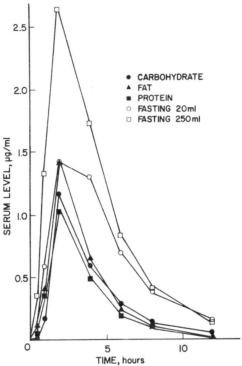

FIG. 4. Mean serum levels of erythromycin in 6 subjects following single 500-mg doses of erythromycin stearate in tablets under fasting and nonfasting conditions. (From Welling et al., ref. 76, with permission.)

CONCLUSIONS

The wide variety of diseases that can afflict the gastrointestinal tract, surgical procedures, infections, and indirect and direct interactions between orally administered drug products and other drugs and substances gives rise to a vast number of circumstances that can alter the absorption of orally administered compounds. Despite the obvious practical importance of this problem in drug therapy, it has received serious attention only recently. The rate of drug absorption may be altered depending on the rate of stomach emptying. The effect of achlorhydria on drug absorption is uncertain, and some forms of intestinal surgery have been shown to have greater effects on drug absorption than others. Diseases that influence the nature of the intestinal epithelium have been studied in some detail, in particular celiac disease and Crohn's disease. The results of various studies do not reveal a simple relationship, but rather a complex pattern dictated by the nature of the drug and its interactions within the gastrointestinal tract. The situation is further complicated by possible changes in drug protein binding and distribution characteristics

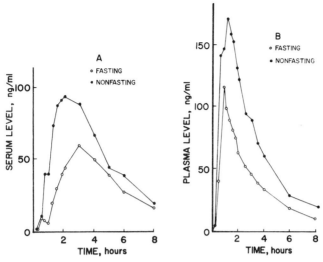

FIG. 5. Concentrations of **(A)** propranolol in serum and **(B)** metoprolol in plasma in 2 subjects following single doses of 80 mg propranolol or 100 mg metoprolol under fasting and nonfasting conditions. (From Melander et al., ref. 60, with permission.)

in various disease conditions, and this is exemplified by the atypical behavior of the highly protein-bound and extensively metabolized drug propranolol. Additional studies incorporating parenteral dosages, in order to separate distribution from absorption phenomena, are needed to resolve these problems.

Diseases of the large bowel, changes in the intestinal microflora, and parasite infestations can also influence drug absorption, but reports have been fragmentary.

Interactions between drugs have been shown to markedly affect drug absorption, often in a predictable manner. Other studies have clearly shown the advantages of giving drugs with large accompanying fluid volumes, and conversely the potential disadvantage of small accompanying fluid volumes, for example, in patients with restricted fluid intake. Food-drug interactions have been shown, as have many gastrointestinal diseases, to have variable effects on drug absorption. It has not been possible to establish general rules and guidelines for optimal drug dosing conditions; each compound and each formulation must be considered separately. Drug interactions are extensively discussed in Chapter 11.

Many diseases and conditions of the gastrointestinal tract, and also interactions, have not been considered here. Diseases and conditions such as pancreatitis, ileus, esophageal stricture, intestinal obstruction, gut ischemia, gastric dumping, and intestinal cancer can have profound effects on drug absorption. However, there is little information available on the influences of these and many other conditions on the absorption efficiency of orally administered compounds. A great deal of work needs to be done. Well-designed clinical studies with appropriate controls are needed to determine the nature, incidence, and severity of factors influencing gastrointestinal drug absorption and also the underlying mechanisms.

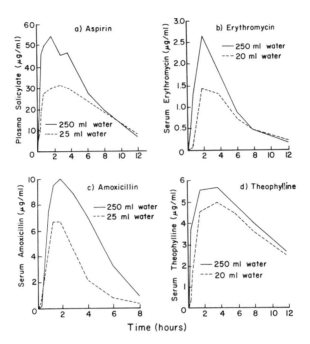

FIG. 6. Mean plasma or serum levels in 6 healthy fasting volunteers who received single oral doses of aspirin (650 mg) tablets, erythromycin stearate (500 mg) tablets, amoxicillin (500 mg) capsules, and theophylline (260 mg) tablets, together with large and small accompanying volumes of water. (From Welling, ref. 1, with permission.)

REFERENCES

1. Welling, P. G. (1980): Drug bioavailability and its clinical significance. In: *Progress in Drug Metabolism*, Vol. 4, edited by J. W. Bridges and L. F. Chasseaud, pp. 131–163. John Wiley & Sons, New York.
2. Bank, S., Saunders, S. J., Marks, I. N., Novis, B. H., and Barbezat, G. O. (1980): Gastrointestinal and hepatic diseases. In: *Drug Treatment Principles and Practice of Clinical Pharmacology and Therapeutics*, edited by G. S. Avery, pp. 193–194, 683–759. ADIS Press, Sydney.
3. Losowsky, M. S., Walker, B. E., and Kelleher, J. (1974): *Malabsorption in Clinical Practice*. Churchill Livingstone, London.
4. Schanker, L. S. Shore, P. A., Brodie, B. B., and Hogben, C. A. M. (1957): Absorption of drugs from the stomach. I. The rat. *J. Pharmacol. Exp. Ther.*, 120:528–539.
5. Nimmo, W. S. (1976): Drugs, diseases and altered gastric emptying. *Clin. Pharmacokinet.*, 1:189–203.
6. Halvorsen, L., Dotevall, G., and Walan, A. (1973): Gastric emptying in patients with achlorhydria or hyposecretion of hydrochloric acid. *Scand. J. Gastroenterol.*, 8:395–399.
7. Bromster, D. (1969): Gastric emptying rate in gastric and duodenal ulceration. *Scand. J. Gastroenterol.*, 4:193–201.
8. Pottage, A., Nimmo, J., and Prescott, L. F. (1974): The absorption of aspirin and paracetamol in patients with achlorhydria. *J. Pharm. Pharmacol.*, 26:144–145.
9. Adjepon-Yamoah, K. K., Scott, D. B., and Prescott, L. F. (1973): Impaired absorption and metabolism of oral lignocaine in patients undergoing laparoscopy. *Br. J. Anaesthesia*, 45:143–147.
10. Otto, U., and Paalzow, L. (1975): Effect of stress on the pharmacokinetics of sodium salicylate and quinidine sulfate in rats. *Acta Pharmacol. Toxicol.*, 36:415–526.
11. Harris, F. C. (1973): Pyloric stenosis: Hold-up of enteric coated aspirin tablets. *Br. J. Surg.*, 60:979–981.

12. Parsons, R. L., Hossack, G., and Paddock, G. (1975): The absorption of antibiotics in adult patients with coeliac disease. *J. Antimicrob. Chemother.*, 1:39–50.
13. Parsons, R. L., Kaye, C. M., and Raymond, K. (1977): Pharmacokinetics of salicylate and indomethacin in coeliac disease. *Eur. J. Clin. Pharmacol.*, 11:473–477.
14. Gibbons, D. O., and Lant, A. F. (1975): Effects of intravenous and oral propantheline and metoclopramide on ethanol absorption. *Clin. Pharmacol. Ther.*, 17:578–584.
15. Nimmo, J., Heading, R. C., Tothill, P., and Prescott, L. F. (1973): Pharmacological modification of gastric emptying: Effects of propantheline and metoclopramide on paracetamol absorption. *Br. Med. J.*, 1:587–589.
16. Morris, J. G. L., Parsons, R. L., Trounce, J. R., and Groves, M. J. (1976): Plasma dopa concentrations after different preparations of levodopa in normal subjects. *Br. J. Clin. Pharmacol.*, 3:983–990.
17. Crammer, J. L., Rosser, R. M., and Crance, G. (1974): Blood levels and management of lithium treatment. *Br. Med. J.*, 3:650–654.
18. Gothini, G., Pentilcainen, P., Vapaatalo, H. I., Hackman, R., and Bjorksten, K. A. (1972): Absorption of antibiotics: Influence of metoclopramide and atropine on serum levels of pivampicillin and tetracycline. *Ann. Clin. Res.*, 4:228–232.
19. Manninen, V., Apajalahti, A., Melin, J., and Karesoja, M. (1973): Altered absorption of digoxin in patients given propantheline and metoclopramide. *Lancet*, 1:398–401.
20. Levy, G., Gibaldi, M., and Procknal, J. A. (1972): Effect of an anticholinergic agent on riboflavin absorption in man. *J. Pharm. Sci.*, 61:279–280.
21. Hurwitz, A., and Schlozman, D. L. (1974): Effects of antacids on gastrointestinal absorption in rat and man. *Am. Rev. Respir. Dis.*, 109:41–47.
22. Hurwitz, A. (1971): The effects of antacids on gastrointestinal drug absorption. II. Effect on sulfadiazine and quinine. *J. Pharmacol. Exp. Ther.*, 179:485–489.
23. Jussila, J., Matilla, M. J., and Takki, S. (1970): Drug absorption during lactose-induced intestinal symptoms in patients with selective lactose malabsorption. *Ann. Medicinae Experimentalis et Biologie Fenniae*, 48:33–37.
24. John, A. H., and Jones, A. (1975): Gastroenteritis causing failure of oral contraception. *Br. Med. J.*, 3:207–208.
25. Davies, J. A., Holt, J. M., and Mullinger, B. (1975): Absorption of cephalexin in diseased and aged subjects. *J. Antimicrob. Chemother. [Suppl.]*, 1:69–70.
26. Kramer, P. A., Chapron, D. J., Benson, J., and Mercik, S. A. (1978): Tetracycline absorption in elderly patients with achlorhydria. *Clin. Pharmacol. Ther.*, 23:467–472.
27. Venho, V. M. K., Aukee, S., Jussila, J., and Mattila, M. J. (1975): Effect of gastric surgery on gastrointestinal drug absorption in man. *Scand. J. Gastroenterol.*, 10:43–47.
28. Antonioli, J. A., Schelling, J. L., Steininger, E., and Borel, G. A. (1971): Effect of gastrectomy and of an anticholinergic drug on the gastrointestinal absorption of a sulfonamide in man. *Int. J. Clin. Pharmacol.*, 5:212–215.
29. Lode, H., Frisch, D., and Naumann, P. (1973): Orale Antibiotikatherapie bie magenresezierten Patienten. *Verh. Dtsch. Gen. Inn. Med.*, 79:837–839.
30. Ritter, U. (1969): Agastrische Dystrophie. *Langenbecks Arch. Chir.*, 325:458–461.
31. Schmid, E., Schandig, H., Meythaler, C., and Bokenkamp, O. (1966): Sur Resorption von Nitrofurantoin bei Magenresezierten. *Z. Gastroenterol.*, 4:276–278.
32. Stoffels, G., Krautheim, J., Schreibe, O., and Schmid, E. (1968): Die Ausscheidung von Nitrofurantoin mit dem Harn nach Applikation eines neuen dragierten Handelspraparates. *Arzneim. Forsch.*, 18:360–362.
33. Ochs, H., Bodem, G., Kodrat, G., Savic, B., and Baur, M. P. (1975): Biologische Verfugbarkeit von Digoxin bei Patienten mit und ohne Magenresektion nach Billroth II. *Dtsch. Med. Wochenschr.*, 100:2430–2434.
34. Ochs, H. R., Greenblatt, D. J., and Dengler, H. J. (1978): Absorption of oral tetracycline in patients with Billroth II gastrectomy. *J. Pharmacokinet. Biopharm.*, 6:295–303.
35. Johansson, E. D. B., and Kral, J. G. (1976): Effectiveness of oral contraceptives after an intestinal by-pass. *J.A.M.A.*, 236:2847.
36. Backman, L., Beermann, B., Groschinsky-Grind, M., and Hallberg, D. (1979): Malabsorption of hydrochlorothiazide following intestinal shunt surgery. *Clin. Pharmacokinet.*, 4:63–68.

37. Andreasen, P. B., Dano, P., Kirk, H., and Griesen, G. (1977): Drug absorption and hepatic drug metabolism in patients with different types of intestinal shunt operation for obesity. A study with phenazone. *Scand. J. Gastroenterol.*, 12:531–535.
38. Klein, H., Kampmann, J., Lumholtz, B., and Hansen, J. (1977): Drug absorption in intestinal shunt operations. *Acta Pharmacol. Toxicol.*, 41(Suppl. 4):58.
39. Elfstrom, J. (1979): Drug pharmacokinetics in the postoperative period. *Clin. Pharmacokinet.*, 4:16–22.
40. Elfstrom, J. (1977): Plasma protein binding of phenytoin after cholecystectomy and neurosurgical operations. *Acta Neurol. Scand.*, 55:455–464.
41. Kunst, M. W., and Mattie, H. (1975): Absorption of pivampicillin in postoperative patients. *Antimicrob. Agents Chemother.*, 8:11–14.
42. Nimmo, W. S., Heading, R. C., Wilson, J., Tothill, P., and Prescott, L. F. (1975): Inhibition of gastric emptying and drug absorption by narcotic analgesics. *Br. J. Clin. Pharmacol.*, 2:509–513.
43. Parsons, R. L., Jusko, W. J., and Young, J. M. (1976): Pharmacokinetics of antibiotic absorption in coeliac disease. *J. Antimicrob. Chemother.*, 2:214–215.
44. Parsons, R. L., and Paddock, G. M. (1975): Absorption of two antibacterial drugs, cephalexin and co-trimoxazole, in malabsorption syndromes. *J. Antimicrob. Chemother. 1 (Suppl.)*: 59–67.
45. Heizer, W. D., Smith, T. W., and Goldfinger, S. E. (1971): Absorption of digoxin in patients with malabsorption syndromes. *N. Engl. J. Med.*, 285:257–259.
46. Parsons, R. L. (1977): Drug absorption in gastrointestinal disease with particular reference to malabsorption syndromes. *Clin. Pharmacokinet.*, 2:45–60.
47. Schneider, R. E., Babb, J., Bishop, H., Mitchard, M., Hoare, A. M., and Hawkins, C. F. (1976): Plasma levels of propranolol in treated patients with coeliac disease and patients with Crohn's disease. *Br. Med. J.*, 2:794–795.
48. Parsons, R. L., Paddock, G. M., Hossack, G. M., and Hailey, D. M. (1976): Antibiotic absorption in Crohn's disease. In: *Chemotherapy, Vol. 4: Pharmacology of Antibiotics*, edited by J. D. Williams and A. M. Geddes, pp. 219–229. Plenum Press, New York.
49. Cooper, B. T., Cooke, W. T., Lucas, M. L., and Blair, J. A. (1976): Propranolol absorption in Crohn's disease and coeliac disease. *Br. Med. J.*, 2:1135.
50. Schneider, R. E., Bishop, H., and Hawkins, C. F. (1979): Plasma propranolol concentrations and the erythrocyte sedimentation rate. *Br. J. Clin. Pharmacol.*, 8:43–47.
51. Kendall, M. J., Quarterman, C. P., Bishop, H., and Schneider, R. E. (1979): Effects of inflammatory disease on plasma oxprenolol concentrations. *Br. Med. J.*, 2:465–468.
52. Piafsky, K. M., Borga, O., Odar-Cederlöf, I., Johansson, C., and Sjöqvist, F. (1978): Increased plasma protein binding of propranolol and chlorpromazine mediated by disease-induced elevations of α_1-acid glycoprotein. *N. Engl. J. Med.*, 299:1435–1439.
53. Bishop, H., Schneider, R. E., and Welling, P. G. (1981): Plasma propranolol concentrations in rats with adjuvant induced arthritis. *Biopharm. Drug Dispos.*, 2:291–297.
54. Mattila, M. J., Jussila, J., and Takki, S. (1963): Drug absorption in patients with intestinal villous atrophy. *Arzneim. Forsch.*, 23:583–585.
55. Nelson, J. D., Shelton, S., Kusmiesz, H. T., and Haltalin, K. C. (1972): Absorption of ampicillin and nalidixic acid by infants and children with acute shigellosis. *Clin. Pharmacol. Ther.*, 13:879–886.
56. Das, K. M., and Dubin, R. (1976): Clinical pharmacokinetics of sulphasalazine. *Clin. Pharmacokinet.*, 1:406–425.
57. Anthonisen, P., Barany, F., Folkenborg, O., Holtz, A., Jarnum, S., Kristensen, M., Riis, P., Walan, A., and Worning, H. (1974): The clinical effect of salazosulphapyridine (Salzopyrin) in Crohn's disease. A controlled double-blind study. *Scand. J. Gastroenterol.*, 9:549–554.
58. Welling, P. G. (1977): Influence of food and diet on gastrointestinal drug absorption. *J. Pharmacokinet. Biopharm.*, 5:291–334.
59. Melander, A. (1978): Influence of food on the bioavailability of drugs. *Clin. Pharmacokinet.*, 3:337–351.
60. Melander, A., Danielson, K., Schersten, B., and Wahlin, E. (1977): Enhancement of the bioavailability of propranolol and metoprolol by food. *Clin. Pharmacol. Ther.*, 22:108–112.
61. Barr, W. H., Adir, J., and Garrettson, L. (1971): Decrease of tetracycline absorption in man by sodium bicarbonate. *Clin. Pharmacol. Ther.*, 12:779–784.
62. Caldwell, J. H., Bush, C. A., and Greenberger, N. J. (1971): Interruption of the enterohepatic circulation of digoxin by cholestyramine. *J. Clin. Invest.*, 50:2638–2644.

63. Beeley, L. (1976): *Safer Prescribing, A Guide to Some Problems in the Use of Drugs*. Blackwell, Oxford.
64. Northcutt, R. C., Steil, J. N., Hollifield, J. W., and Stant, E. G. (1969): The influence of cholestyramine on thyroxine absorption. *J.A.M.A.*, 208:1857–1861.
65. Benjamin, D., Robinson, D. S., and McCormack, J. (1970): Cholestyramine binding of warfarin in man and *in vitro*. *Clin. Res.*, 18:336. (abstr.).
66. Toothaker, R. D., and Welling, P. G. (1980): The effect of food on drug bioavailability. *Annu. Rev. Pharmacol. Toxicol.*, 20:173–199.
67. Welling, P. G. (1980): Effect of food on bioavailability of drugs. *Pharm. Int.*, 1:14–18.
68. Holt, S., Heading, R. C., Clements, J. A., Tothill, P., and Prescott, L. F. (1981): Acetaminophen absorption and metabolism in celiac disease and Crohn's disease. *Clin. Pharmacol. Ther.*, 30:232–238.
69. McLean, A. J., Isbister, C., Bobik, A., and Dudley, F. J. (1981): Reduction of first-pass hepatic clearance of propranolol by food. *Clin. Pharmacol. Ther.*, 30:31–34.
70. Tobert, J. A., De Schepper, P., Tjandramaga, T. B., Mullie, A., Buntinx, A. P., Meisinger, M. A. P., Huber, P. B., Hall, T. L. P., and Yeh, K. C. (1981): Effect of antacids on the bioavailability of diflunisal in the fasting and postprandial states. *Clin. Pharmacol. Ther.*, 30:385–389.
71. Hamilton, R. A., Garnett, W. R., Kline, B. J., and Pellock, J. M. (1981): Effects of food on valproic acid absorption. *Am. J. Hosp. Pharm.*, 38:1490–1493.
72. Pederson, S. (1981): Delay in the absorption rate of theophylline from a sustained release theophylline preparation caused by food. *Br. J. Clin. Pharmacol.*, 12:904–905.
73. Welling, P. G., and Barbhayia, R. H. (1982): Influence of food and fluid volume on chlorothiazide bioavailability: Comparison of plasma and urinary excretion methods. *J. Pharm. Sci.*, 71:32–35.
74. Barbhayia, R. H., Craig, W. A., Corrick-West, H. P., and Welling, P. G. (1982): Pharmacokinetics of hydrochlorothiazide in fasted and non-fasted subjects: A comparison of plasma level and urinary excretion methods. *J. Pharm. Sci.*, 71:245–248.
75. Hunt, J. N., and Stubbs, D. F. (1975): The volume and energy content of meals as determinants of gastric emptying. *J. Physiol.*, 245:209–225.
76. Welling, P. G., Huang, H., Hewitt, P. F., and Lyons, L. L. (1978): Bioavailability of erythromycin stearate: Influence of food and fluid volume. *J. Pharm. Sci.*, 67:764–766.
77. Antal, E. J., Gillespie, W. R., Phillips, J. P., and Albert, K. S. (1982): The effects of food on the bioavailability and pharmacodynamics of tolbutamide in diabetic patients. *Eur. J. Clin. Pharmacol.*, 22:459–462.
78. Black, H. R., Israel, K. S., and Wolen, R. L. (1979): Pharmacology of cinoxacin in humans. *Antimicrob. Agents Chemother.*, 15:165–170.

Pharmacokinetic Basis for Drug Treatment,
edited by L. Z. Benet et al., Raven Press,
New York © 1984

Chapter 3

Effects of Hepatic Disease on Clinical Pharmacokinetics

G. R. Wilkinson and R. A. Branch

Departments of Medicine and Pharmacology, Vanderbilt University, School of Medicine, Nashville, Tennessee 37232

Liver disease in humans encompasses a wide range of pathophysiological disturbances that can lead to reduction in blood flow, extrahepatic or intrahepatic shunting of blood, hepatocyte dysfunction, quantitative and qualitative changes in serum proteins, and changes in bile flow. One expression of these perturbations is altered disposition of some, but not all, drugs in patients with liver disease.

Recent advances in the understanding of some of the physiological determinants of hepatic drug elimination have facilitated interpretation of the large number of studies in which drug handling has been investigated in patients with liver disease. The objective of this review is to briefly describe the involved pharmacokinetic principles and to demonstrate how drugs can be used to provide information on specific aspects of hepatic function. Finally, the heterogeneity of the effects of liver disease on different routes of drug metabolism and the possible therapeutic implications will be discussed. A more encyclopedic tabulation of the effects of liver disease on the disposition of drugs is presented in Chapter 4.

PHARMACOKINETIC PRINCIPLES

The disposition of a drug is governed by the following factors: its clearance by the organs of elimination; the volume of distribution, a reflection of extravascular tissue uptake; the elimination half-life and systemic availability, the fraction of an oral dose that reaches the systemic circulation (see Chapter 1).

Clearance

Systemic clearance *(CL)* is a measure of the efficiency with which a drug is irreversibly removed from the body. Under first-order conditions, clearance is independent of dosage and can be calculated from single-dose studies as

$$CL = \frac{FD}{AUC} = \frac{0.693\,V}{T_{1/2}} \tag{1}$$

where FD is the fraction (F) of the administered dose (D) reaching the systemic circulation unchanged, AUC is the total area under the blood or plasma concentration/time curve, V_{area} is the apparent volume of distribution, and $T_{1/2}$ is the elimination half-life. Clearance can also be estimated under steady-state conditions as

$$CL = \frac{I}{C_B^{ss}} = \frac{D/\tau}{C_B^{avg}} \qquad (2)$$

where I is the infusion rate, C_B^{ss} is the steady state drug concentration in blood, τ is the dosage interval and hence D/τ is the drug delivery rate, and C_B^{avg} is the average drug concentration in the blood during the dosing interval at steady state. Furthermore, individual organ clearance (see Chapter 1) can be measured as

$$\text{Organ clearance} = \frac{Q(C_a - C_v)}{C_a} = QE \qquad (3)$$

where Q is organ blood flow, C_a is the arterial concentration of total drug, C_v is the venous concentration of total drug, and E is the steady-state organ extraction ratio. The sum of individual organ clearances equals systemic clearance, and thus for drugs eliminated entirely by the liver, systemic and hepatic clearances are equivalent. Considering the relationship in Eq. 3, as the extraction ratio approaches unity, the hepatic clearance will approximate and be limited by hepatic blood flow; conversely, when E is very small, hepatic clearance will vary according to hepatic extraction and will be relatively independent of flow Q. This allows a classification of drugs into three major types based on the rate-limiting step of hepatic elimination: those with a high hepatic extraction ratio, where elimination is primarily dependent on blood flow (flow limited or perfusion limited); those with a low hepatic extraction ratio, where elimination is mainly dependent on uptake and metabolism, and clearance is independent of flow (capacity limited); those with an intermediate extraction ratio, where both blood flow and the activity of the removal process contribute to clearance. Table 1 provides guidelines to the physiological, pathological, and pharmacological states that are known to alter hepatic blood flow (1–6).

Intrinsic Clearance

Although both the hepatic clearance and the extraction ratio of a drug are empirical measures of the efficiency of elimination, they are dependent on three independent variables: the rate of delivery of drug to the liver, i.e., total hepatic blood flow; the extent of drug binding to blood constituents expressed as the unbound (free) fraction of drug in blood (fu_B); the rate-limiting step in hepatic uptake from sinusoidal blood, intracellular transport, metabolism, and, where applicable, biliary secretion. The efficiency of this latter removal process can be quantified as free intrinsic clearance (CL_{int}^u), which may be conceptualized as the clearance of drug from liver water. The relationship of these three parameters to hepatic clearance (CL_H) can be defined, using the venous equilibration model, as (7)

TABLE 1. *Some factors that alter hepatic blood flow*

	Increased flow	Decreased flow
Physiological	Chronic respiratory problems Food intake, digestion Supine posture ?[a] Pregnancy (most likely in second and third trimesters)	Acute respiratory problems Thermal stress, exercise Upright posture Decreased systemic blood pressure Portacaval shunt Volume depletion Elderly (>age 65)
Pathological	Viral hepatitis Uncontrolled diabetes mellitus Diarrhea (severe) ? Renal failure ($CL_{cr} < 5$ ml/min)	Congestive heart failure Burns (≥25%, first week) Cirrhosis Circulatory collapse Renovascular hypertension
Pharmacological	Glucagon Low-dosage dopamine Isoproterenol Salbutamol Phenobarbital Phentolamine PGE$_2$ Clonidine	Propranolol High-dosage dopamine Norepinephrine Phenylephrine Dimethylbiguanide Anesthetics Cimetidine, ranitidine Labetalol

[a]Question mark indicates questionable clinical significance.
Adapted from Wilkinson (1), with permission.

$$CL_H = Q \; \frac{fu_B \; CL_{int}^u}{Q + fu_B \; CL_{int}^u} = \frac{Q \; CL_{int}^{tot}}{Q + CL_{int}^{tot}} \qquad (4)$$

Quantitation of the relative contributions of intrinsic clearance and liver blood flow to hepatic extraction helps extend the earlier classification of drugs with high and low extraction ratios to high and low intrinsic clearances. When CL_{int}^u is very high, then E approaches 100%, and hepatic clearance approximates and is dependent on liver blood flow. In addition, changes in fu_B tend not to influence CL_H because the affinity of the removal process far exceeds that for the plasma (nonrestrictive elimination). Conversely, when CL_{int}^u is very low, extraction is inefficient, and CL_H is essentially equal to CL_{int}^{tot} and independent of Q. Under these circumstances, binding in blood tends to hinder elimination, and CL_H is proportional to fu_B (restrictive elimination). Between these extremes, Q, CL_{int}^u, and fu_B all influence CL_H to varying extents (see Chapter 4 also).

Systemic Availability

Assuming complete absorption of a drug across the gastrointestinal tract, a proportion of the dose may be eliminated by the liver before reaching the systemic circulation because of the anatomical arrangement of the portal circulation. Such

presystemic or first-pass elimination is determined by the extraction ratio E, so that the fraction of the dose that is available is equal to $1 - E$.

In this situation, assuming the absorption rate constant is much greater than the terminal elimination rate constant, CL_{int}^{tot} is measured from the oral dose divided by the AUC assuming that elimination is solely hepatic in nature:

$$CL_{int}^{tot} = \frac{D_{oral}}{AUC} \tag{5}$$

In contrast to the situation with intravenously administered drugs, the area under the concentration/time curve following oral administration under these conditions is dependent only on CL_{int}^{u} and fu_B and is independent of blood flow changes.

In liver disease there is the potential for changing the systemic availability of highly extracted drugs, thereby affecting steady state drug concentrations. Two factors contribute to this increase. First, if liver disease causes a modest reduction in the hepatic extraction ratio for a given drug, for example, from 0.95 to 0.90, then the fraction of that orally administered drug reaching the systemic circulation $(1 - E)$ will be doubled. Second, one of the consequences of the pathogenesis of chronic liver disease is the development of portasystemic vascular shunts that may carry drug absorbed from the gastrointestinal tract through the mesenteric veins directly into the systemic circulation. Thus, even in liver diseases in which biochemical hepatic function is relatively well maintained (e.g., schistosomiasis), oral treatment with high-clearance drugs such as niridazole can lead to high blood levels and an increase in adverse neuropsychiatric symptoms (8).

DRUG BINDING

Binding of drugs to the various constituents of blood and tissue varies widely according to the chemical nature of the drug. Both red cells and various plasma proteins can provide binding sites for drugs, but albumin is quantitatively the most important blood constituent involved in binding of acidic drugs, whereas both albumin and α_1-acid glycoprotein bind basic drugs. Liver disease has the potential for affecting drug binding by qualitative or quantitative changes in the binding macromolecules, by alteration of other proteins, and by the accumulation of endogenous substances such as bilirubin and bile acids that may displace drugs from binding sites. See Chapter 10 for further discussion.

The importance of drug binding is central to an understanding of the pharmacokinetic disposition of and pharmacodynamic response to a drug. The free (unbound) fraction of drug in blood is available for distribution to tissues, including receptor sites in the target organ(s), and is the fraction that is immediately available to removal processes.

The venous equilibration model (Eq. 4) allows three major classes of drugs to be distinguished in terms of their hepatic intrinsic clearance and binding (9). In the situation of flow-limited (highly extracted) binding-insensitive drugs (clearance insensitive to changes in protein binding), the high binding of such drugs as pro-

pranolol acts as a carrier to retain a supply of drug in the blood available for delivery to the site of elimination, where it can be stripped in a single passage through a capillary bed, and binding is nonrestrictive. Second, there are capacity-limited (poorly extracted) binding-sensitive drugs, which have a low CL_{int}^u and low fu_B, such as warfarin, where the binding determines the amount of free drug available for metabolism and results in a clearance that is linear with respect to fu_B. For such drugs it is possible that liver disease results in a decrease in CL_{int}^u but also an increase in fu_B; in this instance the resultant CL_H does not only reflect the change in drug metabolizing activity. This has been clearly illustrated with tolbutamide, where patients with hepatitis have an increase in fu_B but no change in CL_{int}^u, and as a result CL is increased and $T_{1/2}$ decreased (10). The change in $T_{1/2}$, therefore, reflects a change in binding, not drug metabolizing activity. Third, there are capacity-limited but binding-insensitive drugs, i.e., low CL_{int}^u and high fu_B. Changes in the CL of such compounds, e.g., antipyrine, fairly accurately reflect changes in CL_{int}^u.

DRUG DISPOSITION AS A PROBE OF HEPATIC FUNCTION

Numerous studies have confirmed that the pharmacokinetic disposition of many drugs is altered in patients with a variety of liver diseases (4,11,12). Furthermore, appropriate study design in many of these studies has permitted a clearer understanding of the mechanisms that produce the observed clearance changes in drug disposition. These studies confirm that each of the four major determinants of drug disposition, namely, CL_{int}^u, fu_B, Q, and hepatic vascular architecture, may be independently altered. This clearer appreciation of the influence of liver disease on drug disposition may be reversed to ask the question whether or not drugs can be used to evaluate specific aspects of hepatic function and architecture in an analogous fashion to the situation in the kidney with respect to renal blood flow, glomerular filtration, and intact tubular function.

The clearances of a large number of drugs, some of which are noted in Table 2, have confirmed that both acute and chronic liver diseases cause impairment of drug elimination. Figure 1 is illustrative of many of these examples and emphasizes two

TABLE 2. *Examples of drugs that could be used in the evaluation of liver function*

High clearance	Low clearance
Bile salts	Aminopyrine
Bromsulfophthalein	Antipyrine
Galactose	Chlordiazepoxide
Indocyanine green	Diazepam
Lidocaine	Lorazepam
Pentazocine	Oxazepam
Phenacetin	
Propoxyphene	
Propranolol	

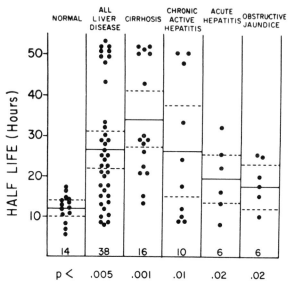

FIG. 1. The half-life of antipyrine in normal subjects and in patients with a variety of liver diseases. (From Branch et al., ref. 13, with permission.)

important points (13). First, although liver disease patients collectively have a clear twofold increase in half-life of antipyrine in comparison with normal subjects, the extent of overlap between the two groups is considerable. Thus, measurement of drug elimination alone does not differentiate between the two populations. Discrimination can be enhanced by considering clearance and relating it to liver volume to yield a measure of specific activity of drug metabolizing activity per unit of liver mass (Fig. 2) (14). Although this approach does considerably improve separation, it must be recognized that drug clearance is a functional measure that should range as a continuous spectrum from high to low values and that mild liver disease, even though histologically apparent, should not be expected to markedly influence drug metabolism. There is now evidence that when hepatic synthetic functions, as judged by serum albumin concentrations and/or prothrombin times, are impaired (i.e., albumin level below 3.0–3.5 mg/dl and/or impaired prothrombin activity of less than 80% normal), then drug metabolism becomes more markedly affected. The second point raised by Fig. 1 is the extensive overlap in antipyrine $T_{1/2}$ between the diagnostic groups of patients with liver disease. Although there are numerous causes of hepatic abnormalities, it appears that the hepatic response to injury is a limited one and that the functional consequences are determined more by the extent of the injury than by the cause.

The development of the concept of high- and low-clearance drugs suggests that drugs with low intrinsic clearances could be used to detect changes in metabolic function, and high-clearance drugs to detect changes in flow. Several groups of investigators have used this approach and compared the clearances of antipyrine, a drug with low intrinsic clearance, with high-intrinsic-clearance drugs like pro-

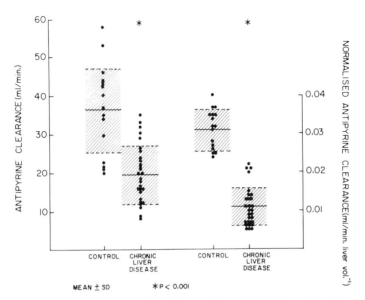

FIG. 2. Antipyrine clearance in normal subjects and in patients with a miscellaneous group of chronic liver diseases. The left two panels are total body clearance; the right two panels are clearances from the same subjects normalized by liver volume measured by ultrasound. (From Branch, ref. 35, with permission.)

pranolol, indocyanine green, galactose, lidocaine, and lorcainide in patients with chronic liver disease (15–18). In each instance there has been a positive correlation. In theory, the positive correlation between high- and low-clearance drugs could arise if there was an association between flow and intrinsic clearance. Based on Eq. 4, if these were the only changes to take place, hepatic extraction should not be reduced. However, direct measurements of the hepatic extraction of indocyanine green, propranolol, bromsulfophthalein, and galactose have demonstrated reductions in the hepatic extraction ratios in patients with liver disease (19–23). These apparently conflicting observations can be explained on the basis of the "intact-hepatocyte theory." This operational hypothesis is based on the assumption that even though liver disease is associated with complex changes of hepatocyte damage, regeneration, and inflammation resulting in disordered blood flow, the changes within the liver can be considered to be due to a reduced mass of cells that function relatively normally and are normally perfused (24–26). The reduced extraction of high-intrinsic-clearance drugs would then be due to the presence of intrahepatic shunts, which have been anatomically demonstrated (27). In the presence of intrahepatic shunts, hepatic clearance may be defined as

$$CL_H = f_m \, Q_T \, E_{\text{true}} \tag{6}$$

where f_m is the fraction of total blood flow (Q_T) that goes to functioning parenchyma that has an extraction ratio that is the same as in normals (E_{true}). The problem is that neither E_{true} nor the degree of shunting can be directly measured. The intact-

hepatocyte theory assumes that even in cirrhosis, E_{true} is normal, and thus the reduced observed extraction ratio is a function of intrahepatic shunts. Two approaches can be used to determine either Q_T or f_m. In the former instance, Q_T can be directly measured from an arterio-hepatic vein concentration difference using the Fick principle (23). In the example shown in Fig. 3, the normal extraction ratio of d-propranolol was measured in a group of patients with hepatic fibrosis. CL_H and Q_T were measured in patients with cirrhosis, and from this f_m could be calculated. The mean results indicate that these patients with cirrhosis had an 83% reduction in CL_{int}^{tot} and a 44% reduction in Q_T (Fig. 3). Application of Eq. 6 indicates that approximately 60% of this flow was passing to functioning hepatocytes and that the remaining 40% was passing through intrahepatic portal shunts.

An alternative approach, which avoids the necessity of hepatic vein catheterization, is to assume that the change in CL_{int}^{tot} of a low-clearance drug such as antipyrine is proportional to the change in flow to functioning hepatocytes, thus providing a measure of f_m. This approach can be applied to the data of Wood et al. (25). In this example (Fig. 4) the total intrinsic clearance and hepatic extraction of propranolol were measured in normal subjects using the systemic availability approach, and systemic clearances of propranolol and antipyrine were measured in patients with cirrhosis (25). Application of the intact-hepatocyte theory as an operational model to these data indicated that the mean Q_T in the patients with cirrhosis was modestly reduced by 37%, and of this flow, 13% was through intrahepatic shunts. In patient G, the most severely affected patient, the reduction in Q_T was greater, as was the proportion of intrahepatic shunting, so that functional flow was reduced to only a quarter of normal.

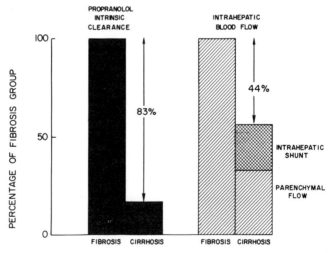

FIG. 3. Changes in intrinsic clearance of *d*-propranolol *(solid bars)* and hepatic blood flow *(hatched and crosshatched bars)* in patients with cirrhosis compared with patients with hepatic fibrosis. The relative proportions of intrahepatic shunt and parenchymal flow have been estimated assuming the intact-hepatocyte hypothesis. (From Branch, ref. 35, with permission.)

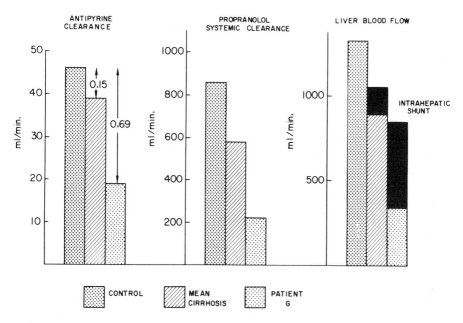

FIG. 4. Antipyrine clearance, propranolol systemic clearance, and estimated intrahepatic blood flow through functioning parenchyma or intrahepatic shunts assuming the intact-hepatocyte hypothesis. Normal subjects are compared with the mean for eight patients with cirrhosis and patient G, the patient with the most severe liver disease. (From Branch, ref. 35, with permission.)

In summary, there is now sufficient information to support the contention that measurement of drug pharmacokinetics can be used to provide quantitative information of hepatic function in patients with liver disease. However, there is debate as to which drug or drug combination is best and which parameters should be measured. There is also a theoretical basis to indicate that drugs can be used as tools not only to define hepatic metabolic function but also to describe abnormal splanchnic blood flow. It remains to be determined whether or not detailed pharmacokinetic studies can provide insight into the natural history of liver diseases and whether or not they can provide measures of the efficacy of therapeutic interventions.

HETEROGENEITY OF ROUTE OF DRUG METABOLISM

Even though the clearances of many drugs that are metabolized by the liver are reduced in liver disease, there are instances where this is not true. A notable example has been observed with the benzodiazepine group of drugs. All of these drugs are highly lipid-soluble and therefore have to be metabolized prior to elimination; in humans they have low CL_{int}^u and are highly plasma-bound. In single-dose studies, the clearances of diazepam and chlordiazepoxide are reduced by both acute and chronic liver disease and in the instance of acute liver disease return to normal on recovery, whereas the clearances of lorazepam and oxazepam remain virtually

unchanged (Table 3).The major difference between the former and latter pairs of drugs is their initial route of metabolism. Both diazepam and chlordiazepoxide are metabolized by phase I mixed-function oxygenase(s) prior to further phase II conjugation and renal elimination. In contrast, lorazepam and oxazepam are directly conjugated with glucuronide, and this latter pathway appears to be well maintained in the presence of liver disease. One possible explanation could be that a significant proportion of glucuronyl transferase activity takes place outside the liver. However, experiments with hepatic microsomal enzyme activity in rats pretreated with either carbon tetrachloride or placebo vehicle indicate that hepatotoxic rats with evidence of decreased microsomal cytochrome P-450 concentration and mixed-function oxidase activity also have an unaltered or even increased capability of glucuronyl transferase activity (32). Similar results have been obtained in investigation of glucuronyl transferase activity in the intact isolated perfused rat liver preparation (33). Thus, it appears that some drug-metabolizing enzymes have a reserve of functional capability. This implies that each specific drug's pharmacokinetics must be evaluated in patients with liver disease rather than be inferred from the limited literature available. A further implication of these findings, namely that lorazepam and oxazepam should be the drugs of choice in patients with liver disease, should be made only with extreme caution. From a pharmacokinetic perspective, this statement is valid; however, the clinical endpoint is the pharmacological response. Patients with liver disease and portasystemic encephalopathy are unusually susceptible to psychotropic drugs, and it is possible that increased receptor sensitivity is more important than modest differences in kinetics.

CLINICAL IMPLICATIONS

Whereas most dispositional studies follow the concentration/time profile of a drug after a single dose, in clinical practice most drugs are administered in repeated doses. Nevertheless, information from acute studies may be extrapolated to chronic studies. In the usual situation of repeated dosing, the time to achieve steady state will depend on the drug's half-life, taking approximately 3 to 5 half-lives to achieve

TABLE 3. *Routes of metabolism and influence of liver disease on elimination of some benzodiazepines*

	Initial route of metabolism	Cirrhosis	Hepatitis	Reference
Diazepam	Oxidation	Decrease	Decrease	Klotz et al. (28)
Chlordiazepoxide	Oxidation	Decrease	Decrease	Roberts et al. (29)
Lorazepam	Glucuronidation	No change	No change	Kraus et al. (30)
Oxazepam	Glucuronidation	No change	No change	Schull et al. (31)

steady state, whereas the actual drug level achieved depends only on clearance. Thus, in liver disease, drug accumulation will take longer and will achieve higher levels than in normal subjects.

Clearly, then, dosage regimens derived from studies obtained in healthy individuals may lead to the accumulation of drug to inappropriately high levels in patients with liver disease, where the disease process is associated with decreased clearance of the drug in question. Such high plasma drug concentrations may lead to unwanted effects such as excessive central nervous system depression in the case of sedative drugs. The situation is more complex, however, when the parent drug is metabolized in the liver to pharmacologically active metabolites. For example, both diazepam and chlordiazepoxide are metabolized to several compounds with pharmacological properties similar to those of the parent drugs, and they accumulate to varying degrees in chronic dosing in healthy individuals. Exactly how liver disease will affect the kinetics of formation and elimination of these metabolites and consequently their steady state levels cannot be predicted from acute studies of the kinetics of the parent drug. One study has shown impaired elimination of the first metabolite of diazepam (desmethyldiazepam) in patients with liver disease, indicating that at least two metabolic steps in diazepam removal may be affected (34).

Further studies of clinical pharmacokinetics in liver disease should be designed to take these and other considerations into account. An ideal approach would involve chronic administration of the drug in question until steady state conditions of the parent drug and metabolites are reached, oral and intravenous clearance measurements before and during chronic dosing to define changes in absorption, distribution, and elimination that could accompany chronic dosing, and the measurement of an appropriate end-organ response before and during chronic dosing to attempt to define the contributions of both parent drug and metabolite(s) to this response.

ACKNOWLEDGMENT

This work was supported in part by USPHS grant GM-15431.

REFERENCES

1. Wilkinson, G. R. (1976): Pharmacokinetics in disease states modifying body perfusion. In: *The Effect of Disease States on Drug Pharmacokinetics*, edited by L. Z. Benet, pp. 13–32. American Pharmaceutical Association, Academy of Pharmaceutical Sciences, Washington, D. C.
2. Richardson, P. D. I., and Withrington, P. G. (1981): Liver blood flow. II. Effects of drugs and hormones on liver blood flow. *Gastroenterology*, 81:356–375.
3. Blaschke, T. F., and Rubin, P. C. (1979): Hepatic first-pass metabolism in liver disease. *Clin. Pharmacokinet*, 4:423–432.
4. George, C. F. (1979): Drug kinetics and hepatic blood flow. *Clin. Pharmacokinet.*, 4:433–448.
5. Feely, J., Wilkinson, G. R., and Wood, A. J. J. (1981): Reduction of liver blood flow and propranolol metabolism by cimetidine. *N. Engl. J. Med.*, 304:692–695.
6. Feely, J., and Guy, E. (1982): Ranitidine also reduces liver blood flow. *Lancet*, 1:169.
7. Wilkinson, G. R., and Shand, D. G. (1975): A physiological approach to hepatic drug clearance. *Clin. Pharmacol. Ther.*, 18:377–390.
8. Faigle, J. W., and Kerberle, H. (1969): Metabolism of niridazole in various species, including man. *Ann. N.Y. Acad. Sci.*, 160:544–557.

9. Blaschke, T. F. (1977): Protein binding and kinetics of drugs in liver disease. *Clin. Pharmacokinet*, 2:32–44.
10. Williams, R. L., Blaschke, T. F., Meffin, P. J., Melmon, K. L., and Rowland, M. (1977): Influence of acute viral hepatitis on disposition and plasma binding of tolbutamide. *Clin. Pharmacol. Ther.*, 21:301–309.
11. Wilkinson, G. R., and Schenker, S. (1975): Drug disposition and liver disease. *Drug Metab. Rev.*, 4:139–175.
12. Williams, R. L., and Mamelok, R. D. (1980): Hepatic disease and drug pharmacokinetics. *Clin. Pharmacokinet.*, 5:528–547.
13. Branch, R. A., Herbert, C. M., and Read, A. E. (1973): Determinants of serum antipyrine half-lives in patients with liver disease. *Gut*, 14:569–573.
14. Homeida, M., Roberts, C. J. C., Halliwell, M., Read, A. E., and Branch, R. A. (1979): Antipyrine clearance per unit volume liver; an assessment of hepatic function in chronic liver disease. *Gut*, 20:596–601.
15. Andreasen, P. B., Ranek, L., Statland, B. E., and Tygstrup, N. (1974): Clearance of antipyrine-dependence of quantitative liver function. *Eur. J. Clin. Invest.*, 4:129–134.
16. Forrest, J. A., Finlayson, N. D. C., Adjepon-Yamoah, K. K., and Prescott, L. F. (1977): Antipyrine, paracetamol and lignocaine elimination in chronic liver disease. *Br. Med. J.*, 1:1384–1387.
17. Branch, R. A., James, J. A., and Read, A. E. (1976): The clearance of antipyrine and indocyanine green in normal subjects and in patients with chronic liver disease. *Clin. Pharmacol. Ther.*, 20:81–89.
18. Klotz, U., Müller-Seydlitz, P., and Heimburg, P. (1978): Pharmacokinetics of lorcainide in man: A new antiarrhythmic agent. *Clin. Pharmacokinet.*, 3:407–418.
19. Bradley, S. E., Ingelfinger, F. J., Bradley, G. P., and Curry, J. J. (1945): The estimation of hepatic blood flow in man. *J. Clin. Invest.*, 24:890–897.
20. Bradley, S. E., Ingelfinger, F. J., and Bradley, G. P. (1952): Hepatic circulation in cirrhosis of the liver. *Circulation*, 5:419–429.
21. Tygstrup, N., and Winkler, K. (1958): Galactose blood clearance as a measure of hepatic blood flow. *Clin. Sci.*, 17:1–9.
22. Redeker, A. G., Geller, H. M., and Reynolds, T. B. (1958): Hepatic wedge pressure, blood flow, vascular resistance and oxygen consumption in cirrhosis before and after end-to-side portacaval shunt. *J. Clin. Invest.*, 37:606–618.
23. Pessayre, D., Lebrec, D., Descatoire, V., Peignoux, M., and Benhamou, J. P. (1978): Mechanism for reduced drug clearance in patients with cirrhosis. *Gastroenterology*, 74:566–571.
24. Branch, R. A., and Shand, D. G. (1976): Propranolol disposition in chronic liver disease: A physiological approach. *Clin. Pharmacokinet*, 1:264–279.
25. Wood, A. J. J., Kornhauser, D. M., Wilkinson, G. R., Shand, D. G., and Branch, R. A. (1978): The influence of cirrhosis on steady-state blood concentrations of unbound propranolol after oral administration. *Clin. Pharmacokinet.*, 3:478–487.
26. Shand, D. G. (1979): Hepatic circulation and drug disposition in cirrhosis. *Gastroenterology*, 77:184–186.
27. Popper, H., Elias, H., and Petty, D. E. (1952): Vascular pattern of the cirrhotic liver. *Am. J. Clin. Pathol.*, 22:717–729.
28. Klotz, U., Avant, G. R., Hoyumpa, A., Schenker, S., and Wilkinson, G. R. (1975): The effects of age and liver disease on the disposition and elimination of diazepam in adult man. *J. Clin. Invest.*, 55:347–359.
29. Roberts, R. K., Wilkinson, G. R., Branch, R. A., and Schenker, S. (1978): Effects of age and parenchymal liver disease on the disposition and elimination of chlordiazepoxide. (Librium). *Gastroenterology*, 75:479–485.
30. Kraus, J. W., Desmond, P. V., Marshall, J. P., Johnson, R. F., Schenker, S., and Wilkinson, G. R. (1978): The effects of aging and liver disease on the disposition of lorazepam in man. *Clin. Pharmacol. Ther.*, 24:411–419.
31. Shull, H. J., Wilkinson, G. R., Johnson, R., and Schenker, S. (1976): Normal disposition of oxazepam in acute viral hepatitis and cirrhosis. *Ann. Intern. Med.*, 84:420–425.
32. Desmond, P. V., James, R., Schenker, S., Gerkens, J. F., and Branch, R. A. (1981): Preservation of glucuronidation in carbon tetrachloride-induced acute liver injury in the rat. *Biochem. Pharmacol.*, 30:993–999.

33. James, R., Desmond, P., Kupfer, A., Schenker, S., and Branch, R. A. (1981): The differential localization of various drug metabolizing systems within the rat liver as determined by the hepatotoxins allyl alcohol, carbon tetrachloride, and bromobenzene. *J. Pharmacol. Exp. Ther.*, 217:127–132.
34. Klotz, U., Antonin, K. H., Brügel, H., and Bieck, P. R. (1977): Disposition of diazepam and its major metabolite desmethyldiazepam in patients with liver disease. *Clin. Pharmacol. Ther.*, 21:430–436.
35. Branch, R. A. (1982): Drugs as indicators of hepatic function. *Hepatology*, 2:97–105.

Pharmacokinetic Basis for Drug Treatment,
edited by L. Z. Benet et al., Raven Press,
New York © 1984

Chapter 4

Drugs and the Liver: Clinical Applications

Roger L. Williams

*Departments of Medicine and Pharmacy, University of California at San Francisco,
San Francisco, California 94143*

Until recently, advice to physicians caring for patients with liver disease could be summarized by the following general statement: Use drugs as infrequently as possible, and use them when necessary at lower doses. The high incidence of primary hepatic disease, the presence of hepatic dysfunction as a result of other pathophysiologic processes (e.g., congestive heart failure), and the availability of a large number of powerful pharmacologic agents to treat patients with hepatic disease demand a more sophisticated approach. The relatively simplistic admonitions regarding pharmacologic therapy for patients with hepatic disease are in contrast to the reasonably well-defined methods to determine drug dosing regimens and drug choice in patients with renal impairment. The success of these latter guidelines is attributable primarily to the good correlations that exist between kinetic parameters of renal function (e.g., creatinine clearance) and pharmacokinetic variables that define the disposition of drugs that are eliminated via the renal route.

In the last 10 years, a number of excellent theoretical and clinical reports of drug disposition in patients with liver disease have appeared, as reviewed in Chapter 3. These investigations have not resolved all issues of drug dosing and effects in patients with liver disease. They have dramatically extended our understanding of how specific physiologic variables can influence drug absorption and disposition in patients with hepatic impairment. They have also provided a substantial amount of information about drug disposition in patients with liver impairment that is directly applicable to specific clinical settings. The goal of these investigations has been to generate data that will allow the health care practitioner to select rational dosing regimens of drugs for patients with liver disease. Using well-established tools and principles of clinical pharmacology and clinical pharmacokinetics, these dosing regimens are designed to produce maximum efficacy and minimum toxicity for drugs that are administered to patients with acute or chronic liver impairment.

Theoretical discussions of drug disposition and the liver have resulted in at least two models of how drugs reach the liver, distribute into liver tissue, and eliminate from the liver, either via biotransformation (metabolism) or via biliary excretion. The most popular of these models, termed either the venous equilibrium model (1)

or the well-stirred model (2) are perfusion models that identify hepatic blood flow (Q), intrinsic clearance of the liver (CL_{int}^u), and binding of drug to blood constituents (fu_B) as principal determinants of hepatic drug clearance (CL_H). The primary equation relating these physiologic variables is

$$CL_H = \frac{Q \cdot fu_B \cdot CL_{int}^u}{Q + fu_B \cdot CL_{int}^u} \tag{1}$$

The implications of Eq. 1 and the model represented by it are discussed in Chapters 1 and 3. Despite inherent difficulties in confirming the validity of the well-stirred (venous equilibrium) model of hepatic drug disposition in humans, the model itself, as exemplified by Eq. 1, has been valuable in focusing attention on specific physiologic variables that can influence hepatic drug disposition. It is important to remember that none of the clinical investigations conducted to date in humans has corroborated the assumptions of the model. Rather, the model itself has been used to elucidate potential mechanisms by which hepatic disease can alter drug absorption and disposition. For a more extensive discussion and analysis of physiologic models in hepatic drug disposition, the reader is referred to earlier reviews (1,3,4).

Descriptive investigations of drug disposition in hepatic disease have been conducted with increasing frequency over the last decade, and when performed correctly they have provided a significant amount of clinical information pertinent to the care of patients with hepatic damage. As a result of these investigations, the ways in which hepatic impairment can alter drug absorption and disposition have been more clearly defined. Whereas earlier investigations provided measurements of drug half-life as the primary parameter of interest in patients with hepatic disease, studies performed over the last decade have attempted to define drug disposition using more sophisticated pharmacokinetic methods. These studies have frequently provided measures of metabolic (hepatic) and nonmetabolic clearance, one or more volumes of distribution and half-lives, and, at times, determination of drug protein binding. To indicate where the values of these variables have differed from those in the healthy state, most descriptive clinical drug investigations have duplicated these determinations in healthy controls, who usually have been age-matched and sex-matched to the study population with hepatic disease. By comparing pharmacokinetic variables in the patient population and those in the control population, dosing regimens can be calculated that will, in the average patient, account for the changes in drug absorption and disposition with hepatic disease.

In Chapter 3, the elements and implications of the venous equilibrium model were discussed. In this chapter, information from selected clinical reports will be presented. These reports define how hepatic impairment can alter the disposition of specific drugs. This clinical information can then be used to design initial dosage regimens for patients with evidence of hepatic impairment. Following the sections in which clinical pharmacokinetic data are presented, this chapter will provide a brief review of pharmacodynamic alterations that can occur in patients with hepatic impairment.

Before proceeding with this discussion, some cautionary statements are in order. Hepatic impairment occurs as a consequence of different insults to the hepatic parenchyma. Although the response by the liver to these insults may be limited, it is nonetheless true that most investigations of the influence of hepatic disease on drug disposition and effect have been performed in patients with chronic cirrhosis. The degree to which other forms of hepatic disease can contribute to alterations in drug pharmacokinetics has been less well studied. Furthermore, hepatic disease undoubtedly is not a static, unvarying clinical entity that results in stable alterations in hepatic function over protracted periods of time; it is more likely a dynamic process that can alter disposition variably, depending on the course of the disease. The numbers provided in the following pages of this chapter should therefore be used as approximations that can vary in a single individual over time, depending on improvement or deterioration in the pathologic processes affecting the liver. Finally, it should be remembered that both the mean alteration in drug disposition and the variance about this mean are important. Consideration of the variance will indicate that there is usually considerable overlap in values for pharmacokinetic parameters measured in healthy individuals and patients with hepatic impairment. Thus, the dose in a single patient required to achieve a desired pharmacologic effect may need to be altered to a significantly greater (or lesser) degree than would be expected from average data. The clinician administering drugs to patients with hepatic disease must rely on carefully selected endpoints for both efficacy and toxicity and, where indicated, plasma drug concentrations to assist in the design of an appropriate dosage regimen.

CLINICAL PHARMACOKINETICS OF DRUGS IN PATIENTS WITH HEPATIC DISEASE

Drugs Highly Extracted by the Liver

As discussed in Chapters 1 and 3, and as indicated by Eq. 1, the disposition of a drug that is efficiently eliminated from the blood (a high-extraction-ratio drug) is sensitive to changes in hepatic blood flow ($CL_H \simeq Q$ when $CL_{int}^u >> Q$). For such a drug, the limiting factor in elimination is the rate at which the hepatic artery and hepatic portal vein can deliver the drug to the hepatic parenchyma. Highly extracted drugs are relatively insensitive to changes in intrinsic metabolic activity of the liver (CL_{int}^u) and to changes in drug binding to blood constituents (fu_B). Although the influences of endogenous and exogenous compounds and disease states on hepatic blood flow are relatively complex, it appears that hepatic blood flow in patients with chronic liver disease is reduced (5–7). In addition, shunting of blood past functioning hepatocytes occurs in acute as well as chronic liver disease (see Chapter 3 for a more complete discussion). These changes in hepatic perfusion suggest that drug clearance of highly extracted drugs, on average, will be reduced in patients with hepatic impairment. Plasma and tissue drug concentrations will therefore be markedly higher at a given dosing regimen in patients with hepatic

disease than in individuals with normal hepatic function. Because the liver is positioned between enteric sites of drug absorption and the systemic circulation, shunting of blood within the liver and reduced hepatic clearance (as a result of reduced hepatic blood flow) may also produce marked increases in drug bioavailability (see Chapters 1 and 3).

In general, clinical investigations of the disposition of highly extracted drugs have corroborated these theoretical concepts (Table 1). Although these changes are probably attributable to a reduction in blood flow, one carefully performed clinical investigation has suggested that the change in hepatic clearance for a highly extracted drug is due as much to a decrease in intrinsic clearance as to a reduction in flow (19). The reduction in hepatic clearance for these drugs is about 50% of that observed in a healthy control population (Table 1). Accordingly, for drugs such as propranolol, lidocaine, and some narcotic analgesics (meperidine, pentazocine), the initial oral dose should be reduced on average by about half in patients with evidence of hepatic impairment. Further reductions may be necessary to account for the increase in bioavailability of these drugs that occurs with hepatic impairment. For most of the drugs in Table 1, the change in clearance is not accompanied by a corresponding change in volume of distribution. Therefore, to achieve a specific blood drug concentration with either an intravenous bolus dose or a rapidly administered intravenous infusion, the amount to be administered for the drugs appearing in Table 1 may be similar to that given to patients without hepatic impairment. However, subsequent dosing to maintain the initial blood concentration will have to be reduced based on the change that occurs in clearance. Changes in drug clearance but not in volume of distribution will result in changes in drug half-life. For many highly extracted drugs, drug half-life is significantly prolonged in patients with hepatic disease (Table 1). Whereas alterations in drug half-life should not per se affect dosing regimens, they do indicate the time required to attain and decay from the steady state. Institution of a dosing regimen of a highly extracted drug in a patient with hepatic disease may require a significantly longer period of time to reach steady state (both in terms of drug concentration in the body and in terms of pharmacologic effect) than would be observed in an individual without evidence of hepatic disease.

Drugs Poorly Extracted by the Liver

The data in Table 2 indicate changes in clinical pharmacokinetic variables that occur in patients with hepatic disease for drugs that are poorly extracted by the liver. The drugs listed in this table represent only a small fraction of the total number of poorly extracted drugs that have been studied in patients with hepatic impairment. The drugs listed in Table 2 are presented because they are commonly used clinically and because adequate amounts of pharmacokinetic data are available to describe their disposition in healthy individuals and patients with hepatic disease. A more complete listing of pharmacokinetic changes of poorly extracted drugs in patients with hepatic dysfunction appears elsewhere (34). The data in Table 2 indicate that acute and chronic hepatic disease can alter the disposition of drugs that are poorly

TABLE 1. *Highly extracted drugs: changes in pharmacokinetics in patients with liver disease*

Drug	Reference	Extraction ratio	Disease[a]	Bioavailability (% change)	Volume[b]	$T_{1/2}$	Clearance
Chlormethiazole	11	0.9	C	+1,000		8.7 ± 4.0 hr (6.6 ± 2.4)[c]	12.8 ± 4.8 ml/min/kg[d] (18.1 ± 2.9)
Labetalol	14	0.7	C	+91	526 ± 31 liters[d] (805 ± 91)(V_{area})	170 ± 24 min (187 ± 26)	
Lidocaine	9	0.7	C		2.22 ± 0.94 liters/kg (1.70 ± 0.21)(V_{area})	343 ± 234 min[d] (108 ± 70)	5.2 ± 2.1 ml/min/kg[d] (9.2 ± 0.8)
	10		AVH		3.10 ± 1.80 liters/kg (2.00 ± 0.5)(V_{ss})	160 min (90)	13.0 ± 3.9 ml/min/kg (20.0 ± 3.9)
Lorcainide	50		C			12.5 ± 4.5 hr (7.7 ± 2.0)	814 ± 144 ml/min[d] (1,002 ± 304)
Meperidine	12	0.5	C	+81	263 ± 28 liters (232 ± 53)(V_{ss})	359 ± 77 min[d] (213 ± 25)	523 ± 158 ml/min[d] (900 ± 316)
	13		AVH		5.56 ± 1.8 liters/kg (5.94 ± 2.65)(V)	6.99 ± 2.74 hr[d] (3.37 ± 0.82)	649 ± 228 ml/min[d] (1,261 ± 527)
Metoprolol	15	0.5	C	+65	4.0 ± 0.3 liters/kg (3.2 ± 0.2)(V)	7.2 ± 1.2 hr (4.2 ± 1.1)	0.61 ± 0.13 liter/min (0.81 ± 0.11)
Morphine	16	0.6–0.8	C		2.3 ± 1.3 liters/kg (2.9 ± 2.4)(V_{ss})	2.2 ± 1.3 hr (2.5 ± 1.5)	1,153 ± 345 ml/min (1,233 ± 427)
Pentazocine	12	0.8	C	+278	356 ± 94 liters (415 ± 107)(V_{area})	396 ± 115 min[d] (230 ± 28)	675 ± 296 ml/min[d] (1,246 ± 236)
Propranolol	8	0.6	C	+42	380 ± 41 liters[d] (290 ± 17)(V_{area})	11.2 ± 3.2 hr[d] (4.0 ± 0.3)	580 ± 140 ml/min (860 ± 90)
Verapamil	17	0.87	C	+140[f]	481 ± 141 liters[d] (296 ± 67)(V_{ss})	815 ± 516 min[d] (170 ± 72)	0.545 ± 0.181 liter/min[d] (1.571 ± 0.405)
	18[e]		C		9.17 liters/kg (6.15)(V_{ss})	840 min (220)	0.62 liter/min (1.26)

[a]C, cirrhosis; AVH, acute viral hepatitis.
[b]V_{ss}, volume of distribution at steady state; V, volume of distribution (one compartment); V_{area} = clearance × $0.693/T_{1/2z}$.
[c]Numbers in parentheses indicate values observed in healthy controls.
[d]Statistically significant differences between patients and healthy controls.
[e]Mean values only reported.
[f]Because of a sixfold variability, caution is suggested in interpretation of this change in bioavailability (52).

TABLE 2. Poorly extracted drugs: changes in pharmacokinetics in patients with liver disease[a-e]

Drug	Reference	Disease	Volume	$T_{1/2}$	Clearance
Ampicillin	20	C	59.1 ± 43.1 liters[d] (19.5 ± 4.6)(V_{ss})	1.90 ± 0.56 hr[d] (1.31 ± 0.15)	280 ± 136 ml/min (342 ± 80)
Chloramphenicol	21	C	49.9 ± 4 liters[d] (65.9 ± 4)(V_{ss})	10.45 ± 1.14 hr[d] (4.6 ± 0.3)	59.2 ± 8.4 ml/min[d] (168.6 ± 9)
Chlordiazepoxide	22	C	428 ± 108 ml/kg (321 ± 77)(V)	40.1 ± 5.1 hr[d] (16.5 ± 3.6)	7.6 ± 1.08 ml/kg/hr[d] (13.8 ± 1.2)
	23	C	0.48 ± 0.14 liter/kg (0.33 ± 0.06)(V_{ss})	62.7 ± 27.3 hr[d] (23.8 ± 11.6)	7.7 ± 2.1 ml/min[d] (15.4 ± 4.4)
Cimetidine	24	L[f]	1.4 ± 0.6 liters/kg (1.1 ± 0.4)(V_{ss})	2.9 ± 1.1 hr (2.3 ± 0.7)	463 ± 145 ml/min (511 ± 93)
Diazepam	25	C	1.74 ± 0.21 liters/kg[d] (1.13 ± 0.28)(V_{ss})	105.6 ± 15.2 hr[d] (46.6 ± 14.2)	13.8 ± 2.4 ml/min[d] (26.6 ± 4.1)
Furosemide	26[e]	C	533 ml/kg[d] (210)(V)	2.2 hr (0.79)	192 ml/min (194)
	27	C	12 ± 3.5 liters (9.3 ± 3.7)(V_{ss})	129 ± 75 min (74 ± 18)	120 ± 36 ml/min (142 ± 42)

Drug	Ref.	Type	Volume of distribution	Half-life	Clearance
Hexobarbital	51	C (compensated)	1.14 ± 0.26 liters/kg (V_{ss}) (1.25 ± 0.24)(V_{ss})	509 ± 174 min[d] (340 ± 110)	1.88 ± 0.70 ml/min/kg[d] (3.32 ± 0.99)
		C (uncompensated)	1.57 ± 0.64 liters/kg (V_{ss}) (1.25 ± 0.24)(V_{ss})	1,017 ± 450 min[d] (340 ± 110)	1.26 ± 0.49 ml/min/kg[d] (3.32 ± 0.99)
Lorazepam	28	C	2.01 ± 0.82 liters/kg (V_{area}) (1.28 ± 0.34)(V_{area})	31.9 ± 9.6 hr[d] (22.1 ± 5.4)	0.81 ± 0.48 ml/min/kg (0.75 ± 0.23)
		AVH	1.52 ± 0.61 liters/kg (V_{area}) (1.28 ± 0.34)(V_{area})	25.0 ± 6.4 hr (22.1 ± 5.4)	0.74 ± 0.34 ml/min/kg (0.75 ± 0.23)
Oxazepam	29	C	60.9 ± 9.5 liters (61.2 ± 12.2)(V_{area})	5.8 ± 1.1 hr (5.6 ± 0.8)	155.5 ± 70.4 ml/min (136.0 ± 46.3)
		AVH	51.7 ± 17.2 liters (47.7 ± 16.7)(V_{area})	5.3 ± 0.7 hr (5.1 ± 1.3)	137.4 ± 51.4 ml/min (113.5 ± 30.7)
Prednisolone	30	CAH[g]	69 ± 13 liters (70 ± 8)(V)	3.0 ± 1.0 hr (3.3 ± 1.0)	278 ± 79 ml/min (256 ± 56)
Ranitidine	53	C	115 ± 32 liters (106 ± 35)	166 ± 41 min (124 ± 16)	476 ± 139 ml/min (543 ± 126)
Theophylline	31	C	0.563 ± 0.08 liter/kg (0.482 ± 0.08)(V)	28.8 ± 14.3 hr[d] (6.0 ± 2.1)	18.8 ± 11.3 ml/hr/kg[d] (63.0 ± 28.5)
Tolbutamide	32	C	0.15 ± 0.03 liter/kg (0.15 ± 0.03)(V)	4.0 ± 0.9 hr[d] (5.9 ± 1.4)	26 ± 5.4 ml/hr/kg[d] (18 ± 2.8)
Warfarin	33	AVH	0.19 ± 0.04 liter/kg (0.21 ± 0.02)(V)	23 ± 5 hr (25 ± 3)	6.1 ± 0.9 liters/hr (6.1 ± 0.7)

a-eFootnotes as for Table 1.
fL, type of liver disease not cited, enhanced CNS penetration of cimetidine.
gCAH, chronic active hepatitis.

extracted by the liver to the same degree and in the same direction as for drugs that are highly extracted by the liver. However, the data for poorly extracted drugs are not nearly so consistent as the data for highly extracted drugs. Hepatic disease can produce no change (warfarin), a decrease (diazepam), or even an increase (tolbutamide) in clearance of poorly extracted drugs. Furthermore, volume and half-life sometimes change (e.g., ampicillin), but clearance does not, whereas at times (as was the case for highly extracted drugs) clearance and half-life change reciprocally (e.g., chlordiazepoxide) but volume does not. The variability in the data in Table 2 precludes general statements about changes that occur for poorly extracted drugs in liver disease. These data, however, are clearly helpful in selecting drugs and in determining dosage regimens for patients with hepatic disease. Assuming equal changes (if any) in pharmacologic effect for the benzodiazepine group of drugs, it will probably be better to select oxazepam or lorazepam rather than diazepam, because the kinetics of the former two drugs do not change appreciably in liver disease (see Chapter 3, p. 58).

Protein Binding Changes in Hepatic Disease

Several reports have now documented that binding of drug to blood constituents is changed in patients with hepatic disease (Table 3). Endogenous displacers (e.g., bilirubin), present as a result of the deranged metabolism that occurs in patients

TABLE 3. *Hepatic disease and drug protein binding*

Drug	Disease[a]	Percentage increase in fraction unbound	Reference
Highly extracted drugs			
Lidocaine	AVH	No change	10
Meperidine	AVH	No change	13
Morphine	AVH/C	15	35
Propranolol	AVH/C	38	36
Poorly extracted drugs			
Amobarbital	AVH/C	38	37
Azapropazone	CAH/C	477	38
Diazepam	C	210	25
Diazepam	C	65	39
Phenybutazone	C	400	40
Phenylbutazone	AVH/C	500	41
Phenytoin	AVH	33	42
Phenytoin	C	40	43
Quinidine	C	300	43
Tolbutamide	AVH	28	32

[a]AVH, acute viral hepatitis; C, cirrhosis; CAH, chronic active hepatitis.
Adapted from Blaschke (44), with permission.

with liver disease, can account for some of these changes in drug protein binding. Changes in drug protein binding for a poorly extracted drug, in the absence of changes in other kinetic parameters, do not necessarily require a change in dosage. Williams et al. (32) demonstrated that although the clearance of tolbutamide increased in patients with acute viral hepatitis, this change could be attributed entirely to a change in protein binding (fu_B). Whereas the fraction of drug unbound increased, as did total plasma clearance, clearance based on unbound drug concentration did not change. In the absence of changes in this latter clearance, the concentration of unbound drug in plasma at a constant dosing regimen should not change. Because unbound drug concentration is presumably the effective (active) drug concentration, no dosage alterations are required for poorly extracted drugs when the only variable that is observed to change is fu_B. Conversely, changes in drug protein binding for drugs that are highly extracted by the liver may not alter clearance based on total drug concentration (because it is dependent primarily on hepatic blood flow), but may alter clearance based on unbound drug concentration. Changes in unbound drug clearance at a constant dosing regimen will result in changes in concentration of unbound drug. These latter changes will, in turn, lead to changes in pharmacologic effect. Changes in binding of a highly extracted drug should therefore dictate a change in dosing regimen in the absence of change in other pharmacokinetic parameters.

PHARMACODYNAMICS

Alterations in drug effect (pharmacodynamics) may accompany alterations in drug absorption and disposition in patients with hepatic impairment. Clinical investigations to document pharmacodynamic changes are difficult to perform, relying as they frequently do on less precise and less easily performed clinical measurements of drug response. To be unambiguous, pharmacodynamic studies in patients with hepatic impairment require concurrent performance of drug pharmacokinetic studies. This is necessary because it is not possible to determine if a change has occurred in the pharmacologic effect of a drug unless it can also be demonstrated that no change has occurred in the absorption and disposition of the drug. The requirement for dual investigation of both drug pharmacokinetics and pharmacodynamics probably accounts for the small number of reports that have described the influence of acute or chronic liver disease on the pharmacologic responses to drugs. A few reports have appeared, however, that suggest that hepatic impairment can increase sensitivity to drugs. For the most part, these investigations have been conducted with drugs acting on the central nervous system. Although pharmacokinetics was not discussed, Laidlaw et al. (45) reported that patients with cirrhosis, particularly those with a history of hepatic coma or precoma, were inordinately sensitive to either 8- or 16-mg doses of morphine. Both Read et al. (46) and Maxwell et al. (47) reported that cirrhotic patients were more sensitive to chlorpromazine-induced CNS depression than healthy subjects. All of these investigators (45–47) also observed that this increased sensitivity was particularly prominent in patients with a

past history of encephalopathy. In both chlorpromazine studies (46,47), pharmacokinetic analysis suggested that drug disposition was unchanged in patients with hepatic impairment. Morgan and Read (48) reported that patients with cirrhosis were more sensitive to the monoamine oxidase inhibitor tranylcypromine and to a lesser degree to the tricylic antidepressant amitriptyline, but they did not comment on alterations in the pharmacokinetics of either drug. Branch et al. (49) reported that the electroencephalographic changes at similar plasma concentrations of diazepam were more pronounced in patients with hepatic impairment, and particularly so in patients with a prior history of hepatic encephalopathy.

These investigations indicate that patients with chronic hepatic disease might be more sensitive to the pharmacologic effects of drugs, particularly those drugs that act on the central nervous system. However, further investigations will be necessary to define adequately the influence of hepatic disease on drug pharmacodynamics.

SUMMARY AND CONCLUSIONS

After more than a decade of intensive investigation, it is now possible to describe the influences of acute and chronic hepatic impairment on drug pharmacokinetics with some precision. Theoretical descriptions based on perfusion models of hepatic drug elimination have identified several physiologic variables (hepatic blood flow, intrinsic hepatic clearance, and protein binding) that are primary determinants of disposition for drugs eliminated by the liver. Derangement in any of these variables as a consequence of hepatic disease or dysfunction should alter hepatic clearance in a predictable fashion. In addition, descriptive pharmacokinetic investigations have provided much useful information about the way in which specific hepatic disease states can alter drug absorption and disposition. These investigations have suggested that clearance of drugs that are highly extracted by the liver is frequently reduced in patients with hepatic impairment because of the associated decreases in blood flow. For drugs that are poorly extracted by the liver, the influence of hepatic disease is more variable and may be manifested in a decrease, no change, or even an increase in drug clearance. The variable effects of hepatic diseases on drug metabolic routes and on drug protein binding (both of which are important determinants of clearance of poorly extracted drugs) appear to account for this variable influence.

Although progress in the last decade has been impressive, further work is necessary to extend our understanding of how liver disease can alter drug disposition and effect. Little information is available to indicate the influences of different forms of hepatic damage on drug disposition. The longitudinal course of hepatic disease relative to drug pharmacokinetics and effect has yet to be defined. Further studies are necessary to define the influence of hepatic disease on drug pharmacodynamics. New pharmacologic products must be tested in patients with hepatic impairment to determine if hepatic disease alters their pharmacologic effect(s) and pharmacokinetics. The information from future investigations must be transmitted in a usable way to health care professionals. The goal in these efforts will be to

supplant the therapeutic nihilism that sometimes attends the care of patients with liver disease. If these patients can benefit from a drug, they should have access to that drug. Carefully performed clinical investigations that define drug pharmacokinetics and pharmacodynamics will improve drug efficacy and reduce drug toxicity in these patients.

ACKNOWLEDGEMENTS

This work was supported by the U.S. Public Health Service (Grant 07546) and by the Drug Studies Unit, School of Pharmacy, University of California, San Francisco.

REFERENCES

1. Wilkinson, G. R., and Shand, D. G. (1975): A physiologic approach to hepatic drug clearance. *Clin. Pharmacol. Ther.* 18:377–390.
2. Rowland, M., Benet, L. Z., and Graham, G. G. (1973): Clearance concepts in pharmacokinetics. *J. Pharmacokinet. Biopharm.*, 1:123–136.
3. Pang, K. S., and Rowland, M. (1977): Hepatic clearance of drugs. I. Theoretical considerations of a "well-stirred" model and a "parallel tube" model. Influence of hepatic blood flow, plasma and blood cell binding, and the hepatocellular enzymatic activity on hepatic drug clearance. *J. Pharmacokinet. Biopharm.*, 5:625–653.
4. Williams, R. L., and Benet, L. Z. (1980): Drug pharmacokinetics in cardiac and hepatic disease. *Annu. Rev. Pharmacol. Toxicol.*, 20:389–413.
5. Richardson, P. D. I., and Withrington, P. G. (1981): Liver blood flow: II. Effects of drugs and hormones on liver blood flow. *Gastroenterology*, 81:356–375.
6. Nies, A. S., Shand, D. G., and Wilkinson, G. R. (1976): Altered hepatic blood flow and drug disposition. *Clin. Pharmacokinet.*, 1:135–156.
7. Daneshmend, T. K., Jackson, L., and Roberts, C. J. C. (1981): Physiological and pharmacological variability in estimated hepatic blood flow in man. *Br. J. Clin. Pharmacol.*, 2:491–496.
8. Wood, A. J. J., Kornhauser, D. M., Wilkinson, G. R., Shand, D. G., and Branch, R. A. (1978): The influence of cirrhosis on steady-state blood concentrations of unbound propranolol after oral administration. *Clin. Pharmacokinet.*, 3:478–487.
9. Thompson, P. D., Melmon, K. L., Richardson, J. A., Cohn, K., Steinbrunn, W., Cudihee, R., and Rowland, M. (1973): Lidocaine pharmacokinetics in advanced heart failure, liver disease, and renal failure in humans. *Ann. Intern. Med.*, 78:499–508.
10. Williams, R. L., Blaschke, T. F., Meffin, P. J., Melmon, K. L., and Rowland, M. (1976): Influence of viral hepatitis on the disposition of two compounds with high hepatic clearance: Lidocaine and indocyanine green. *Clin. Pharmacol. Ther.*, 20:290–299.
11. Pentikainen, P. J., Neuvonen, P. J., Torpila, S., and Syvalahti, E. (1978): Effect of cirrhosis of the liver on the pharmacokinetics of chlormethiazole. *Br. Med. J.*, 2:861–863.
12. Neal, E. A., Meffin, P. J., Gregory, P. B., and Blaschke, T. F. (1979): Enhanced bioavailability and decreased clearance of analgesics in patients with cirrhosis. *Gastroenterology*, 77:96–102.
13. McHorse, T. S., Wilkinson, G. R., Johnson, R. F., and Schenker, S. (1975): Effect of acute viral hepatitis in man on the disposition and elimination of meperidine. *Gastroenterology*, 68:775–780.
14. Homeida, M., Jackson, L., and Roberts, C. J. C. (1978): Decreased first-pass metabolism of labetalol in chronic liver disease. *Br. Med. J.*, 2:1048–1050.
15. Regardh, C. G., Jordo, L., Erik, M., Lundborg, P., Olsson, R., and Rönn, O. (1981): Pharmacokinetics of metoprolol in patients with hepatic cirrhosis. *Clin. Pharmacokinet.*, 6:375–388.
16. Patwardhan, R. V., Johnson, R. F., Hoyumpa, A., Sheehan, J. J., Desmond, P. V., Wilkinson, G. R., Branch, R. A., and Schenker, S. (1981): Normal metabolism of morphine in cirrhosis. *Gastroenterology*, 81:1006–1011.
17. Woodcock, B. G., Rietbrock, I., Vohringer, H. F., and Rietbrock, N. (1981): Verapamil disposition in liver disease and intensive care patients: Kinetics, clearance and apparent blood flow relationships. *Clin. Pharmacol. Ther.*, 29:27–34.

18. Somogyi, A., Albrecht, M., Kliems, G., Schäfer, K., and Eichelbaum, M. (1981): Pharmacokinetics, bioavailability and ECG response of verapamil in patients with liver cirrhosis. *Br. J. Clin. Pharmacol.*, 12:51–60.

19. Pessayre, D., Lebrec, D., Descatoire, V., Peignoux, M., and Benhamou, J. P. (1978): Mechanism for reduced drug clearance in patients with cirrhosis. *Gastroenterology*, 74:566–571.

20. Lewis, G. P., and Jusko, W. J. (1975): Pharmacokinetics of ampicillin in cirrhosis. *Clin. Pharmacol. Ther.*, 18:475–484.

21. Narang, D. P. S., Datta, D. V., Nath, N., and Mathur, V. S. (1981): Pharmacokinetic study of chloramphenicol in patients with liver disease. *Eur. J. Clin. Pharmacol.*, 20:479–483.

22. Morgan, D. D., Robinson, J. D., and Mendenhall, C. L. (1981): Clinical pharmacokinetics of chlordiazepoxide in patients with alcoholic hepatitis. *Eur. J. Clin. Pharmacol.*, 19:279–285.

23. Roberts, R. K., Wilkinson, G. R., Branch, R. A., and Schenker, S. (1978): Effect of age and parenchymal liver disease on the disposition and elimination of chlordiazepoxide (Librium). *Gastroenterology*, 75:479–485.

24. Schentag, J. J., Cerra, F. B., Calleri, G., Leising, M. E., French, M. A., and Bernhard, H. (1981): Age, disease and cimetidine in healthy subjects and chronically ill patients. *Clin. Pharmacol. Ther.*, 29:737–743.

25. Klotz, U., Avant, G. R., Hoyumpa, A., Schenker, S., and Wilkinson, G. R. (1975): The effects of age and liver disease on the disposition and elimination of diazepam in adult man. *J. Clin. Invest.*, 55:347–359.

26. Allgulander, C., Beermann, B., and Sjogren, A. (1980): Furosemide pharmacokinetics in patients with liver disease. *Clin. Pharmacokinet.*, 5:570–575.

27. Sawhney, V. K., Gregory, P. B., Swezey, S. E., and Blaschke, T. F. (1981): Furosemide disposition in cirrhotic patients. *Gastroenterology*, 81:1012–1016.

28. Kraus, J. W., Desmond, P. V., Marshall, J. P., Johnson, R. F., Schenker, S., and Wilkinson, G. R. (1978): Effects of aging and liver disease on disposition of lorazepam. *Clin. Pharmacol. Ther.*, 24:411–419.

29. Shull, H. J., Wilkinson, G. R., Johnson, R., and Schenker, S. (1976): Normal disposition of oxazepam in acute viral hepatitis and cirrhosis. *Ann. Intern. Med.*, 84:420–425.

30. Schalm, S. W., Summerskill, W. H. J., and Go, V. L. W. (1977): Prednisone for chronic active liver disease. *Gastroenterology*, 72:910–913.

31. Mangione, A., Imhoff, T. E., Lee, R. V., Shum, L. Y., and Jusko, W. J. (1978): Pharmacokinetics of theophylline in hepatic disease. *Chest*, 73:616–622.

32. Williams, R. L., Blaschke, T. F., Meffin, P. J., Melmon, K. L., and Rowland, M. R. (1977): Influence of acute viral hepatitis on disposition and plasma binding of tolbutamide. *Clin. Pharmacol. Ther.*, 23:301–309.

33. Williams, R. L., Schary, W. L., Blaschke, T. F., Meffin, P. J., Melmon, K. L., and Rowland, M. R. (1976): Influence of acute viral hepatitis on disposition and pharmacologic effect of warfarin. *Clin. Pharmacol. Ther.*, 20:90–97.

34. Williams, R. L., and Mamelok, R. D. (1980): Hepatic disease and drug pharmacokinetics. *Clin. Pharmacokinet.*, 5:528–547.

35. Olsen, G. D., Bennett, W. M., and Porter, G. A. (1973): Morphine and phenytoin binding to plasma proteins in renal and hepatic failure. *Clin. Pharmacol. Ther.*, 17:677–684.

36. Branch, R. A., Morgan, M. H., James, J., and Read, A. E. (1976): Intravenous administration of diazepam in patients with chronic liver disease. *Gut*, 17:975–983.

37. Mawer, G. E., Miller, N. E., and Turnberg, L. A. (1972): Metabolism of amylobarbitone in patients with chronic liver disease. *Br. J. Pharmacol.*, 44:549–560.

38. Jahnchen, E., Blanck, K. J., Breuing, K. H., Gilfrich, H. J., Meinertz, T., and Trenk, D. (1981): Plasma protein binding of azapropazone in patients with kidney and liver disease. *Br. J. Clin. Pharmacol.*, 2:361–367.

39. Thiessen, J. J., Sellers, E. M., Denbeigh, P., and Dolman, L. (1976): Plasma protein binding of diazepam and tolbutamide in chronic alcoholics. *J. Clin. Pharmacol.*, 16:345–351.

40. Wallace, S., and Brodie, M. J. (1976): Decreased drug binding in serum from patients with chronic hepatic disease. *Eur. J. Clin. Pharmacol.*, 9:429–432.

41. Held, V. H., Eisert, R., and Oldershaussen, H. F. V. (1973): Pharmacokinetics von glymidine (glycodiazine) und tobutamid bei akuten und chronischen Leber Schaden. *Arzneim. Forsch.*, 23:1801–1807.

42. Blaschke, T. F., Meffin, P. J., Melmon, K. L., and Rowland, M. (1975): Influence of acute viral hepatitis on phenytoin kinetics and protein binding. *Clin. Pharmacol. Ther.*, 17:685–691.

43. Affrime, M., and Reidenberg, M. M. (1975): The protein binding of some drugs in plasma from patients with alcoholic liver disease. *Eur. J. Clin. Pharmacol.*, 8:267–269.

44. Blaschke, T. F. (1977): Protein binding and kinetics of drugs in liver disease. *Clin. Pharmacokinet.*, 2:32–44.

45. Laidlaw, J., Read, A. E., and Sherlock, S. (1961): Morphine tolerance in disease. *Gastroenterology*, 40:389–396.

46. Read, A. E., Laidlaw, J., and McCarthy, C. F. (1969): Effects of chlorpromazine in patients with hepatic disease. *Br. Med. J.*, 2:497–499.

47. Maxwell, J. D., Carrella, M., Parkes, J. D., Williams, R., Mould, G. P., and Curry, S. H. (1972): Plasma disappearance and cerebral effects of chlorpromazine in cirrhosis. *Clin. Sci.*, 43:143–151.

48. Morgan, M. H., and Read, A. E. (1972): Antidepressants and liver disease. *Gut*, 13:697–701.

49. Branch, R. A., Morgan, M. H., James, J., and Read, A. E. (1976): Intravenous administration of diazepam in patients with chronic liver disease. *Gut*, 17:975–983.

50. Klotz, U., Fischer, C., Muller-Seydlitz, P., Schulz, J., and Muller, W. A. (1979): Alterations in the disposition of differently cleared drugs in patients with cirrhosis. *Clin. Pharmacol. Ther.*, 26:221–227.

51. Zilly, W., Breimer, D. D., and Richter, E. (1978): Hexobarbital disposition in compensated and decompensated cirrhosis of the liver. *Clin. Pharmacol. Ther.*, 23:525–534.

52. Woodcock, B. G., and Rietbrock, N. (1982): Verapamil bioavailability and dosage in liver disease. *Br. J. Clin. Pharmacol.*, 13:240–241.

53. Young, C. J., Daneshmend, T. K., and Roberts, C. J. C. (1982): Pharmacokinetics of ranitidine in hepatic cirrhosis and in the elderly. *Br. J. Clin. Pharmacol.*, 13:152P.

Pharmacokinetic Basis for Drug Treatment,
edited by L. Z. Benet et al., Raven Press,
New York © 1984

Chapter 5

Pharmacokinetics and Drug Excretion in Bile

Douglas E. Rollins

*Departments of Medicine and Pharmacology, University of Utah School of Medicine,
Salt Lake City, Utah 84132*

Biliary excretion of drugs is unique. Drugs cleared by this route are not simply eliminated from the body but may undergo enterohepatic circulation, metabolism within the intestine, or elimination in the feces. The pharmacokinetics of entero-hepatic circulation are extremely complex and poorly understood. Nevertheless, our knowledge of drugs that are excreted in bile and of the mechanisms involved has increased greatly in the past few years. From this information it is now possible to estimate (at least from a qualitative aspect) the implications of biliary tract disease for drug elimination.

Extrahepatic and intrahepatic cholestatic liver diseases potentially can interrupt biliary excretion of drugs, much as ureteral obstruction or parenchymal renal disease interferes with urinary excretion of drugs. Extrahepatic biliary tract obstruction, such as choledocholithiasis, bile duct carcinoma, strictures, periampullar carcinoma, acute or chronic pancreatitis, or pancreatic carcinoma, can result in complete in-terruption of bile drainage and biliary excretion of endogenous and exogenous substances. The results of intrahepatic cholestasis are more varied, and consequently the effects on biliary drug elimination are more difficult to predict. Furthermore, intrahepatic cholestasis is characterized by functional impairment of bile formation at the biliary canaliculus. As will be emphasized throughout this chapter, most drugs are secreted into bile by specific transport systems. Certain causes of intra-hepatic cholestasis can block these specific transport systems. Thus, it is easy to understand why cholestatic liver disease induced by estrogens, for example, may or may not influence the biliary secretion of a particular drug.

Drug uptake, drug concentrations in the liver and bile, and drug metabolism cannot be controlled in humans; therefore, much of our knowledge about the biliary excretion of drugs originates from animal studies. However, because of the large species variations in biliary excretion that exist among experimental animals, it is impossible at this time to extrapolate these data to humans (1). Furthermore, most biliary excretion studies have been performed in patients with T-tube drainage following cholecystectomy or other biliary tract surgery. Few studies of biliary drug excretion have been performed during acute biliary tract obstruction or during the

acute phase of intrahepatic cholestasis. Nevertheless, with knowledge of how drugs are handled within the hepatobiliary system, it is possible to estimate the consequences of biliary tract disease for drug disposition.

MECHANISMS OF DRUG EXCRETION IN BILE

The liver cell is a polar structure, and drug transport processes are directed to the uptake of drugs across the sinusoidal membrane and their secretion into the bile across the canalicular membrane. Transport systems have been identified within the hepatic sinusoidal and canalicular membranes that are responsible for uptake and secretion of foreign compounds (2). At least three active transport systems exist for the excretion of organic compounds in the bile in rats: one for organic acids, one for organic bases, and another for organic neutral compounds. The presence of these transport systems in the human liver seems likely, given the nature of the substances secreted in human bile. The organic anion indocyanine green (3), the organic base hexafluorenium (4), and the neutral compound digoxin (5) are all excreted into human bile. In addition to active transport systems, it has also been suggested that organic acids might be transferred from plasma to liver cells by binding to the cytoplasmic protein ligandin (6). Another method by which organic compounds might be concentrated in bile is by entrapment within micelles composed of bile salts, cholesterol, and phospholipids (7). This has been shown to occur with imipramine in rat bile (8), and it may possibly occur in human bile with other drugs or drug metabolites. Independent of the mechanism, biliary excretion can be a significant route of elimination for drugs that are highly concentrated in bile. Such compounds achieve bile/plasma concentration ratios greater than unity, and the bile concentrations often are 10 to 1,000 times greater than those in plasma. For example, a bile-to-plasma ratio of 639 and a biliary clearance of 176 ml/hr were observed following a single dose of doxorubicin in a patient with external drainage (9).

Chemical structure, polarity, and molecular weight are characteristics of a drug that are important in determining its excretion in bile. In rats, there is a threshold molecular weight (approximately 325) above which compounds are readily excreted in the bile and below which compounds are less likely to be excreted by this route (10). It is important to understand that molecular size is not an absolute determinant of biliary excretion; it only implies that as molecular weight increases, a larger percentage of an administered dose will appear in the bile. In fact, the hepatobiliary transport systems for drugs carry not only high-molecular-weight drugs but also low-molecular-weight compounds such as N-acetyl-p-aminohippuric acid (MW 236) (2). Nevertheless, the molecular weight of a drug or its metabolites can be useful in predicting its biliary excretion. There is a trend for high-molecular-weight compounds to be excreted in human bile (11). However, interindividual differences, nonspecific analytical techniques, and incomplete bile collections make it difficult to calculate a threshold molecular weight for biliary excretion of drugs in humans at this time.

STUDIES OF DRUG EXCRETION IN HUMAN BILE

Generalizations

Most studies of biliary excretion of drugs in humans have been performed in patients with T-tube drainage following cholecystectomy or other biliary tract surgery. The data obtained from many of these studies are less than ideal, because the disease for which the surgery was performed may have influenced drug excretion, bile flow, and bile composition. Postsurgery, bile flow and bile composition probably are not entirely normal, and T-tube drainage is not designed to totally divert bile flow. The use of multilumen tubes with or without balloon occlusion of the duodenum may improve studies of biliary excretion of drugs in humans, because the enterohepatic circulation of the drug need not be interrupted, and the studies could be performed in healthy volunteers (5,12,13).

The most widely studied drugs to date are the antineoplastic agents, cardiac glycosides, and antibiotics. A list of these and other drugs that have been shown to be excreted in human bile is presented in Table 1. Only studies that have demonstrated biliary excretion in humans have been included in this table. A brief examination of these studies reveals that the data are reported in a variety of ways. Occasionally the bile/plasma ratio has been reported. This is an important figure because the following formula can be used to calculate the biliary clearance of a drug:

$$\text{biliary clearance} = \frac{\text{bile flow} \times \text{concentration in bile}}{\text{concentration in plasma}}$$

Obviously, drugs with larger bile/plasma ratios will have greater biliary clearance. More frequently, however, the percentage of the administered dose excreted in bile over a given period of time has been reported. Unfortunately, these studies have been as short as 2 hr and as long as 7 days, making comparison difficult. Finally, proof that a drug is excreted in bile does not imply that it undergoes enterohepatic circulation. There have been few studies in humans that have actually confirmed the enterohepatic circulation of a drug.

Antineoplastic Drugs

Information about the biliary excretion and enterohepatic circulation of antineoplastic drugs is essential for the development of rational therapeutic regimens. Many of these drugs are high-molecular-weight compounds that are concentrated in bile, and consequently biliary excretion plays an important role in their elimination. Doxorubicin and vincristine have molecular weights of 543 and 825, respectively, and both are extensively eliminated in bile and most likely undergo enterohepatic circulation (9,14). Patients receiving these drugs may have primary tumors or metastatic disease involving the hepatobiliary tree that may limit their elimination, resulting in prolonged high drug concentrations and increased risk of toxicity.

TABLE 1. *Biliary secretion of drugs in humans*

Drug (molecular weight)	Reference	Bile/plasma ratio	Biliary excretion (% dose/time)	Dose
Antibiotics				
Ampicillin (349)	17		0.03%/12 hr	1,000 mg[a] p.o.
	31	8.8		500 mg[b] p.o.
Cefoperazone (667.7)	57		19–36%/24 hr	1,000 mg[a] i.v.
Cefamandole (445)	32	6.4	0.4%/2 hr	500 mg[a] i.v.
Cefazolin (454)	32	0.2	0.13%/12 hr	1,000 mg[a] i.v.
	32	0.5	0.12%/2 hr	1,000 mg[a] i.m.
Cephacetrile (361)	33	0.1	0.02%/10 hr	1,000 mg[a] i.v.
Cephalothin (396)	32	0.4	0.25%/2 hr	1,000 mg[a] i.v.
Cephaloridine (415)	17		0.06%/12 hr	
Chloramphenicol (323)	34	2.0	2.7%/24 hr	3,000 mg[a] p.o.
Chlortetracycline (479)	35	4.0		500 mg[b] i.v.
Clindamycin (425)	19	3.0		600 mg[b] i.v.
Demethylchlortetracycline (465)	36	20–30		500 mg[b] i.v.
Doxycycline (444)	37	8.8	4%/24 hr	200 mg[a] i.v.
Erythromycin estolate (1,056)	17		0.04%/12 hr	500 mg[a] p.o.
Gentamicin (477)	38	0.46		1 mg/kg[a] i.m.
Moxalactam (564)	58	0.4–12		2,000 mg[a] i.v.
Nafcillin (436)	39	19–60		1,000 mg[a] p.o.
Novobiocin (612)	17		0.40%/12 hr	500 mg[a] i.m.
Penicillin G (351)	17		0.08%/12 hr	600 mg[a] i.m.
Pivampicillin (463)	21	2.0 (ampicillin)	1%/5 hr (ampicillin)	700 mg[a] p.o.
Rifamide (811)	17		34%/12 hr	300 mg[a] i.m.
Rifamicin SV (698)	17		25%/12 hr	250 mg[a] i.v.
Tetracycline (444)	17		0.08%/12 hr	200 mg[a] i.m.
Antineoplastic agents				
Doxorubicin (adriamycin) (543)	9		41%/7 days (unchanged and metabolites)	117 mg[a] i.v.

				Tracer dose[a]
5-Fluorouracil (130)	40	2.0	21.7%/24 hr	0.5 mg[a] i.v.
Vincristine (825)	14			
Cardiac glycosides				
Digoxin (781)	15		8.1%/7 days (primarily unchanged)	0.5 mg[a] i.v.
	41	20	8.8%/24 hr	0.6 mg[a] i.v.
	5		30%/24 hr (unchanged and metabolites)	0.5 mg[c] i.v.
	30		16%/24 hr (unchanged)	0.125 mg[a] p.o. (maintenance)
Digitoxin (765)	42		1.5%/24 hr (unchanged and active metabolites)	0.6 mg[a] i.v.
Lanatoside C (985)	12		6.9%/24 hr	0.1 mg[c] p.o.
	43		10%/24 hr (metabolites)	1 mg[c] p.o.
Proscillaridin A (530)	44	10–100	30%/24 hr (conjugates)	1–1.5 mg[a] p.o.
Steroids				
Estradiol (272)	45		52%/12 hr (conjugates)	0.37–0.74 mg[a] i.v.
Testosterone (288)	46		13%/48 hr	0.2–1.0 mg[a] i.v.
Hydrocortisone (362)	47		4%/24 hr	50–500 mg[a] i.v.
Other drugs				
Acebutolol (336)	48	60–100	5.6%/24 hr (unchanged and N-acetyl metabolites)	300 mg[a] p.o.
Terbutaline (225)	49	3.0	0.36–0.73%/24 hr	2 µg/kg[c] i.v.
Practolol (264)	50	4.0	23–40%/48 hr	400 mg[a] p.o.

TABLE 1. (continued)

Drug (molecular weight)	Reference	Bile/plasma ratio	Biliary excretion (% dose/time)	Dose
Other drugs (cont.)				
Diazepam (285)	51		15%/15 days (metabolites)	Tracer dose[a]
	52		0.23%/24 hr (diazepam and N-desmethyl diazepam)	10 mg[a] p.o. × 14 days
Spironolactone (416)	53		5–33%/4 days (metabolites)	300 mg[d]
Indomethacin (358)	54		15%/24 hr (glucuronide)	Not stated[a]
Indocyanine green (775)	3		43–88% (not stated)	0.7 mg/kg[a] i.v.
Carbenoxolone (571)	55		50–70%/48 hr (glucuronide)	100–200 mg[a] p.o.
Ioglycamide (620)	25		Icteric, 3.2%/2 hr; anicteric, 20.6%/2 hr	2 mg/kg/min[a] i.v. × 120 min
Hexafluorenium (662)	4		27–48%/24 hr (unchanged)	5 mg[a] i.v.
Metronidazole (171)	56	1.27		500 mg[a] i.v.

[a]Bile collected by T-tube drainage.
[b]Bile collected from gallbladder at surgery.
[c]Bile obtained by duodenal aspiration.
[d]Bile collected by balloon occlusion of T tube after surgery.

Cardiac Glycosides

Data resulting from studies of biliary excretion of the cardiac glycosides in humans are conflicting. The biliary excretion of digoxin has been reported to range from 8.1% in 7 days in patients with T tubes (15) to 30% in 24 hr in patients with duodenal aspiration (5). It is tempting to suggest that the lower biliary excretion in patients with T tubes was due to their underlying hepatobiliary disease or to the effect of surgery. Whether or not this is the case is not certain. However, the cardiac glycoside digitoxin undergoes significant enterohepatic circulation (24–28%) in humans. Caldwell et al. (16) demonstrated that administration of the organic-acid-binding resin cholestyramine interrupts the enterohepatic circulation of digitoxin, reduces its plasma half-life, and results in a more rapid return to baseline values for the digitoxin-induced changes in cardiac systolic time intervals. This is perhaps the best demonstration in humans of the effect that interruption of the enterohepatic circulation can have on the pharmacokinetics of a drug.

Antibiotics

Because of their potential use in treating infections of the biliary tract, human biliary excretion of antibiotics has received a great deal of attention. The biliary excretion of many antibiotics is quantitatively low, but the bile/plasma ratios indicate that a few are concentrated in the bile (11). For example, biliary excretion of rifamicin SV (MW 698) is extensive, 25% of a 250-mg i.v. dose being excreted in human bile in 12 hr (17). In patients with common duct or cystic duct obstruction, the cephalosporins do not enter bile (18). However, Brown et al. (19) demonstrated that although bile concentrations are low, high concentrations of clindamycin are found in the liver tissue of patients with obstruction of the common bile duct. This information may be helpful in treating pyogenic infections of liver produced by sensitive organisms. Future studies of antibiotic excretion in bile should not be directed toward determining the percentage of a dose excreted but rather toward the question whether or not the concentration of drug in bile is sufficient to inhibit the usual enteric organisms found in bile. Finally, from our knowledge of human biliary excretion of antibiotics, we know that the percentage of an administered dose excreted is small, and it is probably not necessary to change dosages in patients with biliary drainage.

ENTEROHEPATIC CIRCULATION

Enterohepatic circulation can be defined as the secretion of a substance in the bile, followed by reabsorption from the gut and return to the liver via the portal blood. Such recycling may involve the parent drug only or a biotransformation product such as a conjugate that must undergo hydrolysis within the gut prior to reabsorption. Regardless of the biotransformations involved, enterohepatic recycling has the net effect of maintaining a high concentration of drug within the liver, gut, and portal blood, which otherwise would occur only during the initial absorption phase following oral dosage.

For obvious reasons it is difficult to establish that there is enterohepatic circulation of a drug in humans. By sampling blood simultaneously from the portal and peripheral veins, Dencker et al. (20) were able to establish that imipramine does undergo enterohepatic recycling. They were also able to demonstrate that demethylation of imipramine does not occur in the intestinal wall during absorption and that desmethylimipramine formed in the liver also undergoes enterohepatic circulation. In a similar study, Lund et al. (21) have shown that the prodrug pivampicillin is completely hydrolyzed in the intestine and enters the portal vein and is subsequently excreted in bile, as ampicillin.

It is apparent that enterohepatic circulation can result in a delay in drug elimination from the body. As was described earlier with regard to cholestyramine and digitoxin, interruption in the enterohepatic circulation can hasten elimination and lessen the side effects of certain drugs. Furthermore, if the parent drug and/or its metabolic product exhibit toxicity within the liver, biliary tree, or intestine, then enterohepatic circulation is particularly important in determining the accumulative response of these organs. Duggan and Kwan (22) have derived the following equation to express the total or accumulative biliary secretion of a drug as a percentage of the dose:

$$\Sigma\%_{\text{bile}} = \frac{CL_{\text{bile}} \times [0.8(AUC_{\text{port}})_0^\infty + 0.2(AUC_{\text{hep}})_0^\infty] \times 100}{\text{dose}}$$

In this equation, CL_{bile} is biliary clearance of a drug, AUC_{port} and AUC_{hep} are the areas under the plasma concentration/time curves for the drug in the portal vein and hepatic artery, respectively. The total blood supply to the liver comprises 80% portal blood and 20% hepatic arterial blood; thus, each AUC is weighted accordingly. Using this equation, these authors were able to demonstrate in five laboratory species good correlation between the sensitivity to indomethacin-related intestinal lesions and the total exposure of the intestinal mucosa to drug as a consequence of enterohepatic recycling. Similar approximations in humans lead to an estimation of the minimal toxic dosages of 1.25 to 12 mg/kg/day (22). These authors concluded that this high degree of interindividual variation is consistent with the idiosyncratic intestinal sensitivity to indomethacin encountered in clinical use.

INTESTINAL METABOLISM

Drugs or metabolites excreted in bile can be further biotransformed by intestinal bacteria (23). This is most commonly described for glucuronide conjugates that are hydrolyzed by β-glucuronidase present in human intestinal flora (24). The numerous metabolic reactions of the intestinal bacteria can result in the formation of active metabolites with considerable pharmacological or toxicological effects.

CLINICAL IMPLICATIONS OF BILIARY TRACT DISEASE FOR DRUG KINETICS

For many years it has been known that visualization of the gallbladder by means of cholecystographic contrast material is poor if the serum bilirubin level is 3 mg/dl

or greater. Bell et al. (25) studied biliary excretion of the cholecystographic agent ioglycamide in 5 patients with common bile duct T tubes with varying degrees of liver impairment and elevated serum bilirubin levels and 5 similar patients with relatively normal liver function and serum bilirubin levels. Despite similar plasma levels following 2-hr infusion of ioglycamide at 2 mg/kg/min, the biliary excretion was only 3.2% of the dose in the patients with jaundice, compared with 20.6% in anicteric patients. Moreover, urinary excretion of ioglycamide was 42.3% of the administered dose in the jaundiced group, compared with 18.1% in the anicteric group. They also found that in the jaundiced group, 11.9% of the contrast agent was not bound to plasma proteins, compared with 6.4% in the anicteric group. Thus, in jaundiced patients, the concentrations of bilirubin and other substances are elevated in plasma and compete for protein binding and biliary elimination of radiographic contrast material. Similar factors probably are also operative in biliary elimination of other drugs in patients with biliary tract disease. Yam and Roberts (26) have demonstrated that acute bile duct ligation in rats significantly reduces hepatic uptake of organic anions such as sulfobromophthalein, phenol-3,6-dibromo-phthalein disulfonate, and the neutral organic compound ouabain, but not the organic cation procainamide ethobromide. Bile duct ligation for 72 hr has been shown to depress the *in vitro* metabolic activity of the cytochrome-P-450-dependent mixed-function oxidases (27). Thus, extrahepatic bile duct obstruction appears to alter two important steps in the biliary elimination of drugs: hepatic uptake and biotransfor-mation. Whether or not the third step, transport from the liver cell into bile, is also affected is not known.

Only a few studies of drug penetration into the abnormal human biliary tract have been performed. Brown et al. (19) found that patients with patent common bile ducts who had received 600 mg of clindamycin intravenously prior to biliary tract surgery had concentrations of drug in bile and liver tissue greater than in serum. In contrast, patients with obstruction of the common bile duct had no measurable drug in bile. In the obstructed group, however, liver concentrations of clindamycin were higher than those in the group without obstruction. This report confirms the findings of others that the presence of bile duct obstruction markedly decreases the appearance of antibiotics in bile (19,28,29). It is interesting, however, that hepatic uptake of antibiotics in humans appears to be preserved in the presence of biliary tract obstruction. Whether or not these observations can be extrapolated to other drugs is not known at this time.

CONCLUSIONS

As a result of our knowledge of biliary excretion of drugs, changes in drug dosages can be suggested when treating patients with biliary tract obstruction or drainage. This will be particularly true if a significant amount of drug is excreted via the bile or if the therapeutic index is such that a small change in drug elimination will result in a rise of the serum drug concentration to a toxic level. Carruthers and Dujovne (30) observed in a patient with biliary drainage that within an 8-hr period

19.2% of the bioavailable dose of digoxin was excreted in the bile, and the serum digoxin concentration was low. After the T tube was removed and the enterohepatic circulation was intact, the patient developed sinus bradycardia with multiple ventricular ectopic beats, and the serum digoxin concentration was noted to be 2.1 ng/ml. Temporary discontinuation of the digoxin therapy resulted in disappearance of the arrhythmia. These authors concluded that the fluctuations in this patient's digoxin concentration were due to loss of drug during biliary drainage, with a rise in the serum level when the enterohepatic circulation was reinstituted. Serum concentrations of the antineoplastic drugs doxorubicin and vincristine might increase into a toxic range as a result of biliary obstruction. For most drugs, however, this is probably not a significant problem. We are now also aware that toxicity to certain organs such as the intestine or liver might be enhanced by enterohepatic circulation of drugs and/or metabolites.

The present state of our knowledge on this subject makes it clear that further studies of excretion of drugs into human bile are warranted. Where possible, such studies should include minimal interruption of the enterohepatic circulation.

REFERENCES

1. Klassen, C. D. (1977): Biliary excretion. In: *Handbook of Physiology: Reaction to Environmental Agents*, edited by D. H. K. Lee, pp. 537–553. American Physiological Society, Washington, D.C.
2. Rollins, D. E., Freston, J. W., and Woodbury, D. M. (1980): Transport of organic anions into liver cells and bile. *Biochem. Pharmacol.*, 29:1023–1028.
3. Hirom, P. C., Milburn, P., Smith, R. L., and Williams, R. T. (1972): Species variations in the threshold molecular weight factor for the biliary excretion of organic anions. *Biochemistry*, 129:1071–1077.
4. Meijer, D. K. F., Vermeer, G. A., and Kwant, G. (1971): The excretion of hexafluorenium in man and rat. *Eur. J. Pharmacol.*, 14:280–285.
5. Caldwell, J. H., and Cline, C. T. (1976): Biliary excretion of digoxin in man. *Clin. Pharmacol. Ther.*, 19:410–415.
6. Fleischner, G., Robbins, J., and Arias, I. M. (1972): Immunological studies of Y protein. A major cytoplasmic organic anion-binding protein in rat liver. *J. Clin. Invest.*, 51:677–684.
7. Scharschmidt, B. F., and Schmid, R. (1978): The micellar sink. A quantitative assessment of the association of organic anions with mixed micelles and other macromolecular aggregates in rat bile. *J. Clin. Invest.*, 62:1122–1131.
8. Bickel, M. H., and Minder, R. (1970): Metabolism and biliary excretion of the lipophilic drug molecules, imipramine and desmethylimipramine in the rat. II. Uptake into bile micelles. *Biochem. Pharmacol.*, 19:2437.
9. Riggs, C. E., Benjamin, R. S., Serpick, A. A., and Bachur, N. R. (1977): Biliary disposition of adriamycin. *Clin. Pharmacol. Ther.*, 22:234–241.
10. Milburn, P., Smith, R. L., and Williams, R. T. (1967): Biliary excretion of foreign compounds: Biphenyl stilboestrol and phenophthalein in the rat: Molecular weight, polarity and metabolism as factors in biliary excretion. *Biochem. J.*, 105:1275–1281.
11. Rollins, D. E., and Klaassen, C. D. (1979): Biliary excretion of drugs in man. *Clin. Pharmacokinet.*, 4:368–379.
12. Beermann, B., Helstrom, K., and Rosen, A. (1971): Fate of orally administered ^{3}H-digitoxin in man with special reference to the absorption. *Circulation*, 43:852–861.
13. Askin, J. R., Lyon, D. I., Shull, S. D., Wagner, C. I., and Soloway, R. D. (1978): Factors affecting delivery of bile to the duodcnum in man. *Gastroenterology*, 74:560–565.
14. Jackson, D. V., Castle, M. C., and Bender, R. A. (1978): Biliary excretion of vincristine. *Clin. Pharmacol. Ther.*, 24:101–107.

15. Doherty, J. E., Flanigan, W. J., Murphy, M. L., Bulloch, R. I., Dalrymple, G. L., Beard, O. W., and Perkins, W. H. (1970): Tritiated digoxin. XIV. Enterohepatic circulation, absorption and excretion studies in human volunteers. *Circulation*, 42:867–873.

16. Caldwell, J. H., Bush, C. A., and Greenberger, N. J. (1971): Interruption of the enterohepatic circulation of digitoxin by cholestyramine. II. Effect on metabolic disposition of tritium-labeled digitoxin and cardiac systolic intervals in man. *J. Clin. Invest.*, 50:2638–2644.

17. Acocella, G., Mattivssi, R., Nicolis, F. B., Pallanza, R., and Tenconi, L. T. (1968): Biliary excretion of antibiotics in man. *Gut*, 9:536–545.

18. Ratzan, K. R., Ruiz, C., and Irvin, G. L. (1974): Biliary tract excretion of cephazolin, cephalothin and cephaloridine in the presence of biliary tract disease. *Antimicrob. Agents Chemother.*, 6:426–431.

19. Brown, R. B., Martyak, S. N., Barza, M., Curtis, L., and Weinstein, L. (1976): Penetration of clindamycin phosphate into the abnormal human biliary tract. *Ann. Intern. Med.*, 84:168–170.

20. Dencker, H., Dencker, S. J., Green, A., and Nagy, A. (1976): Intestinal absorption, demethylation and enterohepatic circulation of imipramine. *Clin. Pharmacol. Ther.*, 19:584–586.

21. Lund, B., Kampmann, J. P., Lindaho, F., and Hansen, J. M. (1976): Pivampicillin and ampicillin in bile, portal and peripheral blood. *Clin. Pharmacol. Ther.*, 19:587–591.

22. Duggan, D. E., and Kwan, K. C. (1979): Enterohepatic recirculation of drugs as a determinant of therapeutic ratio. *Drug Metab. Rev.*, 9:21–41.

23. Scheline, R. R. (1973): Metabolism of foreign compounds by gastrointestinal microorganisms. *Pharmacol. Rev.*, 25:451–523.

24. Kent, T. H., Fischer, L. J., and Marr, R. (1972): Glucuronidase activity in intestinal contents of rat and man and relationship to bacterial flora. *Proc. Soc. Exp. Biol. Med.*, 140:590–594.

25. Bell, G. D., McMullin, J., Doran, J., Oliver, J., McAllister, J., Ins, F., Monks, A., and Richens, A. (1978): Ioglycamide (Biligram) studies in man—plasma binding, renal and biliary excretion studies in jaundiced and anicteric patients. *Br. J. Radiol.*, 51:251–256.

26. Yam, J., and Roberts, R. J. (1977): Hepatic uptake of foreign compounds: Influence of acute extrahepatic biliary obstruction. *J. Pharmacol. Exp. Ther.*, 200:425–433.

27. Drew, R., and Priestly, B. H. (1976): Hexobarbital sleeping time and drug metabolism in rats with ligated bile ducts: A lack of correlation. *Biochem. Pharmacol.*, 25:1659–1663.

28. Mortimer, P. R., Mackie, D. B., and Haynes, S. (1969): Ampicillin levels in human bile in the presence of biliary tract disease. *Br. Med. J.*, 3:88–89.

29. Sales, J. E. L., Sutcliffe, M., and O'Grady, F. (1972): Cephalexin levels in human bile in the presence of biliary tract disease. *Br. Med. J.*, 3:441–442.

30. Carruthers, G., and Dujovne, C. A. (1978): Digoxin therapy during T-tube drainage in man. *J.A.M.A.*, 240:2756–2757.

31. Ayliff, G. A. J., and Davis, A. (1965): Ampicillin levels in human bile. *Br. J. Pharmacol.*, 24:189–193.

32. Ratzan, K. R., Baker, H. B., and Lauredo, I. (1978): Excretion of cefamandole, cefazolin and cephalothin into T-tube bile. *Antimicrob. Agents Chemother.*, 13:985–987.

33. Brogard, J. M., Haegele, P., Dorner, M., and Lavillaureix, J. (1973): Biliary excretion of a new semisynthetic cephalosporin, cephacetrile. *Antimicrob. Agents Chemother.*, 3:19–23.

34. Glazko, A. J., Wolf, L. M., Dill, W. A., and Bratton, A. C. (1949): Biochemical studies on chloramphenicol (chloromycetin). II. Tissue distribution and excretion studies. *J. Pharmacol. Exp. Ther.*, 96:445–459.

35. Pulaski, E. J., and Fusillo, M. H. (1955): Gallbladder bile concentrations of the major antibiotics following intravenous administration. *Surg. Gynecol. Obstet.*, 100:571–574.

36. Kunin, C. M., and Finland, M. (1959): Excretion of demethylchlortetracycline into the bile. *N. Engl. J. Med.*, 261:1069–1071.

37. Alestig, K. (1974): Studies on the intestinal excretion of doxycycline. *Scand. J. Infect. Dis.*, 6:265–271.

38. Pitt, H. A., Roberts, R. B., and Johnson, W. D. (1973): Gentamicin levels in the human biliary tract. *J. Infect. Dis.*, 127:299–302.

39. Green, G. R., and Geraci, J. E. (1965): A note on the concentration of nafcillin in human bile. *Mayo Clin.*, 40:700–704.

40. Douglass, H. O., and Mittleman, A. (1974): Metabolic studies of 5-fluorouracil. II. Influence of route of administration on the dynamics of distribution in man. *Cancer*, 34:1878–1881.

41. Klotz, U., and Antonin, K. H. (1977): Biliary excretion studies with digoxin in man. *Int. J. Clin. Pharmacol.*, 15:332–334.
42. Storstein, L. (1975): Studies on digitalis. III. Biliary excretion and enterohepatic circulation of digitoxin and its cardioactive metabolites. *Clin. Pharmacol. Ther.*, 17:313–320.
43. Beermann, B. (1972): On the fate of orally administered ^{3}H-Lanatoside C in man. *Eur. J. Clin. Pharmacol.*, 5:11–18.
44. Andersson, K. E., Berdahl, B., and Wettrell, G. (1977): Biliary excretion and enterohepatic recycling of proscillaridin A after oral administration to man. *Eur. J. Clin. Pharmacol.*, 11:273–276.
45. Sandberg, A. A., and Slaunwhite, W. R. (1957): Studies on phenolic steroids in human subjects. II. The metabolic fate and hepatobiliary-enteric circulation of ^{14}C-esterone and ^{14}C-estradiol in women. *J. Clin. Invest.*, 36:1266–1278.
46. Sandberg, A. A., and Slaunwhite, W. R. (1956): Metabolism of 4-^{14}C-testosterone in human subjects. I. Distribution in bile, food, feces and urine. *J. Clin. Invest.*, 35:1331–1339.
47. Peterson, R. E., Wyngaarden, J. B., Guerra, S. L., Brodie, B. B., and Bunim, J. J. (1955): The physiological disposition and metabolic fate of hydrocortisone in man. *J. Clin. Invest.*, 34:1779–1785.
48. Kaye, C. M. (1976): The biliary excretion of acebutolol in man. *J. Pharm. Pharmacol.*, 28:449–450.
49. Nilsson, H. T., Persson, C. G. A., Tegner, K., Ingemarsson, I., and Liedberg, G. (1973): Biliary excretion of ^{3}H-terbutaline in man. *Biochem. Pharmacol.*, 22:3128–3129.
50. Carruthers, S. G., Kelly, J. G., Johnson, G. W., and McDevitt, D. G. (1976): Biliary excretion and enterohepatic recirculation of practolol in man. *Ir. J. Med. Sci.*, 145:187–194.
51. Mahon, W. A., Inaba, T., Umeda, T., Tsutsumi, E., and Stone, R. (1976): Biliary elimination of diazepam in man. *Clin. Pharmacol. Ther.*, 19:443–450.
52. Seliman, R., Hurme, M., and Kanto, J. (1977): Biliary excretion of diazepam and its metabolites in man after repeated oral doses. *Eur. J. Clin. Pharmacol.*, 12:209–212.
53. Abshagen, U., von Grodzicki, U., Hirschberger, U., and Rennekamp, H. (1977): Effect of enterohepatic circulation on the pharmacokinetics of spironolactone in man. *Naunyn Schmiedebergs Arch. Pharmacol.*, 300:281–287.
54. Hucker, H. B., Zacchei, A. G., Cox, S. V., Brodie, D. A., and Cantwell, N. H. R. (1966): Studies on the absorption, distribution and excretion of indomethacin in various species. *J. Pharmacol. Exp. Ther.*, 153:237–249.
55. Downer, H. D., Galloway, R. W., Horwich, L., and Parke, D. V. (1970): The absorption and excretion of carbenoxolone in man. *J. Pharm. Pharmacol.*, 22:449–487.
56. Nielsen, M. L., and Justesen, T. (1977): Excretion of metronidazole in human bile. *Scand. J. Gastroenterol.*, 12:1003–1008.
57. Brogden, R. N., Carmie, A., Heel, R. C., Morley, P. A., Speight, T. M., and Avery, G. S. (1981): Cefoperazone: A review of its in-vitro antimicrobial activity, pharmacological properties and therapeutic efficacy. *Drugs*, 22:423–460.
58. Martinez, O. V., Levi, J. U., Livingstone, A., Malinin, T. I., Zeppa, R., Hutson, D., and Einkorn, N. (1981): Biliary excretion of moxalactam. *Antimicrob. Agents Chemother.*, 20:231–234.

Pharmacokinetic Basis for Drug Treatment,
edited by L. Z. Benet et al., Raven Press,
New York © 1984

Chapter 6

Effects of Cardiac Disease on Pharmacokinetics: Pathophysiologic Considerations

Neal L. Benowitz

Clinical Pharmacology Unit, Medical Service, San Francisco General Hospital Medical Center, and Department of Medicine, University of California at San Francisco, San Francisco, California 94143

Occurrence of important adverse effects to drugs in patients with cardiac disease is not uncommon. Although differences in sensitivity to drugs between healthy persons and those with cardiac disease may contribute, it is likely that abnormal pharmacokinetics account for much of the increased incidence of drug toxicity in cardiac patients. The intent of this review is to discuss how pathophysiological disturbances in cardiac disease states can influence pharmacokinetics. This chapter updates a 1976 review of this subject (1).

PATHOPHYSIOLOGY OF CARDIAC FAILURE

Cardiac failure, the pathological state in which abnormal cardiac function results in insufficient blood flow to meet the requirements of body tissues at rest and during normal activity, will be discussed as the prototype cardiac disease. The spectrum of cardiac failure ranges from mild congestive failure to cardiogenic shock.

In response to reduced cardiac function, a number of compensatory or primary disturbances occur (2). Renal sodium and water retention results in blood volume expansion and increased cardiac filling pressures. Increased filling pressures lead to increased stroke volume by the Frank-Starling mechanism, but they also lead to increased pulmonary and systemic venous pressures. Myocardial muscle mass enlarges, and the sympathetic nervous system increases myocardial contractility. When these compensatory mechanisms become inadequate, cardiac output falls.

There are significant consequences of or secondary disturbances owing to cardiac failure. As a consequence of sympathetic nervous stimulation, blood flow is redistributed. Disproportionately higher fractions of cardiac output go to brain and heart; smaller fractions go to kidney, skin, and splanchnic tissues (1,3). Redistribution of blood flow within organs, such as kidney and lung, may also occur. Reduced blood flow due to reduced cardiac output and/or local vasoconstriction

may reduce organ perfusion and result in tissue hypoxia. Increased systemic venous pressures may result in visceral congestion and disturbed organ function. Alterations in autonomic nervous system activity may result in abnormalities of gastrointestinal motility.

EFFECTS OF CARDIAC FAILURE ON DRUG DISTRIBUTION

The effects of cardiac failure on pharmacokinetics will be discussed in terms of effects on the processes of distribution, clearance, and absorption. Potential circulatory effects on drug distribution are listed in Table 1 and Fig. 1. Autonomic nervous responses to cardiac failure may result in altered drug distribution. Autoregulation of blood flow occurs so that relatively more of a given amount of drug in the blood goes to brain and myocardium and relatively less to kidney, muscle, and splanchnic organs (1,3). Within the kidney, blood flow is shifted from cortical to juxtamedullary nephrons. Musculoskeletal tissue, because of its large mass, is a major uptake organ for many drugs. Reduced blood flow will significantly reduce the rate and possibly the extent of drug uptake by musculoskeletal tissue. A few drugs are water-soluble and, because of expansion of extracellular fluid volume, may be distributed to a larger-than-normal volume.

TABLE 1. *Circulatory effects on drug distribution:*
general considerations

Altered distribution pattern
  Autoregulation
  Increased brain and myocardial blood flow
  Decreased kidney, muscle, and splanchnic blood flow
  Intrarenal redistribution: cortical to juxtamedullary

Decreased distribution volume
  Reduced rate and possibly extent of musculoskeletal uptake

Increased distribution volume
  Expanded extracellular fluid volume

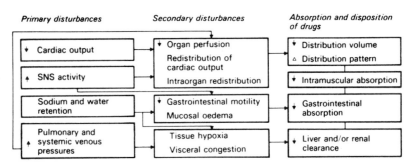

FIG. 1. Pathophysiology of cardiac failure and its effects on pharmacokinetics. (From Benowitz and Meister, ref. 1, with permission.)

As an example of the effects of circulatory disturbances on distribution kinetics of drugs to tissues, the effects of hypovolemia on lidocaine distribution will be considered. A computer simulation, based on a perfusion model, of the time course of concentration of lidocaine in various tissues after intravenous injection is shown in Fig. 2. Lidocaine concentrations are initially high in venous blood, and a significant percentage of the drug is taken up in the first pass through the lung. The lung dampens the bolus and transforms it into a short infusion as seen by tissues in the systemic circulation. After the lung, lidocaine is distributed to well-perfused, rapidly equilibrating tissues (RET). As blood concentrations fall, lidocaine redistributes from well-perfused tissue back to the blood pool and then to more slowly perfused, slowly equilibrating tissues (SET), such as muscle and adipose.

Hypovolemic shock resembles cardiac failure in that tissue hypoperfusion, intense sympathetic nervous stimulation, and the pattern of redistribution of cardiac output are similar (4). The effects of hemorrhage on tissue lidocaine concentrations are simulated in Fig. 3. Blood lidocaine concentrations in the early minutes (after 2 min) following injection are higher during hemorrhage because of the decreased rates of perfusion of other tissues. This is reflected clinically as a decreased initial

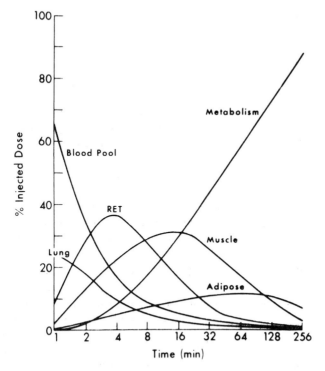

FIG. 2. Perfusion-model simulation of the distribution of lidocaine in various tissues and its elimination following intravenous infusion of 100 mg for 1 min in a 70-kg man. RET represents rapidly equilibrating tissue and includes heart and kidney. (From Benowitz et al., ref. 39, with permission.)

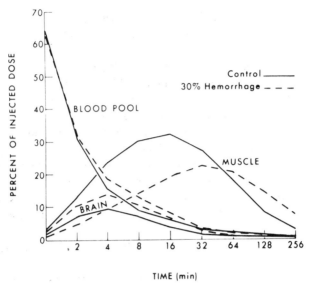

FIG. 3. Perfusion-model simulation of the distribution of lidocaine into various tissues after a 1-min injection of 100 mg in a 70-kg man, showing the effect of hemorrhage. (From Benowitz et al., ref. 4, with permission.)

volume of distribution. Preservation of blood flow to the brain and heart in the presence of higher concentrations of drug in the blood leads to a higher concentration of lidocaine in these organs soon after injection. Thus, adverse effects of lidocaine affecting the central nervous system, particularly convulsions, and the heart are likely to occur shortly after administration in the presence of shock or cardiac failure. The rate of presentation of drug to more slowly perfused tissues is markedly reduced in circulatory insufficiency states and leads to delayed and reduced total tissue uptake.

Tissue distribution of digoxin has been examined directly during hemorrhage in the conscious dog (5). Five minutes after intravenous injection, digoxin concentrations in blood and in myocardium were higher during hemorrhage than in control animals. The effect is analogous to what was simulated for lidocaine in Fig. 3. The myocardial/plasma concentration ratio was unchanged at 5 min, but at 60 min the ratio was increased more than twofold in hemorrhaged animals as compared with controls. Thus, myocardial digoxin content may be greater than expected on the basis of blood concentration of digoxin in the shock state.

Although not a consequence of circulatory disturbance per se nor a feature of cardiac failure, abnormal protein binding has been described in cardiac diseases. Myocardial infarction produces an inflammatory response, with increased circulating acute-phase reactants, including α_1-acid glycoproteins (6) (see Chapter 10). The latter bind basic drugs, such as lidocaine. Increased lidocaine binding is responsible, at least in part, for the progressively increasing lidocaine blood concentrations observed for as long as 48 hr during constant infusion of lidocaine in myocardial infarction patients.

The effects of cardiac failure on the volume of distribution for specific drugs in humans are summarized in Table 2 (the data in this table are representative rather than comprehensive). For the antiarrhythmic drugs, the initial volumes of distribution (V_1) are reduced by an average of 25% to 42%, a change that can clearly be clinically significant and, if ignored, could result in early drug toxicity. The volume of distribution estimated from the terminal decline phase (V_{area}) is frequently reported to be reduced in cardiac failure. However, this may be at least in part due to the influence of a prolonged terminal half-life because of reduced clearance (7). Thus, the steady state volume of distribution (V_{ss}) is a better indicator of altered tissue distribution (see Chapter 1). Although circulatory insufficiency would not be expected to influence V_{ss}, reduced V_{ss} for lidocaine has been reported in cardiac failure patients; the mechanism is yet unknown. The increased volume of distribution for aminopyrine (8) illustrates how cardiac failure can increase the volume of distribution of a water-soluble drug as a consequence of fluid retention.

CARDIAC FAILURE AND HEPATIC CLEARANCE

Cardiac disease can influence both hepatic and renal drug clearance. Circulatory influences on hepatic drug clearance have been discussed previously in Chapter 3. For those drugs whose intrinsic metabolic clearance is very high (extraction ratio > 70%), clearance is primarily determined by liver blood flow (see Chapters 3 and 4). Lidocaine elimination has been considered, at least in healthy persons and animals, to be primarily determined by liver blood flow (9,10). Thus, maneuvers that increase liver blood flow, such as isoproterenol infusion (Fig. 4A), also increase lidocaine clearance; whereas, those that decrease hepatic blood flow, such as propranolol (11,12) (Fig. 5) or norepinephrine infusion (Fig. 4B), decrease lidocaine clearance.

For those drugs whose liver metabolic capacity is much lower than liver blood flow, hepatic clearance is largely independent of blood flow and is determined by

TABLE 2. *Effects of cardiac failure on drug distribution for specific drugs*

Drug	Percentage change in volume of distribution	Reference
Aminopyrine	↑ 20 (V_{area})	Hepner et al. (8)
Dihydroquinidine	↓ 43 (V_1)	Ueda and Dzindzio (34)
	↓ 60 (V_{area})	Ueda and Dzindzio (34)
Disopyramide	↓ 12 (V_{area})	Landmark et al. (35)
Lidocaine	↓ 42 (V_1)	Thomson et al. (32)
	↓ 33 (V_{ss})	Thomson et al. (32)
Procainamide	↓ 25[a]	Koch-Weser (28)
Quinidine	↓ 41 (V_1)	Ueda and Dzindzio (33)
	↓ 32 (V_{area})	Ueda and Dzindzio (33)
Theophylline	No change	Powell et al. (36)

[a]Volume term not described.

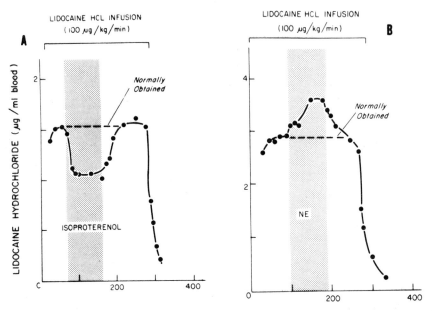

FIG. 4. Arterial lidocaine blood concentrations in the rhesus monkey showing the effects of **(A)** isoproterenol and **(B)** norepinephrine (NE) infusion on lidocaine levels during constant infusion. (From Benowitz et al., ref. 4, with permission.)

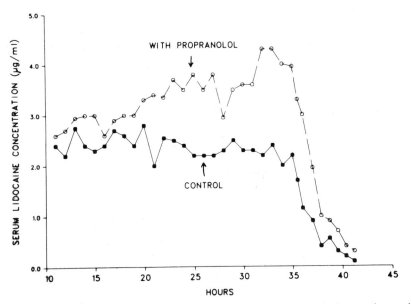

FIG. 5. Serum lidocaine concentrations in a healthy subject during and after continuous infusion of lidocaine in control state and during coadministration of propranolol (80 mg every 8 hr). (From Ochs et al., ref. 12, with permission.)

intrinsic metabolic capacity (see Chapters 1 and 3). Both hepatic blood flow and metabolism can be affected in cardiac failure. Blood flow to the liver is reduced and appears to change in proportion to cardiac index (9). Cardiac disease might influence the metabolic capacity of the liver either by (a) hepatocellular damage resulting from hepatic congestion or hypoperfusion or (b) hypoxemia with impaired microsomal drug oxidation. For some drugs, as has been suggested for lidocaine, there may be a time- or dose-dependent metabolism such that over the course of continued infusion and with increasing blood concentrations, hepatic clearance decreases (13). The mechanisms of this effect are unclear; metabolite inhibition has been suggested as one possibility. How this phenomenon interacts with other metabolic effects of cardiac failure is unclear.

As seen in Fig. 6, lidocaine clearance is substantially lower and blood concentrations higher during constant infusion in myocardial infarction patients with cardiac failure, as compared with those without. The prolonged time course of accumulation in patients with myocardial infarction, with and without cardiac failure, may be due in part to time- or dose-dependent reduction in clearance, but may also be due to increases in α_1-acid glycoprotein binding of lidocaine (6). Following discontinuation of infusion, the half-life of lidocaine is also longer in patients with myocardial infarction and cardiac failure (10.2 ± 2.0 hr $\pm$ SE), as compared with myocardial infarction without cardiac failure (4.3 ± 0.8) and compared with healthy individuals (1.4 ± 0.1) (14). The prolonged half-life in patients with myocardial infarction cannot be explained on the basis of increased protein binding, however, because the latter would be expected to reduce the volume of distribution and, if anything, shorten half-life.

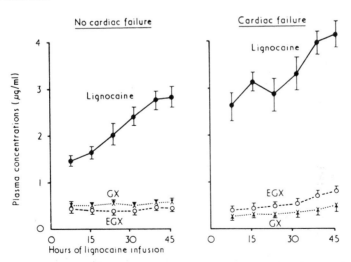

FIG. 6. Mean ($\pm$ SE) plasma concentrations of lidocaine, monoethyl glycine xylidide (EGX) and glycine xylidide (GX) in patients in coronary care unit with ($N = 7$) and without ($N = 6$) cardiac failure during constant infusion of lidocaine, 1.4 mg/min. (From Prescott et al., ref. 14, with permission.)

Investigators have tried to relate changes in lidocaine clearance to changes in indocyanine green clearance, assuming that the latter is a measure of hepatic blood flow. As seen in Fig. 7, in patients with cardiac failure, lidocaine and indocyanine green clearances are reduced (15). The magnitude of reduction reflects the severity of the cardiac failure. Clearances of lidocaine and indocyanine green correlate well with each other, and these authors have proposed that indocyanine green clearance, which can be determined in a relatively short period of time, might be predictive of lidocaine dosing requirements. Unfortunately, in a recent report by another group of investigators, no correlation between lidocaine and indocyanine green clearances in cardiac patients was found (16). It is unlikely that indocyanine green will have clinical utility as a guide to lidocaine dosing.

CIRCULATORY INFLUENCES ON RENAL DRUG CLEARANCE

Cardiac disease may affect renal clearance by several mechanisms (17). Reduced kidney blood flow may result in reduced glomerular filtration rate. Redistribution of blood flow from cortical to juxtamedullary nephrons may result in increased tubular reabsorption or reduced urine flow, or both. Little has been published with respect to the effects of disease states on tubular secretion. A question of current interest is whether urea clearance, which is more sensitive to both glomerular filtration and urine flow rates, might be a better predictor of clearance that creatinine for certain drugs like digoxin (18). Although not experimentally demonstrated, one might predict that reduced cardiac output, with reduced renal blood flow and/or intrarenal shunts, might result in decreased tubular secretion of drugs.

Not only cardiac failure itself but also therapy for cardiac failure can have hemodynamic effects that affect renal clearance of drugs. We have noted such interactions between diuretics and vasodilators, and digoxin (19). Table 3 sum-

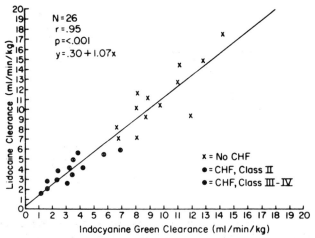

FIG. 7. Lidocaine and indocyanine green clearances in patients with and without congestive heart failure (CHF). (From Zito and Reid, ref. 15, with permission.)

TABLE 3. *Clinical data and digoxin pharmacokinetic parameters in decompensated cardiac failure (phase A) and after diuretic therapy (phase B)*

	Case 1		Case 2	
	Phase A	Phase B	Phase A	Phase B
Weight (kg)	90	84	67	60
Blood urea nitrogen (BUN) (mg/dl)	20	51	17	27
Serum creatinine (mg/dl)	1.8	2.0	1.3	1.5
Ratio BUN/serum creatinine	11.1	25.5	13.1	18.0
Ratio urea/creatinine clearance	0.55	0.31	0.37	0.27
Digoxin terminal half-life (hr)	52	71	44	71
Total digoxin clearance (ml/min)	103	54	86	44
Renal digoxin clearance (ml/min)	81	43	52	30
Nonrenal digoxin clearance (ml/min)	22	11	34	15
Ratio renal digoxin clearance/ creatinine clearance	0.96	0.83	1.10	0.91
Predicted mean plasma concentration (ng/ml) for an i.v. daily dose of 0.25 mg digoxin	0.8	1.3	1.4	2.3

marizes clinical data for 2 patients at the time of hospital admission in acute pulmonary edema (phase A) and after extensive diuresis (phase B). The reduction in body weight, increased blood urea/creatinine ratio, and decreased urea/creatinine renal clearance ratio suggested excessive diuresis with prerenal azotemia. The pharmacokinetics of digoxin were studied in these patients by simultaneous administration of intravenous radiolabeled and oral cold digoxin. After diuresis, digoxin half-life was substantially increased, primarily because of a reduction in clearance. Of interest was that both renal and extrarenal digoxin clearances were reduced. Renal digoxin clearance was decreased proportionally more than creatinine clearance. Both digoxin and creatinine are excreted in part by tubular secretion. It appears, therefore, that after overdiuresis, either digoxin tubular secretion is reduced or tubular reabsorption, the presence of which is not established, is increased. As expected, predicted serum digoxin concentrations are substantially higher in the postdiuresis state, and in 1 patient apparent digitalis intoxication was observed.

Another type of digoxin interaction is illustrated in Fig. 8. Patients with severe cardiac failure (New York Heart Association, classes 3 and 4) were treated with intravenous nitroprusside and hydralazine for the purpose of afterload reduction (20). During vasodilator drug administration, glomerular filtration rate (GFR) (measured as iothalamate clearance), renal blood flow (estimated from PAH clearance), renal digoxin clearance, and digoxin secretory clearance were determined. During vasodilator treatment, there was no significant change in GFR, but a substantial increase in renal blood flow. Renal digoxin clearance increased by about 50%. Because GFR did not significantly change, it appears that tubular secretion of digoxin was increased by vasodilator therapy. Possibly, this is a consequence of

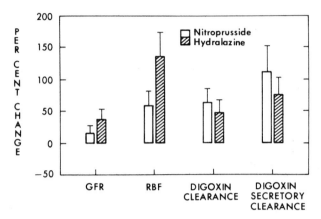

FIG. 8. Effects of vasodilators on renal hemodynamics and digoxin excretion (mean ± 1 SE). Changes in renal blood flow (RBF), digoxin renal clearance, and digoxin secretory clearance were significant ($p < 0.05$), whereas changes in glomerular filtration rate (GFR) were not. (From Cogan et al., ref. 20, with permission.)

TABLE 4. *Circulatory effects on drug clearance for specific drugs*

Drug	Disease state[a]	Percentage change in clearance	Reference
Aminopyrine	CF	↓ 76	Hepner et al. (8)
Dihydroquinidine	CF	↓ 53	Ueda and Dzindzio (34)
		↓ 49 (CL_R)	Ueda and Dzindzio (34)
Disopyramide	CF	↓ 65	Landmark et al. (35)
	MI	↓ 31	Bryson et al. (41)
Lidocaine	CF	↓ 37	Thomson et al. (32)
Mexiletine	CF	No change	Vozeh et al. (42)
Prazosin	CF	↓ 53 ($CL_{p.o.}$)	Jaillon et al. (25)
	CF	↓ 54 ($CL_{p.o.}$)	Baughman et al. (40)
Procainamide	MI	↓ 38	Lalka et al. (37)
	MI, CF	No change[b]	Wyman et al. (38)
Quinidine	CF	↓ 36	Ueda and Dzindzio (33)
		↓ 49 (CL_R)	Ueda and Dzindzio (33)
Theophylline[c]	CF	↓ 40	Powell et al. (36)

[a]CF, cardiac failure; MI, myocardial infarction.
[b]Comparison between MI patients with and without CF.
[c]See also Appendix A.

increased renal blood flow and/or redistribution of renal blood from juxtamedullary to cortical nephrons.

The effects of cardiac disease on the clearance of specific drugs are summarized in Table 4. Average decreases in total clearance of 36% to 53% are reported for the various antiarrhythmic drugs, indicating that reductions in rate of administration during continuous infusion or maintenance therapy are necessary for safe dosing of cardiac patients.

CARDIAC INFLUENCES ON DRUG ABSORPTION

Cardiac disease might be expected to alter the rate or extent of drug absorption. Reduced muscle blood flow due to sympathetically mediated vasoconstriction would reduce the rate of drug absorption from intramuscular sites in cardiac failure patients. Autonomic nervous disturbances (increased sympathetic and decreased parasympathetic activity) and/or tissue hypoperfusion could reduce gastrointestinal motility and increase transit time. This would result in delayed oral absorption and, depending on the drug, could increase or decrease bioavailability.

Cardiac failure is also associated with reduced mesenteric and presumably intestinal villus blood flow (21). Theoretically, for drugs that are highly permeable to the intestinal mucosa, reduced villus blood flow could delay diffusion and, therefore, rate of absorption. The absorption rate for digoxin, for example, has been shown in experimental animals to be affected by changes in intestinal blood flow (22). Mucosal edema might reduce epithelial permeability and thereby affect drug absorption, which has been speculated to account for abnormal fat (^{131}I-triolein) absorption in patients with cardiac failure (23,24).

As discussed previously, hepatic drug-metabolizing activity may be reduced in cardiac failure patients, which, in addition to altering systemic clearance, could by reducing first-pass metabolism increase the bioavailability of drugs with high hepatic extraction ratios. For example, the area under the blood concentration/time curve for oral prazosin is substantially greater in patients with cardiac failure than in normals (25,40). Likewise, the bioavailability of oral hydralazine, another drug that undergoes extensive first-pass metabolism and that is used for afterload reduction in patients with severe cardiac failure, might be predicted to be increased in the disease state.

Data regarding absorption kinetics of drugs in humans with cardiac disease are sparse and often inadequate to reach any conclusion. A recent study by Korhonen et al. (26) (Fig. 9) did demonstrate slowed absorption with lower peak concentrations of digoxin after ingestion of tablets in patients with myocardial infarction, as compared with age-matched controls. The bioavailability, as judged by the area under the blood concentration curve at 24 hr, was unaffected by myocardial infarction and cardiac failure. It must be noted, however, that 5 of the 12 patients reported had received morphine, which has been shown to slow gastric emptying and absorption of other drugs. Applefeld et al. (27) found that marked right-side congestive heart failure was associated with higher serum digoxin concentrations *(AUC)* during daily oral dosing, as compared with the same subjects after treatment. Without comparison to kinetics after intravenous dosing, the bioavailability of digoxin cannot be determined from these data. But it does appear, based on the two studies discussed earlier and other studies, that, in contrast to predictions from animal studies, digoxin absorption is not reduced by cardiac failure to the extent that higher-than-usual doses should be administered to achieve therapeutic concentrations. It has been reported that absorption of procainamide is erratic in patients with myocardial infarction (28).

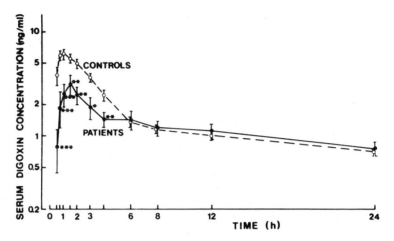

FIG. 9. Mean (±SEM) serum digoxin concentrations after a single oral dose of 0.75 mg in patients with myocardial infarction (N = 12) and healthy controls (N = 9). $^*p < 0.05$; $^{**}p < 0.01$; $^{***}p < 0.001$. (From Korhonen et al., ref. 26, with permission.)

CARDIAC FAILURE AND ACTIVE METABOLITES

Accumulation of active metabolites with resultant toxicity may occur in circulatory insufficiency states. It has been demonstrated, for example, that during constant infusion of lidocaine, blood concentrations of its major and active metabolite, monoethyl glycine xylidide (MEGX), are higher in patients with cardiac failure than in those without (29). One patient with neurological symptoms suggesting lidocaine toxicity, but with a therapeutic lidocaine concentration and an elevated MEGX concentration, has been described (30). Procainamide is metabolized to N-acetylprocainamide (NAPA), which has some pharmacologic activity and potential toxicity (31). Elimination of some metabolites, such as NAPA, depends to a major extent on renal clearance, and therefore it might be expected to accumulate in circulatory insufficiency states when complicated by renal insufficiency.

RECOMMENDATIONS FOR THERAPY IN PATIENTS WITH CARDIAC DISEASE

Based on the preceding considerations, several recommendations for therapy in patients with cardiac disease are suggested (Table 5):

1. Because of potentially incomplete or delayed oral or intramuscular absorption, drugs that are critically necessary should be administered intravenously. Conversely, reduced first-pass metabolism may lead to unexpectedly greater effects for certain drugs such as prazosin, and initial oral doses should be small.

2. Because of higher initial blood concentrations and altered distribution patterns, drugs are likely to reach brain and heart in higher concentrations in patients with cardiac failure. Rapid injection may produce toxicity immediately following the

TABLE 5. *Cardiac disease and drug kinetics: therapeutic implications*

Potential incomplete or delayed oral or i.m. absorption → administer intravenously
Brain and/or cardiac toxicity following rapid injection → infuse slowly
Reduced volume of distribution → reduce loading dose
Reduced metabolic clearance → reduce infusion rate; monitor blood concentration;
  potential usefulness of hemodynamic monitoring
Reduced renal clearance → reduce infusion rate; dose according to creatinine
  clearance; monitor blood concentration
Prolonged half-life and time course of accumulation → reduce infusion rate once effect
  is achieved
Accumulation of active metabolites → use specific assays; consider in understanding
  adverse effects
Consider hemodynamic consequences of therapy

---

dose. Slow intravenous infusion, over 1 to 2 min, will avoid this type of toxicity in most cases.

3. Because of the reduced initial volume of distribution, blood concentrations will be higher after loading doses in patients with cardiac failure. Loading doses should be reduced (preferentially based on data given in Table 2) by approximately 50%.

4. Metabolic clearance of several drugs is reduced in cardiac failure patients. Continuous infusion rates and maintenance daily oral doses should be lower in cardiac failure patients. A 50% reduction in maintenance dosage is a reasonable approximation (based on the data summarized in Table 3). However, because interindividual variability in clearance is so great, monitoring blood concentrations of drugs, if rapidly available, is extremely helpful. Hemodynamic monitoring and the use of test drugs, like indocyanine green, have been proposed as possible guides to adjust infusion rates for drugs, such as lidocaine in cardiac failure patients, but their practical utility has yet to be demonstrated.

5. Reduced renal clearance of drugs, particularly digoxin and procainamide, requires that rates of administration for these drugs also be reduced. Creatinine clearance may provide a useful first approximation in predicting doses (see Chapter 8). Hemodynamic consequences of diuretic-induced hypovolemia and vasodilator therapy in cardiac failure patients should also be considered as possible causes of altered renal clearance of other drugs.

6. For many drugs, elimination half-life will be prolonged, resulting in accumulation of drug over long periods of time during infusion or repetitive dosing. In the early hours of a constant infusion, when only a fraction of the steady state concentration has been achieved, supplemental injections of drugs may be required to achieve therapeutic concentrations. Once effective antiarrhythmic control has been achieved during infusion, infusion rates may need to be reduced in order to maintain constant blood concentrations of the drug. Because changes in protein binding of drugs may occur, especially during myocardial infarction, resulting in higher bound drug concentrations, monitoring of free-drug concentrations may be more appropriate.

7. Accumulation of active metabolites of various drugs should be considered in understanding unexpected therapeutic or toxic responses. Nonspecific assays for drugs such as procainamide or quinidine may measure metabolites as well as parent drug. When available, specific assays should be used.

ACKNOWLEDGMENT

Preparation of manuscript supported in part by USPHS grant DA-01696.

REFERENCES

1. Benowitz, N. L., and Meister, W. (1976): Pharmacokinetics in patients with cardiac failure. *Clin. Pharmacokinet.*, 1:389–405.
2. Braunwald, E., Ross, J., Jr., and Sonnenblick, E. H. (1976): *Mechanisms of Contraction of the Normal and Failing Heart*, 2nd Ed., pp. 309–356. Little, Brown, Boston.
3. Zelis, R., Nellis, S. H., Longhurst, J., Lee, G., and Mason, D. T. (1975): Abnormalities in the regional circulations accompanying congestive heart failure. *Prog. Cardiovasc. Dis.*, 18:181–199.
4. Benowitz, N., Forsyth, R. P., Melmon, K. L., and Rowland, M. (1974): Lidocaine disposition kinetics in monkey and man. II. Effects of hemorrhage and sympathomimetic drug administration. *Clin. Pharmacol. Ther.*, 16:99–109.
5. Lloyd, B. L., and Taylor, R. R. (1975): Augmentation of myocardial digoxin concentration in hemorrhagic shock. *Circulation*, 51:718–722.
6. Routledge, P. A., Stargel, W. W., Wagner, G. S., and Shand, D. G. (1980): Increased alpha-1-acid glycoprotein and lidocaine disposition in myocardial infarction. *Ann. Intern. Med.*, 93:701–704.
7. Riegelman, S., Loo, J., and Rowland, M. (1968): Concept of a volume of distribution and possible errors in evaluation of this parameter. *J. Pharm. Sci.*, 57:128–133.
8. Hepner, G. W., Vesell, E. S., and Tantum, K. R. (1978): Reduced drug elimination in congestive heart failure. Studies using aminopyrine as a model drug. *Am. J. Med.*, 65:271–276.
9. Stenson, R. E., Constantino, R. E., and Harrison, D. C. (1971): Interrelationships of hepatic blood flow, cardiac output, and blood levels of lidocaine in man. *Circulation*, 43:205–211.
10. Shand, D. G., Kornhauser, D. M., and Wilkinson, G. R. (1975): Effects of route of administration and blood flow on hepatic drug elimination. *J. Pharmacol. Exp. Ther.*, 195:424–432.
11. Branch, R. A., Shand, D. G., Wilkinson, G. R., and Nies, A. S. (1973): The reduction of lidocaine clearance by *dl*-propranolol: An example of hemodynamic drug interaction. *J. Pharmacol. Exp. Ther.*, 184:515–519.
12. Ochs, H. R., Carstens, G., and Greenblatt, D. J. (1980): Reduction in lidocaine clearance during continuous infusion and by coadministration of propranolol. *N. Engl. J. Med.*, 303:373–377.
13. LeLorier, J., Moisan, R., Gagne, J., and Caille, G. (1977): Effect of the duration of infusion on the disposition of lidocaine in dogs. *J. Pharmacol. Exp. Ther.*, 203:507–511.
14. Prescott, L. F., Yamoah-Adjepon, K. K., and Talbot, R. G. (1976): Impaired lignocaine metabolism in patients with myocardial infarction and cardiac failure. *Br. Med. J.*, 1:939–941.
15. Zito, R. A., and Reid, P. R. (1978): Lidocaine kinetics predicted by indocyanine green clearance. *N. Engl. J. Med.*, 298:1160–1163.
16. Bax, N. D. S., Tucker, G. T., and Woods, H. F. (1980): Lignocaine and indocyanine green kinetics in patients following myocardial infarction. *Br. J. Clin. Pharmacol.*, 10:353–361.
17. Cannon, P. J. (1977): The kidney in heart failure. *N. Engl. J. Med.*, 296:26–32.
18. Halkin, H., Sheiner, L. B., Peck, C. C., and Melmon, K. L. (1975): Determinants of the renal clearance of digoxin. *Clin. Pharmacol. Ther.*, 17:385–394.
19. Meister, W., Benowitz, N. L., and Benet, L. Z. (1983): Impaired elimination of digoxin after diuretic therapy for cardiac failure *(submitted for publication)*.
20. Cogan, M. J., Humphreys, M. H., Carlson, C. J., Benowitz, N. L., and Rappaport, E. (1981): Acute vasodilator therapy increases the renal clearance of digoxin in patients with congestive heart failure. *Circulation*, 64:973–976.
21. Higgins, C. B., Vatner, S. F., Franklin, D., and Braunwald, E. (1974): Pattern of differential vasoconstriction in response to acute and chronic low-output states in the conscious dog. *Cardiovasc. Res.*, 8:92–98.

22. Haass, A., Lullmann, H., and Peters, T. (1972): Absorption rate of some cardiac glycosides and portal blood flow. *Eur. J. Pharmacol.*, 19:336–370.
23. Hakkila, J., Makela, T. E., and Halonen, P. I. (1960): Absorption of ^{131}I-triolein in congestive heart failure. *Am. J. Cardiol.*, 5:295–299.
24. Berkowitz, D., Droll, M. N., and Likoff, W. (1963): Malabsorption as a complication of congestive heart failure. *Am. J. Cardiol.*, 11:43–47.
25. Jaillon, P., Rubin, P., Yee, Y.-G., Ball, R., Kates, R., Harrison, D., and Blaschke, T. (1979): Influence of congestive heart failure on prazosin kinetics. *Clin. Pharmacol. Ther.*, 25:790–794.
26. Korhonen, U. R., Jounela, A. J., Pakarinen, A. J., Pentikainen, P. J., and Takkunen, J. T. (1979): Pharmacokinetics of digoxin in patients with acute myocardial infarction. *Am. J. Cardiol.*, 44:1190–1194.
27. Applefeld, M. M., Adir, J., Crouthamel, W. G., and Roddman, D. S. (1981): Digoxin pharmacokinetics in congestive heart failure. *J. Clin. Pharmacol.*, 21:114–120.
28. Koch-Weser, J. (1971): Pharmacokinetics of procainamide in man. *Ann. N.Y. Acad. Sci.*, 179:370–382.
29. Halkin, H., Meffin, P., Melmon, K. L., and Rowland, M. (1975): Influence of congestive heart failure on blood levels of lidocaine and its active monodeethylated metabolite. *Clin. Pharmacol. Ther.*, 17:385–394.
30. Strong, J. M., Parker, M., and Atkinson, A. J., Jr. (1973): Identification of glycinexylidide in patients treated with intravenous lidocaine. *Clin. Pharmacol. Ther.*, 14:67–72.
31. Elson, J., Strong, J. M., Lee, W.-K., and Atkinson, A. J., Jr. (1975): Antiarrhythmic potency of *N*-acetylprocainamide. *Clin. Pharmacol. Ther.*, 17:134–140.
32. Thomson, P. D., Melmon, K. L., Richardson, J. A., Cohn, K., Steinbrunn, W., Cudihee, R., and Rowland, M. (1973): Lidocaine pharmacokinetics in advanced heart failure, liver disease, and renal failure in humans. *Ann. Intern. Med.*, 78:499–508.
33. Ueda, C. T., and Dzindzio, B. S. (1978): Quinidine kinetics in congestive heart failure. *Clin. Pharmacol. Ther.*, 23:158–164.
34. Ueda, C. T., and Dzindzio, B. S. (1979): Pharmacokinetics of dihydroquinidine in congestive heart failure patients after intravenous quinidine administration. *Eur. J. Clin. Pharmacol.*, 16:101–105.
35. Landmark, K., Bredesen, J. E., Thaulow, E., Simonsen, S., and Amlie, J. P. (1981): Pharmacokinetics of disopyramide in patients with imminent to moderate cardiac failure. *Eur. J. Clin. Pharmacol.*, 19:187–192.
36. Powell, J. R., Vozeh, S., Hopewell, P., Costell, J., Sheiner, L. B., and Riegelman, S. (1978): Theophylline disposition in acutely ill hospitalized patients. *Am. Rev. Respir. Dis.*, 118:229–238.
37. Lalka, D., Wyman, M. G., Goldreyer, B. N., Ludden, T. M., and Cannom, D. S. (1978): Procainamide accumulation kinetics in the immediate postmyocardial infarction period. *J. Clin. Pharmacol.*, 18:397–401.
38. Wyman, M. G., Goldreyer, B. N. ,Cannom, D. S., Ludden, T. M., and Lalka, D. (1981): Factors influencing procainamide total body clearance in the immediate post myocardial infarction period. *J. Clin. Pharmacol.*, 21:20–25.
39. Benowitz, N. L., Forsyth, R. P., Melmon, K. L., and Rowland, M. (1974): Lidocaine disposition kinetics in monkey and man. I. Prediction by a perfusion model. *Clin. Pharmacol. Ther.*, 16:87–98.
40. Baughman, R. A., Jr., Arnold, S., Benet, L. Z., Lin, E. T., Chatterjee, K., and Williams, R. L. (1980): Altered prazosin pharmacokinetics in congestive heart failure. *Eur. J. Clin. Pharmacol.*, 17:425–428.
41. Bryson, S. M., Cairns, C. J., and Whiting, B. (1982): Disopyramide pharmacokinetics during recovery from myocardial infarction. *Br. J. Clin. Pharmacol.*, 13:417–421.
42. Vozeh, S., Katz, G., Steiner, V., and Follath, F. (1982): Population pharmacokinetic parameters in patients treated with oral mexiletine. *Eur. J. Clin. Pharmacol.*, 23:445–451.

Pharmacokinetic Basis for Drug Treatment,
edited by L. Z. Benet et al., Raven Press,
New York © 1984

Chapter 7

The Lungs and Metabolic Drug Clearance in Health and Disease

Robert A. Roth, Jr.

*Department of Pharmacology and Toxicology, Michigan State University,
East Lansing, Michigan 48824*

The liver is commonly held to be the organ of drug metabolism par excellence. This view is based primarily on the liver invariably having a higher content of drug-metabolizing enzymes than do other organs. Although their metabolic capacity is far less than that of liver, many extrahepatic organs are now known to possess some ability to metabolize drugs. The lung, for example, contains enzymes capable of metabolizing therapeutic agents, environmental toxicants such as benzo[a]pyrene (BP), and endogenous agents, such as biogenic amines, prostaglandins, and peptide hormones. Although the lungs may act on agents of several chemical classes, basic amino compounds have perhaps been studied most extensively and seem to be commonly acted on by lung. Certain of these compounds are metabolized by lung, whereas others are removed from the circulation and accumulate in lung tissue (Table 1).

Despite the potential of lung to modify the concentrations of circulating agents, this organ has often been ignored in the development of pharmacokinetic models of drug clearance *in vivo*. Recent studies suggest that the lung may be more important than heretofore recognized in the total body clearance of circulating agents (39). In this chapter, evidence supporting this hypothesis is presented, and the effects of disease states on the capacity of lung to clear circulating agents are discussed. The participation of the lung in the elimination of volatile drugs is well known and will not be reviewed here; instead, discussion will be confined to the role of the lung in metabolic drug clearance.

THE IMPORTANCE OF RELATIVE TISSUE PERFUSION AND INTRINSIC CLEARANCE

The perfusion-limited model of metabolic clearance as it relates to the hepatic clearance of drugs has been studied extensively in recent years (40–44). This model relates drug clearance (CL_0) by an organ to organ blood flow (Q_0) and intrinsic free clearance (CL^u_{int}), the maximal metabolic clearance of drug from the organ

TABLE 1. *Drugs and other agents acted on by intact lung[a]*

Agent	Species	Disposition[b]	Reference
1-α-Acetylmethadol	Monkey	ACC	1
	Rat	ACC	2
Aldrin	Rabbit	ACC, MET	3
α-Naphthol	Rabbit	MET	4
Amphetamine	Rabbit	ACC	5
Benzo[a]pyrene	Rat	MET	6, 7
	Rabbit	MET	8
Biphenyl	Rabbit	ACC, MET	9
Carbaryl	Rabbit	ACC, MET	10
Chlorcyclizine	Rabbit	ACC	5
Chlorphentermine	Rabbit	ACC	11
	Rat	ACC	12
Chlorpromazine	Rat	ACC, MET	13
Clozapine	Rat	ACC	14
Dieldrin	Rabbit	ACC	3
Estradiol	Rat	MET	15
Ibuterol	Rat, guinea pig	MET	16
Imipramine	Rabbit	ACC	5, 17
	Rat	ACC	18
Lidocaine	Rat	ACC	19
1-(+)-Mepivacaine	Rabbit	ACC	20
Mescaline	Rabbit	ACC, MET	21
d-Methadone	Rabbit	ACC	22
	Rabbit	ACC, MET	5, 23, 24
Methylaniline	Cat, rat	MET	25
4-Methylumbelliferone	Rat	MET	26
Morphine	Rabbit	ACC	27
p-Nitroanisole	Rat, rabbit	MET	28
Nortriptyline	Dog	ACC, MET	29
Pentobarbital	Rabbit	MET	24
Phenol	Rat	MET	30–32
Progesterone	Rat	MET	33
Propranolol	Rat	ACC	34, 35
	Rat, dog, monkey	ACC	36
	Rat	ACC	37
Trifluoperazine	Rat	ACC	38

[a]All entries made on the basis of studies performed *in vivo* or in the isolated perfused lung.
[b]ACC indicates accumulation by lung tissue; MET indicates pulmonary metabolism of drug by intact lung.

water when blood flow is not limiting. These parameters are related to organ clearance, as described in Chapter 1, by the following equation:

$$CL_0 = \frac{Q_0 \cdot fu_B \cdot CL^u_{int}}{Q_0 + fu_B \cdot CL^u_{int}} \qquad (1)$$

where fu_B is that fraction of drug that is unbound in the blood. This equation describes a parabolic relationship between organ clearance and blood flow. The intrinsic

clearance term (CL^u_{int}) relates to the amount and character of the enzyme(s) of disposition for any given drug. Thus, Eq. 1 indicates in theory that an organ with less dispositional enzymatic capacity but with higher blood flow could contribute as much to total body metabolic clearance of a drug as an organ with higher enzyme content but lower blood flow. Because the lung receives all of the cardiac output, whereas liver blood flow is only approximately one-fourth of this value, one might infer from this perfusion-limited model that the lung, despite its relative paucity of enzyme(s), will contribute substantially to the total body clearance of certain circulating compounds.

Benzo[a]pyrene (BP) Clearance

With this in mind, we have begun to examine the flow dependence of pulmonary clearance of certain agents and to compare the clearance of drugs by isolated lungs and livers perfused at flows that occur *in vivo*. For example, circulating BP is eliminated from the body by metabolism mediated by mixed-function oxidase(s) (MFO). Arylhydrocarbon hydroxylase (AHH) mediates the first step in the metabolism of BP. AHH activity may be increased markedly in rat tissues by pretreating animals with 3-methylcholanthrene (3MC). In both untreated and 3MC-treated animals, however, the total content of AHH in lung is less than 1% of that in liver (45,46; D. A. Wiersma and R. A. Roth, *unpublished observations*). We have recently measured BP clearance by isolated lungs and liver perfused at relevant flows (47,48). Cardiac output in rats of the size used in this study is approximately 45 ml/min, whereas liver blood flow is approximately one-fourth of this value (49). Studies in which lungs and livers were perfused at these flows indicate that clearance of BP by lungs of untreated rats is very small compared with that by liver. However, clearance of isolated lungs of 3MC-pretreated rats (perfused at 45 ml/min) was 8.8 ± 0.5 ml/min, whereas hepatic clearance (livers perfused at 10 ml/min) was 6.4 ± 0.6 ml/min. Thus, lung and liver probably contribute almost equally to the total body clearance of circulating BP in 3MC-induced animals. Moreover, any large effect of induction of AHH on total body clearance of BP likely results from effects on enzyme(s) in extrahepatic rather than hepatic tissue, because hepatic BP clearance cannot be increased a great deal without increasing hepatic blood flow. That is, despite the fact that AHH activity was increased more than sevenfold in both organs, this resulted in a marked elevation in BP clearance only in lung, as would be expected, because liver clearance approaches blood flow (see Chapters 3 and 4). In this regard, it is of particular interest that exposure of rats to cigarette smoke results in stimulation of pulmonary AHH activity, whereas AHH activity in liver remains unchanged (50). Thus, such agents that have different effects on drug-metabolizing activities in pulmonary and hepatic tissue may enhance further the contribution of lung to total body clearance.

In a related study, Smith and Bend (51) recently reported a high pulmonary extraction of benzo[a]pyrene-4,5-oxide by isolated rabbit lungs perfused at a flow approaching cardiac output. This suggests that pulmonary metabolic clearance of some xenobiotic agents is substantial even in animals unexposed to stimulators of MFOs.

Pulmonary Amine Clearance

The lungs efficiently remove many amino compounds from the circulation, some of which are taken into lung by carrier-mediated transport processes. These amino compounds include drugs such as chlorphenteramine (12), propranolol (37), imipramine (18), clozapine (14), and others (Table 1), as well as endogenous amines such as 5-hydroxytryptamine (5HT, serotonin) (52) and norepinephrine (NE). Some of these are merely accumulated by lung without metabolism, whereas others are metabolized to various degrees. The transport process for 5HT, for example, has been localized to vascular endothelial cells in lung. Following uptake, 5HT is extensively metabolized by monoamine oxidase (MAO) and aldehyde dehydrogenase to 5-hydroxyindoleacetic acid (52,53). We measured the clearance of 5HT under first-order conditions in isolated rat lungs and livers perfused at physiologically relevant flows (54). Under these conditions the clearance by both organs was flow-dependent, and at flows occurring *in vivo*, clearance by lung was 19 ml/min, whereas hepatic clearance was 7 ml/min. Thus, in the rat, lung clears 5HT nearly three times as rapidly as liver, even though it contains less than 8% as much MAO. In fact, at all flows tested, clearance of 5HT by lung was greater than that by liver, a finding that was not predicted from the kinetics of MAO in these organs *(vide infra)*. It is likely, therefore, that the carrier-mediated uptake process for 5HT, present in lung but apparently not in liver, is largely responsible for the greater clearance by lung.

These studies in rats suggest that the lung is the predominant organ in the total body clearance of 5HT *in vivo*. In these experiments, the pulmonary extraction ratio for 5HT in lungs perfused at a flow approximating cardiac output in the rat was 0.43. Studies by others indicate that the pulmonary extraction ratio in humans may be somewhat greater. For example, Gillis et al. (55) reported that the pulmonary 5HT extraction ratio in anesthetized human patients was 0.61 ± 0.03. Cardiac output in these patients was 5.0 ± 0.7 liters/min, as measured by indicator dilution. Thus, their pulmonary 5HT clearance was approximately 3.0 liters/min. Hepatic 5HT clearance has not been reported in humans, but total hepatic blood flow is approximately 1.5 liters/min (56). Accordingly, even if the hepatic extraction ratio for 5HT were as high as 1.0, hepatic clearance of this substrate would be only half as great as pulmonary clearance. Failure to account for this pulmonary first-pass effect for drugs injected intravenously may lead to large errors in the estimation of certain pharmacokinetic parameters (e.g., volume of distribution), as emphasized by Chiou for circulating prostaglandins (57).

The lungs may also influence the pharmacokinetics of certain therapeutic agents. For example, lungs of animals extensively accumulate circulating propranolol, with little or no metabolism (5,37). Accumulation of other amines such as octylamine (58) and lidocaine (59) in lungs of humans has also been demonstrated. Geddes et al. (60) recently measured first-pass uptake of ^{14}C-propranolol by lungs of patients undergoing cardiac catheterization for ischemic heart disease. In patients who had not previously taken the drug, $75 \pm 13\%$ of an intravenous bolus dose was removed on first passage through the pulmonary vasculature. In other patients who had been

receiving regular oral treatment with propranolol, this value was only 33 ± 12%. This study suggests that pulmonary extraction of propranolol in humans is of considerable magnitude and that the binding to lung is partly saturable by normal therapeutic doses. In this study, the increase in aortic blood concentration was far greater in the patients who had previously received propranolol. Thus, the same dose given intravenously might result in either a therapeutically useful or a toxic aortic drug concentration, depending on the previous treatment that the patient had received. Because other basic drugs, for example, the tricyclic antidepressants (37), inhibit pulmonary accumulation of propranolol, previous treatment with these would likely have the same effect on initial aortic propranolol concentrations and might thereby bring about cardiac arrhythmia. In this regard, injection of lidocaine has been shown to displace nortriptyline from lung *in vivo* (61). Thus, pulmonary first-pass effects may be significant for certain drugs when administered intravenously, and in some cases drug-drug interactions occurring in lung may precipitate unwanted pharmacological responses.

The intrinsic free clearance (CL^u_{int}) of drugs eliminated by hepatic metabolism can be predicted from enzyme kinetic parameters using the following relationship (62):

$$CL^u_{int} = V_{max}/K_m \qquad (2)$$

where V_{max} is the maximum rate of metabolism and K_m is the apparent Michaelis-Menten constant of the enzyme responsible for disposition. The clearance of a drug by an organ at any given blood flow can then be predicted by substitution into Eq. 1. Our recent studies showed that BP clearance by lungs of 3MC-pretreated rats could be predicted adequately from kinetic parameters of AHH determined in subcellular fractions of lung.

We used this model to predict the pulmonary clearance of circulating mescaline. Mescaline is taken into rabbit lung apparently by passive diffusion and metabolized by an amine oxidase (21). Although mescaline disposition by isolated rabbit lung has been studied at low perfusion, studies performed at flows approaching cardiac output (approximately 350 ml/min in the rabbit) are lacking. Although rabbit lung possesses only 13% as much mescaline oxidase activity as liver, the foregoing model suggests that clearance of mescaline by lung *in vivo* is 70% of that by liver (63). Thus, despite its relative lack of mescaline oxidase content, the lung may contribute substantially to the total body clearance of mescaline in the rabbit.

Although many of the studies in animals mentioned earlier are preliminary and require further study as well as confirmation in humans, they suggest that the lung may be more important than has been recognized in the total body clearance of certain drugs that are eliminated from the circulation by metabolism.

EFFECTS OF ALTERED PULMONARY PHYSIOLOGY ON DRUG CLEARANCE

Changes in alveolar gas exchange, airway resistance, or control of breathing, as occur in divers disease states, may precipitate tissue hypoxia and/or changes in

plasma pH. Such changes could result in altered metabolic drug clearance by the lungs and other organs.

Plasma pH and Pulmonary Amine Clearance

Because the basic amines represent an important class of drugs that are removed from the circulation by lung, we chose mescaline as a model amino drug in a study of pH effects on clearance. Rabbit lungs were perfused with a buffer of pH 7.4, and mescaline clearance was measured. Increasing the pH of the perfusion medium to 7.9 resulted in a 50% increase in mescaline clearance (64). Conversely, lowering the pH of the perfusion medium reduced mescaline clearance. Similar effects could be produced by ventilating the isolated lungs with different gas mixtures. For example, isolated rabbit lungs perfused in a single-pass system and ventilated with 95% air/5% CO_2 had a lower pH of the effluent perfusion medium and cleared mescaline much less rapidly than did lungs ventilated with room air. Because mescaline enters lung presumably by passive diffusion of its nonionized form across pulmonary cell membranes, these effects may be attributed to changes in the ionization of this amine. Under conditions such that intracellular free drug concentration is low, the rate of passive diffusion of drug from the vasculature into lung tissue will depend on the concentration of the nonionized form in the plasma. Application of the Henderson-Hasselbalch equation indicates that when pH is changed from 7.4 to 7.8, a 2.5-fold increase in the nonionized form of mescaline ($pK_a = 9.56$) occurs. Similarly, decreased pH lowers the uptake of lidocaine into slices of lung (65).

Although data are lacking, the clearance of other basic drugs that enter lung by passive diffusion would be expected to change similarly with alterations in plasma pH. Indeed, when hyperventilation or hypoventilation leads to a change in arterial pH, drug disposition by other organs may be affected as well. Interestingly, large increases in perfusion-medium pH had only minimal effects on the pulmonary clearance of 5HT and NE, amines that are taken into lung by carrier-mediated transport rather than by passive diffusion (64).

Alveolar Hypoxia and Drug Clearance

Diseases of the lung that result in alveolar hypoxia may also result in depressed clearance of circulating substances. For example, clearance of 5HT by isolated lungs was markedly reduced when the lungs were ventilated with gas mixtures of low Po_2 (18).

Because adequate oxygenation of all tissues *in vivo* ultimately depends on proper functioning of the lungs, pulmonary diseases that result in arterial hypoxia will also affect extrapulmonary drug kinetics. Acute exposure of rats, for example, to atmospheres of lowered Po_2 (hypoxic hypoxia) resulted in a depressed rate of absorption of hexobarbital following intraperitoneal administration. In addition, disappearance of this drug from the plasma, which occurs primarily by hepatic metabolism, was also markedly depressed (66,67). That such effects may alter pharmacologic responses was confirmed by the observation that hexobarbital sleep-

ing time was markedly prolonged by hypoxic hypoxia. Hepatic hexobarbital clearance is blood-flow-dependent in the rat, and hypoxic hypoxia markedly reduces hepatic blood flow (43). Thus, effects of alveolar hypoxia on hepatic drug clearance may occur not only as a result of decreased oxygen content of blood perfusing the liver but also from decreased hepatic blood flow (i.e., drug delivery) to this organ. In chronically hypoxic human patients, significant redistribution of blood flow away from the splanchnic region occurs (68). In this regard, it is of interest that in some species, including humans, hypoxic hypoxia also results in substantial increases in cardiac output. Accordingly, the contribution of lung to total body clearance might be increased for certain drugs for which pulmonary and/or hepatic clearance is flow-dependent.

Deficiencies in pulmonary gas exchange may also lead to alterations in binding of drugs to plasma macromolecules. This, in turn, could produce changes in drug clearance, as predicted by Eq. 1. These effects, as well as the little that is known about the effects of gas-exchange deficits on drug disposition in humans, have been recently reviewed by du Souich et al. (69).

Pulmonary Drug Disposition and Prostaglandin Biosynthesis

Recent studies indicate that certain xenobiotic agents may be co-oxidized by prostaglandin hydroperoxyendoperoxides (e.g., prostaglandin G_2) formed during prostaglandin biosynthesis. For example, prostaglandin endoperoxide synthetase preparations from guinea pig lung co-oxidized BP-7,8-diol to derivatives that bind covalently to cellular macromolecules (70). Certain conditions, including hyperinflation of lungs (71) or antigenic challenge of lungs of sensitized individuals (72), are known to cause the production in lung tissue of large amounts of prostaglandins formed by this pathway. Thus, it seems possible that hyperventilation or other conditions resulting in increased synthesis of prostaglandins may be associated with both qualitative and quantitative alterations in the production of metabolites from drug substrates that enter lung. This possibility apparently has not yet been tested in intact lung, but it is one that merits study.

EFFECTS OF DISEASE STATES ON PULMONARY DRUG CLEARANCE

Although the lungs may be important in the total body clearance of certain drugs and circulating endogenous agents, the effects of disease states on pharmacokinetic properties of lung have not been extensively studied. Diseases resulting in altered pulmonary physiology may be associated with altered drug clearance, as described earlier. In addition, animal studies indicate that toxicants that cause cellular injury in lung interfere with the ability of the lungs to clear circulating agents.

Hyperoxia and Paraquat

Exposure to atmospheres of high P_{O_2}, for example, results in extensive injury to capillary endothelial cells in lung. Isolated lungs of rats exposed to 1-atm O_2

were impaired in their ability to clear perfused NE or 5HT, amines that are removed from the circulation by transport into pulmonary endothelium (73,74). In similar studies, pulmonary imipramine clearance was unaffected by O_2 exposure (74). Significantly depressed 5HT clearance occurred after only 18 hr of O_2 exposure, whereas ultrastructural changes in rat lungs occurred only after 2 days of breathing 1-atm O_2 (75). Thus, 5HT clearance may be a sensitive index of early injury to pulmonary endothelium. In this regard, paraquat toxicity in rats results in only modest changes in pulmonary endothelium and is associated with much smaller decreases in 5HT clearance by lung (76).

Pulmonary Hypertension and Pyrrolizidine Alkaloids

Pyrrolizidine alkaloids occur in small plants of several families and intoxicate both humans and grazing animals (77). Monocrotaline (MCT) is one such alkaloid that produces hepatic and pulmonary lesions. Ingestion of MCT by young rats results in pulmonary vascular injury, including thrombosis, lesions of the arterial media, and swelling of pulmonary capillary endothelial cells (78–80). These changes are accompanied by depressed removal of 5HT and NE by rat lungs (81,82). Pulmonary lesions from MCT are associated also with pulmonary hypertension and right ventricular hypertrophy (83). Interestingly, morphologic alterations in pulmonary vascular endothelium have also been described in humans with pulmonary hypertension (84). Moreover, Sole et al. (85) have reported that lungs of patients with either primary or secondary pulmonary hypertension are markedly impaired in their ability to remove NE, although conflicting results have also been reported (86). The pulmonary clearance of therapeutic agents in patients with pulmonary hypertension has not been reported.

Systemic Hypertension

It is possible that other diseases are associated with elevated, rather than depressed, pulmonary clearance. We have recently found that clearance of perfused NE was markedly higher in isolated lungs of spontaneously hypertensive rats (SHR) than in those of Kyoto-Wistar controls (87). The elevated NE extraction in adult SHR does not seem to result directly from elevations in systemic arterial pressure, because elevated NE extraction was also observed in young SHR, in which arterial pressure is not yet elevated. Also, no difference in NE clearance was observed between other, nongenetic models of hypertension in the rat and their respective controls (R. A. Roth and G. D. Fink, *unpublished observations*).

Altered Nutrition

Hypovitaminosis A results in decreased ability of rat lung slices to accumulate certain basic drugs such as imipramine and chlorpromazine (88). The degree of uptake of agents into lung is of interest in light of enhanced susceptibility of lung to chemical carcinogenesis in animals deficient in vitamin A (89). In addition, low

dietary intake of vitamin A has been associated in humans with a high incidence of cancer of the respiratory system (90). Potential relationships among altered nutritional states, pulmonary disease, and disposition of agents by lung have received little attention.

Development and Pulmonary Clearance

Because the lungs mature relatively late in development, age-related differences in pulmonary clearance may also be expected. Indeed, isolated lungs of 7-day-old rats clear perfused angiotension I and 5HT less efficiently than those of adults (91,92). In humans, the ability of minced lung samples to interconvert cortisol and cortisone changes during gestation and infancy (93). Such studies raise the possibility that the effects of disease states on pulmonary drug clearance may be different in young and adult individuals.

CONCLUSION

Much work obviously needs to be done to elucidate fully the role of the lung in total body metabolic drug clearance in humans and to understand the effects of disease states on drug disposition by lung. The limited studies that have been reported suggest that (a) the lung may play an important role in the metabolic clearance of certain substances from the circulation, (b) altered ventilatory function of lung may cause changes in pulmonary and extrapulmonary drug disposition by altering blood and tissue pH, Po_2, etc., and (c) diseases associated with altered cell function in lung may influence pulmonary disposition of circulating agents.

REFERENCES

1. Misra, A. L., Mule, S. J., Block, R., and Bates, T. R. (1978): Physiological disposition and biotransformation of 1-α-[2-³H]acetylmethadol (LAAM) in acutely and chronically treated monkeys. *J. Pharmacol. Exp. Ther.*, 206:475–491.
2. Roerig, D. L., Hasegawa, A. T., and Wang, R. H. (1977): Effect of alteration of metabolism on the analgesic activity, toxicity, distribution and excretion of 1-α-acetylmethadol in the rat. *J. Pharmacol. Exp. Ther.*, 203:377–387.
3. Mehendale, H. M., and El-Bassiouni, E. A. (1975): Uptake and disposition of aldrin and dieldrin by isolated perfused rabbit lung. *Drug Metab. Dispos.*, 3:543–556.
4. Wilson, A. G. E., Hirom, P. C., and Kung, H. C. (1979): Pharmacokinetics of uptake and metabolism of α-naphthol by the isolated perfused lung. Abstracts of papers, Society of Toxicology, 18th annual meeting, p. A161.
5. Orton, T. C., Anderson, M. W., Pickett, R. D., Eling, T. E., and Fouts, J. R. (1973): Xenobiotic accumulation and metabolism by isolated perfused rabbit lungs. *J. Pharmacol. Exp. Ther.*, 186:482–497.
6. Vahakangas, K., Nevasaari, K., Pelkonen, O., and Karki, N. T. (1977): The effects of cigarette smoke on the metabolism of benzo(a)pyrene in perfused rat lung. *Acta Pharmacol. Toxicol.*, 41 *(Suppl. 4)*:78.
7. Vahakangas, K., Nevasaari, K., Pelkonen, O., and Karki, N. T. (1977): The metabolism of benzo(a)pyrene in isolated perfused lungs from variously-treated rats. *Acta Pharmacol. Toxicol.*, 41:129–140.
8. Bingham, E., Niemeier, R., and Dalbey, W. (1976): Metabolism of environmental pollutants by the isolated perfused lung. *Fed. Proc.*, 35:81–84.
9. Hook, G. E. R., and Bend, J. R. (1976): Pulmonary metabolism of xenobiotics. *Life Sci.*, 18:279–290.

10. Blase, B. W., and Loomis, T. A. (1976): The uptake and metabolism of carbaryl by isolated perfused rabbit lung. *Toxicol. Appl. Pharmacol.*, 37:481–490.
11. Angevine, L. S., and Mehendale, H. M. (1980): Chlorphenteramine uptake by isolated perfused rabbit lung. *Toxicol. Appl. Pharmacol.*, 52:336–346.
12. Minchin, R. F., Madsen, B. W., and Ilett, K. F. (1979): Effect of desmethylimipramine on the kinetics of chlorphenteramine accumulation in isolated perfused rat lung. *J. Pharmacol. Exp. Ther.*, 211:514–518.
13. Ohmiya, Y., and Mehendale, H. M. (1980): Uptake and metabolism of chlorpromazine by rat and rabbit lungs. *Drug Metab. Dispos.*, 8:313–318.
14. Gardiner, T. H., Lewis, J. M., and Shore, P. A. (1978): Distribution of clozapine in the rat: Localization in lung. *J. Pharmacol. Exp. Ther.*, 206:151–157.
15. Hartalia, J., Uotila, P., and Nienstedt, U. (1980): Metabolism of estradiol in isolated perfused rat lungs. *J. Steroid Biochem.*, 13:571–572.
16. Ryrfeldt, A., and Nilsson, E. (1978): Uptake and biotransformation of ibuterol and terbutaline in isolated perfused rat and guinea pig lung. *Biochem. Pharmacol.*, 27:301–305.
17. Eling, T. E., Pickett, R. D., Orton, T. C., and Anderson, M. W. (1975): A study of the dynamics of imipramine accumulation in the isolated perfused rabbit lung. *Drug Metab. Dispos.*, 3:389–399.
18. Junod, A. F. (1972): Accumulation of ^{14}C-imipramine in isolated perfused rat lungs. *J. Pharmacol. Exp. Ther.*, 183:182–187.
19. Post, C., Andersson, R. G. G., Ryrfeldt, A., and Nilsson, E. (1978): Transport and binding of lidocaine by lung slices and perfused lung of rats. *Acta Pharmacol. Toxicol.*, 43:156–163.
20. Aberg, G. (1972): Toxicological and local anaesthetic effects of optically active isomers of two local anaesthetic compounds. *Acta Pharmacol. Toxicol.*, 31:273–286.
21. Roth, R. A., Roth, J. A., and Gillis, C. N. (1977): Disposition of ^{14}C-mescaline by rabbit lung. *J. Pharmacol. Exp. Ther.*, 200:394–401.
22. Swanson, B. N., Gordon, W. P., Lynn, R. K., and Gerber, N. (1978): Seminal excretion, vaginal absorption, distribution and whole blood kinetics of *d*-methadone in the rabbit. *J. Pharmacol. Exp. Ther.*, 206:507–514.
23. Wilson, A. G. E., Law, F. C. P., Eling, T. E., and Anderson, M. W. (1976): Uptake, metabolism and efflux of methadone in "single-pass" isolated perfused rabbit lungs. *J. Pharmacol. Exp. Ther.*, 199:360–367.
24. Law, F. C. P., Eling, T. E., Bend, J. R., and Fouts, J. R. (1974): Metabolism of xenobiotics by the isolated perfused lung. Comparison with *in vitro* incubations. *Drug Metab. Dispos.*, 2:433–442.
25. Uehleke, H. (1969): Extrahepatic microsomal drug metabolism. In: *International Congress Series 181; Sensitization to Drugs*, edited by de C. Baker and Tripod, pp. 94–100. Excerpta Medica, Amsterdam.
26. Aitio, A., Hartiala, J., and Uotila, P. (1976): Glucuronide synthesis in the isolated perfused rat lung. *Biochem. Pharmacol.*, 25:1919–1920.
27. Davis, M. E., and Mehendale, H. M. (1979): Absence of metabolism of morphine during accumulation by isolated perfused rabbit lung. *Drug Metab. Dispos.*, 7:425–428.
28. Norio, I., Fisher, A. B., and Thurman, R. G. (1977): Cytochrome P450-linked *p*-nitroanisole *O*-demethylation in the perfused lung. *J. Appl. Physiol.*, 43:238–245.
29. Whitnack, E., Knapp, D. R., Holmes, J. C., Fowler, N. O., and Gaffney, T. E. (1972): Demethylation of nortriptyline by the dog lung. *J. Pharmacol. Exp. Ther.*, 181:288–291.
30. Cassidy, M. K., and Houston, J. B. (1980): *In vivo* assessment of extrahepatic conjugative metabolism in first pass effects using the model compound phenol. *J. Pharm. Pharmacol.*, 32:57–59.
31. Cassidy, M. K., and Houston, J. B. (1980): Phenol conjugation by lung *in vivo*. *Biochem. Pharmacol.*, 29:471–474.
32. Hogg, S. I., Curtis, C. G., Upshall, D. G., and Powell, G. M. (1981): Conjugation of phenol by rat lung. *Biochem. Pharmacol.*, 30:1551–1555.
33. Hartalia, J., Uotila, P., and Nienstedt, W. (1979): Metabolism of progesterone in the isolated perfused rat lung. *J. Steroid Biochem.*, 11:1539–1541.
34. Black, J. W., Duncan, W. A. M., and Shanks, R. G. (1965): Comparison of some properties of pronethalol and propranolol. *Br. J. Pharmacol. Chemother.*, 25:577–591.
35. Schneck, D. W., Pritchard, J. F., and Hayes, A. H. (1977): Studies on the uptake and binding of propranolol by rat tissues. *J. Pharmacol. Exp. Ther.*, 203:621–629.

36. Hayes, A., and Cooper, R. G. (1971): Studies on the absorption, distribution and excretion of propranolol in the rat, dog and monkey. *J. Pharmacol. Exp. Ther.*, 176:302–311.
37. Dollery, C. T., and Junod, A. F. (1976): Concentration of (±)-propranolol in isolated, perfused lungs of rat. *Br. J. Pharmacol.*, 57:67–71.
38. Schmalzing, G. (1977): Metabolism and disposition of trifluoperazine in the rat. II. Kinetics after oral and intravenous administration in acutely and chronically treated animals. *Drug Metab. Dispos.*, 5:104–115.
39. Roth, R. A., and Wiersma, D. A. (1979): Role of the lung in total body clearance of circulating drugs. *Clin. Pharmacokinet.*, 4:355–367.
40. Wilkinson, G. R., and Shand, D. G. (1975): A physiological approach to hepatic drug clearance. *Clin. Pharmacol. Ther.*, 18:377–390.
41. Pang, K. S., and Rowland, M. (1977): Hepatic clearance of drugs. III. Additional experimental evidence supporting the "well-stirred" model, using metabolite (MEGX) generated from lidocaine under varying hepatic blood flow rates and linear conditions in the perfused liver *in situ* preparation. *J. Pharmacokinet. Biopharm.*, 5:681–699.
42. Nies, A. S., Shand, D. G., and Wilkinson, G. R. (1976): Altered hepatic blood flow and drug disposition. *Clin. Pharmacokinet.*, 1:135–155.
43. Roth, R. A., and Rubin, R. J. (1976): Role of blood flow in carbon monoxide- and hypoxic hypoxia-induced alterations in hexobarbital metabolism in rats. *Drug Metab. Dispos.*, 4:460–467.
44. Rowland, M., Benet, L. Z., and Graham, G. G. (1973): Clearance concepts in pharmacokinetics. *J. Pharmacokinet. Biopharm.*, 1:123–136.
45. Vadi, H., Jernstrom, B., and Orrenius, S. (1976): Recent studies on benzo(a)pyrene metabolism in rat liver and lung. *Carcinogen*, 1:45–61.
46. Zampaglione, N. G., and Mannering, G. J. (1973): Properties of benzpyrene hydroxylase in the liver, intestinal mucosa and adrenal of untreated and 3-methylcholanthrene-treated rats. *J. Pharmacol. Exp. Ther.*, 183:676–685.
47. Wiersma, D. A., and Roth, R. A. (1980): Clearance of benzo(a)pyrene by rat lung: Importance of tissue perfusion. *Pharmacologist*, 22:278.
48. Wiersma, D. A., and Roth, R. A. (1981): The metabolic clearance of benzo(a)pyrene by rat lung and liver. *Fed. Proc.*, 40:620.
49. Sapirstein, L. A., Sapirstein, E., and Bredemeyer, A. (1960): Effect of hemorrhage on the cardiac output and its distribution in the rat. *Circ. Res.*, 8:135–148.
50. Bilimoria, M. H., and Echobicon, D. J. (1980): Responses of rodent hepatic, renal and pulmonary arylhydrocarbon hydroxylase following exposure to cigarette smoke. *Toxicology*, 15:83–89.
51. Smith, B. R., and Bend, J. R. (1980): Prediction of pulmonary benzo(a)pyrene 4,5-oxide clearance: A pharmacokinetic analysis of epoxide-metabolizing enzymes in rabbit lung. *J. Pharmacol. Exp. Ther.*, 214:478–482.
52. Junod, A. F. (1972): Uptake, metabolism and efflux of ¹⁴C-5-hydroxytryptamine in isolated perfused rat lungs. *J. Pharmacol. Exp. Ther.*, 183:341–355.
53. Alabster, V. A., and Bahkle, Y. S. (1970): Removal of 5-hydroxytryptamine in the pulmonary circulation of isolated rat lungs. *Br. J. Pharmacol.*, 40:468–482.
54. Wiersma, D. A., and Roth, R. A. (1980): Clearance of 5-hydroxytryptamine in rat lung and liver: The importance of relative perfusion and intrinsic clearance. *J. Pharmacol. Exp. Ther.*, 212:97–102.
55. Gillis, C. N., Cronau, L. H., Mendel, S., and Hammond, G. L. (1979): Indicator dilution measurement of 5-hydroxytryptamine clearance by human lung. *J. Appl. Physiol.*, 46:1178–1183.
56. Guyton, A. C. (1971): *Textbook of Medical Physiology*, p. 369. W. B. Saunders, Philadelphia.
57. Chiou, W. L. (1979): Potential pitfalls in the conventional pharmacokinetic studies: Effects of the initial mixing of drug in blood and the pulmonary first-pass elimination. *J. Pharmacokinet. Biopharm.*, 7:527–536.
58. Gallagher, B., Christman, D., Fowler, J., McGregor, R., Wolf, A. P., Som, P., Ansari, A. M., and Atkins, H. (1977): Radioisotope scintigraphy for the study of dynamics of amine regulation by the human lung. *Chest*, 71:282–284.
59. Post, C., Andersson, R. G. G., Ryrfeldt, A., and Nilsson, E. (1979): Physico-chemical modification of lidocaine uptake in rat lung tissue. *Acta Pharmacol. Toxicol.*, 44:103–109.
60. Geddes, D. M., Nesbitt, K., Traill, T., and Blackburn, J. P. (1979): First-pass uptake of ¹⁴C-propranolol by the lung. *Thorax*, 34:810–813.
61. Post, C., and Lewis, D. H. (1979): Displacement of nortriptyline and uptake of ¹⁴C-lidocaine in the lung after administration of ¹⁴C-lidocaine to nortriptyline intoxicated pigs. *Acta Pharmacol. Toxicol.*, 45:218–224.

62. Rane, A., Wilkinson, G. R., and Shand, D. G. (1977): Prediction of hepatic extraction ratio from *in vitro* measurement of intrinsic clearance. *J. Pharmacol. Exp. Ther.*, 200:420–424.
63. Hilliker, K. S., and Roth, R. A. (1980): Prediction of mescaline clearance by rabbit lung and liver from enzyme kinetic data. *Biochem. Pharmacol.*, 29:253–255.
64. Roth, R. A., and Gillis, C. N. (1978): Effect of ventilation and pH on removal of mescaline and biogenic amines by rabbit lung. *J. Appl. Physiol.*, 44:553–558.
65. Post, C. (1979): Studies on the pharmacokinetic function of the lung with special reference to lidocaine. *Acta Pharmacol. Toxicol.*, 44 (Suppl. I):1–53.
66. Roth, R. A., and Rubin, R. J. (1976): Comparison of the effect of carbon monoxide and of hypoxic hypoxia. I. *In vivo* metabolism, distribution and action of hexobarbital. *J. Pharmacol. Exp. Ther.*, 199:53–60.
67. Roth, R. A., and Rubin, R. J. (1976): Comparison of the effect of carbon monoxide and of hypoxic hypoxia. II. Hexobarbital metabolism in the isolated, perfused rat liver. *J. Pharmacol. Exp. Ther.*, 199:61–66.
68. Kirby, B. J., Cooke, N. J., and Fenley, D. C. (1976): Tissue oxygenation and regional blood flow in chronic respiratory failure. *Clin. Sci.*, 49:11P.
69. du Souich, P., McLean, A. J., Lalka, D., Erill, S., and Gibaldi, M. (1978): Pulmonary disease and drug kinetics. *Clin. Pharmacokinet.* 3:257–266.
70. Sivarajah, K., Anderson, M. W., and Eling, T. (1978): Metabolism of benzo(a)pyrene to reactive intermediate(s) via prostaglandin biosynthesis. *Life Sci.*, 23:2571–2578.
71. Said, S. I. (1977): Release induced by physical and chemical stimuli. In: *Metabolic Functions of the Lung*, edited by Y. S. Bakhle and J. R. Vane, pp. 297–320. Marcel Dekker, New York.
72. Piper, P. J. (1977): Release induced by anaphylaxis. In: *Metabolic Functions of the Lung*, edited by Y. S. Bakhle and J. R. Vane, pp. 261–295. Marcel Dekker, New York.
73. Block, E. R., and Fisher, A. B. (1977): Depression of serotonin clearance by rat lungs during oxygen exposure. *J. Appl. Physiol.*, 42:33–38.
74. Block, E. R., and Cannon, J. K. (1978): Effect of oxygen exposure on lung clearance of amines. *Lung*, 155:287–295.
75. Kistler, G. S., Caldwell, P. R. B., and Weibel, E. R. (1967): Development of fine structural damage to alveolar and capillary lining cells in oxygen-poisoned rat lungs. *J. Cell. Biol.*, 32:605–628.
76. Roth, R. A., Wallace, K. B., Alper, R. H., and Bailie, M. D. (1979): Effect of paraquat treatment of rats on disposition of 5-hydroxytryptamine and angiotensin I by perfused lung. *Biochem. Pharmacol.*, 28:2349–2355.
77. McLean, E. K. (1970): The toxic actions of pyrrolizidine alkaloids. *Pharmacol. Rev.*, 22:429–483.
78. Schoental, R., and Head, M. A. (1955): Pathological changes in rats as a result of treatment with monocrotaline. *Br. J. Cancer*, 9:229–237.
79. Merkow, L., and Kleinerman, J. (1966): An electron microscopic study of pulmonary vasculitis induced by monocrotaline. *Lab. Invest.*, 15:547–564.
80. Valdiva, E., Lalich, J. J., Hayashi, Y., and Sonnad, J. (1967): Alterations in pulmonary alveoli after a single injection of monocrotaline. *Arch. Pathol.*, 84:64–76.
81. Gillis, C. N., Huxtable, R. J., and Roth, R. A. (1978): Effects of monocrotaline pretreatment of rats on removal of 5-hydroxytryptamine and noradrenaline by perfused lung. *Br. J. Pharmacol.*, 63:435–443.
82. Roth, R. A., Dotzlaf, L. A., Baranyi, B., Kuo, C.-H., and Hook, J. B. (1981): Effect of monocrotaline ingestion on liver, kidney and lung of rats. *Toxicol. Appl. Pharmacol.*, 60:193–203.
83. Huxtable, R., and Chubb, J. (1977): Adrenergic stimulation of taurine transport by the heart. *Science*, 198:409–411.
84. Walcott, G., Burchell, H. B., and Brown, A. L. (1970): Primary pulmonary hypertension. *Am. J. Med.*, 49:70–79.
85. Sole, M. J., Drobac, M., Schwartz, L., Hussain, M. N., and Vaughn-Neil, E. F. (1979): The extraction of circulating catecholamines by the lungs in normal man and in patients with pulmonary hypertension. *Circulation*, 60:160–163.
86. Gillis, C. N., Cronau, L. H., Green, N. M., and Hammond, G. L. (1974): Removal of 5-hydroxytryptamine and norepinephrine from the pulmonary vascular space of man: Influence of cardiopulmonary bypass and pulmonary arterial pressure on these processes. *Surgery*, 76:608–616.
87. Roth, R. A., and Wallace, K. B. (1980): Disposition of biogenic amines and angiotensin I by lungs of spontaneously hypertensive rats. *Am. J. Physiol.*, 239:H736–H741.

88. Siddik, Z. H., Trush, M. A., and Gram, T. E. (1980): Pulmonary accumulation of drugs in vitamin A deficiency. *Lung*, 157:209–217.
89. Sporn, M. B., Dunlop, N. M., Newton, D. L., and Smith, J. M. (1976): Prevention of chemical carcinogenesis by vitamin A and its synthetic analogs (retinoids). *Fed. Proc.*, 35:1332–1338.
90. Bjelke, E. (1975): Dietary vitamin A and human lung cancer. *Int. J. Cancer*, 15:561–565.
91. Hook, J. B., and Roth, R. A. (1980): Disposition of 5-hydroxytryptamine in lungs of developing rats. *Am. J. Physiol.*, 239:401–406.
92. Wallace, K. B., Roth, R. A., Hook, J. B., and Bailie, M. D. (1980): Age-related differences in angiotensin I metabolism by isolated perfused rat lungs. *Am. J. Physiol.*, 238:R395–R399.
93. Pearson-Murphy, B. E. (1978): Cortisol production and inactivation by the human lung during gestation and infancy. *J. Clin. Endocrinol. Metab.*, 47:243–248.

Pharmacokinetic Basis for Drug Treatment,
edited by L.Z. Benet et al., Raven Press,
New York © 1984

Chapter 8

Effects of Renal Disease: Pharmacokinetic Considerations

D. Craig Brater and Polavat Chennavasin*

Department of Pharmacology, The University of Texas Health Science Center at Dallas, Dallas, Texas 75235

This chapter will focus on excretion pathways for drugs and on dosing regimens. The effects of renal dysfunction on absorption, distribution, metabolism, and accumulation of active metabolites will be discussed in Chapter 9.

RENAL BLOOD FLOW

By far the most important excretory route, when considering both parent drug and metabolites, is the kidney. It is easiest to consider renal modes of elimination of drugs in terms of the kidney's physiologic functions of filtration, secretion, and reabsorption. All of these functions can be influenced by renal blood flow. Documented changes in renal blood flow are reviewed in Table 1. Changes in renal blood flow will have more pronounced effects on secretory and reabsorption processes. However, consideration must also be given to urinary pH, drug polarity, and lipid solubility. Drugs that are eliminated by the kidney and that have high renal extraction ratios (i.e., penicillins, sulfates, glucuronides) are more dependent on renal blood flow than those that have low extraction ratios (i.e., chlorpropamide, digoxin, furosemide, gentamicin, tobramycin, tetracycline, sulfisoxazole, acetazolamide, diazoxide).

Depending on the change and the extent of the underlying abnormality, changes in renal blood flow can have pronounced effects on the former group of drugs. One must also consider that (a) a further increase in renal blood flow does not necessarily dictate an increased secretory rate, and (b) an increase or a decrease in renal blood flow often is (but may not be) expressed as an equal change in glomerular filtration rate when implementing dosage adjustments for drugs with significant renal elimination.

FILTRATION

The determinants of a drug's capacity to be filtered are protein binding, molecular size, glomerular integrity ("leaky" glomerulus), and the number of filtering nephrons.

---

*Deceased.

TABLE 1. *Factors that influence kidney blood flow*[a]

	Decreased renal blood flow (RBF)	Increased renal blood flow

Physiological	Volume
	  Restricted salt intake
	Vasoconstrictor
	  Fright
	  Exercise
	  Assuming upright position
	  Thromboxane A_2
	  Stress (of greater clinical relevance in hypertensive
	    patients)
	Age
	  Old age (?preferential inner cortex flow)
	  Arteriosclerosis
	  Neonates ↓ GFR, which increases after the 1st week
	    and proceeds from inner to outer cortex
		PGE_2, PGD_2, PGI_2 at certain doses[b]
		Pregnancy (2nd to 8th months)
		Expansion of intravascular fluid volume (i.e., high-salt
		  diet, fluids)
		Recumbent
		Kallikrein[c] if infused in renal artery only
		Acetylcholine

Pathological	Decreased effective circulation resulting from:
	  Abdominal ascites without cirrhosis
	  Severe dehydration (i.e., burns, GI loss)
	  Rapid hemorrhage[c] (i.e., hemolysis, operation)
	  Shock,[c] sudden hypotension
	Vascular glomerular process resulting from:
	  Malignant hypertension
	  Renovascular hypertension
		Pyrogens
		Acute volume expansion

Scleroderma
Rhabdomyolysis
Advanced polyarteritis nodosa
Pre-eclampsia
Hepatorenal syndrome
Severe cirrhosis[c]
Cardiac failure[c] (CHF, MI, tamponade)

Pharmacological	Tubular interstitial nephropathies (e.g., toxins, lead, cadmium, chemicals)	Progesterone, corticosteroids
	Norepinephrine,[c] enflurane (?)	Captopril, phentolamine
	Alprenolol	Minoxidil[c,d,f]
	Propranolol,[d] verapamil?	Low-dose dopamine *or* isoproterenol
	Indomethacin,[d,e] meclofenamate	Hydralazine,[d] ethacrynic acid,[c,d] bumetanide[c,d]
	Clonidine,[d] alfacalcidol	Nadolol[d,f]
	Chlorothiazide[d]	
	Guanethidine,[d] bethanidine, debrisoquine, reserpine, dyazide (early decrease, then to normal)	
	Angiotensin II[d] (tachyphylaxis develops quickly)	
	Oral contraceptives (estrogen & progestin)	

[a]General references (1,2); specific references (3–18).
[b]Perhaps only at pharmacological doses is there a notable change.
[c]Renal redistribution of blood flow from cortical to medullary area.
[d]Some reports indicate no change in RBF.
[e]The decrease in RBF by prostaglandin inhibitors such as indomethacin is of greater significance in patients who already have a decrease in RBF (i.e., severe cirrhosis, stress, restricted salt intake). For example, a patient in acute CHF would have a much greater decrease in RBF while on indomethacin.
[f]Some reports indicate a decrease in RBF.

Because only that amount of drug free in plasma can pass a normal glomerulus, displacement of highly bound drugs (>90%) from serum proteins may increase the amount available for filtration and thereby be eliminated in the urine. This phenomenon occurs with phenytoin (90% bound), valproic acid (99% bound), and warfarin (99% bound), the clinical importance of which relates to proper interpretation of the concentration of drug in blood. Chapter 10 provides a listing of drugs that are commonly prescribed and more than 90% protein-bound.

Effective molecular size has been shown to be a limiting factor for excretion of mixed and high-molecular-weight dextrans. For example, Dextran 40 used clinically is actually a mixture of species of different molecular weights; the high-molecular-weight species (MW approximately 70,000) is selectively retained, because it cannot be filtered (19). Consequently, these preparations remain in patients for weeks. Most drugs are of molecular size sufficiently small that there are essentially no size limitations to filtration.

The integrity of the glomerulus as a sieve is disrupted in nephrotic syndrome. As hypoalbuminemia develops, there is a decrease in the binding of a variety of drugs (see Chapter 10). In addition, drugs bound to albumin can be carried with the protein into the urine, enhancing renal elimination. This phenomenon has been shown to occur with phenytoin and clofibrate, but in the four patients studied, the excretion rate was not increased enough to be important compared with overall elimination (20).

Most studies and clinical attention have been directed toward influences of decreased numbers of functioning nephrons on the renal elimination of drugs. The effect of decreased creatinine clearance on the elimination of digoxin and aminoglycoside antibiotics is particularly well known (21–26). A number of different approaches have been taken in coping with the burgeoning literature regarding the effects of changes in glomerular filtration rate (GFR) on drug excretion. Bennett and co-workers, for example, published an updated series of tables listing a large number of drugs with recommendations for dosage adjustments (27–32). Dettli has devised a system using rate constants (33–36). Anderson et al. (37) have also published guidelines in a book, the abridged version of which is a chapter in the nephrology text of Brenner and Rector (1).

Interindividual variability mandates that therapy be tailored to each individual patient. Consequently, one must assume from the outset that guidelines from these general sources are starting points and that the individual patient must be closely monitored, where possible, for endpoints of efficacy and toxicity. It is likely that with close scrutiny one will need to adjust the dosage in an individual patient differently than suggested in general guidelines.

RENAL SECRETION

The renal tubule can both actively secrete and actively reabsorb a variety of substrates. Active reabsorption appears to be inconsequential, except for iodipamide (a cholecystographic agent), which presumably decreases the active reabsorption

of uric acid in the proximal tubule (38). The uricosuria could be etiologic to the acute renal failure occasionally reported with this contrast agent. The same mechanism accounts for the uricosuria caused by probenecid, high-dose salicylates, and high-dose phenylbutazone.

The uptake by pinocytosis from the proximal tubular lumen of gentamicin and other aminoglycoside antibiotics might be considered as an example of active reabsorption. Different capacities for uptake, or egress from the tubular cells after uptake, apparently contribute to the potential for nephrotoxicity of aminoglycosides, those that tend to accumulate within the cell being most toxic (39).

The pars recta (straight segment) of the proximal tubule actively secretes into the tubular lumen a variety of organic acids and bases (40). The transport system for acids is more fully characterized than is that for bases, although our understanding of even the organic acid transport system is fragmentary. The *sine qua non* of an actively secreted drug is a renal excretion rate greater than the GFR. However, drugs with excretion rates less than GFR may also be actively secreted if the secretory capacity is low or if a portion of the secreted drug is reabsorbed more distally in the tubule.

Active secretion of drugs by the kidney is usually considered in terms of those compounds that are organic acids and those that are organic bases (41). The pathways for acids and for bases appear to be separate, but within a group there is lack of specificity such that a variety of organic acids can compete with each other for transport, as can a variety of organic bases. (Pharmacokinetic interactions of this type are discussed in Chapter 11.)

Table 2 shows a short list of organic acids with potentially important renal secretions. All acids listed have the potential to compete with each other. However, the degree to which they will compete is impossible to predict, as illustrated by a study that showed a wide spectrum of effects of a variety of organic acids on the elimination half-life of penicillin (42).

Competition for secretion can be important clinically. The use of the probenecid-penicillin combination for gonorrhea is well known. Most clinicians are aware of the need to decrease the dose of methotrexate if probenecid is administered. Few are aware, with potentially disastrous consequences, of a possible similar need if other acids listed in Table 2 are administered with methotrexate (43). One might speculate that "idiopathic sensitivity" to methotrexate might well be due in some cases to coadministration of inhibitors of the active secretion of methotrexate. A similar scenario could be postulated for combinations of any of the acids listed in Table 2.

Table 2 also lists bases that have been shown to undergo potentially clinically important active secretion (44–46). It has been assumed that organic bases can compete with each other for secretion as do acids, but such interaction has never been documented clinically (for further discussion, see Chapter 11). Consequently, its importance in humans is unknown. A collation of studies appears to indicate that there may be several different base transport systems that do not show cross-competition. Because our understanding of the base transport system is so rudi-

TABLE 2. *Drugs actively transported by the kidney*

Organic acids
Acetazolamide
p-Aminohippurate
Cephalosporins (most)
Chlorpropamide
Indomethacin
"Loop" diuretics
Methotrexate
Nitrofurantoin
Penicillins
Phenylbutazone
Probenecid
Salicylates
Sulfonamides
Thiazide diuretics
Organic bases
Amantadine
Amiloride
Cimetidine
Dopamine
Ethambutol
Mecamylamine
Meperidine (pethidine)
N-methylnicotinamide
Morphine
Procainamide
d-Pseudoephedrine
Quinacrine
Tetraethylammonium
Triamterene

mentary, it is impossible to speculate about its importance, although clinicians should be aware of the potential for interactions of drugs within this group.

A clinically important drug transport that is not of acids or bases is the secretory component of digoxin elimination, which can be altered by spironolactone, amiloride, verapamil, and quinidine (47–50). Some patients coadministered these drugs may need less digoxin. The site of digoxin transport in the kidney appears to be the distal nephron.

REABSORPTION

Weak acids and bases can be passively reabsorbed along the nephron. For this to occur, these drugs must gain entry to the tubular lumen in the proximal portion of the nephron, either at the glomerulus or by active secretion by the proximal tubule. Even drugs with high rates of proximal entry can be almost completely reabsorbed in the collecting duct. Passive reabsorption is affected by urinary pH and flow rate (41,51–54).

Urinary pH

The effect of urinary pH is related to the principle of passive nonionic diffusion, which is based on the premise that a nonionized molecule more readily passes across a lipid membrane than does its ionized congener. Consequently, the effect of urinary pH on the relative amount of ionized versus un-ionized drug can determine the extent of reabsorption. For weak acids (pK_a = 3.0–7.5), as the pH increases, the ionized component increases, and excretion increases, whereas for weak bases (pK_a = 7.5–10), as the pH increases, the ionized component decreases, and excretion decreases.

Not all weak acids and bases demonstrate urine-pH-dependent elimination. Part of the lack of effect with some drugs probably relates to the drug's pK_a and the lipid solubility of the congeners. For example, if even the nonionized species is poorly soluble in lipid, its ability to cross the tubular plasma membrane can not be enhanced. Another modulator of the ability of the nonionized congener to pass across the lipid membrane may be antidiuretic hormone. In a series of elegant *in vitro* studies, antidiuretic hormone increased by 50 to 100% the ability of lipophilic compounds to pass across the toad urinary bladder, a structure functionally analogous to the mammalian collecting duct (55). These findings have not been extrapolated to studies in humans.

It is important to keep the influence of urinary pH or flow in clinical perspective. For drugs in which only a small amount is eliminated by the kidney (<20%), such as quinidine, although passive reabsorption may be demonstrable in experimental settings, it is unimportant clinically. In addition, extremes of pH and urine flow at which important changes in overall elimination occur may only rarely, if ever, be achieved in a patient.

Urinary pH has been shown to be a clinically important determinant of elimination for the drugs shown in Table 3 (54–62). That it is important for weak acids, particularly phenobarbital and salicylate, is well known. Alkalinization of the urine, by favoring excretion of the ionized congener of phenobarbital or salicyclates, is

TABLE 3. *Compounds with clinically important urine-pH-dependent elimination*

Weak acids	pK_a	Weak bases	pK_a
Phenobarbital	7.2	Acebutolol	9.4
Salicylates	3.5	Amphetamine	9.8
Sulfa derivatives	4.9–7.4	Atenolol	9.6
		Ephedrine	9.4
		Mexiletine	9.0
		Phencyclidine (PCP)	9.4
		d-Pseudoephedrine	9.3
		Quinine	4.1 & 8.4
		Tocainide	
		Tricyclic antidepressants	8–9.7

a mainstay of therapy for toxicity due to these agents. It has also been demonstrated by Levy et al. (63) that the small changes in urinary pH caused by modest doses of antacids can enhance the elimination rate of salicylate sufficiently to prevent attaining concentrations in blood necessary for the antiinflammatory effect of salicylates.

The effect of urinary pH on the elimination of amphetamine may be better known to abusers of this drug than to clinicians. Because amphetamine is a weak base, alkalinizing the urine increases the amount un-ionized, favoring reabsorption. Amphetamine abusers regularly ingest baking soda before "shooting" to prolong the "high." Therapeutically, it would be important to assure an acid urine in a patient with an overdose of amphetamines.

Recently, a similar importance of urinary pH has been demonstrated with phencyclidine (PCP or "angel dust"), the abuse of which in some areas is at epidemic proportions. Toxicity can last for days, and it has been shown that acidification of the urine can increase excretion and shorten the period of toxicity.

The supposedly nontoxic *d*-pseudoephedrine has been shown to accumulate to toxic levels in children with renal tubular acidosis in whom a persistently alkaline urine favored passive reabsorption of the drug (54). A similar phenomenon occurs with tocainide, an orally available lidocaine-like agent, where the administration of bicarbonate decreased the elimination rate (60).

Urine Flow Rate

Urine flow rate can affect excretion of some drugs by two proposed mechanisms: (a) by decreasing the concentration gradient for reabsorption because the urine is dilute and (b) by decreasing the time for drug to diffuse out of the urine.

Urine flow rate has been shown to be an important determinant of elimination of theophylline, phenobarbital, chloramphenicol, *d*-pseudoephedrine, and ephedrine (51,54,62,64). This phenomenon would probably be clinically important only in patients with high urinary flow rates for prolonged periods of time. The flow rate may be more important than inducing an alkaline urine in enhancing elimination of phenobarbital, although one should clearly attempt to alkalinize the urine.

Clinicians seem to pay little attention to the importance of urinary pH and flow rate except in the case of salicylate or barbiturate overdose. As discussed earlier, more thought should be given to the importance of the urine pH for excretion of a broader gamut of drugs, as well as for clinical diagnosis.

DOSING REGIMENS

The medical literature is replete with guidelines for dosing drugs in patients with renal disease. Several different methods have been proposed, with advocates and criticisms of all. At one extreme are publications testifying to the accuracy and predictability of a particular nomogram in allowing attainment of a desired concentration of drug. At the other extreme are examples of inaccuracies and poor predictability, leaving the clinician with little confidence in the ability of nomograms

to allow attainment of desired concentrations in the individual patient. As a result, the clinician is left with the dilemma of not knowing which nomogram to use, and if he uses one, how much he can trust it. Clearly, measuring concentrations of drug facilitates attainment of desired concentrations in individual patients (see Chapters 21 and 22).

As stated in Chapter 1, the steady state concentration of a drug is an inverse function of dosing interval and clearance and is directly related to dose. If drug clearance decreases as a result of decreased renal function, a new steady state will be attained where the average plasma concentration, Cp_{ave}, is increased by the same order of magnitude as the decrease in clearance. Changes in dose or in dosing interval or both can be used to compensate for changes in clearance and thus maintain Cp_{ave} at the same level as in patients with normal drug clearance. Dosing nomograms provide guidelines for changes in dose and dosing interval, but additionally many guidelines attempt to quantitatively correlate an index of renal function such as serum creatinine or creatinine clearance with drug clearance at that level of renal function.

Two other pharmacokinetic parameters are important in considering dosing regimens, namely Cp_{max}, the maximum or peak concentration, and Cp_{min}, the minimum or trough concentration. Both can be important determinants of efficacy and toxicity, as will be discussed in more detail subsequently. Additionally, in a patient receiving intermittent multiple dosing, Cp_{max} and Cp_{min} are the usual values measured when monitoring the patient with determinations of concentrations of drug in serum. Methods for calculating Cp_{max}, Cp_{min}, and Cp_{ave} are provided in Chapter 1. Dosing nomograms can be designed to obtain a desired Cp_{max} or Cp_{min} as well as Cp_{ave}.

As demonstrated in Fig. 1, drug accumulation occurs in patients with renal failure and may cause toxicity. Quantitative dose adjustment is mandatory to avoid toxicity from a drug with a low therapeutic index, and it involves three steps: (a) evaluation and quantitative estimation of renal function, i.e., GFR; (b) estimation or prediction of the clearance of the chosen drug in that patient based on the estimated GFR and data from the literature relating drug clearance to renal function; (c) choice of an appropriate dosing regimen of the drug with selection of dose and dosing interval to produce the desired predicted concentrations of drug in serum and the desired time course of these concentrations. The reliability of a dosing nomogram is limited by the inherent error in each of these steps, which we shall consider in sequence.

Creatinine Clearance as an Index of Renal Function

Serum creatinine or creatinine clearance is generally used clinically to estimate GFR. Clinical laboratories usually use one of three methods for measuring creatinine: total chromogen, "true" creatinine, or an autoanalyzer method. Measurement of total chromogen includes that which is due to creatinine plus noncreatinine chromogen, which accounts for 10 to 15% of the total chromogen in serum of patients with normal renal function. No noncreatinine chromogen is measured in

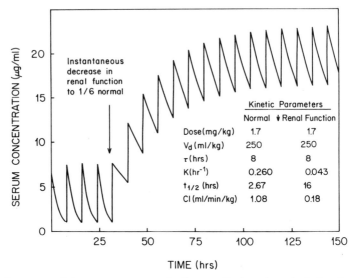

FIG. 1. Schematic of the serum concentration/time profile for a hypothetical patient administered gentamicin in whom an instantaneous decrease in renal function to one-sixth normal occurs *(arrow)*. Kinetic parameters for gentamicin as derived by Hull and Sarubbi (89,90) are listed. Volume of distribution was assumed to remain constant. Intravenous bolus administration is depicted for illustrative purposes only. (From Chennavasin and Brater, ref. 33, with permission.)

the urine. As a consequence, methods utilizing total chromogen result in a serum creatinine 10 to 15% higher and a creatinine clearance the same percent lower than methods utilizing "true" creatinine. Results from the autoanalyzer method are similar to those measuring "true" creatinine (65). Creatinine clearance is not an ideal measure of GFR, for 10 to 15% of urinary creatinine in patients with normal renal function derives from tubular secretion, in contrast to inulin or iothalamate, which are solely filtered. Consequently, with GFR determined from measures of "true" creatinine, the overestimate in GFR or inulin clearance because of the 10 to 15% error in the serum measurement cancels the error of the same magnitude in the urine, and creatinine clearance equals GFR or inulin clearance. However, this canceling effect does not hold in patients with decreased renal function, because the noncreatinine chromogen becomes quantitatively minor relative to the elevated serum creatinine. Consequently, serum measurements as "true" creatinine or as total chromogen become virtually identical. In addition, the contribution of secretion to creatinine in urine becomes relatively greater. Thus, some authors have indicated that in renal impairment, creatinine clearance may exceed GFR or inulin clearance by as much as 50 to 100% (65). Clearly, considerable error can occur because of the discrepancies between creatinine clearance and GFR.

Because of the inherent difficulties and errors of urine collection, serum creatinine, rather than direct measurement of creatinine clearance, has been commonly used to estimate renal function. Several limitations are associated with this use of

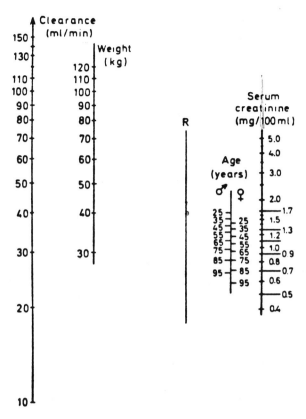

FIG. 2. Nomogram for rapid evaluation of endogenous creatinine clearance. With a ruler, join weight to age. Keep ruler at crossing-point of line marked R. Then move the right-hand side of the ruler to the appropriate serum creatinine value, and read the patient's clearance from the left side of the nomogram. (From Siersbaek-Nielsen et al., ref. 71, with permission.)

serum creatinine. Patients with the same serum creatinine may have widely varying renal function, which relates in part to age and body size, because endogenous creatinine production relates directly to lean body mass and inversely to age. Several nomograms and formulas that consider age, sex, and body weight are available to convert serum creatinine to creatinine clearance. Other nomograms have not considered these variables and are generally less accurate predictors of creatinine clearance than the nomograms accounting for age and weight of patients (66–70). A simple nomogram (Fig. 2) for bedside use to obtain creatinine clearance based on serum creatinine, age, sex, and weight of a patient was published by Siersbaek-Nielsen and colleagues (71). This nomogram was presented in graphic form and was based on data from 149 male and 219 female adult patients aged 20 to 99 years. This nomogram is widely used and appears to be very reliable. Creatinine clearance normalized to 70 kg body wt, which is similar to a normalized 1.73-m²

body surface area, can also be obtained directly from their nomogram. Cockcroft and Gault (66) have published a formula estimating creatinine clearance from serum creatinine in an adult male:

$$CL_{cr} = \frac{(140 - age) \times wt \text{ in kg}}{72 \times cr(mg/dl)} \quad ml/min$$

or

$$CL_{cr} = \frac{140 - age}{cr} \quad ml/min/72 \text{ kg body wt}$$

The creatine clearance for females is 85% of that for males. The method was derived from data from 249 adult males, aged 18 to 92 years. Creatinine clearances from this method are almost identical with those from the Siersbaek-Nielsen nomogram. The variability of values derived by this method compared with those from creatinine clearance determined with a urine collection was no greater than the variability between two separate, direct measurements of creatinine clearance. This formula has been tested by other groups in over 100 patients and found to be extremely reliable.

Schwartz et al. (72) published a formula designed for the pediatric age group (6 months to 16 years) derived from data from 186 children:

$$CL_{cr} = \frac{0.55 \times body \text{ length}}{cr} \quad ml/min/1.73 \text{ m}^2$$

A limitation of using serum creatinine and these nomogarms is that serum creatinine can correctly relate to renal function only during steady state with a stable serum creatinine (73). Creatinine, not unlike any drug or exogenous compound, can be described by basic pharmacokinetics. Thus, the half-life of creatinine in normal humans is approximately 3 hr (69,74). When renal function declines, the half-life increases proportionally. For example, if the GFR instantaneously decreased to 25% of normal, the creatinine half-life would quadruple and be 12 hr. Because it takes four to five half-life periods before the serum creatinine will reach a new steady state, a lag time of 2 to 3 days occurs before serum creatinine reaches the level that will correctly predict the GFR. These considerations make it extremely difficult to accurately predict GFR from serum creatinine during changes in renal function, as commonly occur in extremely ill patients. For practical purposes, one can assume a stable creatinine when clinical evaluation so indicates and if two separate determinations of serum creatinine (obtained preferably 24 hr apart) have values within 0.2 mg/dl (69). If the second serum creatinine is taken before 24 hr, any change may merely be a reflection of circadian rhythm or laboratory variability. Serum creatinine in most patients peaks in the afternoon (see Chapter 12, Table 2).

It is important to note that many clinicians may need to reorient their thinking regarding magnitudes of change in creatinine clearance. For example, when considering the patient whose creatinine clearance decreases by 50% from 100 to 50 ml/min/1.73 m², the clinician readily recognizes the magnitude of this decrement and its importance to therapy and drug dosing. On the other hand, a comparable percentage decrease from 10 to 5 ml/min/1.73 m² may be less readily appreciated, for both levels of renal function represent severe impairment, and therapy would differ only a small amount if at all. However, such a change, when used in a dosing nomogram, mandates a large change in recommended dose or dosing interval, the neglect of which could result in toxicity or inadequacy of treatment.

In summary, by using the Siersbaek-Nielsen nomogram or the Cockcroft and Gault formula, one may estimate clearance from serum creatinine with a degree of reliability sufficient for clinical settings, assuming serum creatinine is at steady state. However, creatinine clearance in many circumstances may not be an accurate measure of GFR and cannot be used. For example, some drugs, such as cimetidine, amiloride, triamterene, spironolactone, cefoxitin, and trimethoprim, as well as vitamin C (>6 g/day), levodopa (>4 g/day), and ASA (>3 g/day), may interfere with either the laboratory assay or the secretory component of creatinine's elimination. In addition, disease states such as severe burns, severe uremia, muscle-wasting syndrome, extreme obesity, and gross ascites, as well as dialysis or the post-renal-transplantation condition, may cause creatinine clearance to be an inaccurate measure of renal function (75–78). (The effects of pregnancy and old age on creatinine clearance are discussed in Chapters 13 and 15, respectively.) Competition by drugs for tubular creatinine secretion should always be taken into consideration.

Choice of an Appropriate Dosing Regimen

After the clearance of the drug in an individual patient is predicted from published data, one must select a dosing regimen to produce the desired predicted concentration and the desired time course of the concentration of drug for that patient.

As with any dosing regimen, the objective is to achieve efficacy without toxicity. Precisely defining the pattern of concentration of drug versus time that accomplishes this objective is difficult, for with some types of drugs the goal is not well defined even in patients with normal renal function. For example, it is debated in the infectious disease literature whether the objective of a dosing regimen is to maintain concentrations of antibiotic continually above the minimum inhibitory concentration (MIC) or to allow wide swings in concentrations from peak to trough, with periods of time in which concentrations of antibiotic are less than the MIC. With cardiac glycosides, antiarrhythmics, antiepileptics, and theophylline, the objective is more clearly to maintain trough concentration. Consequently, a dosing regimen in a patient with decreased renal function will not produce a serum concentration/time curve identical with that for a subject with normal renal function (with the exception of a continuous intravenous infusion).

Several methods have been used to obtain a serum concentration profile close to that in uncompromised patients (79,80). All assume the attainment of steady state during stable renal function. One method of dose adjustment is commonly referred to as the variable frequency regimen. This method in particular has been widely used for aminoglycoside dosing adjustment (81,82). McHenry et al. (83), in a commonly cited nomogram, used this method by recommending the same dose of gentamicin in patients with decreased renal function as in the uncompromised patient, administered at an increased dosing interval in direct relation to the prolongation of the half-life of elimination. Thereby, Cp_{max}, Cp_{ave}, and Cp_{min} remained the same as in patients with normal renal function (Fig. 3). Implicit in this treatment is the assumption that the change in clearance due to renal insufficiency (RI) is inversely related to the change in half-life:

$$\frac{CL_{RI}}{CL_{normal}} = \frac{T_{1/2normal}}{T_{1/2\,RI}}$$

That is, a change in half-life reflects only a change in elimination, not a change in volume of distribution (see Chapter 1); i.e., renal insufficiency has no effect on the volume of distribution. (Note that many of the nomograms for dosage adjustment in renal failure were developed prior to our understanding of clearance concepts and are based exclusively on changes in half-life, implicitly assuming no change in the volume of distribution.)

In Fig. 3 we have assumed pharmacokinetic parameters identical with those in Fig. 1 in a patient with normal renal function and in a patient with renal function one-sixth of normal. This method of dosing interval adjustment prevents toxicity caused by accumulation of drug in serum in patients with renal impairment, because the total dose administered is decreased in proportion to the decrease in renal function. However, for a considerable amount of time during the dosing interval, the serum concentration of the drug may be below the minimally effective concentration. This phenomenon normally occurs with gentamicin and other aminoglycoside antibiotics. Using this method of dose adjustment, the duration of time in which the concentration is below the effective concentration increases with increasing half-life and consequent increasing dosing interval, as illustrated in Table 4. The calculations in this table used data from McHenry et al. (83) for gentamicin administration to a group of patients with varying degrees of renal function receiving gentamicin at different dosing intervals based on the estimated elimination half-life for gentamicin for each patient. Because a peak serum concentration of gentamicin above 4 μg/ml is necessary for treating serious Gram-negative systemic infections (84), we chose this serum concentration as a minimal effective concentration. However, the same general conclusion can be drawn for any selected effective concentration. The time during a dosing interval in which the serum drug concentration remains above or below the therapeutic level was calculated by assuming first-order kinetics. As one can see in patients with the worst renal impairment, serum concentrations remain below the effective concentration for prolonged periods

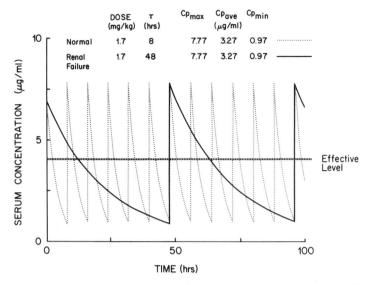

FIG. 3. Schematic of the serum concentration profile for gentamicin in a patient with normal renal function *(dotted line)* and in a patient with renal function one-sixth normal in whom the variable frequency regimen has been used for dose adjustment *(solid line)*. A serum concentration of 4 μg/ml was selected as the "effective level." Derived values for each hypothetical patient assuming intravenous bolus administration are shown in the figure. (From Chennavasin and Brater, ref. 33, with permission.)

TABLE 4. *Effects of dosing interval on time of serum concentrations of gentamicin above and below a therapeutic level (4 μg/ml) in patients with different degrees of renal failure*

CL_{cr} (ml/ min)	$T_{1/2}$(hr)	Dose (mg/kg)	τ (hr)	Cp_{max} (μg/ml)	Cp_{min} (μg/ml)	Time above 4 μg/ml (hr)	Time below 4 μg/ml (hr)
90	3.0	1.0	8	5.9	0.9	1.7	6.3
48	3.9	1.0	10	4.1	0.7	0.1	9.9
49	3.7	1.0	14	3.3	0.5	0	14.0[b]
20	12.2	1.2	32	5.0	0.6	3.4	28.6
17	16.6	1.1	46	5.8	0.6	7.4	37.6
19	22.9	1.3	64	8.0	1.0	21.3	42.7
90[a]	3.0	1.7	8	10.0	1.5	3.9	4.1

[a]Predicted values if the first patient is administered doses of 1.7 mg/kg rather than 1 mg/kg.
[b]The serum concentration in this patient was below the effective concentration at all times.
Data taken from McHenry et al. (83).

of time. Despite the increased absolute amount of time with serum concentrations above the effective level, the very long continuous time at subtherapeutic concentrations must be of concern to the clinician. In fact, its importance may be demonstrated by a recent study describing the occurrence of "breakthrough" bacteremia

during trough serum concentrations of antibiotics (85). Clearly, a longer period of time "subtherapeutic" might increase the likelihood of persistent infection when considering antibiosis or the likelihood of exacerbation of signs and symptoms of disease when considering other agents.

As a basic pharmacokinetic principle, the time during which the serum concentration is higher or lower than a fixed effective level is a function not only of half-life but also of dose. Increasing the dose of a drug will not only increase absolute serum concentrations but also increase the amount of time spent above a chosen concentration. For example, in the first patient in Table 4, if one increases the dose of gentamicin from 1.0 to 1.7 mg/kg, the time for serum concentration above the minimal effective concentration will increase from 1.7 to 3.9 hr, and the time below will decrease from 6.3 to 4.1 hr. However, increasing the dose to vary the amount of time above a selected effective level is limited by the narrow therapeutic ratio of many drugs, including gentamicin. It is not known what duration of subeffective concentrations becomes critical for continued efficacy of the regimen. Clearly, however, most clinicians would feel uncomfortable with the prolonged subtherapeutic concentrations of drug that occur in patients with wide dosing intervals.

In contrast to the variable frequency method, several authors have suggested a variable dosage regimen: maintaining the dosing interval as in patients with normal renal function and compensating for the decreased clearance of drug by decreasing the dose. If the dose of a drug is reduced proportionally to the increase in half-life, as suggested by Wagner (86), then in renal insufficiency (RI), $dose_{RI} = dose_{normal} (T_{1/2\ normal}/T_{1/2RI})$.

This regimen results in the same Cp_{ave}, but Cp_{max} is lower and Cp_{min} higher than in patients with normal renal function. This regimen, like the variable frequency regimen, prevents drug accumulation, but, in contrast, it avoids great fluctuations of serum concentration and theoretically could thereby avoid the prolonged duration of subeffective serum concentrations. However, as illustrated in Fig. 4, the serum concentration may actually remain below the effective concentration at all times in patients with severe renal failure. This phenomenon occurs with a drug like gentamicin, in which the dosing regimen in patients with normal renal function produces wide swings of serum concentration, with a Cp_{ave} below the effective concentration.

Another important consideration when using a variable dose regimen is that a loading dose is necessary to avoid a delay in time before the serum concentration reaches steady state. Figure 4 demonstrates a serum concentration profile of this regimen when beginning administration with a maintenance dose (lower curve), as opposed to first administering a dose identical with a dose used in patients with normal renal function, a loading dose (upper curve). It is important to note that with a loading dose there will be a delay before the patient becomes "subtherapeutic."

Chan et al. (87), in a frequently cited gentamicin nomogram, proposed an approach similar to the varying dose regimen. Theoretical calculations of serum drug concentrations from this nomogram would result in subtherapeutic drug levels in

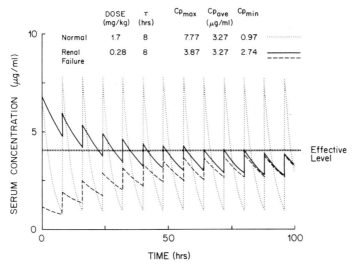

FIG. 4. Schematic of the serum concentration profile of gentamicin using the variable dose regimen for dose adjustment. The format is as in Fig. 3. The solid curve represents the profile when a loading dose is administered to the patient with renal impairment, and the dashed curve represents the profile when the patient receives a maintenance dose throughout. (From Chennavasin and Brater, ref. 33, with permission.)

patients with severe renal dysfunction. However, in clinical use, this does not appear to occur. One explanation for the discordance between actual and predicted results is that the Chan nomogram, by assuming a normal gentamicin half-life in patients with creatinine clearance of 70 ml/min/1.73 m² (as opposed to 100 ml/min/1.73 m²), may underestimate the actual elimination half-life. This underestimation would then, in effect, result in giving a higher gentamicin dose and attainment of therapeutic drug concentrations.

In another so-called variable dosage regimen approach, one can calculate a dose that will attain a serum concentration of Cp_{max} in patients with renal disease similar to that of a patient with normal renal function. Many nomograms, in fact, are calculated to achieve the same Cp_{max} in patients with decreased renal function as in those without renal impairment. The dose used in patients with renal failure will not decrease in proportion to decreased clearance of the drug, because the dose also depends on the magnitude of the chosen dosing interval relative to half-life.

Figure 5 depicts a serum concentration/time curve for a dosing regimen calculated to obtain a Cp_{max} similar to that for patients with normal renal function and maintaining the same dosing interval. Again the importance of the loading dose is depicted in the figure. Using this regimen, one can avoid subtherapeutic serum concentrations for patients with severe renal failure. However, using this regimen, the patient with compromised renal function is exposed to a greater concentration of drug over time, because the Cp_{min} is higher the worse the patient's renal function.

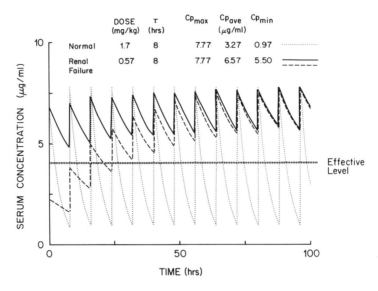

FIG. 5. Schematic of the serum concentration profile of gentamicin using a variable dose approach to dose adjustment but with maintenance of Cp_{max} in the patient with decreased renal function the same as in the "normal" patient. The format is as in Fig. 3. Note the difference in this profile compared to Fig. 3, in which the variable dose regimen targeted the same Cp_{ave} in both sets of patients. (From Chennavasin and Brater, ref. 33, with permission.)

Consequently, to increase the amount of time with therapeutic concentrations of drug, one may have to subject the patient to greater risk, assuming risk is related to total drug exposure or related to trough concentration of drug in serum (88).

Another method of dosing, originally proposed by Kunin (24), suggests one-half of the dose usually administered to patients with normal renal function given to the patient with renal failure at a dosing interval equal to the drug half-life. Figure 6 shows the serum concentration/time curve using this method, with the first dose of the drug being similar to that for normal subjects, i.e., a modified loading dose. This method of dosing regimen provides fixed Cp_{max}, Cp_{ave}, and Cp_{min} regardless of renal function. However, the manner in which the serum concentration profile obtained by this method differs from that of a patient with normal renal function depends on whether the dosing interval used in normal patients is longer or shorter than the normal half-life. For example, if a drug is normally administered at a dosing interval longer than twice the half-life, such as gentamicin, which is normally given every third half-life, Kunin's method provides total doses higher than those in the variable frequency regimen. This may result in increased toxicity. In patients with very severe renal impairment, with a markedly prolonged half-life, a prolonged subtherapeutic serum concentration may occur similar to that of the standard variable frequency regimen. On the other hand, for drugs in which the dosing interval used normally is shorter than the normal half-life, this method will result in a lower dose than the variable frequency regimen.

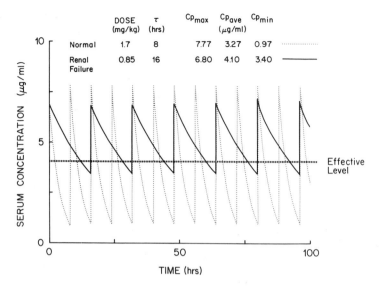

FIG. 6. Schematic of the serum concentration profile of gentamicin using Kunin's method of dose adjustment in which one-half of the dose used normally is administered every half-life. The format is as in Fig. 3.

A combination approach has been suggested by Dettli (34,35) for a number of drugs. Likewise, Hull and Sarubbi (89,90) have designed a nomogram specifically for aminoglycosides, suggesting for mild renal dysfunction a variable dose regimen to obtain a Cp_{max} similar to that in normals and a modified regimen in patients with more severe renal failure, by increasing dosing interval, still maintaining Cp_{max} but avoiding sustained, high trough levels of drug that may cause toxicity.

Derived values from the Hull and Sarubbi nomogram demonstrate that as renal function worsens, the magnitude of difference between Cp_{max} and Cp_{min} becomes less, but Cp_{max} remains the same as in patients with normal renal function. The authors appropriately recommend increasing the dosing interval at severe degrees of renal impairment to avoid sustained high trough concentrations. We believe this feature of the Hull and Sarubbi nomogram to be its main advantage, and we recommend that the dosing interval not be greater than 24 hr, to avoid long durations of subtherapeutic serum concentrations.

In summary, different dosage regimens have advantages and disadvantages. There is no one universal dosing method that is applicable to all situations. A regimen is the best regimen for one drug at one renal function. In Table 5 we list some of the advantages and disadvantages of the various general approaches. Dosing nomograms are subject to the errors of their assumptions and their data base, as discussed previously. We cannot, therefore, overemphasize the need for close following of individual patients with measures of serum concentrations of drugs and evaluation of clinical endpoints of pharmacologic effect.

TABLE 5. *Advantages and disadvantages of general approaches of dosing nomograms*

Method	Advantages	Disadvantages
Variable frequency (Fig. 2)	1. Same Cp_{ave}, Cp_{max}, Cp_{min} 2. "Normal" dose 3. Ease of calculation	1. Possibly deleterious length of time subtherapeutic 2. "Odd" dosing interval causes potential for administration errors
Variable dose with fixed Cp_{ave} (Fig. 3)	1. Same Cp_{ave} 2. "Normal" dosing interval 3. Ease of calculation	1. Decreased Cp_{max} that may be continually subtherapeutic 2. "Odd" doses may lead to medication errors 3. Increased Cp_{min}; increased toxicity
Variable dose with fixed Cp_{max} (Fig. 4)	1. Same Cp_{max}; attains therapeutic concentrations 2. "Normal" dosing interval	1. Increased Cp_{ave}, Cp_{min}; increased toxicity 2. More difficult to compute dose
Kunin method (Fig. 5)	1. Same Cp_{max}; attains therapeutic concentrations 2. Ease of calculation of both dose (fixed as ½ normal) and dosing interval (every half-life)	1. "Odd" dosing interval 2. Increased dose for drug with half-life shorter than dosing interval in subjects with normal renal function 3. Decreased dose for drug with half-life longer than dosing interval in subjects with normal renal function
Combination	1. Can target same Cp_{max} 2. Can simultaneously change dosing interval and lessen impact of increased Cp_{ave} and Cp_{min} and possible toxicity	1. Need specific regimen for level of renal function and for each drug

We believe that the approach of Dettli, in general, and that of Hull and Sarubbi, for aminoglycosides, are preferable, for they individualize therapy at different levels of renal dysfunction in an effort to maximize theoretical benefit and lessen the risk of potentially toxic serum concentrations. This approach can be utilized with a measure of the fraction of drug excreted unchanged *(fe)* in a normal individual and the change in renal function observed in the patients; that is:

$$\frac{CL_{RI}}{CL_{normal}} = 1 - fe(1 - \frac{CL_{cr,RI}}{CL_{cr,normal}})$$

As stated earlier, clearance will be inversely related to half-life. To obtain the same Cp_{ave}, the dose should vary in direct proportion to clearance.

$$\frac{dose_{RI}}{dose_{normal}} = \frac{CL_{RI}}{CL_{normal}}$$

Table 6 (pp. 140–141) contains values for fe and $T_{1/2normal}$ for a wide variety of drugs. The values with standard deviations were compiled by Benet and Sheiner (91) and are referenced to the original source. Other values were obtained from Dettli's 1979 compilation (33). With these values and the foregoing equations, initial dosage adjustments may be made for patients with different degrees of renal function.

The clinician must be aware of the limitations of dosing guidelines. Nomograms cannot be used to relieve the clinician of his responsibility to evaluate clinical endpoints to pharmacologic effect in each patient. He must realize the nomograms should be used as approximations. Their usefulness has limits, particularly in the patient with severe renal failure or in the patient with changing renal function when the patient may never be at steady state. When available, previous individual patient pharmacokinetic data or measurements of serum concentrations of drugs should be used frequently but judiciously, for their use can clearly facilitate attaining a desired serum concentration (25,92–94). What concentration is desired may be yet another question and may vary among patients or disease states, thereby mandating frequent clinical assessment. Nomograms and measures of serum concentrations of drugs are clearly helpful but must be viewed as input data to be assimilated into the individual patient's overall clinical picture, from which the clinician must make quantitative estimates using his overall fund of knowledge and experience.

EFFECTS OF UREMIA ON DISTRIBUTION OF DRUGS TO TISSUES

Changes in the distribution of a drug that affect the relationship between dose and the drug concentration in blood were discussed previously. This section will consider changes in distribution of a drug in which the concentration is altered. This phenomenon should not be construed as a change in "sensitivity" to the drug, for it probably more represents a change in distribution of drug in peripheral tissues that favors more drug reaching its site of action, the relationship between concentration at the site of action and effect remaining the same.

Uremia or alterations in systemic pH appear capable of changing access of a drug to its site of action. In uremia, the change in albumin binding of diazoxide increased the antihypertensive effect, although the total concentration of diazoxide in blood remained the same as in nonuremic patients (95). A similar phenomenon occurred with thiopental anesthesia (96).

TABLE 6. *Mean urinary excretion of unchanged drug and overall elimination half-life in patients with normal renal function*

Drug	fe	$T_{1/2\ normal}$ (hr)[a]	Drug	fe	$T_{1/2\ normal}$ (hr)[a]
Acebutolol	0.44 ± 0.11	2.7 ± 0.4	Kanamycin	0.9	2.1 ± 0.2
Acetaminophen	0.03 ± 0.01	2.0 ± 0.4	Lidocaine	0.02 ± 0.01	1.8 ± 0.4
Acetohexamide	0.4	1.3	Lincomycin	0.6	5
Allopurinol	0.1	2–8	Lithium	0.95 ± 0.15	22 ± 8
Active metabolite		16–30	Lorazepam	0.01	14 ± 5
Alprenolol	0.005	3.1 ± 1.2	Meperidine	0.04–0.22	3.2 ± 0.8
Amantadine	0.85	10	Methadone	0.2	22
Amikacin	0.98	2.3 ± 0.4	Methicillin	0.88 ± 0.17	0.85 ± 0.23
Amiloride	0.5	8 ± 2	Methotrexate	0.94	8.4
Amoxicillin	0.52 ± 0.15	1.0 ± 0.1	Methyldopa	0.63 ± 0.10	1.8 ± 0.2
Amphetamine	0.4–0.45	12	Metronidazole	<0.25	8.2
Amphotericin B	0.03	360	Mexiletine	0.1	12
Ampicillin	0.90 ± 0.08	1.3 ± 0.2	Mezlocillin	0.75	0.8
Atenolol	0.85	6.3 ± 1.8	Minocycline	0.1 ± 0.02	18 ± 4
Azlocillin	0.6	1.0	Minoxidil	0.1	4
Bacampicillin	0.88	0.9	Moxalactam	0.82–0.96	2.5–3.0
Baclofen	0.75	3–4	Nadolol	0.73 + 0.04	16 ± 2
Bleomycin	0.55	1.5–8.9	Nafcillin	0.27 ± 0.05	0.9–1.0
Bretylium	0.8 ± 0.1	4–17	Nalidixic acid	0.2	1.0
Bumetanide	0.33	3.5	Netilmicin	0.98	2.2
Carbenicillin	0.82 ± 0.09	1.1 ± 0.2	Neostigmine	0.67	1.3 ± 0.8
Cefalothin	0.52	0.6 ± 0.3	Nitrazepam	0.01	29 ± 7
Cefamandole	0.96 ± 0.03	0.77	Nitrofurantoin	0.5	0.3
Cefoperazone	0.2–0.3	2.0	Nomifensine	0.15–0.22	3.0 ± 1.0
Cefotaxime	0.5–0.6	1–1.5	Oxacillin	0.75	0.5
Cefoxitin	0.88 ± 0.08	0.7 ± 0.13	Oxprenolol	0.05	1.5
Cefuroxime	0.92	1.1	Pancuronium	0.5	3.0
Cephalexin	0.96	0.9 ± 0.18	Pentazocine	0.2	2.5
Cephazolin	0.80 ± 0.13	1.8 ± 0.4	Phenobarbital	0.2 ± 0.05	86 ± 7
Chloramphenicol	0.05	2.7 ± 0.8	Pindolol	0.41	3.4 ± 0.2
Chlorphentermine	0.2	120	Pivampicillin	0.9	0.9
Chlorpropamide	0.2	36	Polymyxin B	0.88	4.5

Drug		
Chlorthalidone	0.65 ± 0.09	44 ± 10
Cimetidine	0.77 ± 0.06	2.1 ± 1.1
Clindamycin	0.09–0.14	2.7 ± 0.4
Clofibrate	0.11–0.32	13 ± 3
Clonidine	0.62 ± 0.11	8.5 ± 2.0
Colistin	0.9	3
Cytarabine	0.1	2
Cyclophosphamide	0.3	5
Dapsone	0.1	20
Dicloxacillin	0.60 ± 0.07	0.7 ± 0.07
Digitoxin	0.33 ± 0.15	166 ± 65
Digoxin	0.72 ± 0.09	42 ± 19
Disopyramide	0.55 ± 0.06	7.8 ± 1.6
Doxycycline	0.40 ± 0.04	20 ± 4
Erythromycin	0.15	1.1–3.5
Ethambutol	0.79 ± 0.03	3.1 ± 0.4
Ethosuximide	0.19	33 ± 6
Flucytosine	0.63 – 0.84	5.3 ± 0.7
Flunitrazepam	0.01	15 ± 5
Furosemide	0.74 ± 0.07	0.85 ± 0.17
Gentamicin	0.98	2–3
Griseofulvin	0	15
Hydralazine	0.12–0.14	2.2–2.6
Hydrochlorothiazide	0.95	2.5 ± 0.2
Indomethacin	0.15 ± 0.08	2.6–11.2
Isoniazid		
Rapid acetylators	0.07 ± 0.02	1.1 ± 0.2
Slow acetylators	0.29 ± 0.05	3.0 ± 0.8
Isosorbide dinitrate	0.05	0.5
Prazosin	0.01	2.9 ± 0.8
Primidone	0.42 ± 0.15	8.0 ± 4.8
Procainamide	0.67 ± 0.08	2.9 ± 0.6
Propranolol	0.005	3.9 ± 0.4
Quinidine	0.18 ± 0.05	6.2 ± 1.8
Rifampin	0.16 ± 0.04	2.1 ± 0.3
Salicylic acid	0.2	3
Sisomicin	0.98	2.8
Sotalol	0.6	6.5–13
Streptomycin	0.96	2.8
Sulfisoxazole	0.53 ± 0.09	5.9 ± 0.9
Sulfinpyrazone	0.45	2.3
Tetracycline	0.48	9.9 ± 1.5
Thiamphenicol	0.9	3
Thiazinamium	0.41	
Theophylline	0.08	9 ± 2.1
Ticarcillin	0.86	1.2
Timolol	0.2	3–5
Tobramycin	0.98	2.2 ± 0.1
Tocainide	0.20–0.70 (0.40 mean)	1.6–3
Tolbutamide	0	5.9 ± 1.4
Triamterene	0.04 ± 0.01	2.8 ± 0.9
Trimethoprim	0.53 ± 0.02	11 ± 1.4
Tubocurarine	0.43 ± 0.08	2 ± 1.1
Valproic acid	0.02 ± 0.02	16 ± 3
Vancomycin	0.97	5–6
Warfarin	0	37 ± 15

[a] Half-life is a derived parameter that changes as a function of both clearance and volume of distribution. It is independent of body size, because it is a function of these two parameters (CL, V_d), each of which is proportional to body size. It is important to consider that half-life is the time to eliminate 50% of the "drug" from the body (plasma), not the time in which 50% of the effect is lost.
Data from various sources (33,34,91).

Changes in systemic pH can also affect distribution of a drug to a site of activity without changing concentrations in blood, as has been demonstrated with salicylates, phenobarbital, and mecamylamine. Salicylates and phenobarbital demonstrate increased distribution into the central nervous system during acidemia. Central nervous system toxicity at any given blood concentration of either of these drugs is increased during acidemia (97–104). It appears that acidemia favors the nonionized species, allowing diffusion of more drug into the CNS. This phenomenon has been documented in pediatric patients, in whom acidemia causes increased delivery of salicylate into the cerebrospinal fluid. Consequently, an important part of therapy for salicylate or phenobarbital toxicity would be correction of systemic acidemia.

A similar phenomenon occurs with mecamylamine, a weak base, the site of action of which is extracellular. Acidemia favors the ionized congener, increasing amounts of mecamylamine extracellularly at its site of action and increasing the drug's hypotensive effect (105). This phenomenon has not been investigated in humans.

EFFECTS OF RENAL FUNCTION ON RESPONSES TO DRUGS

Whether or not renal function can modulate intrinsic drug activity is unclear. Supposed instances in increased sensitivity may, in fact, represent changes in distribution or access of drug to its site of action. For example, the effect described earlier of thiopental in patients with uremia was originally believed to represent changes in sensitivity, but further scrutiny showed the effect to be one of distribution rather than of changing the relationship between drug concentration at the active site and response.

The acidemia of uremia or renal tubular acidosis, or both, may cause resistance to the pressor effects of catecholamines. This phenomenon may be a true example of a change in sensitivity (106).

Electrolyte and acid-base abnormalities due to renal dysfunction can change sensitivity to drugs that affect the cardiovascular system. Hyperkalemia slows conduction throughout the heart and predictably increases the similar effects on conductivity of digitalis glycosides, quinidine, procainamide, phenothiazines, and tricyclic antidepressants. Alkalosis, magnesium or potassium depletion, and hypercalcemia increase sensitivity to the toxic effects of digitalis glycosides (107,108). Some investigators believe that decreased plasma potassium concentrations increase digoxin availability to its site of action; if this is the case, sensitivity has not changed, but the relationship has changed between the amounts of digoxin in blood and amounts at the active site. Whether or not the other conditions predisposing to digitalis toxicity represent true changes in sensitivity is unclear. Uremia appears to increase the sensitivity to pindolol in that blockade of exercise-induced tachycardia occurs at lower serum concentrations of pindolol than required in normals (109).

The exact mechanism by which changes occur in response to a given concentration of drug in blood is minor compared with the importance of realizing that it may occur in clinical settings. If the drug concentration in blood does not closely relate

to response, clinicians cannot rely on measures of serum or plasma drug concentrations as therapeutic guidelines. One must follow clinical endpoints to assess response.

CONCLUSION

The kidney can influence the disposition of drugs and response to drugs in many ways. Categorizing and cataloging these effects are helpful in sorting out the complexities of the kidney's role in handling of drugs. A better understanding of the multiplicity of effects of the kidney should help clinicians recognize and anticipate deviations from the norm with respect to drug effect and disposition. By so doing, they should be able to improve drug efficacy and decrease toxicity. Because changes in renal function can affect handling of a drug in many different ways, the clinician must understand not only the pathophysiology of his patient's disease but also the pharmacology of the drugs being used so that he can assess clinical endpoints of efficacy and toxicity as a guide to therapy.

ACKNOWLEDGMENTS

During the development of this chapter, the authors were supported by the following: National Institutes of Health Award 1-RO1-AM27059, Food and Drug Administration Grant 1-RO1-FDO11O4, General Clinical Research Center Grant USPHS 1-MO1-RRO5531, and clinical pharmacology training Grant 5-T32-GMD-7247-04.

REFERENCES

1. Brenner, B. M., and Rector, F. C. (1981): *The Kidney*, ed. 2, pp. 2659–2708. W. B. Saunders, Philadelphia.
2. Block, D., and Jones, N. F. (1979): *Renal Disease*, ed. 4, pp. 30–63. Blackwell Scientific, Oxford.
3. Lifschitz, M. D. (1981): Prostaglandins and renal blood flow: In vivo studies. *Kidney Int.*, 19:781–785.
4. Levinsky, N. G. (1979): The renal kallikrein-kinin system. *Circ. Res.*, 4:441–450.
5. Mitas, J. A., Levey, S. B., Holle, R., Frigon, R. P., and Stone, R. A. (1978): Urinary kallikrein activity in the hypertension of renal paraenchymal disease. *N. Engl. J. Med.*, 299:162–165.
6. Brunner, H. R., Gavras, H., Waeber, B., Kershaw, G. R., Turini, G. A., Vukovich, R. A., McKinstry, D. N., and Gavras, I. (1979): Oral angiotensin-converting enzyme inhibitor in long-term treatment of hypertensive patients. *Ann. Intern. Med.*, 90:19–23.
7. George, C. R. P. (1974): Non-specific enhancement of glomerular filtration by corticosteroids. *Lancet*, 2:728.
8. Pettinger, W. A. (1975): Clonidine, a new antihypertensive drug. *N. Engl. J. Med.*, 293:1179–1180.
9. Woosley, R. L., and Nies, A. S. (1975): Guanethidine. *N. Engl. J. Med.*, 295:1053–1057.
10. Campese, V. M. (1981): Minoxidil: A review of its pharmacological properties and therapeutic use. *Drugs*, 22:257–278.
11. Bauer, J. H., and Brooks, C. S. (1976): The long-term effect of propranolol therapy on renal function in the nephrotic syndrome. *Acta Med. Scand.*, 199:111–115.
12. Pedersen, E. B. (1975): Glomerular filtration rate and renal plasma flow in patients with essential hypertension before and after treatment with alprenolol. *Acta Med. Scand.*, 198:365–371.

13. Arisz, L., Donker, A. J. M., Brentjens, J. R. H., and Van der Hem, G. K. (1976): The effect of indomethacin on proteinuria and kidney function in the nephrotic syndrome. *Acta Med. Scand.*, 199:121–125.
14. Gary, N. E., Dodelson, R., and Eisinger, R. P. (1980): Indomethacin-associated acute renal failure. *Am. J. Med.*, 69:135–136.
15. McDonald, R. H., Jr., Goldberg, L. I., McNay, J. L., and Tutle, E. P. (1964): Effects of dopamine in man: Augmentation of sodium excretion, glomerular filtration rate, and renal plasma flow. *J. Clin. Invest.*, 43:1116–1123.
16. Wilkinson, S. P., Williams, R., Bernardi, M., Wheeler, P. G., and Smith, I. K. (1979): Diuretic-induced renal impairment without volume depletion in cirrhosis: Changes in the renin-angiotensin system and the effect of β-adrenergic blockade. *Postgrad. Med. J.*, 55:862–867.
17. Anon. (1981): The role of a new blocker in the management of hypertension. *Br. J. Clin. Pharmacol.*, 12(Suppl)1S–140S.
18. Heel, R. C., Brogden, G. E., Pakes, T. M., Speight, T. M., and Avery, G. S. (1980): Nadolol: A review of its pharmacological properties and therapeutic efficacy in hypertension and angina pectoris. *Drugs*, 20:1–23.
19. Data, J. L., and Nies, A. S. (1974): Dextran 40. *Ann. Intern. Med.*, 81:500–504.
20. Gugler, R., Shoeman, D. W., Huffman, D. H., Cohlimia, J. D., and Azarnoff, D. L. (1975): Pharmacokinetics of drugs in patients with the nephrotic syndrome. *J. Clin. Invest.*, 55:1182–1189.
21. Halkin, H., Sheiner, L. B., Peck, C. C., and Melmon, K. L. (1975): Determinants of the renal clearance of digoxin. *Clin. Pharmacol. Ther.*, 17:385–392.
22. Jackson, E. A., and McLeod, D. C. (1974): Pharmacokinetics and dosing of antimicrobial agents in renal impairment. *Am. J. Hosp. Pharm.*, 31:36–55, 137–148.
23. Jelliffee, R. W., and Brooker, G. (1974): A nomogram for digoxin therapy. *Am. J. Med.*, 57:53–68.
24. Kunin, C. M. (1967): A guide to use of antibiotics in patients with renal disease. *Ann. Intern. Med.*, 57:121–158.
25. Sheiner, L. B., Halkin, H., Peck, C., Rosenberg, B., and Melmon, K. L. (1975): Improved computer assisted digoxin therapy. A method using feedback of measured serum digoxin concentrations. *Ann. Intern. Med.*, 82:619–627.
26. Van Scoy, R. E., and Wilson, W. R. (1977): Antimicrobial agents in patients with renal insufficiency. *Mayo Clin. Proc.*, 52:704–706.
27. Bennett, W. M. (1978): Drug therapy in patients with chronic renal failure. *Kidney*, 11:5–9.
28. Bennett, W. M., Porter, G. A., Bagby, S. P., and McDonald, W. J. (1978): *Drugs and Renal Disease*, pp. 9–10. Churchill Livingstone, New York.
29. Bennett, W. M., Singer, I., and Coggins, C. J. (1973): Guide to drug usage in adult patients with impaired renal function. A supplement. *J.A.M.A.*, 223:991–997.
30. Bennett, W. M., Singer, I., and Coggins, C. J. (1974): A guide to drug therapy in renal failure. *J.A.M.A.*, 120:1544–1553.
31. Bennett, W. M., Singer, I., Golper, T., Peig, P., and Coggins, C. J. (1977): Guidelines for drug therapy in renal failure. *Ann. Intern. Med.*, 85:754–783.
32. Bennett, W. M., Muther, R. S., Parker, R. A., Feig, P., Morrison, G., Golper, T. A., and Singer, I. (1980): Drug therapy in renal failure: Dosing guidelines for adults. *Ann. Intern. Med.*, 93:62–89, 286–325.
33. Chennavasin, P., and Brater, D. C. (1981): Nomograms for drug use in renal disease. *Clin. Pharmacokinet.*, 6:193–214.
34. Dettli, L. (1976): Drug dosage in renal disease. *Clin. Pharmacokinet.*, 1:126–134.
35. Dettli, L. (1977): Elimination kinetics and dosage adjustment of drugs in patients with kidney disease. *Prog. Pharmacol.*, 1:1–32.
36. Dettli, L., Spring, P., and Tyter, S. (1971): Multiple dose kinetics and drug dosage in patients with kidney disease. *Acta Pharmacol. Toxicol.*, 29:211–224.
37. Anderson, R. J., Gambertoglio, J. G., and Schrier, R. W. (1981): *Clinical Use of Drugs in Renal Failure.* Charles C Thomas, Springfield, Ill.
38. Mudge, G. H. (1971): Uricosuric action of cholecystographic agents. *N. Engl. J. Med.*, 284:929–933.
39. Silverblatt, F. J., and Kuehn, C. (1979): Autoradiography of gentamicin uptake by the rat proximal tubule cell. *Kidney Int.*, 15:335–345.

40. Woodhall, P. B., Tisher, C. C., Simonton, C. A., and Robinson, R. R. (1978): Relationship between para-aminohippurate secretion and cellular morphology in rabbit proximal tubules. *J. Clin. Invest.*, 61:1320–1329.
41. Weiner, I. M., and Mudge, G. H. (1964): Renal tubular mechanisms for excretion of organic acids and bases. *Am. J. Med.*, 36:743–762.
42. Kampmann, J., Hansen, J. M., Siersbaek-Nielsen, K., and Laursen, H. (1972): Effect of some drugs on penicillin half-life in blood. *Clin. Pharmacol. Ther.*, 13:516–519.
43. Aherne, G. W., Piall, E., Marks, V., Mould, G., and White, W. F. (1978): Prolongation and enhancement of serum methotrexate concentrations by probenecid. *Br. Med. J.*, 1:1097–1099.
44. Galeazzi, R. L., Sheiner, L. B., Lockwood, T., and Benet, L. Z. (1976): The renal elimination of procainamide. *Clin. Pharmacol. Ther.*, 19:55–62.
45. Lee, C. S., Gambertoglio, J. G., Brater, D. C., and Benet, L. Z. (1977): Kinetics of oral ethambutol in the normal subject. *Clin. Pharmacol. Ther.*, 22:615–621.
46. Weily, H. S., and Genton, E. (1972): Pharmacokinetics of procainamide. *Arch. Intern. Med.*, 120:366–369.
47. Hager, W. D., Fenster, P., Mayersohn, M., Perrier, D., Graves, P., Marcus, F. I., and Goldman, S. (1979): Digoxin-quinidine interaction: Pharmacokinetic evaluation. *N. Engl. J. Med.*, 300:1238–1241.
48. Pedersen, K. E., Dorph-Pedersen, A., Hvidt, S., Klitgaard, N. A., and Nielsen-Kudsk, F. (1981): Digoxin-verapamil interaction. *Clin. Pharmacol. Ther.*, 30:311–316.
49. Waldorff, S., Hansen, P. B., Kjaergard, H., Bush, J., Egeblad, H., and Steiness, E. (1981): Amiloride-induced changes in digoxin dynamics and kinetics: Abolition of digoxin-induced inotropism with amiloride. *Clin. Pharmacol. Ther.*, 30:172–176.
50. Waldorff, S., Andersen, J. D., Heeboll-Nielsen, N., Nielsen, O. G., Moltke, E., Sorensen, U., and Steiness, E. (1978): Spironolactone-induced changes in digoxin kinetics. *Clin. Pharmacol. Ther.*, 24:162–167.
51. Gutman, A. B., Dayton, P. G., Yu, T. F., Berger, L., Chen, W., Sican, L. E., and Burns, J. J. (1960): A study of the inverse relationship between pKa and rate of renal excretion of phenylbutazone analogs in man and dog. *Am. J. Med.*, 28:1017–1033.
52. Milne, M. D., Scribner, B. H., and Crawford, M. A. (1968): Non-ionic diffusion and the excretion of weak acids and bases. *Am. J. Med.*, 24:709–729.
53. Mudge, G. H., Silva, P., and Stibitz, G. R. (1975): Renal excretion by non-ionic diffusion (the nature of the disequilibrium). *Med. Clin. North Am.*, 59:681–698.
54. Scribner, B. H., Crawford, M. A., and Dempster, W. J. (1959): Urinary excretion by non-ionic diffusion. *Am. J. Physiol.*, 196:1135–1140.
55. Levine, S. D., Franki, N., Einhorn, R., and Hays, R. M. (1976): Vasopressin-simulated movement of drugs and uric acid across the toad urinary bladder. *Kidney Int.*, 9:30–35.
56. Gerhardt, R. E., Knouss, R. F., Thyrum, P. T., Luchi, R. J., and Morris, J. J. (1969): Quinidine excretion in aciduria and alkaluria. *Ann. Intern. Med.*, 71:927–933.
57. Haag, H. B., Larson, P. S., and Schwartz, J. J. (1943): The effect of urinary pH on the elimination of quinine in man. *J. Pharmacol. Exp. Ther.*, 79:136–139.
58. Kostenbauder, H. B., Portnoff, J. B., and Swintosky, J. V. (1962): Control of urine pH and its effect on sulfaethidole excretion in humans. *J. Pharm. Sci.*, 51:1084–1089.
59. Kuntzman, R. G., Tsai, I., Brand, L., and Mark, L. C. (1970): The influence of urinary pH on the plasma half-life of pseudoephedrine in man and dog and a sensitive assay for its determination in human plasma. *Clin. Pharmacol. Ther.*, 12:62–67.
60. Lalka, D., Meyer, M. B., Duce, B. R., and Elvin, A. T. (1976): Kinetics of the oral antiarrhythmic lidocaine congener, tocainide. *Clin. Pharmacol. Ther.*, 19:757–766.
61. Wadell, W. J., and Butler, T. C. (1957): The distribution and excretion of phenobarbital. *J. Clin. Invest.*, 36:1217–1226.
62. Wilkinson, G. R., and Beckett, A. H. (1978): Absorption, metabolism and excretion of the ephedrines in man. I. The influence of urinary pH and urine volume output. *J. Pharmacol. Exp. Ther.*, 152:139–147.
63. Levy, G., Lampman, T., Kamath, L., and Garrettson, L. K. (1975): Decreased serum salicylate concentrations in children with antacids. *N. Engl. J. Med.*, 293:323–325.
64. Levy, G., and Koysooko, R. (1976): Renal clearance of theophylline in man. *J. Clin. Pharmacol.*, 15:329–332.

65. Kassirer, J. P. (1971): Clinical evaluation of kidney function-glomerular function. *N. Engl. J. Med.*, 285:385–389.
66. Cockcroft, D. W., and Gault, M. H. (1976): Prediction of creatinine clearance from serum creatinine. *Nephron*, 15:31–41.
67. Edwards, K. D. G., and White, H. M. (1959): Plasma creatinine level and creatinine clearance as tests of renal function. *Austral. Ann. Med.*, 8:218–233.
68. Jelliffe, R. W. (1971): Estimation of creatinine clearance when urine cannot be collected. *Lancet*, 1:975–976.
69. Lott, R. S., and Hayton, W. L. (1978): Estimation of creatinine clearance from serum creatinine concentration. *Drug Intel. Clin. Pharm.*, 12:140–150.
70. Wagner, J. G. (1971): *Biopharmaceutics and Relevant Pharmacokinetics*, pp. 222–233. Drug Intelligence Publications, Hamilton, Ill.
71. Siersbaek-Nielsen, K., Hansen, J. M., Kampmann, J., and Kristensen, M. (1971): Rapid evaluation of creatinine clearance. *Lancet*, 1:1133–1134.
72. Schwartz, G. J., Haycock, G. B., Edelmann, C. M., Jr., and Spitzer, A. (1976): A simple estimate of glomerular filtration rate in children derived from body length and plasma creatinine. *Pediatrics*, 58:259–263.
73. Traub, S. L., and Johnson, C. E. (1980): Comparison of methods of estimating creatinine clearance in children. *Am. J. Hosp. Pharm.*, 37:195–201.
74. Chiou, W. L., and Hsu, F. H. (1975): Pharmacokinetics of creatinine in man and its implications in the monitoring of renal function and in dosage regimen modifications in patients with renal insufficiency. *J. Clin. Pharmacol.*, 15:427–434.
75. Kampmann, J. P., and Hansen, J. M. (1981): Glomerular filtration rate and creatinine clearance. *Br. J. Clin. Pharmacol.*, 12:7–14.
76. Loirat, P., Rohan, J., Baillet, A., Beaufils, F., David, R., and Chapman, A. (1978): Increased glomerular filtration rate in patients with major burns and its effect on the pharmacokinetics of tobramycin. *N. Engl. J. Med.*, 299:915–919.
77. Lott, R. S., Uden, D. L., Wargin, W. A., Strate, R. G., and Zaske, D. F. (1978): Correlation of predicted versus measured creatinine clearance values in burn patients. *Am. J. Hosp. Pharm.*, 35:717–720.
78. Saah, A. J., Koch, T. R., and Drusano, G. L. (1982): Cefoxitin falsely elevates creatinine levels. *J.A.M.A.*, 247:205–206.
79. Fabre, J., and Balant, L. (1976): Renal failure, drug pharmacokinetics and drug action. *Clin. Pharmacokinet.*, 1:99–120.
80. O'Grady, F. (1971): Antibiotics in renal failure. *Br. Med. J.*, 27:142–147.
81. Cutler, R. E., and Orme, B. M. (1969): Correlation of serum creatinine concentration and kanamycin half-life. *J.A.M.A.*, 209:539–542.
82. Cutler, R. E., Gyselynck, A. M., Fleet, P., and Forrey, A. W. (1972): Correlation of serum creatinine concentration and gentamicin half-life. *J.A.M.A.*, 219:1037–1041.
83. McHenry, M. C., Gavan, T. L., Gifford, R. W., Jr., Guerkink, N. A., Van Ommen, R. A., Town, M. A., and Wagner, J. G. (1971): Gentamicin dosages for renal insufficiency. *Ann. Intern. Med.*, 74:192–197.
84. Jackson, G. G., and Riff, L. J. (1971): Pseudomonas bacteremia: Pharmacologic and other bases for failure of treatment with gentamicin. *J. Infect. Dis.*, 124(Suppl):185–191.
85. Anderson, E. T., Young, L. S., and Hewitt, W. L. (1976): Simultaneous antibiotic levels in "breakthrough" gram-negative rod bacteremia. *Am. J. Med.*, 61:493–497.
86. Wagner, J. G. (1974): Relevant pharmacokinetics of antimicrobial drugs. *Med. Clin. North Am.*, 58:479–492.
87. Chan, R. A., Benner, E. J., and Hoeprich, P. D. (1972): Gentamicin therapy in renal failure: A nomogram for dosage. *Ann. Intern. Med.*, 76:773–778.
88. Dahlgren, J. G., Anderson, E. T., and Hewitt, W. L. (1975): Gentamicin blood levels: A guide to nephrotoxicity. *Antimicrob. Agents Chemother.*, 8:58–62.
89. Hull, J. G., and Sarubbi, F. A., Jr. (1976): Gentamicin serum concentrations: Pharmacokinetic predictions. *Ann. Intern. Med.*, 85:183–189.
90. Sarubbi, F. A., and Hull, J. H. (1978): Amikacin serum concentrations: Prediction of levels and dosage guidelines. *Ann. Intern. Med.*, 89:612–618.

91. Benet, L. Z., and Sheiner, L. B. (1980): Design and optimization of dosage regimens: Pharmacokinetic data. In: *Pharmacological Basis of Therapeutics*, edited by A. G. Gilman, L. S. Goodman, and A. Gilman, pp. 1675–1737. Macmillan, New York.
92. Noone, P., Beale, D. F., Pollock, S. S., Perera, M. R., Amirak, I. D., Fernando, O. N., and Moorhead, J. F. (1978): Monitoring aminoglycoside use in patients with severely impaired renal function. *Br. Med. J.*, 2:470–473.
93. Noone, P., Parsons, T. M. C., and Pattison, J. R. (1974): Experience in monitoring gentamicin therapy during treatment of serious gram-negative sepsis. *Br. Med. J.*, 1:477–481.
94. Peck, C. C., Sheiner, L. B., Martin, C. M., Combs, D. T., and Melmon, K. L. (1973): Computer-assisted digoxin therapy. *N. Engl. J. Med.*, 289:441–446.
95. Pearson, R. M., and Breckenridge, A. M. (1976): Renal function, protein binding and pharmacological response to diazoxide. *Br. J. Clin. Pharmacol.*, 3:169–175.
96. Dundee, J. W., and Richards, R. K. (1954): Effect of azotemia upon the action of intravenous barbiturate anesthesia. *Anesthesiology*, 15:333–346.
97. Buchanan, N., and Rabinowitz, L. (1974): Infantile salicylism: A reappraisal. *J. Pediatr.*, 84:391–395.
98. Feuerstein, R. D., Finberg, L., and Fleishman, E. (1960): The use of acetazolamide in the therapy of salicylate poisoning. *Pediatrics*, 25:215–227.
99. Goldberg, M. A., Barlow, C. F., and Roth, L. J. (1961): The effects of carbon dioxide on the entry and accumulation in the central nervous system. *J. Pharmacol. Exp. Ther.*, 121:308–318.
100. Hill, J. B. (1971): Experimental salicylate poisoning observations on the effects of altering blood pH on tissue and plasma salicylate concentrations. *Pediatrics*, 47:658–665.
101. Hill, J. B. (1973): Salicylate intoxication. *N. Engl. J. Med.*, 288:1110–1113.
102. Liddell, N. E., and Maren, T. H. (1975): CO_2 retention as a basis for increased toxicity of salicylate with acetazolamide: Avoidance of increased toxicity with benzolamide. *J. Pharmacol. Exp. Ther.*, 195:1–7.
103. Morgan, A. G., and Polak, A. (1969): Acetazolamide and sodium bicarbonate in treatment of salicylate poisoning in adults. *Br. Med. J.*, 1:16–19.
104. Reimold, E. W., Worthen, H. G., and Reilly, T. P. (1973): Salicylate poisoning; comparison of acetazolamide administration and alkaline diuresis in the treatment of experimental salicylate intoxication in puppies. *Am. J. Dis. Child.*, 125:668–674.
105. Payne, J. P., and Rowe, G. G. (1957): The effects of mecamylamine in the cat as modified by the administration of carbon dioxide. *Br. J. Pharmacol.*, 12:457–460.
106. Nash, C. W., and Heath, C. (1961): Vascular responses to catecholamines during respiratory changes in pH. *Am. J. Physiol.*, 200:755–782.
107. Binnion, P. F. (1978): Drug interactions with digitalis glycosides. *Drugs*, 15:369–380.
108. Brater, D. C., and Morrelli, H. F. (1977): Cardiovascular drug interactions. *Ann. Rev. Pharmacol. Toxicol.*, 17:293–309.
109. Galeazzi, R. L., Gugger, M., and Weidmann, P. (1979): Beta blockade with pindolol. Differential cardiac and renal effects despite similar plasma kinetics in normal and uremic man. *Kidney Int.*, 15:661–668.

Pharmacokinetic Basis for Drug Treatment,
edited by L. Z. Benet et al., Raven Press,
New York © 1984

Chapter 9

Effects of Renal Disease: Altered Pharmacokinetics

John G. Gambertoglio

Division of Clinical Pharmacy, School of Pharmacy, University of California at San Francisco, San Francisco, California 94143

There is a large and increasing number of patients with kidney disease. These patients have a multiplicity of medical problems, many of which require some form of drug therapy. Figure 1 illustrates the numerous complications commonly associated with chronic renal disease. In addition, many of these patients are in the older age range, and some may also have additional diseases along with their impaired kidney function (see Chapter 15). Thus, the administration of drugs to this patient population can obviously predispose to adverse effects.

Patients with renal dysfunction are administered many drugs for treatment of their underlying disease and for other associated conditions. Recently we performed a survey of the drugs that are given to patients on chronic dialysis, mostly hemodialysis. The medical and drug records of 266 patients were reviewed. The percentages of males and females were almost equal, and approximately 75% were 45 years of age or older, with an age range of 19 to 87 years. The average number of drugs these patients were receiving was 8.4, with no differences between the older and younger groups. Table 1 gives the details of the various types of drugs being administered.

Because of the physiological and biochemical changes associated with uremia, renal failure patients may respond to a given dose of a drug differently than patients with normal renal function. It is generally believed that there is an increased frequency of adverse drug reactions in patients with renal failure. Data from the Boston Collaborative Drug Surveillance Program show that the incidence of adverse reactions to several drugs (e.g., ampicillin, chloral hydrate, flurazepam, chlorothiazide, digoxin, methyldopa, prednisone) was higher in patients with elevated blood urea nitrogen levels on admission (1). Although this type of study provides only a gross estimate of the role of decreased renal function in drug toxicity, it does serve to identify certain drugs of particular importance with respect to toxicity in renal failure patients.

The causes of drug toxicity in renal failure patients may arise either from increased sensitivity to the drug because of uremia-induced alterations in target organs or

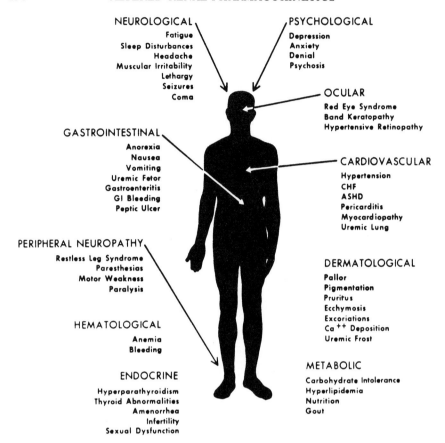

NEUROLOGICAL
Fatigue
Sleep Disturbances
Headache
Muscular Irritability
Lethargy
Seizures
Coma

PSYCHOLOGICAL
Depression
Anxiety
Denial
Psychosis

OCULAR
Red Eye Syndrome
Band Keratopathy
Hypertensive Retinopathy

GASTROINTESTINAL
Anorexia
Nausea
Vomiting
Uremic Fetor
Gastroenteritis
GI Bleeding
Peptic Ulcer

CARDIOVASCULAR
Hypertension
CHF
ASHD
Pericarditis
Myocardiopathy
Uremic Lung

PERIPHERAL NEUROPATHY
Restless Leg Syndrome
Paresthesias
Motor Weakness
Paralysis

DERMATOLOGICAL
Pallor
Pigmentation
Pruritus
Ecchymosis
Excoriations
Ca^{++} Deposition
Uremic Frost

HEMATOLOGICAL
Anemia
Bleeding

METABOLIC
Carbohydrate Intolerance
Hyperlipidemia
Nutrition
Gout

ENDOCRINE
Hyperparathyroidism
Thyroid Abnormalities
Amenorrhea
Infertility
Sexual Dysfunction

FIG. 1. Schematic representation of problems associated with uremia. (From Schoenfeld and Humphreys, ref. 101, with permission.)

from increased plasma drug concentrations due to altered pharmacokinetics of the drug. An example of the first cause is the increased sensitivity of uremic patients to the central nervous system depressant effects of sedative-hypnotic- and narcotic-type drugs. These drugs may potentiate the depressant effect of uremia on the central nervous system. However, it may be that uremia may alter the blood-brain barrier, which would allow for increased concentrations of drug into the central nervous system. Thus, uremia might cause a change in drug distribution, favoring a greater amount of drug reaching its site of action. In the second case, changes in the pharmacokinetics of a drug may lead to drug toxicity in renal failure. Because many drugs or their metabolites, which may be active or toxic, are excreted by the kidney, accumulation may occur with repeated doses and lead to unwanted effects. However, reduced renal excretion is not the only abnormality that occurs in renal failure. There may be alterations in drug bioavailability, protein binding, volume of distribution, or metabolism that determine the pharmacologic or toxic response to a drug.

TABLE 1. *Medications received by chronic dialysis patients*

Drug	Percentage of patients
Vitamins	96
Antacids	93
Antihypertensives	70
Fecal softeners/laxatives	50
Calcium supplements	41
Vitamin D preparations	36
Anabolic steroids	35
Antihistamines	26
Antianginal agents	23
Narcotic analgesics	22
Iron supplements	20
Hypnotics	19
Antianxiety agents	18
Digoxin	18
Acetaminophen	12

The objective of this chapter is to describe what effect renal dysfunction has on drug disposition. This information should form the basis and rationale for dosage regimen adjustment in these patients, in order to achieve the desired therapeutic effect and avoidance of toxicity.

ALTERED PHARMACOKINETICS IN UREMIA

Bioavailability

In terms of drug absorption and bioavailability, adequate information is lacking in patients with renal failure. Several factors, such as gastrointestinal disturbance, altered gastric pH, and antacid administration, could affect drug availability in the uremic setting. The gastrointestinal disturbances of renal failure, such as nausea, vomiting, diarrhea, and edematous changes of the gastrointestinal tract, may alter drug bioavailability (see Chapter 2). These patients may also have uremic gastritis, colitis, and even pancreatitis, which may also affect drug availability.

Uremic patients have elevated salivary urea levels (resulting from elevated blood urea concentrations) that when acted on by gastric ureases cause an increase in gastric ammonia. This serves to buffer hydrochloric acid in the stomach and thereby increases gastric pH. Therefore, iron, as well as other drugs whose absorption is favored in an acidic medium, may have impaired absorption. Patients with renal failure commonly take antacids, usually the aluminum type for treating gastrointestinal symptoms and for lowering serum phosphate levels. (The effects of antacids on drug bioavailability are described in Chapters 2 and 11.)

The availability of many drugs can be affected by the extent of their metabolism during the first pass through the gastrointestinal tract and the liver (see Chapters 3 and 4). A drug that has been studied in this regard in uremic patients is propranolol. Studies by Lowenthal et al. (2) and Bianchetti et al. (3) have suggested that the first-pass hepatic metabolism of orally administered propranolol is reduced in patients with renal failure. Figure 2 shows the blood levels of propranolol following a single oral dose of 40 mg in healthy volunteers, uremic patients not on dialysis, and patients on chronic dialysis. Note the much higher plasma levels and area under the curve seen in the uremic subjects as compared with the controls (4). These data were interpreted by the authors to indicate increased bioavailability of propranolol in uremia, suggested to be the result of decreased hepatic extraction. However, Wood et al. (5) found no change in the bioavailability or clearance of unbound drug in renal failure. These authors concluded that the increased levels result from a significant elevation of the blood/plasma ratio in patients with renal failure. There were no changes in propranolol plasma protein binding. This latter study (5) reemphasizes the importance of examining drug binding, distribution, and free clearance in interpreting the effects of disease states (see Chapters 1, 3, 4, and 10).

Propoxyphene is another drug that has been shown to have an apparently greater systemic oral availability in renal failure. This is believed to be the result of decreased presystemic biotransformation in renal failure patients (6).

Another drug whose bioavailability has been studied in renal failure is digoxin (7). Following oral administration of 0.5 mg in patients with severe chronic renal failure, maximal plasma concentrations were significantly higher (4.1 $\pm$ 1.0 ng/ml)

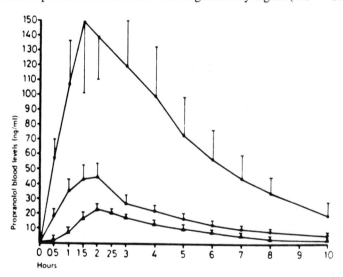

FIG. 2. Average ($\pm$ SEM) blood levels after a single oral dose of 40 mg propranolol to healthy volunteers *(lower curve)*, uremic patients not receiving dialysis treatment *(upper curve)*, and uremic patients receiving regular dialysis treatment *(middle curve)*. (From Bianchetti et al., ref. 3, with permission.)

and were reached at 2 hr, as compared with healthy volunteers, in which the peak level was only 2.3 ± 0.1 ng/ml at 1 hr. In addition, the patients with renal failure had significantly lower absorption rate constants. The mean was 0.76 ± 0.3 hr^{-1} in patients and 2.8 ± 0.6 hr^{-1} in volunteers. However, determination of absolute bioavailability showed no significant differences between the two groups, with a mean value of $70 \pm 13\%$ in renal failure patients, similar to that found in healthy volunteers ($76 \pm 4\%$). It should also be noted that the volume of distribution, determined from an intravenous dose, was significantly smaller in the renal failure group, explaining the higher maximal plasma levels observed. This will be described in greater detail in a subsequent section of this chapter.

Protein Binding

It is generally believed that the intensity of drug effect is related to the concentration of free (unbound) drug in plasma water. The protein binding of a drug to plasma and tissue proteins will thus affect the intensity of its pharmacological action, as well as its distribution and elimination from the body.

Renal failure has been shown to alter the plasma protein binding of many drugs (8) (see Chapter 10). Generally, the plasma protein binding of acidic drugs is decreased in uremia (Table 2), whereas the binding of basic drugs is usually normal, or may be decreased (Table 3).

The exact reasons for the decreased protein binding of drugs in uremia have not been determined. However, several explanations have been proposed. First, decreased binding may be caused, in part, by the hypoalbuminemia that may occur in association with uremia. The lower the albumin concentration, the greater the percentage of free drug available. Second, there is evidence that suggests the existence of a competitive inhibitor or displacer. Renal failure results in the accumulation of a number of acidic metabolites, and it is primarily acidic-type drugs that exhibit decreased binding in uremia. *In vivo* and *in vitro* dialysis improves the protein binding of some drugs, but in others there is no effect (35,43). The addition of an ultrafiltrate of plasma from uremic patients to normal plasma proteins may decrease drug binding in some cases, but not all. The adsorption of uremic serum with charcoal or an anion-exchange resin at pH 3 can normalize the binding of a number of drugs (44). There is some evidence to suggest that some small or medium-size molecule may bind very tightly at pH 7, but is more loosely bound at pH 3. Thus, the major cause of altered binding may be due to an inhibitor or displacer that is not a small, loosely bound molecule, but rather more tightly or highly bound. This corresponds with the fact that addition of urea, creatinine, and other nitrogenous waste products known to accumulate in uremia to normal plasma fails to affect drug binding. Free fatty acids can bind tightly to serum albumin and are well known to affect the interaction between protein and drugs. However, free fatty acid levels in renal failure are usually normal (44).

The third case of altered drug protein binding in renal failure could be related to an alteration in the conformation or structural arrangement of albumin, resulting

TABLE 2. *Plasma protein binding of acidic drugs in renal failure*

Drug	Normal	Renal failure	Change[a]	Comments	Refs.
Azapropazone	99	97	D	CL_{cr} mean 12 ml/min (range 1–52 ml/min)	9
Benzylpenicillin	66	44	D	Uremic patients on chronic hemodialysis	10
Captopril	30	No data	D		14
Cefazolin	85	69	D		11
Cefoxitin	73	22	D		12
Clofibrate	97	91	D	All CL_{cr} below 20 ml/min	13
Cloxacillin	95	80	D		15
Diazoxide	94	84	D		16
Dicloxacillin	97	91	D	Uremic patients on chronic hemodialysis	10
Diflunisal	88	56	D		17
Flucloxacillin	94	92	D	CL_{cr} in uremics <15 ml/min	102
Furosemide	96	94	D		18
Indomethacin	90	90	U		19
Metolazone	95	90	D		20
Moxalactam	52	36	D		22
Naproxen	99.8	99.2	D		24
Pentobarbital	66	59	D	Scr mean 10.1 ± 3.1 mg/dl	23
Phenylbutazone	93–96	82–86	D		21
Phenytoin	88	74	D		26
	93	84	D	Uremic patients on chronic hemodialysis	10
Piretanide	94	88	D		25
Salicylate	87	74	D		27
	97	84	D	Uremic patients on chronic hemodialysis	10
Sulfamethoxazole	66	42	D	Uremic patients on chronic hemodialysis	10
Valproic acid	92	77	D	Scr > 5 mg/dl	28
Warfarin	99	98	D	CL_{cr} 30 ± 8 ml/min/1.73 m²	29

[a]U, unchanged; D, decreased.

in a reduced number or affinity of binding sites for drugs (45). It has been shown from studies of normal and uremic albumin that differences exist in amino acid composition and in the protein content of the two albumin bands determined from isoelectric focusing. Thus, decreased binding of drugs in uremia may partly be related to an alteration in albumin composition.

An additional factor relating to drug binding in renal failure is the accumulation of high levels of metabolites of drugs that could interfere with protein binding, although this appears to be rather unimportant.

Another interesting consideration relating to protein binding of drugs in renal failure is the effect of dialysis and renal transplantation on drug binding. Studies with phenytoin, warfarin, morphine, salicylate, and sulfisoxazole have shown that

TABLE 3. *Plasma protein binding of basic drugs in renal failure*

Drug	Normal	Renal failure	Change[a]	Comments	Refs.
Carbamazepine	82	78	U	Scr > 7 mg/dl	30
Chloramphenicol	51	46	U		31
Chlorpromazine	98	98	U		33
Clorazepate (desmethyldiazepam)	98	95	D		32
Dapsone	82	74	U		34
Desipramine	90	88	U		35
Diazepam	98	92	D		32
Morphine	35	29	D		36
Prazosin	93	91	U	Scr 4.8 ± 1.6 mg/dl	37
Propoxyphene	76	80	U		38
Propranolol	89	89	U		33
Quinidine	85–97	77–97	U		39
Triamterene	81	57	D		34
Trimethoprim	67	66	U		40
d-Tubocurarine	44	41	U		41
Verapamil	89	88	U		42

[a]D, decreased; U, unchanged.

the decreased plasma protein binding present in the uremic state (prior to transplantation) increase toward normal values rapidly following transplantation (36,46,47). The effect of a rejection episode on the protein binding of salicylate and sulfisoxazole is shown in Fig. 3 (48). Rejection caused a decrease in plasma protein binding, which reverted to normal when the rejection subsided. In fact, the percentage of free drug increased several days before the rejection episode occurred.

One would expect the effect of hemodialysis to restore the abnormal plasma protein binding of drugs to normal. *In vitro* dialysis of plasma obtained from patients with acute renal failure increased the protein binding of several acidic-type drugs (49). However, most other studies have shown that *in vitro* and *in vivo* dialysis does not improve the plasma protein binding of drugs. In fact, hemodialysis of patients with chronic renal failure can result in a decrease in drug binding. Measurement of the plasma protein binding of phenytoin before, during, and after hemodialysis indicates that hemodialysis does not increase phenytoin protein binding as would be anticipated if dialysis removed competing substances for binding sites (50,51). Instead, the percentage of unbound drug tends to increase. This has also been demonstrated for other drugs, such as digitoxin (49,52). Because heparin is routinely administered during hemodialysis, the decrease in protein binding has been attributed to heparin-induced release of free fatty acids causing displacement of drug from albumin binding sites.

Little is known of the effect of peritoneal dialysis on drug protein binding. Although heparin is not administered during peritoneal dialysis, there is loss of albumin and other proteins associated with the procedure. This might alter drug

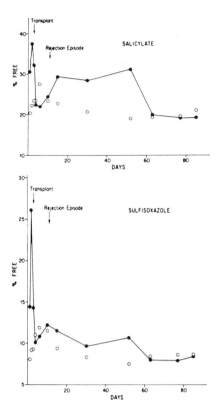

FIG. 3. Top: Percentage free salicylate in serum from donor *(open circles)* and renal transplant recipient *(filled circles)* relative to time. **Bottom:** Percentage free sulfisoxazole in serum from donor *(open circles)* and renal transplant recipient *(filled circles)* relative to time. (From Levy et al., ref. 48, with permission.)

binding. Further study is needed in this area, especially since the recent advent of chronic ambulatory peritoneal dialysis (CAPD), which is performed continuously, rather than on an intermittent basis as with standard peritoneal dialysis.

Volume of Distribution

Renal failure may cause an alteration in the distribution volume of drugs (53,54). Table 4 gives some examples of drugs whose volumes of distribution have been determined in patients with severe renal failure in comparison with subjects with normal kidney function. The volume of distribution may be increased, decreased, or unchanged. Because the plasma protein binding of some drugs is impaired in renal failure, as with phenytoin, this results in an increase in the apparent volume of distribution, in addition to a larger clearance for total drug. Other drugs that are not highly protein-bound, such as gentamicin, isoniazid, and cefamandole, have generally shown unchanged distribution volumes in renal impairment. Digoxin is a unique example, because it has been shown to have a decreased volume of distribution in renal failure.

The apparent volume of distribution of digoxin is decreased in the presence of renal failure (63,76–80). It averages 8.5 ± 3.0 liter/kg in patients with normal

TABLE 4. *Effect of renal failure on drug distribution volume*

Drug	Volume of distribution		Change[e]	Refs.
	Normal	Renal failure		
Amikacin	0.21 ± 0.08 liter/kg[a]	0.28 ± 0.09 liter/kg[a]	U	55
Azapropazone	10.6 ± 3.3 liters[b,d]	10.3 ± 1.5 liters[b,d]	U	56
Atenolol	1.2 ± 0.2 liter/kg[b]	0.9 ± 0.3 liter/kg[b]	U	57
Bezafibrate	0.38 ± 0.14 liter/kg[b,d] (CL_{cr} 50–69 ml/min)	0.31 ± 0.1 liter/kg[b,d]	U	58
Bretylium	3.58 ± 0.25[b]	4.48 ± 0.61[b] (CL_{cr} 1–12 ml/min)		103
Cefamandole	0.134 ± 0.045 liter/kg[a]	0.16 ± 0.05 liter/kg[a]	U	59
Cefazolin	0.13 ± 0.04 liter/kg	0.17 ± 0.03 liter/kg[b,c]	I	60
Clofibrate	0.14 ± 0.02 liter/kg[b,d]	0.24 ± 0.04 liter/kg[b,d]	I	13
Cyclophosphamide	0.73 ± 0.12 liter/kg[a]	0.58 ± 0.17 liter/kg[a] (CL_{cr} 18–51 ml/min)	U	61
Diazepam	2.8 ± 0.4 liter/kg	2.1 ± 0.3 liter/kg	U	65
Digitoxin	33 liters[c]	30 liters[c]	U	62
Digoxin	513 ± 104 liters	280 ± 87 liters	D	63
Disopyramide	0.6 liter/kg[b,d]	0.57 liter/kg[b,d]	U	64
5-Flucytosine	0.58 liter/kg	0.594 liter/kg	U	66
Furosemide	0.11 ± 0.01 liter/kg	0.18 ± 0.03 liter/kg	I	18
Gentamicin	0.28 liter/kg	0.24 liter/kg	U	67
Lidocaine	1.3 liter/kg[b]	1.20 liter/kg[b]	U	68
Lincomycin	0.57 ± 0.1 liter/1.73 m²[a]	0.58 ± 0.19 liter/1.73 m²[a]	U	67
Minoxidil	194 ± 86 liters[d]	214 ± 162 liters[d]	U	69
Moxalactam	9.1 ± 1.7 liter/1.73 m²[a]	21.4 ± 6.2 liter/1.73 m²[a]	I	70
Nafcillin	1.1 ± 0.3 liter/kg[a]	0.8 ± 0.1 liter/kg[a]	U	71
N-Acetyl-procainamide	1.4 ± 0.2 liter/kg[a]	1.7 ± 0.3 liter/kg[a]	U	72
Naproxen	8.3 ± 1.9 liters[b,d]	11.9 ± 2.1 liters[b,d]	I	24
Oxacillin	13.0 liters[a]	13.0 liters[a]	U	67
Phenobarbital	62 ± 25 liters[a]	58 ± 24 liters[a]	U	23
Phenytoin	0.64 ± 0.03 liter/kg[b]	1.4 ± 0.3[b] liter/kg[b]	I	26
Pyridostigmine	1.1 ± 0.3 liter/kg[b]	1.0 ± 0.1 liter/kg[b]	U	73
Procainamide	1.9 ± 0.3 liter/kg[b]	1.7 ± 0.3 liter/kg[b]	U	67
Propranolol	308 ± 28 liters[b]	255 ± 22 liters[b]	U	5
Quinidine	3.0 ± 0.5 liter/kg[a]	2.5 liter/kg[a]	U	74
Sisomicin	0.2 ± 0.03 liter/kg[b]	0.22 ± 0.03 liter/kg[b]	U	67,75
Sotalol	1.6 ± 1.1 liter/kg[d]	1.3 ± 0.6 liter/kg[d] (CL_{cr} 8.5–22.6 ml/min)	U	76

[a] V_{ss}.
[b] V_{area}.
[c]Estimated.
[d]Data from oral dose.
[e]D, decreased; I, Increased; U, unchanged.

renal function and declines as a function of creatinine clearance according to the relationship $V = 3.1CL_{cr} + 3.8$, where CL_{cr} is the patient's creatinine clearance (ml/min/kg) and V is volume of distribution (liter/kg) (79,80). Thus, a 70-kg patient with a creatinine clearance of 10 ml/min (0.14 ml/min/kg) would have a distribution volume as low as 4.2 liter/kg or approximately 300 liters. Consistent with these

pharmacokinetic data are the interesting observations of Jusko and Weintraub (81), who determined digoxin concentrations in serum and in left ventricular tissue measured at autopsy in relationship to antemortem creatinine clearances. It was noted that the myocardial/serum concentration ratio of digoxin decreases with decreasing creatinine clearance (Fig. 4) (81), thus demonstrating that myocardial tissue uptake of digoxin is diminished in renal failure patients.

Because of this decreased distribution volume of digoxin in renal failure, a 30 to 50% reduction in the normal loading dose has been recommended by some for patients with severe renal insufficiency (63). This seems appropriate if the pharmacologic effect of digoxin is a function of its plasma concentration. However, others suggest that no reduction in the usual loading dose is warranted, assuming that the amount of drug in the tissue compartment, i.e., myocardium, correlates better with drug effect (82). Administration of the same loading dose of digoxin to patients with renal failure having a decreased distribution volume as compared with those with normal kidney function will result in higher plasma levels. Presently there is no indication that uremic patients require higher plasma concentrations to achieve a comparable therapeutic effect from digoxin. However, this specific question has not been examined in detail.

A comparison of the total plasma concentrations of phenytoin following intravenous administration of a single 250-mg dose to uremic patients and epileptic patients with normal renal function is shown in Fig. 5 (83). The levels of phenytoin are much lower over the whole time course in the uremic group (83). This suggests an increased distribution volume in renal failure. In a comparative study (26), the volume of distribution for phenytoin in normal subjects ranged from 0.6 to 0.7 liter/kg and increased to 1.0 to 1.8 liter/kg in uremic patients. This is believed to be due to a decrease in the plasma protein binding of phenytoin, changing from

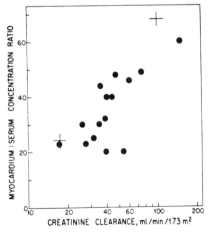

FIG. 4. Relationship between the digoxin myocardial/serum concentration ratio at autopsy and the estimated premorbid creatinine clearance in 15 patients. (From Jusko and Weintraub, ref. 81, with permission.)

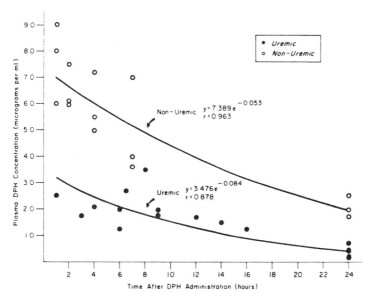

FIG. 5. Plasma phenytoin concentration in five uremic *(filled circles)* and three nonuremic epileptic *(open circles)* patients following 250 mg phenytoin intravenously. (From Letteri et al., ref. 83, with permission.)

approximately 12% to 25% unbound drug, leaving more free drug available for distribution. In addition, because of this altered protein binding, the apparent half-life becomes shorter (11–16 hr, normals; 6–10 hr, uremics), and the total clearance of phenytoin increases (28–41 ml/hr/kg, normals; 64–225 ml/hr/kg, uremics). Thus, in patients with impaired renal function, total plasma phenytoin levels are lower than in normals given the same dose. However, because of the increase in unbound fraction, the concentration of free plasma phenytoin is the same as in normals. The therapeutic plasma concentration range for phenytoin is 10 to 20 µg/ml. With approximately 10% unbound drug, the free drug level is 1.0 to 2.0 µg/ml. In severe renal failure, because the percentage unbound increases to about 25 to 30%, the therapeutic total plasma levels would have to be decreased to about 3 to 7 µg/ml in order to achieve the same level of free drug as in normals. Thus, the therapeutic total concentration range decreases with decreasing kidney function (8). The dose of phenytoin given to renal failure patients is usually the same as that given to patients with normal kidney function, but the therapeutic and toxic plasma levels, as usually determined from total drug levels, are lower.

Drug Elimination and Metabolism

Drugs are eliminated from the body through a number of processes, but principally through metabolism, primarily by the liver, and renal excretion.

The degree to which impaired renal function affects drug elimination depends on the percentage of unchanged drug normally cleared by the kidney. For many

drugs, relationships have been established between some parameter of drug elimination (i.e., half-life, elimination rate constant, or clearance) and some parameter of renal function (i.e., serum creatinine or creatinine clearance). (The details of these relationships and their clinical importance and utility in determination of drug dosage regimens are provided in Chapter 8.)

The various modes of metabolism generally function to convert drugs to more polar, water-soluble compounds that can more readily be eliminated from the body. Usually the metabolites found are inactive or much less active than the parent drug, and metabolism is considered a detoxification process.

Recently, a number of drugs have been shown to form metabolites with significant pharmacologic or toxicologic activity. What is important relative to renal failure patients is that these active metabolites may be primarily excreted by the kidney and thus accumulate in the body. Some examples of drugs that possess active or toxic metabolites partially excreted by the kidney are shown in Table 5 (84–86).

The oral hypoglycemic agents acetohexamide and chlorpropamide may lead to prolonged hypoglycemia in renal failure patients, secondary to a buildup of active metabolites. Accumulation of a toxic metabolite of nitrofurantoin has led to peripheral neuritis in patients with impaired renal function. Meperidine forms a metabolite, normeperidine; although possessing less analgesic potency, it has greater convulsant activity. After repeated doses of meperidine to patients with renal failure,

TABLE 5. *Drugs with active or toxic metabolites*
excreted by the kidney[a]

Drug	Metabolite
Acebutolol	N-Acetyl analog
Acetohexamide	Hydroxyhexamide
Adriamycin	Adriamycinal
Allopurinol	Oxipurinol
Cephalothin	Desacetylcephalothin
Chlorpropamide	Hydroxy metabolites
Clofibrate	Chlorophenoxyisobutyric acid
Daunorubicin	Daunorubicinol
Digoxin	Digoxigenin-*mono*-digitoxiside
	Digoxigenin-*bis*-digitoxiside
Meperidine	Normeperidine
Mephobarbital	Phenobarbital
Methyldopa	Methyl-*o*-sulfate-α-methyldopamine
Naltrexone	6-β-Hydroxynaltrexone
Phenylbutazone	Oxyphenbutazone
Primidone	Phenobarbital
Procainamide	N-Acetylprocainamide
Propoxyphene	Norpropoxyphene
Rifampicin	Desacetylated metabolite
Sodium nitroprusside	Thiocyanate
Sulfonamides	Acetylated metabolites
Nitrofurantoin	Toxic metabolite

[a]For an additional listing of drugs with active or toxic metabolites, see Chapter 21.

normeperidine has been shown to accumulate in plasma and may lead to central nervous system excitation (87).

One very impressive example of active metabolite accumulation is that of the antiarrhythmic agent procainamide, which is partly excreted unchanged in the urine (approximately 50%) and partly metabolized by hepatic N-acetyltransferase to N-acetylprocainamide (NAPA). This metabolite accounts for 7 to 34% of a dose of procainamide excreted in the urine, the greater amounts occurring in fast acetylators. Following direct administration of NAPA, 80% is recovered unchanged. Of special importance is that NAPA possesses substantial pharmacological activity and accumulates in patients with renal failure, achieving plasma levels that can greatly exceed those of procainamide. In Fig. 6, this is demonstrated by data from Gibson et al. (88) in an anephric patient receiving hemodialysis who was given a single dose of 6.5 mg/kg procainamide orally. NAPA levels are much higher than those of procainamide and show very little decline during interdialysis intervals, because of NAPA's continued formation from procainamide and lack of renal excretion.

Because both procainamide and NAPA accumulate in the patient with renal failure, dose reduction (by increasing the dosage interval) is necessary, and close monitoring is essential. Subsequent reduction in dosage from an initial dosage regimen may be necessary as NAPA accumulates because its half-life in renal failure is in the 30- to 40-hr range. In addition, measurement of plasma levels of both procainamide and NAPA (if available) are advocated in patients with impaired renal function and those on dialysis because both are substantially removed by dialysis.

Another area of interest regarding the effects of renal failure on drug kinetics is the effect of uremia on the process of drug biotransformation (89). Dosage regimen

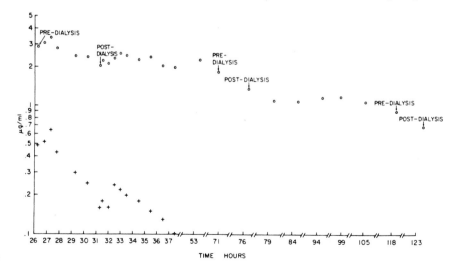

FIG. 6. Serum concentrations of procainamide *(crosses)* and N-acetylprocainamide *(open circles)* versus time in an anephric patient (rapid INH acetylator) following 6.5 mg/kg procainamide hydrochloride orally. (From Gibson et al., ref. 88, with permission.)

adjustments for renal failure generally assume that nonrenal mechanisms of elimination are unaltered. In theory, if metabolism (e.g., nonrenal elimination) were the only route of elimination for a drug, its rate of removal from the body should not be altered in renal failure (assuming other parameters, i.e., protein binding and volume of distribution, do not change because of uremia). However, the uremic state may have effects on the metabolic transformation of drugs. Table 6 shows some examples of drugs for which renal excretion of unchanged drug is negligible, or at least minimal, and the effect of renal failure on their elimination. Drugs undergoing oxidation reactions appear for the most part to have normal elimination. However, antipyrine and phenytoin have been shown to have increased elimination. The accelerated metabolism for phenytoin in uremia can be explained in part by its decreased plasma protein binding. Antipyrine has a very low degree of protein binding, and the reason for its increased elimination in renal failure is unclear.

Reduction reactions may be slowed in uremia, and the reduction of cortisol has been shown to decrease in renal failure. Synthesis reactions, such as with chloramphenicol (glucuronide conjugation) and acetaminophen (glucuronide and sulfate conjugation), appear to be unchanged. However, for acetylation reactions, some

TABLE 6. *Effects of renal failure on drug elimination for drugs primarily excreted by nonrenal routes*

Drug	Elimination
Oxidation	
Antipyrine	Increased
Clonidine	Unchanged/decreased
Lidocaine	Unchanged
Meperidine	Unchanged
Morphine	Unchanged/decreased
Pentobarbital	Unchanged
Phenytoin	Increased
Propranolol	Unchanged/decreased
Quinidine	Unchanged
Tolbutamide	Unchanged
Reduction	
Cortisol	Decreased
Synthesis	
Acetaminophen	Unchanged
Chloramphenicol	Unchanged
Indomethacin	Unchanged
Isoniazid	Unchanged/decreased
Hydrolysis	
Diflunisol	Unchanged/decreased
Insulin	Unchanged/decreased
Procaine	Decreased

have reported the acetylation of isoniazid to be normal in renal failure, and others have found it to be decreased. Finally, hydrolysis reactions (e.g., procaine) may be slowed in renal failure. It should be pointed out, however, that this area regarding the effect of uremia on drug metabolism has not been well studied. For many of the drugs listed in Table 6, half-life was the only parameter of elimination used. As described in Chapters 1, 3, and 4, half-life does not reflect as accurately an alteration in drug elimination as does clearance because half-life is not an independent pharmacokinetic parameter and it is influenced by distribution volume as well as clearance.

DRUG DIALYZABILITY

An ever-increasing number of patients with end-stage renal disease require dialysis in order to sustain life. The great majority of these patients are receiving hemodialysis; only a small percentage are on peritoneal dialysis, although its popularity is growing. Because these patients are on many drugs, as stated earlier, it is important to know what effect dialysis has on drug removal because dose supplementation may be needed in order to maintain adequate amounts of drug in the body. The purpose of this section is to review some of the problems encountered in assessing dialysis removal of drugs. Second, it will be illustrated how pharmacokinetic principles can be used to predict the dialyzability of a drug. This has utility not only in the therapeutic situation but also in the overdose setting. In the latter case, the use of pharmacokinetics may provide an important piece of information that, along with certain clinical information, will aid in the decision whether or not dialysis should be used in the treatment of drug overdose (90,91).

There are several problems encountered in assessing drug removal by dialysis. The literature is mostly qualitative in nature and commonly anecdotal. For example, in some overdose cases the effectiveness of dialysis in removing drug has been based on clinical response alone. In one instance, a patient was comatose prior to dialysis, and after the procedure was completed the patient awoke; drug levels in plasma or dialysate were not even determined to allow a proper assessment of drug removal. The type of dialysis system used is commonly not specified. Because of advances in dialysis technology, it is important to be able to compare different dialyzers. There is generally a lack of adequate patient data (such as weight and renal or hepatic function) that are useful in assessing the patient's ability to eliminate drug. The methods used for calculation of dialysis clearance are commonly unspecified. It is not stated if clearance was calculated using arterial-venous drug concentrations across the dialyzer or by the amount of drug recovered in the dialysate (92,93). It is common to determine drug concentrations before and after dialysis and to use this as a measure of drug removal by dialysis. However, this may not always be interpreted correctly because declining plasma drug levels during dialysis represent elimination by the body (renal and/or hepatic) as well as dialysis removal. On the other hand, if the plasma drug concentrations during a dialysis run remain constant, it is likely that insignificant removal by dialysis occurs. This is true

provided that drug absorption is complete. In cases of drug overdose, some drugs may have prolonged gastrointestinal absorption, thus maintaining blood levels when drug is being removed from the body by dialysis. For many drugs there is a lack of correlation between plasma drug concentrations and clinical response. This is partly due to the role of active metabolites. For example, glutethimide has an active metabolite (4-hydroxy-2-ethyl-2-phenylglutarimide) that contributes significantly to the toxic effects of the drug (94). Other drugs, such as phenothiazines, have many metabolites for which activity and toxicity are unknown. Finally, it should be noted that the pharmacokinetics of a drug may be different in the overdose situation. Most data used for prediction of a drug's dialyzability are obtained from normal healthy subjects. However, during an overdose, where there are suprapharmacological amounts of drug in the body, changes may occur in metabolism, protein binding, or volume of distribution for drugs exhibiting concentration-dependent kinetics (90). Drug metabolism and protein binding may become saturated, and volume of distribution may increase. These changes can affect drug removal by dialysis.

There are several properties of a drug that are important in predicting its dialyzability (67). Small molecules (MW < 500) do cross the dialyzer, the degree of which is dependent on blood flow, dialysate flow, and effective membrane surface area. The dialyzability of larger molecules is more dependent on membrane surface area. Large molecules, such as vancomycin (MW 3,300), amphotericin B (MW 924), and heparin (MW 6,000–20,000), are not effectively removed by dialysis. Drugs that are water-soluble are more readily removed by the aqueous dialysate. Lipid-soluble drugs, such as glutethimide, are dialyzed with difficulty. Furthermore, lipid-soluble drugs generally have larger distribution volumes and thus are less concentrated in the blood from which dialysis takes place. Drugs with large distribution volumes (e.g., digoxin, 600 liters) are not substantially dialyzed because most of the drug is not in the plasma or blood compartment but rather in tissue storage sites. Another important factor is protein binding because only the free (unbound) drug can cross dialysis membranes (95). Drugs with a high degree of protein binding, e.g., propranolol (90–94%) and warfarin (98–99%), are not significantly removed by dialysis.

Finally, when determining the dialyzability of a drug, the dialysis clearance of the drug must be compared to the body's clearance of the drug (90). Clearance terms are additive, as shown in Eq. 1:

$$CL + CL_D = CL_T \tag{1}$$

Thus, the clearance by the body *(CL)* and by dialysis *(CL$_D$)* can be added together to give a total combined clearance *(CL$_T$)*. Furthermore, half-life can be calculated from the relationship shown in Eqs. 2 and 3:

$$T_{1/2 \text{ off}} = \frac{0.693}{CL} \cdot V \qquad \text{(off dialysis)} \tag{2}$$

$$T_{1/2 \text{ on}} = \frac{0.693}{CL + CL_D} \cdot V \quad \text{(on dialysis)} \tag{3}$$

Thus, the half-life can be calculated for the off-dialysis and on-dialysis situations and compared. As a further extension of these relationships, Eq. 4 shows that one can calculate the fraction of drug in the body lost during a dialysis period:

$$\text{Fraction lost} = 1 - e^{-(CL + CL_D)\tau/V} \tag{4}$$

The information required includes the drug clearance by the body and by dialysis, the volume of distribution, and the duration of dialysis (τ). Again, it should be kept in mind that the clearance and volume terms may change under different conditions (e.g., overdose, renal failure).

Several hypothetical examples, shown in Table 7, will illustrate the use of the foregoing concepts in predicting the effect of hemodialysis on the removal of drugs. In the case of a patient overdosed on digoxin with normal renal function, using a distribution volume of 560 liters and a body clearance of 150 ml/min, with a dialysis clearance of 20 ml/min, the half-life off dialysis would be approximately 43 hr, and on dialysis it would decrease to only 38 hr. The fraction of drug lost during 4 hr of dialysis would be only 7%. Thus, dialysis would not be very useful in treating digoxin overdose, being limited primarily by the drug's large volume of distribution. If the same patient had no kidney function, then the values for volume and clearance would be decreased, and the half-life off dialysis would exhibit a larger decrease, from 86 hr to 58 hr. This would mean that the patient would need to be dialyzed for 58 hr in order to remove half the drug from the body, with only 5% being lost in 4 hr of dialysis.

In an overdose with phenobarbital, because dialysis clearance adds substantially to the total body clearance, the decrease in half-life is large, declining to about 8 hr with dialysis. Thus, this drug would be substantially removed with hemodialysis.

TABLE 7. *Predicted effects of hemodialysis on drug half-life and removal in the overdose setting*

Drug	V (liters)	CL (ml/min)	CL_D (ml/min)	$T_{1/2 \text{ off}}$ (hr)	$T_{1/2 \text{ on}}$ (hr)	FL[a]
Digoxin[b]	560	150	20	43	38	0.07
Digoxin[c]	300	40	20	86	58	0.05
Ethchlorvynol	300	35	60	99	36	0.07
Phenobarbital	50	5	70	115	8	0.30
Phenytoin	100	5	10	231	77	0.04
Salicylic acid	40	20	100	23	4	0.51

[a]FL = fraction lost during a dialysis period of 4 hr.
[b]Parameters for a patient with normal renal function.
[c]Parameters for a patient with no renal function.

TABLE 8. *Commonly used drugs removed by hemodialysis*

Acebutolol	Lithium
Acetaminophen	Methotrexate
Actinomycin D	Methyldopa
Aminoglycosides	Metronidazole
Ampicillin/amoxicillin	N-Acetylprocainamide
Azolocillin	Nitrofurantoin
Carbenicillin	Nitroprusside
Cephalosporins	Penicillin G
Chloral hydrate	Phenobarbital
Chloramphenicol	Procainamide
Cimetidine	Salicylate
Disopyramide	Sotalol
Ethambutol	Sulfamethoxazole
Flucytosine	Sulfisoxazole
5-Fluorouracil	Theophylline
Gallamine	Ticarcillin
Isoniazid	Trimethoprim

The next three drugs have all been shown to exhibit concentration-dependent kinetics. Thus, values for volume of distribution, clearance, and half-life would be expected to be altered in the overdose situation. Ethchlorvynol has a half-life of 25 hr after normal therapeutic doses, but during an overdose its half-life may increase to 100 hr or more. This is probably related to decreased metabolic clearance at high drug concentrations. The half-life change with dialysis is shown in Table 7, and only 7% of the drug would be lost from the body during 4 hr of dialysis. Additionally, ethchlorvynol appears to show a postdialysis rebound in plasma concentrations because of redistribution of drug back into the blood from fatty tissues.

Phenytoin has a half-life of 18 to 36 hr in the therapeutic concentration range, whereas in the overdose situation it may be greatly prolonged because of a decrease in the total body clearance from the normal value of 15 to 30 ml/min. The usual volume of distribution of about 50 liters and degree of protein binding of 90% would increase and decrease, respectively, at high plasma concentrations. Thus, a patient who has overdosed on phenytoin would have a change in half-life with dialysis, as shown in Table 7. With this very long half-life on dialysis, it appears that dialysis would be of limited value for detoxification of overdosed patients.

In patients overdosed on aspirin with a plasma salicylic acid concentration of about 100 mg/dl, the estimated parameters for salicylic acid are shown in Table 7. The dialysis clearance of salicylic acid is 100 ml/min and adds significantly to total body clearance, so that the half-life on dialysis is about 4 hr. Thus, an 8-hr period of hemodialysis could remove approximately 75% of the drug from the body.

Another approach to the removal of drugs from the body in the treatment of drug toxicity is the use of resins or activated charcoal (96,97). These act by adsorbing or binding the drug from the patient's blood. Resin hemoperfusion is advocated mostly for drugs that are more lipid-soluble and whose removal by conventional

dialysis procedures is limited. Generally, drug concentrations in blood show a dramatic decrease over the period of hemoperfusion, and drug clearances usually are much larger than those seen with hemodialysis. However, because lipid-soluble drugs commonly have large distribution volumes, their removal, even by hemoperfusion, is limited, because the majority of drug resides in peripheral tissues. This, then, serves as a depot from which the drug returns to the blood once hemoperfusion is discontinued.

Overall, the use of hemodialysis or hemoperfusion in the drug overdose setting should be restricted to more severe cases, and its risks and benefits need to be compared with the use of conservative management alone.

Table 8 lists some commonly used drugs that are substantially removed by hemodialysis (98,100).

CONCLUSION

Administration of drugs to patients with impaired renal function is a complex task. This is due to the multiplicity of medical problems in these patients, the large number of drugs they receive, the altered disposition of many drugs in uremia, and the effect of dialysis on drug removal. The clinician needs to be aware of these various factors in the patient with renal disease in order to create a drug therapy plan with optimal therapeutic effect and minimal toxicity.

REFERENCES

1. Jick, H. (1977): Adverse drug effects in relation to renal function. *Am. J. Med.*, 62:514–517.
2. Lowenthal, D. T. (1977): Pharmacokinetics of propranolol, quinidine, procainamide and lidocaine in chronic renal disease. *Am. J. Med.*, 62:532–538.
3. Bianchetti, G., Graziani, G., Brancaccio, D., Morganti, A., Leonetti, G., Manfrin, M., Sega, R., Gomeni, R., Ponticelli, C., and Morselli, P. L. (1978): Pharmacokinetics and effects of propranolol in terminal uraemic patients and in patients undergoing regular dialysis treatment. *Clin. Pharmacokinet.*, 1:373–384.
4. Lowenthal, D. T., Briggs, W. A., Gibson, T. P., Nelson, H., and Cirkesena, W. J. (1974): Pharmacokinetics of oral propranolol in chronic renal disease. *Clin. Pharmacol. Ther.*, 16:761–796.
5. Wood, A. J. J., Vestal, R. E., Spannuth, C. L., Stone, W. J., Wilkinson, G. R., and Shand, D. G. (1980): Propranolol disposition in renal failure. *Br. J. Clin. Pharmacol.*, 10:561–655.
6. Gibson, T. P., Giacomini, K. M., Briggs, W. A., Whitman, W., and Levy, G. (1980): Propoxyphene and norpropoxyphene plasma concentrations in the anephric patient. *Clin. Pharmacol. Ther.*, 27:665–670.
7. Ohnhaus, E. E., Vozeh, S., and Nuesch, E. (1979): Absolute bioavailability of digoxin in chronic renal failure. *Clin. Nephrol.*, 11:302–306.
8. Reidenberg, M. M. (1977): The binding of drugs to plasma proteins and the interpretation of measurements of plasma concentrations of drugs in patients with poor renal function. *Am. J. Med.*, 62:466–470.
9. Jahnchen, E., Blanck, K. J., Breuing, K. H., Gilfrich, H. J., Meinertz, T., and Trenk, D. (1981): Plasma protein binding of azapropazone in patients with kidney and liver disease. *Br. J. Clin. Pharmacol.*, 11:361–367.
10. Craig, W. A., Evenson, M. A., Sarver, K. P., and Wgnild, J. P. (1976): Correction of protein binding defect in uremic sera by charcoal treatment. *J. Lab. Clin. Med.*, 87:637–647.
11. Welling, P. G., Craig, W. A., Amidon, G. L., and Kunin, C. M. (1973): Pharmacokinetics of cefazolin in normal and uremic subjects. *Clin. Pharmacol. Ther.*, 15:344–353.

12. Garcia, J. J., Dominguez-Gil, A., Tabernero, J. M., and Sanchez Tomero, J. A. (1979): Pharmacokinetics of cefoxitin in patients with normal or impaired renal function. *Eur. J. Clin. Pharmacol.*, 16:119–124.
13. Gugler, R., Kurten, J. W., Jensen, C. J., Klehr, U., and Hartlapp, J. (1979): Clofibrate disposition in renal failure and acute and chronic liver disease. *Eur. J. Clin. Pharmacol.*, 15:341–347.
14. Rommel, A. J., Pierides, A. M., and Heald, A. (1980): Captopril elimination in chronic renal failure. *Clin. Pharmacol. Ther.*, 27:282.
15. Nauta, E. H., Mattie, H., and Goslings, W. R. O. (1973): Pharmacokinetics of cloxacillin in patients on chronic intermittent haemodialysis and in healthy subjects. *Chemotherapy*, 19:261–271.
16. Pearson, R. M., and Breckenridge, A. M. (1976): Renal function, protein binding and pharmacological response to diazoxide. *Br. J. Clin. Pharmacol.*, 3:169–175.
17. Verbeeck, R. K., and De Schepper, P. J. (1980): Influence of chronic renal failure and hemodialysis on diflunisal plasma protein binding. *Clin. Pharmacol. Ther.*, 27:628–634.
18. Rane, A., Villeneuve, J. P., Stone, W. J., Nies, A. S., Wilkinson, G. R., and Branch, R. A. (1978): Plasma binding and disposition of furosemide in the nephrotic syndrome and in uremia. *Clin. Pharmacol. Ther.*, 24:199–207.
19. Hvidberg, E., Lausen, H. H., and Jansen, J. A. (1972): Indomethacin: Plasma concentration and protein binding in man. *Eur. J. Clin. Pharmacol.*, 4:119–124.
20. Tilstone, W. J., Dargie, H., Dargie, E. N., Morgan, H. G., and Kennedy, A. C. (1974): Pharmacokinetics of metolazone in normal subjects and in patients with cardiac or renal failure. *Clin. Pharmacol. Ther.*, 16:322–329.
21. Aarbakke, J. (1978): Clinical pharmacokinetics of phenylbutazone. *Clin. Pharmacokinet.*, 3:369–380.
22. Peterson, L. R., Bean, B., Fasching, C. E., Korchik, W. P., and Gerding, D. N. (1981): Pharmacokinetics, protein binding, and predicted extravascular distribution of moxalactam in normal and renal failure subjects. *Antimicrob. Agents Chemother.*, 20:378–381.
23. Reidenberg, M. M., Lowenthal, D. T., Briggs, W., and Gasparo, M. (1976): Pentobarbital elimination in patients with poor renal function. *Clin. Pharmacol. Ther.*, 20:67–71.
24. Anttila, M., Haataja, M., and Kasanen, A. (1980): Pharmacokinetics of naproxen in subjects with normal and impaired renal function. *Eur. J. Clin. Pharmacol.*, 18:263–268.
25. Elliott, H. L., Ansari, A. F., Campbell, B. C., and Lawrence, J. R. (1982): Protein binding of piretanide in normal and uraemic serum. *Eur. J. Clin. Pharmacol.*, 21:311–313.
26. Odar-Cederlof, I., and Borga, O. (1974): Kinetics of diphenylhydantoin in uraemic patients: Consequences of decreased plasma protein binding. *Eur. J. Clin. Pharmacol.*, 7:31–37.
27. Lowenthal, D. T., Briggs, W. A., and Levy, G. (1974): Kinetics of salicylate elimination by anephric patients. *J. Clin. Invest.*, 54:1221–1226.
28. Gugler, R., and Mueller, G. (1978): Plasma protein binding of valproic acid in healthy subjects and in patients with renal disease. *Br. J. Clin. Pharmacol.*, 5:441–446.
29. Bachmann, K., Shapiro, R., and MacKiewicz, J. (1976): Influence of renal dysfunction on warfarin plasma protein binding. *J. Clin. Pharmacol.*, 16:468–472.
30. Hooper, W. D., Dubetz, D. K., Bochner, F., Cotter, L. M., Smith, G. A., Eadie, M. J., and Tyrer, J. H. (1975): Plasma protein binding of carbamazepine. *Clin. Pharmacol. Ther.*, 17:433–440.
31. Grafnetterova, J., Vodrazka, Z., Jandova, D., Schuck, O., Tomasek, R., and Lachmanova, J. (1976): The binding of chloramphenicol to serum proteins in patients with chronic renal insufficiency. *Clin. Nephrol.*, 6:448–450.
32. Kangas, L., Kanto, J., Forsstrom, J., and Iisalo, E. (1976): The protein binding of diazepam and N-desmethyldiazepam in patients with poor renal function. *Clin. Nephrol.*, 5:114–118.
33. Piafsky, K. M., Borga, O., Odar-Cederlof, I., Johansson, C., and Sjoquist, F. (1978): Increased plasma protein binding of propranolol and chlorpromazine mediated by disease-induced elevations of plasma α_1 acid glycoprotein. *N. Engl. J. Med.*, 299:1435–1440.
34. Reidenberg, M. M., and Affrime, M. (1973): Influence of disease on binding of drugs to plasma proteins. *Ann. N.Y. Acad. Sci.*, 226:115–126.
35. Reidenberg, M. M., Odar-Cederlof, I., von Bahr, C., Borga, O., and Sjoqvist, F. (1971): Protein binding of diphenylhydantoin and desmethylimipramine in plasma from patients with poor renal function. *N. Engl. J. Med.*, 285:264–268.
36. Olsen, G. D., Bennett, W. M., and Porter, G. A. (1975): Morphine and phenytoin binding to plasma proteins in renal and hepatic failure. *Clin. Pharmacol. Ther.*, 17:677–684.

37. Lowenthal, D. T., Hobbs, D., Affrime, M. B., Twomey, T. M., Martinez, E. W., and Onesti, G. (1980): Prazosin kinetics and effectiveness in renal failure. *Clin. Pharmacol. Ther.*, 27:779–783.

38. Giacomini, K. M., Gibson, T. P., and Levy, G. (1978): Plasma protein binding of *d*-propoxyphene in normal subjects and anephric patients. *J. Clin. Pharmacol.*, 18:106–109.

39. Kessler, K. M., Leech, R. C., and Spann, J. F. (1979): Blood collection techniques, heparin and quinidine protein binding. *Clin. Pharmacol. Ther.*, 25:204–210.

40. Craig, W. A., and Kunin, C. M. (1973): Trimethoprim-sulfamethoxazole: Pharmacodynamic effects of urinary pH and impaired renal function. *Ann. Intern. Med.*, 78:491–497.

41. Ghoneim, M. M., Kramer, E., Bannow, R., Pandya, H., and Routh, J. I.: Binding of *d*-tubocurarine to plasma proteins in normal man and in patients with hepatic or renal disease. *Anesthesiology*, 39:410–415.

42. Keefe, D. L., Yee, Y. G., and Kates, R. E. (1981): Verapamil protein binding in patients and in normal subjects. *Clin. Pharmacol. Ther.*, 29:21–26.

43. Andreasen, F. (1974): The effect of dialysis on the protein binding of drugs in the plasma of patients with acute renal failure. *Acta Pharmacol. Toxicol.*, 34:284–294.

44. Craig, W. A., Evenson, M. A., and Ramgopal, V. (1976): The effect of uremia, cardiopulmonary bypass and bacterial infection on serum protein binding. In: *The Effect of Disease States on Drug Pharmacokinetics*, edited by L. Z. Benet, pp. 125–136. American Pharmaceutical Association, Washington, D.C.

45. Boobis, S. W. (1977): Alteration of plasma albumin in relation to decreased drug binding in uremia. *Clin. Pharmacol. Ther.*, 22:147–153.

46. Levy, G., Baliah, T., and Procknal, J. A. (1976): Effect of renal transplantation on protein binding of drugs in serum of donor and recipient. *Clin. Pharmacol. Ther.*, 20:512–516.

47. Odar-Cederlof, I. (1977): Plasma protein binding of phenytoin and warfarin in patients undergoing renal transplantation. *Clin. Pharmacokinet.*, 2:147–153.

48. Levy, G., Baliah, T., and Procknal, J. A. (1976): Effect of renal transplantation on protein binding of drugs in serum of donor and recipient. *Clin. Pharmacol. Ther.*, 20:512–516.

49. Storstein, L., and Janssen, H. (1976): Studies on digitalis. VI. The effect of heparin on serum protein binding of digitoxin and digoxin. *Clin. Pharmacol. Ther.*, 20:15–23.

50. Adler, D. S., Martin, E., Gambertoglio, J. G., Tozer, T. N., and Spire, J. P. (1975): Hemodialysis of phenytoin in a uremic patient. *Clin. Pharmacol. Ther.*, 18:65–69.

51. Martin, E., Gambertoglio, J. G., Adler, D. S., Tozer, T. N., Roman, L. A., and Grausz, H. (1977): Removal of phenytoin by hemodialysis in uremic patients. *J.A.M.A.*, 238:1750–1753.

52. Storstein, L. (1976): Studies on digitalis. V. The influence of impaired renal function, hemodialysis, and drug interaction on serum protein binding of digitoxin and digoxin. *Clin. Pharmacol. Ther.*, 20:6–14.

53. Gibaldi, M. (1977): Drug distribution in renal failure. *Am. J. Med.*, 62:471–474.

54. Klotz, U. (1976): Pathophysiological and disease-induced changes in drug distribution volume: Pharmacokinetic implications. *Clin. Pharmacokinet.*, 1:104–218.

55. Pijck, J., Hallynck, T., Solp, H., Baert, L., Daneels, R., and Boelaert, J. (1976): Pharmacokinetics of amikacin in patients with renal insufficiency; relation of half-life and creatinine clearance. *J. Infect. Dis. [Suppl.]*, 134:331–341.

56. Breuing, K. H., Gilfrich, H. J., Meinertz, T., Wiegand, U. W., and Jahnchen, E. (1981): Disposition of azapropazone in chronic renal and hepatic failure. *Eur. J. Clin. Pharmacol.*, 20:147–155.

57. Kirch, W., Kohler, H., Mutschler, E., and Schafer, M. (1981): Pharmacokinetics of atenolol in relation to renal function. *Eur. J. Clin. Pharmacol.*, 19:65–71.

58. Anderson, P., and Norbeck, H. E. (1981): Clinical pharmacokinetics of bezafibrate in patients with impaired renal function. *Eur. J. Clin. Pharmacol.*, 21:209–214.

59. Gambertoglio, J. G., Aziz, N. S., Lin, E. T., Grausz, H., Naughton, J. L., and Benet, L. Z. (1979): Cefamandole kinetics in uremic patients undergoing hemodialysis. *Clin. Pharmacol. Ther.*, 26:592–599.

60. Czerwinski, A. W., Pederson, J. A., and Barry, J. P. (1974): Cefazolin plasma concentrations and urinary excretion in patients with renal impairment. *J. Clin. Pharmacol.*, 14:560–566.

61. Juma, F. D., Rogers, H. J., and Trounce, J. R. (1981): Effect of renal insufficiency on the pharmacokinetics of cyclophosphamide and some of its metabolites. *Eur. J. Clin. Pharmacol.*, 19:443–451.

62. Storstein, L. (1974): Studies on digitalis. II. The influence of impaired renal function on the renal excretion of digitoxin and its cardioactive metabolites. *Clin. Pharmacol. Ther.*, 16:25–33.

63. Reuning, R. H., Sams, R. A., and Notari, R. E. (1973): Role of pharmacokinetics in drug dosage adjustment. 1. Pharmacologic effect kinetics and apparent volume of distribution of digoxin. *J. Clin. Pharmacol.*, 13:127–141.

64. Johnston, A., Henry, J. A., Warrington, S. J., and Hamer, N. A. J. (1980): Pharmacokinetics of oral disopyramide phosphate in patients with renal impairment. *Br. J. Clin. Pharmacol.*, 10:245–248.

65. Ochs, H. R., Greenblatt, D. J., Abernethy, D. R., and Divoll, M. (1981): Diazepam kinetics in chronic renal failure. *Clin. Pharmacol. Ther.*, 29:270.

66. Dawborn, J. D., Page, M. D., and Schiavone, D. J. (1973): Use of 5-fluorocytosine in patients with impaired renal function. *Br. Med. J.*, 4:382–384.

67. Gibson, T. P., and Nelson, H. A. (1977): Drug kinetics and artificial kidneys. *Clin. Pharmacokinet.*, 2:403–426.

68. Thomson, P. D., Melmon, K. L., Richardson, J. A., Cohn, K., Steinbrunn, W., Cudihee, R., and Rowland, M. (1973): Lidocaine pharmacokinetics in advanced heart failure, liver disease, and renal failure in humans. *Ann. Intern. Med.*, 78:499–508.

69. Gottlieb, T. B., Thomas, R. C., and Chidsey, C. A. (1972): Pharmacokinetic studies of minoxidil. *Clin. Pharmacol. Ther.*, 13:436–441.

70. Leroy, A., Humbert, G., and Fillastre, J. P. (1981): Pharmacokinetics of moxalactam in subjects with normal and impaired renal function. 19:965–970.

71. Rudnick, M., Morrison, G., Walker, B., and Singer, I. (1976): Renal failure, hemodialysis, and nafcillin kinetics. *Clin. Pharmacol. Ther.*, 20:413–422.

72. Strong, J. M., Dutcher, J. S., Lee, W.-K., and Atkinson, A. J., Jr. (1975): Pharmacokinetics in man of the *N*-acetylated metabolite of procainamide. *J. Pharmacokinet. Biopharm.*, 3:223–231.

73. Cronnelly, P., Stanski, D. R., Miller, R. D., and Sheiner, L. B. (1980): Pyridostigmine kinetics with and without renal function. *Clin. Pharmacol. Ther.*, 28:78–81.

74. Conrad, K. A., Molk, B. L., and Chidsey, C. A. (1977): Pharmacokinetic studies of quinidine in patients with arrhythmias. *Circulation*, 55:1–7.

75. Naber, K., Roth, S., and Lange, H. (1979): Sisomicin: Pharmacokinetics and therapy in patients with normal and reduced renal function. *Infection*, 7 (Suppl. 3):275.

76. Blair, A. D., Burgess, E. D., Maxwell, B. M., and Cutler, R. E. (1981): Sotalol kinetics in renal insufficiency. *Clin. Pharmacol. Ther.*, 29:457–462.

77. Jusko, W. J., Szefler, S. J., and Goldfarb, A. L. (1974): Pharmacokinetic design of digoxin dosage regimens in relation to renal function. *J. Clin. Pharmacol.*, 14:525–535.

78. Koup, J. R., Jusko, W. J., Elwood, C. M., and Kohli, R. K. (1975): Digoxin pharmacokinetics: Role of renal failure in dosage regimen design. *Clin. Pharmacol. Ther.*, 18:9–21.

79. Sheiner, L. B., Rosenberg, B., and Marathe, V. V. (1977): Estimation of population characteristics of pharmacokinetic parameters from routine clinical data. *J. Pharmacokinet. Biopharm.*, 5:445–479.

80. Sheiner, L. B., Benet, L. Z., and Pagliaro, L. A. (1981): A standard approach to compiling clinical pharmacokinetic data. *J. Pharmacokinet. Biopharm.*, 9:59–127.

81. Jusko, W. J., and Weintraub, M. (1974): Myocardial distribution of digoxin and renal function. *Clin. Pharmacol. Ther.*, 16:449–454.

82. Wagner, J. G. (1974): Loading and maintenance doses of digoxin in patients with normal renal function and those with severely impaired renal function. *J. Clin. Pharmacol.*, 14:329–338.

83. Letteri, J. M., Mellk, H., Louis, S., Kutt, H., Durante, P., and Glazko, A. (1971): Diphenylhydantoin metabolism in uremia. *N. Engl. J. Med.*, 285:648–652.

84. Drayer, D. E. (1976): Pharmacologically active drug metabolites: Therapeutic and toxic activities, plasma, and urine data in man, accumulation in renal failure. *Clin. Pharmacokinet.*, 1:426–443.

85. Drayer, D. (1977): Active drug metabolites and renal failure. *Am. J. Med.*, 62:486–489.

86. Verbeeck, R. K., Branch, R. A., and Wilkinson, G. K. (1981): Drug metabolites in renal failure. *Clin. Pharmacokinet.*, 6:329–345.

87. Szeto, H. H., Inturrisi, C. E., Houde, R., Saal, S., Cheigh, J., and Reidenberg, M. M. (1977): Accumulation of normeperidine, an active metabolite of meperidine, in patients with renal failure or cancer. *Ann. Intern. Med.*, 86:738–741.

88. Gibson, T. P., Matusik, E. J., and Briggs, W. A. (1976): *N*-acetylprocainamide levels in patients with end-stage renal failure. *Clin. Pharmacol. Ther.*, 19:206–212.

89. Reidenberg, M. M. (1977): The biotransformation of drugs in renal failure. *Am. J. Med.*, 62:482–485.

90. Takki, S., Gambertoglio, J. G., Honda, D., and Tozer, T. N. (1978): Pharmacokinetic evaluation of hemodialysis in acute drug overdose. *J. Pharmacokinet. Biopharm.*, 6:427–442.

91. Tilstone, W. J., Winchester, J. F., and Reavey, P. C. (1979): The use of pharmacokinetic principles in determining the effectiveness of removal of toxins from blood. *Clin. Pharmacokinet.*, 4:23–37.

92. Lee, C. S., Marbury, T. C., and Benet, L. Z. (1980): Clearance calculations in hemodialysis: Application to blood, plasma, and dialysate measurements for ethambutol. *J. Pharmacokinet. Biopharm.*, 8:69–81.

93. Gibson, T. P., Matusik, E., Nelson, L. D., and Briggs, W. A. (1976): Artificial kidneys and clearance calculations. *Clin. Pharmacol. Ther.*, 20:720–726.

94. Hansen, A. R., Kennedy, K. A., Ambre, J. J., and Fisher, L. J. (1975): Glutethimide poisoning. A metabolite contributes to morbidity and mortality. *N. Engl. J. Med.*, 292:250–252.

95. Gwilt, P. R., and Perrier, D. (1978): Plasma protein binding and distribution characteristics of drugs as indices of their hemodialyzability. *Clin. Pharmacol. Ther.*, 24:154–161.

96. Winchester, J. F., and Gelfand, M. C. (1978): Hemoperfusion in drug intoxication: Clinical and laboratory aspects. *Drug Metab. Rev.*, 8:69–104.

97. Pond, S., Rosenberg, J., Benowitz, N. L., and Takki, S. (1979): Pharmacokinetics of haemoperfusion for drug overdose. *Clin. Pharmacokinet.*, 4:329–354.

98. Bennett, W. M., Muther, R. S., Parker, R. A., Feig, P., Morrison, G., Golper, T. A., and Singer, I. (1980): Drug therapy in renal failure: Dosing guidelines for adults. Part I: Antimicrobial agents, analgesics. *Ann. Intern. Med.*, 93:62–89.

99. Bennett, W. M., Muther, R. S., Parker, R. A., Feig, P., Morrison, G., Golper, T. A., and Singer, I. (1980): Drug therapy in renal failure: Dosing guidelines for adults. Part II: Sedatives, hypnotics, and tranquilizers; cardiovascular, antihypertensive, and diuretic agents; miscellaneous agents. *Ann. Intern. Med.*, 93:286–325.

100. Anderson, R. J., and Schrier, R. W. (1981): *Clinical Use of Drugs in Patients with Kidney and Liver Disease.* W. B. Saunders, Philadelphia.

101. Schoenfeld, P., and Humphreys, M. H. (1976): In: *The Kidney*, edited by B. M. Brenner and F. L. Rector, Jr., Chapter 33. W. B. Saunders, Philadelphia.

102. Thijssen, H. H. W., and Wolters, J. (1982): The metabolic disposition of flucloxacillin in patients with impaired kidney function. *Eur. J. Clin. Pharmacol.*, 22:429–434.

103. Josselson, J., Narang, R. K., Adir, J., Yacobi, A., and Sadler, J. H. (1983): Bretylium kinetics in renal insufficiency. *Clin. Pharmacol. Ther.*, 33:144–150.

Pharmacokinetic Basis for Drug Treatment,
edited by L. Z. Benet et al., Raven Press,
New York © 1984

Chapter 10

Implications of Altered Plasma Protein Binding in Disease States

Thomas N. Tozer

*Department of Pharmacy, School of Pharmacy, University of California
at San Francisco, San Francisco, California 94143*

For a drug that acts reversibly, its effects are believed to be closely related to its unbound concentration at the site of action. This concentration is difficult to measure; the more readily determined total drug concentration in plasma is commonly used instead. The relationship between these concentrations depends on nonspecific binding to plasma proteins and on the time required for drug in plasma to equilibrate with that at the active site. Were binding always the same, ignoring the equilibration time, the total concentration in plasma should provide correlations with activity that would be equally as good as those that would be observed using drug at the active site. A major problem exists, however, because of variability in binding to plasma proteins. This problem is compounded in situations in which drug absorption and elimination are affected by alterations in protein binding. Thus, there is clearly a need to measure drug-protein binding and to understand the pharmacokinetic and therapeutic consequences of such alterations.

Disease is a principal cause of variability in binding. Several reviews (1–9) have been published on this subject. The major emphasis of this chapter is to examine the implications of altered plasma protein, particularly that associated with disease, for interpretation of drug concentrations and for dosage requirements. The implications will be examined in terms of (a) the proteins to which drugs bind, (b) how binding depends on protein and drug concentrations, (c) the causes of altered binding, and (d) the effects of altered binding on drug absorption and disposition.

BINDING PROTEINS

Plasma contains many proteins. Albumin, the most abundant of all, has received the greatest attention, but other proteins also bind drugs. The three most common drug-binding proteins are listed in Table 1.

Albumin primarily accounts for the binding of acidic drugs in plasma. Basic drugs, on the other hand, often associate more avidly with other proteins, particularly α_1-acid glycoprotein and lipoproteins, than with albumin (9). Proteins such as

TABLE 1. *Major proteins to which drugs bind in plasma*

| Protein | Molecular weight | Normal range of concentrations | |
		(g/liter)	(molar)
Albumin	65,000	35–50	$5–7.5 \times 10^{-4}$
α_1-Acid glycoprotein	44,000	0.4–1.0	$0.9–2.2 \times 10^{-5}$
Lipoproteins	200,000–3,400,000	Variable	

gammaglobulin, transcortin, fibrinogen, and thyroid-binding globulin also bind drugs; they tend to be more specific with respect to the drugs they bind, and they usually have a much smaller capacity for binding. There is, however, a great lack of information in this area.

DEPENDENCE OF BINDING ON PROTEIN AND DRUG CONCENTRATIONS

The effects of diseases and other conditions on drug binding are complex. Binding depends on the protein involved, the affinity between drug and protein, the drug concentration, the protein concentration, and the presence of other substances. Thus, diseases can alter binding in a number of ways.

Affinity

The extent of binding is, in large part, a function of the affinity of a protein for the drug. It is sometimes difficult to express affinity in a simple manner because each protein molecule often has multiple binding sites, each of which shows a different affinity. To demonstrate the role of affinity in determining the extent of binding however, we shall assume a simple interaction of a drug, D, with a protein, at a set of n equivalent sites to form a drug-protein complex, DP:

$$D + P = DP \tag{1}$$

From the law of mass action, it follows that

$$K = \frac{(DP)}{(D) \cdot (P)} \tag{2}$$

where (D), (P), and (DP) are the concentrations of drug, unbound sites on the protein, and the drug-protein complex, respectively, and K is the association equilibrium (or affinity) constant.

The extent of binding is most often expressed by the fraction of drug present that is bound to protein. It is the ratio of the bound concentration to the total concentration, bound plus unbound:

$$\text{fraction bound} = \frac{(DP)}{(D) + (DP)} \qquad (3)$$

On substituting Eq. 3 into Eq. 2 and rearranging,

$$\text{fraction bound} = \frac{K \cdot (P)}{1 + K(P)} \qquad (4)$$

It is apparent that the extent of binding depends on both the affinity constant, a measure of the avidity or strength of the association, and the concentration of unbound sites to which the drug can bind.

In pharmacokinetics, the fraction unbound, fu, is more useful than the fraction bound, and because $fu = (1 - \text{fraction bound})$, it follows that

$$fu = \frac{1}{1 + K \cdot (P)} \qquad (5)$$

Protein Concentration

With n sites on each protein molecule, the concentration of total sites $n \cdot (P_t)$ is

$$n \cdot (P_t) = (P) + (DP) \qquad (6)$$

where (P_t) is the total protein concentration. At low drug concentrations, that is, when (DP) is much smaller than $n \cdot (P_t)$, the concentration of unbound sites is virtually equal to $n \cdot (P_t)$; therefore,

$$fu = \frac{1}{1 + n \cdot K \cdot (P_t)} \qquad (7)$$

Figure 1 shows the fraction unbound of propranolol in patients with various diseases and in healthy volunteers as a function of the plasma concentration of α_1-acid glycoprotein, the protein to which this drug principally binds. From these data, it appears that the fraction unbound varies inversely with the protein concentration, as predicted by Eq. 7. Indeed, most of the variability in the fraction unbound (range 0.04–0.18) can be accounted for by the concentration of this protein. It is also apparent that elevated protein concentrations and reduced fractions unbound are common to those patients with Crohn's disease and arthritis. A number of conditions are known to alter protein concentrations, as listed in Table 2.

The extent of binding also depends on the drug concentration, as shown by Eq. 6. As the bound concentration (DP) approaches the total concentration of binding sites, the concentration of unbound sites (P) decreases, and, from Eq. 5, the fraction unbound increases. This change occurs because of a limited capacity of the protein to bind the drug. The capacity itself depends on the concentration of the protein and the number of binding sites per molecule.

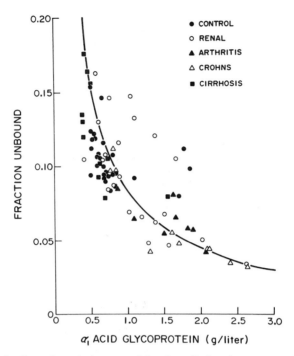

FIG. 1. The fraction unbound of propranolol varies with the plasma concentration of α_1-acid glycoprotein in 78 patients with various diseases and in healthy volunteers. The line, drawn through the data of Piafsky et al. (10), represents the relationship expected from Eq. 7, using a value of 11 liters g^{-1} (4.84 × 10^5 liters mole^{-1}) for nK. This relationship appears to account for most of the observed variability in the fraction unbound.

Figure 2 shows how the fraction unbound is expected to change with total drug concentration for a drug that is bound to albumin only (curve on right) and one that is bound to α_1-acid glycoprotein only (curve on left). One binding site per molecule and a fraction unbound of 0.05 at low concentrations are assumed for each drug. Clearly, when the total drug concentration approaches that of the protein, or, more accurately, that of the total binding sites, the fraction unbound is increased. When there is more than one binding site per molecule, the curve is shifted to the right by a factor of n.

Although both drugs shown in Fig. 2 have the same fraction unbound at low concentrations, it should be noted that the drug bound to α_1-acid glycoprotein has a greater affinity for this protein ($K = 1.27 \times 10^6$ liter mole^{-1}) than does the drug bound to albumin ($K = 3.17 \times 10^4$ liter mole^{-1}). As seen from Eq. 7, they are bound to the same extent at low concentrations because the concentration of albumin is 40 times greater than that of α_1-acid glycoprotein.

A change in the fraction unbound with concentration is referred to as concentration-dependent binding. It occurs for all drugs that bind to proteins. Whether or

TABLE 2. *Physiologic and pathologic conditions altering protein concentrations in plasma[a]*

	Albumin	α_1-Glycoprotein	Lipoprotein
Decreasing	Age (geriatric, neonate)	Fetal concentrations	Hyperthyroidism
	Bacterial pneumonia	Nephrotic syndrome	Injury
	Burns	Oral contraceptives	? Liver disease
	Cirrhosis of liver		Trauma
	Cystic fibrosis		
	GI Disease		
	Histoplasmosis		
	Leprosy		
	Liver abscess		
	Malignant neoplasms		
	Malnutrition (severe)		
	Multiple myeloma		
	Nephrotic syndrome		
	Pancreatitis (acute)		
	Pregnancy		
	Renal failure		
	Surgery		
	Trauma		
Increasing	Benign tumor	Age (geriatric)	Diabetes
	Exercise	Celiac disease	Hypothyroidism
	Hypothyroidism	Crohn's disease	? Liver disease
	? Neurological disease	Injury	Nephrotic
	Neurosis	Myocardial infarction	syndrome
	Paranoia	Renal failure	
	Psychosis	Rheumatoid arthritis	
	Schizophrenia	Stress	
		Surgery	
		Trauma	

[a]In the conditions listed, the protein concentrations are altered, on average, by 30% or more, and in some cases by more than 100%.
Data compiled from Jusko and Gretch (25), and from Friedman (43).

not it is expected in the usual therapeutic range of concentrations can be predicted if one knows the protein to which the drug binds and the therapeutic concentration range. For example, phenytoin binds to albumin (usual concentration 6×10^{-4} M), and the therapeutic range is 10 to 20 mg/liter ($0.4-0.8 \times 10^{-4}$ M); thus, therapeutic drug concentrations are an order of magnitude below the protein concentration, and virtually no concentration dependence is expected. Salicylate, on the other hand, has a therapeutic concentration range of 100 to 300 mg/liter ($7-22 \times 10^{-4}$ M) and because it is bound to albumin, concentration dependence is expected.

Figure 3 shows the influences of both protein and drug concentrations on the binding of salicylate. The rheumatoid arthritis patient has a lower albumin concentration than the volunteers in the other study. On correcting for the albumin

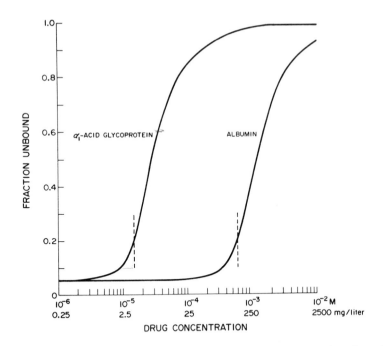

FIG. 2. The fraction unbound depends on the total plasma drug concentration, shown here in molarity and in milligrams per liter for a drug of molecular weight 250. For drugs bound to albumin, concentration-dependent binding is expected when the total concentration *(curve on right)* approaches the concentration of albumin (0.6 mM, *vertical dashed line on right*). Such behavior is observed at lower concentrations for drugs bound to α_1-acid glycoprotein *(curve on left)*, because the concentration, shown here, of this protein is only 0.015 mM *(vertical dashed line on left)*. With higher protein concentrations, or when there is more than one binding site per molecule of protein, the curves are shifted to the right. Note that the fraction unbound is independent of concentration at all values less than approximately one-tenth that of the protein to which the drug binds.

levels, much of the observed difference in binding is accounted for. This suggests that decreased binding in the patient is mainly a result of disease-associated hypoalbuminemia.

A number of additional factors must be considered to evaluate and predict binding of drugs to protein in plasma.

Multiple Proteins and Binding Sites

More than one protein often is involved. This is particularly the case for basic drugs, which have been shown to bind to more than just albumin. Sometimes three or more proteins contribute, as in the case of prednisolone.

On inspecting the data in Fig. 4 for prednisolone, it is apparent that neither binding to α_1-acid glycoprotein nor binding to albumin (Fig. 2) can explain the observed concentration dependence at a concentration of 0.1 to 0.5 mg/liter. This behavior may be explained by capacity-limited binding to transcortin, the glucocorticoid binding protein, in addition to both albumin and α_1-acid glycoprotein (12).

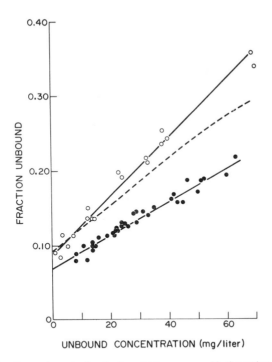

FIG. 3. The fraction unbound of salicylic acid increases with the unbound concentration in healthy volunteers *(filled circles)* and in a patient with rheumatoid arthritis *(open circles)*. The heavy lines are from linear least-squares regression. Note that the unbound concentration of 30 mg/liter corresponds to total values (C_u/fu) of 222 and 146 mg/liter in the volunteers and the arthritis patient, respectively. Much of the observed difference between these studies can be accounted for by the albumin concentrations. The volunteers had a serum albumin (mean 4.8 g/dl, range 4.5–5.2) quite different from that of the rheumatoid arthritis patient (3.6 g/dl). The dashed line is that predicted from Eq. 9 for the arthritis patient based on the serum albumin and the binding data in the volunteers. The data for the volunteers and the arthritis patient are from Furst et al. (11) and Rowland (6), respectively.

Frequently there is more than one binding site on a given protein. For example, using a model with two classes of sites for salicylic acid, albumin has been shown (13) to have an average of 2.2 sites of high affinity and 4.4 sites of weaker affinity per albumin molecule. In reality, there probably is a series of binding sites of varying affinity, but a model for such binding is complex and of questionable value because of the lack of accuracy in estimating the increased number of parameter values required. In such a model, the extent of binding can be expressed by

$$\frac{1 - fu}{fu} = (P_t) \cdot \left[\frac{K_1}{1 + K_1 \cdot (D)} + \frac{K_2}{1 + K_2 \cdot (D)} + \dots + \frac{K_n}{1 + K_n \cdot (D)} \right] \quad (8)$$

where $K_1, K_2, \dots, K_n$ are the affinity constants for each of the respective binding sites. At a given unbound concentration, the quantity in parentheses, K', is constant, and therefore a relationship similar to that of Eq. 5 is obtained:

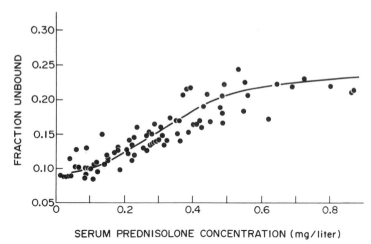

SERUM PREDNISOLONE CONCENTRATION (mg/liter)

FIG. 4. The fraction unbound of prednisolone increases at concentrations of 0.1 to 0.5 mg/liter in eight normal volunteers, suggesting that this drug binds to a protein at a much lower concentration than either albumin or α_1-acid glycoprotein. Data from Fig. 4 of Jusko and Rose (12).

$$fu = \frac{1}{1 + K' \cdot (P_t)} \tag{9}$$

The relationship is valid even if the concentration is in the range in which concentration dependence occurs or if there is more than one binding site. This is the basis of the comparison made in Fig. 3.

Displacement

Endogenous or exogenous substances can compete with a drug for binding sites on a protein. Such competition results in displacement and a decrease in the apparent affinity of the drug.

Coadministration of a drug may produce displacement, but for this to occur, the concentration of the displacing drug must approach the molar concentration of the sites on the binding protein; that is, it must appreciably reduce the sites available for binding. This is seen from the relationship

$$(P) = n \cdot (P_t) - (DP) - (XP) \tag{10}$$

when (XP) is the bound concentration of the displacer. In theory, any substance that shows concentration-dependent binding at usual therapeutic concentrations will also cause displacement of drugs that bind to the same site. For this reason, salicylate, phenylbutazone, and several sulfonamides are common displacers of drugs that bind to albumin. Drugs that bind to the same sites on α_1-acid glycoprotein, lipoprotein, or any other plasma protein and that show concentration dependence should also show displacement behavior (see Chapter 11).

Endogenous fatty acids have been shown to alter the binding of many drugs. For example, ingestion of fatty foods (14) reduces the binding of diazepam. Heparin,

frequently used to permit sampling of blood from indwelling catheters by preventing clotting, has been shown (15,16) to activate lipoprotein lipase, resulting in a decrease in plasma triglycerides and an increase in free fatty acids.

Decreased binding of propranolol (16) and quinidine (17) has been observed with the administration of heparin *in vivo*; however, as suggested by Piafsky (9), this may not be a consequence of elevated fatty acids, but rather a decrease in the concentration of lipoproteins, proteins to which these drugs also bind. Nonetheless, the use of heparin *in vivo* is a complication in binding studies and may be important, in specific situations, in terms of the continued activity of lipase *in vitro*, producing an increase in free fatty acids and decreased binding of drug.

Artifacts in binding studies, particularly for drugs binding to α_1-acid glycoprotein, can be introduced by the use of Vacutainer tubes, as recently reviewed by Piafsky (9). Plasticizers within the cap appear to displace a number of basic drugs from this protein (see Chapter 22).

Displacement by accumulation of drug metabolites can produce a change in binding, as has been suggested for phenylbutazone and its metabolite oxyphen-butazone (6), which are believed to bind to the same site on albumin, and for disopyramide and its monodealkylated metabolite (18), which bind to α_1-acid glycoprotein, although the latter is probably of little importance at the concentrations observed therapeutically. Whenever the concentration of a metabolite approaches that at which concentration-dependent binding occurs, altered binding of the drug should be anticipated. This may be at a relatively low concentration if either α_1-acid glycoprotein or another protein of limited capacity is primarily responsible for the binding. Renal and hepatic diseases are situations in which one might more frequently expect altered binding as a result of the accumulation of either drug metabolites or endogenous substances.

Other conditions are known to play roles in altering binding. For example, cooperative binding, produced perhaps by an allosteric change in protein structure, may alter the extent of binding. For example, free fatty acids, at low concentrations, increase binding of acidic drugs, presumably by a cooperative mechanism, but decrease binding at high concentrations, probably by displacement (7).

CONDITIONS ASSOCIATED WITH ALTERED BINDING

Many diseases and other conditions are known to alter plasma protein binding. Enough information is now available in some cases to make limited generalizations.

Renal Disease

The binding of virtually all acidic drugs that are primarily bound to albumin is decreased in renal disease, often by a factor of two to three (see Chapter 9). Part of this decrease is associated with hypoalbuminemia, but a decrease in the apparent affinity is mostly responsible and presumably is caused by accumulation of endogenous competitors (19).

Most of the studies on the effects of renal disease have compared binding in patients with uremia or the nephrotic syndrome with that in controls. There is currently insufficient information to draw any conclusions with regard to changes in renal function. The data in Fig. 5 for phenytoin suggest that, at least for this drug, the fraction unbound varies linearly with the serum creatinine.

With few exceptions, notably diazepam (21) and triamterene (22), the binding of bases does not appear to be altered in renal disease (9). This is probably a consequence of bases also binding to other plasma proteins. Although the concentration of albumin is decreased, α_1-acid glycoprotein is sometimes increased. This has led to the observation of increased binding for propranolol and chlorpromazine in those renal failure patients with associated inflammatory disease (10).

Hepatic Disease

As reviewed by Blaschke (1), large increases in the fraction unbound have been observed for a number of acidic drugs (e.g., tolbutamide, phenylbutazone, phenytoin, and thiopental) and for the basic drugs quinidine and diazepam in patients with liver disease. Two preliminary observations may be made. First, binding is primarily affected in chronic liver disease, especially cirrhosis, with only minor changes in acute viral hepatitis. Second, the decreased serum albumin in chronic liver disease probably explains the decreased binding of diazepam (23), but it may not account for all of the decreased binding observed for other drugs (22). Because of the variability observed in binding of drugs in hepatic disease however, it is difficult to generalize what changes are anticipated, except that chronic, rather than acute, disease appears to be more important.

Other Diseases

In the acute phases of many diseases, such as rheumatoid arthritis, Crohn's disease, myocardial infarction (see Chapter 6), malignancy, and ulcerative colitis,

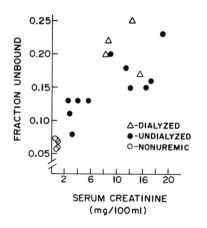

FIG. 5. The fraction unbound of phenytoin appears to be related to the serum creatinine in 15 uremic patients and 5 normal volunteers. (From Reidenberg et al., ref. 20, with permission.)

and in stress conditions, such as surgery and renal transplantation, the concentrations of α_1-acid glycoprotein (9) and other acute-phase proteins increase. The binding of basic drugs that interact with these proteins is expected to increase in these conditions, as has been observed for propranolol in patients with Crohn's disease and rheumatoid arthritis (10) and for quinidine in postsurgical patients (24).

Other Conditions

Many conditions are known, in addition to renal and hepatic disease, in which hypoalbuminemia occurs (25). As shown in Fig. 6, the serum albumin concentration decreases during pregnancy. In the absence of other complications, the binding of acidic drugs is therefore expected to be less in pregnant women (especially late in pregnancy) than in nonpregnant women (see Chapter 13 for more detailed discussion).

Severe burns may produce a pronounced decrease in serum albumin by movement of the protein to extravascular fluids and by loss through the burned area (26). Other conditions producing hypoalbuminemia include surgery, acute febrile infections, neoplastic disease, chronic bronchitis, and cystic fibrosis (25). Elevations of serum albumin have been observed in anxiety, neuroses, and psychoses (27), but these increases, although statistically significant, are generally not important.

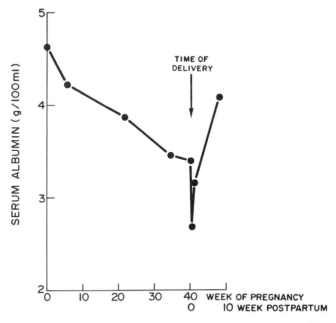

FIG. 6. The serum albumin concentration decreases during pregnancy and immediately after delivery, but quickly returns toward the value observed before pregnancy. These changes have implications with regard to the binding of acidic drugs to albumin. (Data from *Document Geigy, Scientific Tables*, 5th ed. S. Karger, New York, 1959, p. 273.)

ALTERED BINDING AND DRUG DISPOSITION

Because, on average, about 60% of the total albumin in the body is located outside plasma (25), more than just binding to proteins in plasma must be considered in evaluating and predicting the kinetic consequences of altered binding. Concurrent alterations may also occur in the binding to other constituents of the body. The following discussion, however, will be limited to changes in binding to the proteins located in plasma, lymph, and interstitial fluid.

Volume of Distribution

Øie and Tozer (28) have developed a model for the apparent volume of distribution V that takes into account the extravascular distribution of proteins and the intravascular, extravascular/extracellular, and intracellular fluid volumes, as follows:

$$V = V_p(1 + R_{E/l}) + fu \cdot V_p \cdot \left(\frac{V_E}{V_p} - R_{E/l} \right) + \frac{V_R \cdot fu}{fu_R} \qquad (11)$$

where V_P, V_E, and V_R are the volumes of plasma, extracellular fluid outside plasma, and fluids in the rest of the body, respectively; $R_{E/l}$ is the ratio of plasma protein within and outside the circulatory system; and fu_R is the fraction unbound outside the extracellular fluids.

For a drug bound to albumin, the relationship can be simplified. Using an average value of 1.4 for $R_{E/l}$ (25) and 3, 12, and 27 liters for V_P, V_E, and V_R, respectively, the equation becomes

$$V \text{ (in liters)} = 7.2 + 7.8fu + \frac{27fu}{fu_R} \qquad (12)$$

From this relationship it is apparent that the volume of distribution varies linearly with the fraction unbound. Furthermore, for a drug that is extensively bound to plasma proteins ($fu \to 0$) but not in the tissues ($fu_R \to 1$), the volume of distribution has a lower limit of about 7 liters, a value that is relatively insensitive to changes in the fraction unbound. Other consequences of this model have been examined by Tozer (29).

Figure 7 demonstrates the relationship between volume of distribution and the fraction unbound in plasma for propranolol, a drug that is extensively tissue-bound (i.e., fu_R is a small value). The volume here varies virtually in proportion to the value of the fraction unbound, as predicted by Eq. 12.

Clearance

The effect of altered plasma protein binding on clearance depends on the extraction ratio of the drug in the eliminating organ (31) (as discussed in detail in Chapters 1 and 3). Briefly, clearance, measured across the organ of elimination, is the product of blood flow and extraction ratio:

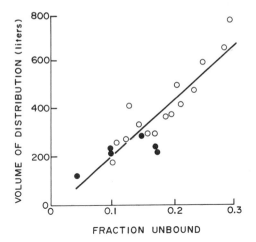

FIG. 7. The volume of distribution of (+)-propranolol varies with the fraction unbound in 6 control subjects *(filled circles)* and in 15 patients *(open circles)* with chronic liver disease. (Adapted from Branch et al., ref. 30, with permission.)

$$\text{clearance} = \text{blood flow} \times \text{extraction ratio} \qquad (13)$$

For a drug with an extraction ratio close to unity, clearance approaches blood flow, and virtually all of the drug is extracted, whether bound or not. For such a drug, clearance is not affected by changes in binding. On the other hand, if a drug is poorly extracted, has a low extraction ratio, then clearance, CL, depends on protein binding (31) as follows:

$$CL = fu \cdot CL_u \qquad (14)$$

where CL_u is the unbound clearance. The clearance of warfarin, an example of a low-extraction drug, has been shown (32) to vary with the fraction unbound. Other examples include disopyramide (33) and phenprocoumon (34).

Half-life

Half-life is an important measure of the speed of drug elimination, an index of the time required to approach steady state on continuous drug administration, and a determinant of the fluctuation of concentrations following intermittent dosing at fixed time intervals. The value of the half-life, $T_{1/2}$, depends on the values of clearance and the volume of distribution, as described in Chapter 1:

$$T_{1/2} = \frac{0.693 \cdot V}{CL} \qquad (15)$$

Changes in the half-life on altering binding can be anticipated from the dependence of these two parameters on plasma protein binding. In the extremes, drugs can be placed in four categories, in which they have either a large volume or low clearance, with dependence on protein binding, or a small volume or high clearance,

with little or no dependence on protein binding. Table 3 lists hypothetical drugs with these four combinations and the changes expected in the volume of distribution, clearance, and half-life on decreasing binding (increased fraction unbound). The two cases in which the half-life is altered deserve further attention.

Table 4 illustrates a drug typical of drug *B* in Table 3. The half-life of (+)-propranolol is increased in patients with reduced plasma protein binding. The explanation is an increase in volume of distribution and only a small change in clearance.

Drug *C*, for which a decrease in half-life is expected with a decrease in binding, is exemplified by the active clofibrate metabolite, *p*-chlorophenoxyisobutyric acid (36). In healthy individuals, 3.6% of the metabolite is unbound, whereas in patients with the nephrotic syndrome the value is 11%. The half-life of the metabolite is considerably shorter (12 hr) in the nephrotic patients than in the controls (21 hr). Although no volume of distribution was given, the value is probably close to 10 liters, a condition approaching that of drug *C*. Such an observation of a decreased half-life could easily be interpreted as an increased metabolism in renal disease, when, in reality, the decrease is simply a function of decreased plasma protein binding.

TABLE 3. *Pharmacokinetic consequences of decreased binding to plasma proteins*

	Characteristics of drug		Changes in		
Drug	Clearance	Volume of distribution (liters)	Volume of distribution	Clearance	Half-life
A	High[a]	8	↔[b]	↔	↔
B	High	100	↑	↔	↑
C°	Low[c]	8	↔	↑	↓
D	Low	100	↑	↑	↔

[a]Extraction ratio close to 1.0.
[b]Symbols: ↔, little or no change; ↑, increase; ↓, decrease.
[c]Extraction ratio less than 0.1.

TABLE 4. *Relationship between half-life and fraction unbound for propranolol*

	Subject					
	1	2	3	4	5	6
Fraction unbound	0.049	0.058	0.065	0.070	0.085	0.090
Half-life (min)	204	240	216	288	360	336

From Evans and Shand (35), with permission.

For drugs showing saturable binding, the values of clearance, volume, and half-life change with drug concentration in plasma. The theoretical pharmacokinetic consequences of saturable binding, following single intravenous doses, have been simulated by McNamara et al. (37) and Øie et al. (38).

ALTERED BINDING AND DRUG AVAILABILITY

Altered binding to plasma proteins, of itself, is not expected to alter drug availability, with one exception, that is, when extensive metabolism occurs in the liver or gut wall. Drugs with this characteristic have, in common, low availabilities because of the loss on first passing through these organs, the first-pass effect (see Chapter 3).

Binding to plasma proteins impedes the removal of drug from blood as it passes through the liver. Because it is the fraction escaping loss that becomes available to the rest of the body, a small decrease in the extraction, because of increased binding, can produce a large increase in the amount available. The increased availability is accompanied, however, by decreases in the volume of distribution and half-life (see Table 4). The therapeutic consequences of this situation in maintenance therapy probably are minor because the increased availability after oral administration is compensated for by decreased distribution to the tissues and an increased elimination rate constant for the drug, as reflected by a shortened half-life (31).

Figure 8 shows the plasma concentrations of propranolol in patients with Crohn's disease and in volunteers after a single 40-mg oral dose. The increased peak concentration in the diseased patients suggests increased availability or decreased vol-

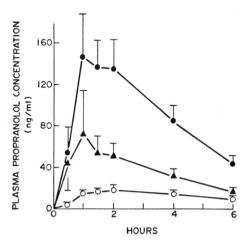

FIG. 8. The mean (± SE) plasma propranolol concentrations following a 40-mg oral dose are much higher and more variable in 16 patients with Crohn's disease than in 13 healthy volunteers *(open circles).* The concentrations are greater in patients with erythrocyte sedimentation rates >20 mm/hr *(filled circles)* than in patients with values ≤20 mm/hr *(filled triangles).* (Adapted from Schneider et al., ref. 39, with permission.)

ume, or both. The observation is probably a result of an elevated concentration of α_1-acid glycoprotein, the acute-phase protein to which propranolol primarily binds. An increased availability, a decreased volume of distribution, and a shortened half-life are consistent with the data, but, unfortunately, protein binding was not measured in these studies to verify the mechanism of the alteration. This study emphasizes the importance of performing protein binding measurements to properly interpret data.

Following parenteral administration, availability is unaffected by increased binding, and because of the increase in the elimination rate constant for the drug, the average unbound concentration following chronic administration is expected to be lowered.

DOSAGE REQUIREMENTS

Altered dosage requirements are anticipated in a few situations in which binding is altered. First, for a highly extracted drug like propranolol, dosage requirements are expected to be diminished on parenteral administration if binding is decreased (and the converse if binding is increased), as noted earlier for patients with acute inflammatory disease. The same applies to a highly extracted drug with a small volume of distribution, drug A in Table 3. Here, however, the half-life does not change with binding. Decreased chronic dosage requirements with decreased binding are anticipated because of a decrease in the unbound clearance (see Eqs. 13 and 14).

For a drug like drug C in Table 3, decreased binding shortens the half-life, but the unbound clearance remains unchanged. Here, the rate of administration, oral or parenteral, to maintain the same average unbound concentration, is unchanged; however, because of the shortened half-life, the drug may need to be administered more frequently if large fluctuations in the unbound concentration or amount in the body are unacceptable.

Loading dose requirements may be altered for a drug with a small volume of distribution and a low clearance, drug C in Table 3. For such a drug, most of that in the body is bound to plasma protein throughout extracellular fluid. Although a change in binding will not appreciably affect the volume of distribution or the total concentration, the unbound concentration for a given dose will be much greater if the binding is decreased, and vice versa. This is seen from Eq. 12 and the relationship

$$V = Vu \cdot fu \qquad (16)$$

The volume of distribution based on the unbound drug, Vu, is then

$$Vu = \frac{7.2}{fu} + 7.8 + \frac{27}{fu_R} \qquad (17)$$

For a drug with $fu = 0.01$ and $fu_R = 1.0$, the unbound volume is 755 liters. On increasing fu to 0.02, the unbound volume decreases to 395 liters. The same argument applies to drug A in Table 3, if it is parenterally administered. On oral

administration, however, decreased availability with decreased binding tends to compensate for the smaller apparent unbound volume of distribution produced.

In Table 5, protein binding values are presented for selected drugs for which the fraction bound to plasma proteins is greater than 90%, a condition in which changes in binding might be expected to have the greatest impact. Selected drugs are classified according to their clearance and volume characteristics as defined in Table 3. Drugs with more than one letter designation are intermediate between the categories. One must keep in mind that many factors besides protein binding are altered in diseases and other conditions. The foregoing discussion assumes changes in plasma protein binding only.

MONITORING PLASMA CONCENTRATIONS

In conditions of altered binding, how total plasma concentrations are interpreted is critical. Because the unbound drug is assumed to be active, it follows that equivalent therapeutic activity will be found when

$$fu \cdot C = fu' \cdot C' \tag{18}$$

where fu and fu' and C and C' are the fractions unbound and total plasma concentrations in conditions of normal and altered binding, respectively. To determine C', information on the change in fu is required, as follows:

$$C' = \frac{fu}{fu'} \cdot C \tag{19}$$

Considerable data are now available for a few drugs on the change in fu in various diseases, especially renal failure, and other conditions. For example, knowing that the usual therapeutic range of phenytoin is 10 to 20 mg/liter and that the fraction unbound in patients with uremia is 0.25, compared with 0.1 in the presence of normal renal function, the therapeutic range in uremic patients is then, on average, 4 to 8 mg/liter (see Chapter 9, pp.158–159).

The fraction unbound depends on the concentration of the binding protein, and, in uremia, there often is great variability in the serum albumin, the protein to which phenytoin binds. Changes in both apparent affinity of albumin for the drug and protein concentration can be taken into account. Because phenytoin binding does not show concentration dependence in the therapeutic range, Eq. 9 can be used to approximate its binding. Using a value of 4.3 g/dl for normal serum albumin, the fraction unbound is

$$fu = \frac{1}{1 + 2.1(P_t)} \tag{20}$$

where 2.1 is the value of $n \cdot K$ that gives a fraction unbound of 0.1 at the usual albumin concentration. Similarly, using a serum albumin of 3.4 g/dl for a typical uremic patient and a value of 0.25 for the fraction unbound, we obtain

TABLE 5. Selected drugs exhibiting greater than 90% plasma protein binding in healthy volunteers classified according to clearance and volume characteristics as defined in Table 3[a]

Drug	% Bound	Category (based on Table 3)	Drug	% Bound	Category (based on Table 3)	Drug	% Bound	Category (based on Table 3)
Acetazolamide	90		Digitoxin	90 ± 2	C,D	Nifedipine	≥90	
Alclofenac	90		Diphenhydramine	98		Nitrazepam	90	
Amitriptyline	96 ± 8	B	Doxycycline	82–93	D	Nortriptyline	94.5 ± 0.6	B,D
Amphotericin B	>90	D	Etidocaine	94		Oxazepam	90	
Atenolol	96	C,D	Fenoprofen	99		Perphenazine	97	
Azapropazone	95		Flurbiprofen	99.5		Phenylbutazone	98–99	
Bromocriptine	96		Furosemide	95.9 ± 2.0	C	Phenytoin	89 ± 23	C
Bumetanide	95		Fusidic acid	96		Pimozide	97	
Bupivacaine	96		Glibenclamide	99		Prazosin	93 ± 2	B,D
Buprenorphine	96		Glibornuride	95		Propranolol	93.3 ± 1.2	B
Carbenoxolone	99		Glipizide	92		Protriptyline	92 ± 0.6	D
Chlordiazepoxide	96		Haloperidol	92		Quinacrine	90	
Chlorothiazide	94.6 ± 1.3	C	Heparin	95		Spironolactone	98	
Chlorpromazine	95–98	B	Hydralazine	90		Sulfisoxazole	88–92	C
Clindamycin	93.6 ± 0.2	B,D	Hydrocortisone	90–95		Sulindac	93	
Clofibrate	96.5 ± 2.0	C	Ibuprofen	99		Sulfinpyrazone	98.5	
Clotrimazole	93		Imipramine	89–94	B,D	Thioridazine	96	
Cloxacillin	95		Indomethacin	90		Thyroxine	99	
Desipramine	92 ± 1	B	Ketoprofen	92		Tolamolol	90	
Diazoxide	90		Loperamide	97		Tolbutamide	93 ± 1	C
Diazepam	98.7 ± 0.2	D	Lorazepam	93 ± 2	D	Tolmetin	90	
Diclofenac	99.7		Metolazone	95		Valproic acid	93 ± 4	C
Dicloxacillin	94.4 ± 1.9	C	Miconazole	98		Verapamil	90	
Dicoumarol	99		Nalidixic acid	93		Warfarin	99	C
Diflunisol	98		Naproxen	98–99				

[a]Selected drugs are classified according to their clearance and volume characteristics as defined in Table 3. Data compiled from Benet and Sheiner (44), and from Heel and Avery (45).

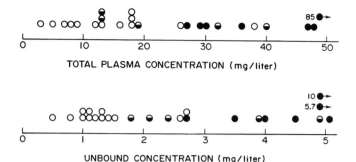

FIG. 9. Less overlap occurs in the unbound concentrations than in the total concentrations that are associated with no toxicity *(open circles)*, mild toxicity *(half-filled circles)*, and more severe toxicity *(filled circles)* with phenytoin. Mild toxicity includes horizontal and vertical nystagmus; severe toxicity includes ataxia, mental confusion, and slurred speech. (Adapted from Booker and Darcey, ref. 41, with permission.)

$$fu' = \frac{1}{1 + 0.9(P_t')} \qquad (21)$$

and the ratio of the fraction unbound in the uremic patient to the normal value is

$$\frac{fu'}{fu} = \frac{10}{1 + 0.9(P_t')} \qquad (22)$$

Thus, both the presence of severe renal function impairment and the serum albumin can be used to interpret a measured phenytoin concentration.

Similar rules for adjusting a measured total concentration can be developed for other drugs. Sheiner and Tozer (40) have suggested that plasma concentrations can, in general, be adjusted using the relationship

$$\frac{fu'}{fu} = \frac{1}{fu + (1 - fu)(P_t'/P_t)} \qquad (23)$$

when a change in binding is due solely to a change in albumin concentration. The information needed is the usual fraction unbound, the serum albumin in the patient (P_t'), and the usual serum albumin, 4.3 g/dl. It should be emphasized, however, that such rules do not preclude the need for a rapid, accurate, and inexpensive means of determining the unbound concentration.

The value of using unbound concentrations is illustrated in Fig. 9. The overlap of total concentrations showing no toxicity, mild toxicity, and more severe toxicity is much greater than that observed for the unbound concentrations. Variability in protein binding simply adds to the variability in the observed effect-concentration relationship.

If the use of unbound concentrations were to become routine, the need for an understanding of the implications of altered binding would be greatly reduced,

except perhaps for the few cases in which changes in dosage requirements are anticipated.

REFERENCES

1. Blaschke, T. F. (1977): Protein binding and kinetics of drugs in liver disease. *Clin. Pharmacokinet.*, 2:32–44.
2. Gugler, R., and Azarnoff, D. L. (1976): Drug protein binding and the nephrotic syndrome. *Clin. Pharmacokinet.*, 1:25–35.
3. Jusko, W. J. (1976): Pharmacokinetics in disease states changing protein binding. In: *The Effect of Disease States on Drug Pharmacokinetics*, edited by L. Z. Benet, pp. 99–124. American Pharmaceutical Association, Washington, D.C.
4. Keen, P. (1971): Effect of binding to plasma proteins on the distribution, activity, and elimination of drugs. In: *Concepts in Biochemical Pharmacology*, Part 1, edited by B. Brodie and J. Gillette, pp. 212–233. Springer-Verlag, New York.
5. Klotz, U. (1976): Pathophysiological and disease-induced changes in drug distribution volume: Pharmacokinetic implications. *Clin. Pharmacokinet.*, 1:204–218.
6. Rowland, M. (1980): Plasma protein binding and therapeutic drug monitoring. *Ther. Drug Monitor.*, 2:29–37.
7. Tillement, J. P., Lhoste, F., and Giudicelli, J. F. (1978): Disease and drug protein binding. *Clin. Pharmacokinet.*, 3:144–154.
8. Vallner, J. J. (1977): Binding of drugs by albumin and plasma protein. *J. Pharm. Sci.*, 66:447–465.
9. Piafsky, K. M. (1980): Disease-induced changes in the plasma binding of basic drugs. *Clin. Pharmacokinet.*, 5:246–262.
10. Piafsky, K. M., Borga, O., Odar-Cederlof, I., Johansson, C., and Sjoqvist, F. (1978): Increased plasma protein binding of propranolol and chlorpromazine mediated by disease-induced elevations of plasma α_1-acid glycoprotein. *N. Engl. J. Med.*, 299:1435–1439.
11. Furst, D. E., Tozer, T. N., and Melmon, K. L. (1979): Salicylate clearance, the resultant of protein binding and metabolism. *Clin. Pharmacol. Ther.*, 26:380–389.
12. Jusko, W. J., and Rose, J. Q. (1980): Monitoring prednisone and prednisolone. *Ther. Drug Monitor.*, 2:169–176.
13. Borga, O., Odar-Cederlof, I., Ringsberger, V., and Norlin, A. (1976): Protein binding of salicylate in uremic and normal plasma. *Clin. Pharmacol. Ther.*, 20:464–475.
14. Colburn, W. A., and Gibaldi, M. (1978): Plasma protein binding of diazepam after a single dose of sodium oleate. *J. Pharm. Sci.*, 67:891–892.
15. Asmal, A. C., Leary, W. P., Thandroyen, F., Botha, J., and Watrus, S. (1979): A dose-response study of the anticoagulant and lipolytic activities of heparin in normal subjects. *Br. J. Clin. Pharmacol.*, 7:531–533.
16. Wood, M., Shand, D. G., and Wood, A. J. J. (1979): Altered drug binding due to the use of indwelling heparinized cannulas (heparin lock) for sampling. *Clin. Pharmacol. Ther.*, 25:103–107.
17. Kessler, K. M., Leech, R. C., and Spann, J. F. (1979): Blood collection techniques, heparin, and quinidine protein binding. *Clin. Pharmacol. Ther.*, 25:204–210.
18. Hinderling, P. H., Bres, J., and Garrett, E. R. (1974): Protein binding and erythrocyte partitioning of disopyramide and its monodealkylated metabolite. *J. Pharm. Sci.*, 63:1684–1690.
19. Sjoholm, I., Kober, A., Odar-Cederlof, I., and Borga, O. (1976): Protein binding of drugs in uremic and normal serum: The role of endogenous inhibitors. *Biochem. Pharmacol.*, 25:1205–1213.
20. Reidenberg, M. M., Odar-Cederlof, I., von Bahr, C., Borga, O., and Sjoqvist, F. (1971): Protein binding of diphenylhydantoin and desmethylimipramine in plasma from patients with poor renal function. *N. Engl. J. Med.*, 285:264–267.
21. Kober, A., Sjoholm, I., Borga, O., and Odar-Cederlof, I. (1979): Protein binding of diazepam and digitoxin in uremic and normal serums. *Biochem. Pharmacol.*, 28:1037–1042.
22. Reidenberg, M. M., and Affrime, M. (1973): Influence of disease on binding of drugs to plasma proteins. *Ann. N.Y. Acad. Sci.*, 226:115–126.
23. Thiessen, J. J., Sellers, E. M., Denbeigh, P., and Dolman, L. (1976): Plasma protein binding of diazepam and tolbutamide in chronic alcoholics. *J. Clin. Pharmacol.*, 16:345–351.

24. Fremstad, O., Bergerud, K., Huffner, J. F. W., and Lunde, P. K. M. (1976): Increased plasma binding of quinidine after surgery: A preliminary report. *Eur. J. Clin. Pharmacol.*, 10:441–444.
25. Jusko, W. J., and Gretch, M. (1976): Plasma and tissue protein binding of drugs in pharmacokinetics. *Drug Metab. Rev.*, 5:43–140.
26. Birke, G., Liljedahl, S. O., Plantin, L. O., and Wetterfors, J. (1960): Albumin catabolism in burns and following surgical procedures. *Acta Chir. Scand.*, 118:353–366.
27. Casey, A. E., Gilbert, F. E., Copeland, H., Downey, E. L., and Casey, J. G. (1973): Albumin, alpha 1, 2, beta, and gamma globulin in cancer and other diseases. *South. Med. J.*, 66:179–185.
28. Øie, S., and Tozer, T. N. (1979): Effect of altered plasma protein binding on apparent volume of distribution. *J. Pharm. Sci.*, 68:1203–1205.
29. Tozer, T. N. (1981): Concepts basic to pharmacokinetics. *Pharmacol. Therap.*, 12:109–131.
30. Branch, R. A., Jones, J., and Reed, A. E. (1976): A study of factors influencing drug disposition in chronic liver disease, using the model drug (±)-propranolol. *Br. J. Clin. Pharmacol.*, 3:243–249.
31. Wilkinson, G. R., and Shand, D. G. (1975): A physiological approach to hepatic drug clearance. *Clin. Pharmacol. Ther.*, 18:377–390.
32. Levy, G., and Yacobi, A. (1974): Effect of plasma protein binding on elimination of warfarin. *J. Pharm. Sci.*, 63:805–806.
33. Meffin, P. J., Robert, E. W., Winkle, R. A., Harapat, S., Peters, F. A., and Harrison, D. C. (1979): Role of concentration-dependent plasma protein binding in disopyramide disposition. *J. Pharmacokinet. Biopharm.*, 7:29–46.
34. Trenk, D., and Jahnchen, E. (1980): Effect of serum protein binding on pharmacokinetics and anticoagulant activity of phenprocoumon in rats. *J. Pharmacokinet. Biopharm.*, 8:177–191.
35. Evans, G. H., and Shand, D. G. (1975): Disposition of propranolol. VI. Independent variation in steady-state circulating drug concentrations and half-life as a result of plasma drug binding in man. *Clin. Pharmacol. Ther.*, 14:494–500.
36. Gugler, R., Shoeman, D. W., Huffman, D. H., Cohlmia, J. B., and Azarnoff, D. L. (1975): Pharmacokinetics of drugs in patients with the nephrotic syndrome. *J. Clin. Invest.*, 55:1182–1189.
37. McNamara, P. J., Levy, G., and Gibaldi, M. (1979): Effect of plasma protein and tissue binding on the time course of drug concentration in plasma. *J. Pharmacokinet. Biopharm.*, 7:195–206.
38. Øie, S., Guentert, T. W., and Tozer, T. N. (1980): Effect of saturable binding on the pharmacokinetics of drugs: A simulation. *J. Pharm. Pharmacol.*, 32:471–477.
39. Schneider, R. E., Bishop, H., and Hawkins, C. F. (1979): Plasma propranolol concentrations and the erythrocyte sedimentation rate. *Br. J. Clin. Pharmacol.*, 8:43–47.
40. Sheiner, L. B., and Tozer, T. N. (1978): Clinical pharmacokinetics: The use of plasma concentrations of drugs. In: *Clinical Pharmacology: Basic Principles in Therapeutics*, 2nd ed., edited by K. L. Melmon and H. F. Morelli, pp. 71–109. Macmillan, New York.
41. Booker, H. E., and Darcey, B. (1973): Serum concentrations of free diphenylhydantoin and their relationship to clinical intoxication. *Epilepsia*, 14:177–184.
42. LeLorier, J., Moisan, R., Gagne, J., and Caille, G. (1977): Effect of the duration of infusion on the disposition of lidocaine in dogs. *J. Pharmacol. Exp. Ther.*, 203:507–511.
43. Friedman, R. B., Anderson, Eutine, S. M., and Hirshberg, S. B. (1980): Effects of diseases on clinical laboratory tests. *Clin. Chem.*, 26.
44. Benet, L. Z., and Sheiner, L. B. (1980): Design and optimization of dosage regimens: Pharmacokinetic data. In: *The Pharmacological Basis of Therapeutics*, 6th ed., edited by A. G. Gilman, L. S. Goodman, and A. Gilman, pp. 1675–1737. Macmillan, New York.
45. Heel, R. C., and Avery, G. S. (1980): Drug data information. In: *Drug Treatment: Principles and Practice of Clinical Pharmacology and Therapeutics*, 2nd ed., edited by G. S. Avery, pp. 1211–1223. ADIS Press, New York.

Pharmacokinetic Basis for Drug Treatment,
edited by L. Z. Benet et al., Raven Press,
New York © 1984

Chapter 11

Pharmacokinetic Drug Interactions

Susan M. Pond

*Medical Service and Division of Clinical Pharmacology, San Francisco General Hospital
Medical Center, and Department of Medicine, University of California at San Francisco,
San Francisco, California 94110*

Strictly speaking, the word *interaction* implies a mutual effect. Thus, a drug-drug interaction occurs when two drugs given together both affect the pharmacokinetics or pharmacodynamics, or both, of each other. In reality, an interaction may only be unidirectional in that one drug is affected and the other is unaffected.

Drugs may interact on a pharmaceutical, pharmacodynamic, or pharmacokinetic basis. Pharmaceutical interactions may occur when drugs are mixed inappropriately in syringes and in infusion fluids before administration and are inactivated. Pharmacodynamic interactions arise when drugs act on the same receptors, sites of action, or physiologic systems. Pharmacokinetic interactions occur when one drug interferes with the absorption, transport, distribution, or elimination of another. More than one primary pharmacokinetic parameter (rate of absorption, unbound serum drug concentration, volume of distribution, systemic clearance, and renal clearance) may be altered. For example, quinidine decreases the volume of distribution and the renal and nonrenal clearances of digoxin (1,2). Phenylbutazone displaces warfarin from plasma protein-binding sites but also inhibits its metabolism (3,4).

INCIDENCE

The potential for drug interactions to occur in clinical practice is limitless. Polypharmacy, which increases the likelihood of drug interactions, is common medical practice. A hospitalized patient is likely to be treated with five or more drugs simultaneously (5,6). Polypharmacy is not restricted to hospital patients. Outpatients also receive prescriptions for a number of drugs at the same time (7,8). Some of the drug combinations are prescribed intentionally to take advantage of interactions to increase therapeutic effect. For example, the efficacy of penicillin is enhanced by concurrent administration of probenecid; standard drug combinations are used to treat anxiety/depressive states and phobic anxieties.

Despite the sometimes therapeutic advantages of drug combinations, most attention has been directed toward the public health hazards of drug interactions that

195

cause unexpected toxicity, heightened pharmacologic response, or therapeutic failure. Epidemiologic studies (Fig. 1) have demonstrated clearly that the rate of adverse reactions to drugs increase with an increase in the number of drugs prescribed simultaneously (9,10). Many of the adverse drug reactions can be ascribed to adverse drug interactions. Talley and Laventurier (11), who surveyed 42,000 patients receiving prescribed drugs, estimated that 7.6% were given drugs known to interact. Stewart and Cluff (12) interviewed 75 patients taking prescription and nonprescription drugs and found that 51.7% of the patients had taken a combination known to interact. Potential drug interactions were identified in 24.2% of 662 patients by Mitchell et al. (13). Robinson (14) estimated that a drug formulary limited to 200 drugs had theoretically 19,900 pairs of combinations. Even if a small fraction of these drug combinations resulted in clinically important drug interactions, the ability of the clinician to commit them to memory or to be alert to their recognition would be exceeded. The problem of their recognition is also compounded by the many over-the-counter nonprescription drugs that patients take, as well as tobacco, alcohol, and food, all of which can potentially interact with prescribed drugs.

The likelihood of a drug interaction is easier to define than is the actual number of interactions that have clinically important consequences. Recognition that an adverse drug reaction is due to an interaction is hampered by many factors. New symptoms during treatment may be attributed to underlying disease or to a reaction to a single drug; these also may be caused by an idiosyncratic response by the patient rather than by an interaction. Furthermore, therapeutic failure may not be easily recognized if an intermittent manifestation of a disease, such as an epileptic seizure or arrhvthmia, is being "treated." Despite the difficulties in recognizing

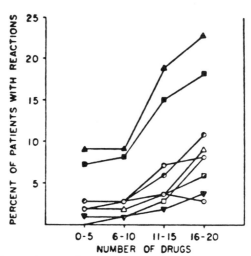

FIG. 1. Rate of adverse drug reactions in relationship to number of drugs prescribed for nine groups of drugs: analgesic *(filled inverted triangles)*, antacid *(half-filled circles)*, antiarrhythmic *(open circles)*, anticoagulant *(filled squares)*, antihypertensive *(filled triangles)*, antiinflammatory *(half-filled squares)*, antimicrobic *(open circles with dot)*, diuretic *(open triangles)*, sedative-tranquilizer *(open squares)*. (From May et al., ref. 9, with permission.)

consequences of drug interactions, clinical awareness of drug interactions has increased. One has only to review the literature on drug interactions to realize that the published reports of animal and human studies and anecdotal case reports form an enormous compilation. How does a clinician wade through this information to identify those interactions that are important for patient management? The answer to this question is complex. Major problems arise when one reviews the data bases. Many of the studies of drug interactions have had limitations. Some of the human reports are based on a single case and are not substantiated by adequate pharmacokinetic or pharmacodynamic studies in additional patients. Some of the reports are based on studies done in healthy volunteers receiving drugs under conditions that are not relevant to the usual clinical situation of the patient. It is not uncommon to find that the dosage regimen used in experimental studies differs from the usual regimen given to a patient. Some interactions occur only when two drugs are given at the same time. For example, a significant impairment of the absorption of tetracycline was observed in five healthy male students who concurrently took ferrous sulfate (15). Gothoni et al. (16) later demonstrated that iron did not interfere with tetracycline absorption if it was given more than 3 hr before or 2 hr after tetracycline. Some studies relate to drugs that are not frequently prescribed together, and on this ground they can be regarded as clinically insignificant. Some purported drug interactions have not been substantiated by other investigators. Often differences between studies, such as in different types of experimental subjects; insufficient numbers of subjects; lack of control for age, sex, and concurrent intake of other drugs; use of marijuana, tobacco, or alcohol; and presence or absence of disease; create apparent differences in results. Animal studies in many cases are not of predictive value for humans because of species differences in drug responses and pharmacokinetics and because of difficulty in assessing which drug response in animals is relevant to patients. The interaction recognized recently in humans between digoxin and quinidine was studied in the dog (17). In humans, serum digoxin concentrations are increased when quinidine is added to the therapeutic regimen (1,2). In part, the increase in digoxin concentration is due to a decrease in digoxin clearance. No such alteration in digoxin clearance was observed in eight dogs (17). Many pharmacokinetic drug interactions do not describe accurately the primary pharmacokinetic parameters. For example, the interpretation of some studies is based on changes in plasma half-life, which may be influenced by both volume of distribution and clearance (see Chapter 1). These studies are at best descriptive and cannot lead to the definition of mechanisms of purported interactions. Even when a pharmacokinetic interaction is demonstrated experimentally, the alteration in pharmacokinetics may not lead to an alteration in clinical response or to enhanced drug toxicity. For example, in one study, although verapamil increased the steady state plasma concentrations of digoxin to levels that would be considered toxic for most patients, no increase in the incidence of digoxin toxicity was observed (18); verapamil may have protected against expression of digoxin toxicity in these patients. In another study, probenecid caused marked changes in the pharmacokinetics

of furosemide but did not alter the latter drug's 8-hr natriuretic or diuretic effect (19).

To enable the clinician to anticipate and prevent undesired interactions without relying on memory or cumbersome lists, two general approaches have been taken. The first approach is to focus on short lists of drugs, such as warfarin, theophylline, tolbutamide, salicylate, digoxin, lidocaine, methotrexate, and lithium, which have steep dose–response curves or low therapeutic indices. Interactions with such drugs are potentially lethal, either by enhanced toxicity or prevention of therapeutic effect. The second approach is to use the basic pharmacologic knowledge of mechanisms of drug action, physiologic alterations produced by a drug, or pharmacokinetic characteristics to predict potential drug interactions. A recent editorial (20) called for the clinician to use such knowledge by being "the prepared observer." The remainder of this chapter will focus on pharmacokinetic drug interactions, discussing sites of interaction, describing mechanisms, when known, and highlighting well-documented, clinically important examples of drug combinations that interact. The common thread of the discussion will be the effect of the interaction on the unbound drug concentration that may predict an alteration in pharmacologic effect.

CLASSIFICATION

Pharmacokinetic interactions can be classified in many ways. One frequent classification describes the sites at which interactions occur; this classification is listed in Table 1. The second approach is to describe the interaction in terms of alteration in a primary pharmacokinetic parameter, i.e., rate and extent of availability, volume of distribution, hepatic and renal clearance. The lists are not mutually exclusive; for example, altered gastrointestinal absorption may lead to an altered absorption rate and altered bioavailability of a drug, each having possible therapeutic consequences. Hepatic clearance of certain drugs can be altered by both the change in drug-metabolizing enzymes and the hepatic blood flow. Renal clearance can be altered by changing plasma protein binding, urinary pH and flow, and renal blood flow. This discussion follows the more usual classification of describing the sites of interaction.

TABLE 1. *Sites of pharmacokinetic drug interactions*

---

1. Gastrointestinal tract
2. Plasma protein- or tissue-binding sites
3. Drug-metabolizing enzyme systems
   a. Enzymes
   b. Organ blood flow
4. Biliary excretion and enterohepatic circulation
5. Renal excretion

Gastrointestinal Absorption

An important distinction must be made between the extent of drug absorption (bioavailability) and the rate of drug absorption (see Chapter 2). Pharmacokinetically, an interaction may increase or decrease either the rate or extent of drug absorption. The attainment of an early or late peak plasma concentration of drug will have no clinical significance if the ultimate pharmacologic effect of the drug is dependent on the total area under the blood or plasma concentration/time curve during a dosing interval. Clinical consequences could result if the pharmacologic effect is dependent on the rate of drug entry into the systemic circulation. For example, a delay in the rate but not extent of absorption of aspirin may delay the onset of pain relief. On the other hand, a similar interaction when the drug has been administered for its antiinflammatory effects may not have clinical significance. Prescott (21) has outlined the many potential mechanisms of drug interactions during absorption, as listed in Table 2.

The three major factors that determine drug absorption are the physicochemical characteristics of the drug and its dosage form, the nature of the biologic membrane that the drug has to cross, and the physiologic characteristics near the site of drug absorption. (These factors are reviewed more extensively in Chapter 2.)

To be absorbed from the gastrointestinal tract, a drug must dissolve in gastrointestinal fluids. The properties of gastrointestinal fluids can influence blood absorption by affecting dissolution rate. An example is provided by the reduction in absorption of tetracycline caused by coadministration of sodium bicarbonate (Fig. 2) (22). For this drug, the extent of absorption is decreased when the solid drug is administered in the capsule dosage form together with sodium bicarbonate, but not when the tetracycline is administered in solution together with the antacid (22).

According to the pH partition hypothesis, only nonionized, lipophilic drug penetrates the intestinal mucosa. Therefore, gastrointestinal pH could also influence drug absorption by influencing the rate and extent of penetration of the drug across the lipid-absorptive membrane. However, this theoretic effect has been difficult to demonstrate in humans. Drugs, such as antacids, that can alter gastric and intestinal pH, have complex and unpredictable effects on the absorption of other drugs (23–

TABLE 2. *Some mechanisms of drug absorption interactions*

---

pH Effects on drug ionization and dissolution
Changes in gastrointestinal motility
Modification of gastric emptying rate
Complex, ion pair, and chelate formation
Interference with active transport
Disruption of lipid micelles
Changes in splanchnic blood flow
Toxic effects on gastrointestinal mucosa
Changes in volume, composition, and viscosity of secretions
Effects on mucosal and bacterial drug metabolism

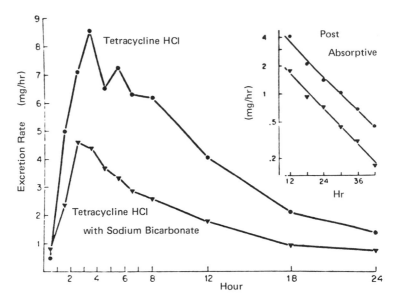

FIG. 2. Effect of sodium bicarbonate on absorption of tetracycline hydrochloride. Filled circles indicate mean urinary excretion rates in subjects receiving a 250-mg tetracycline HCl capsule with 200 ml water. Filled triangles indicate results in same subjects receiving tetracycline in 200 ml water containing 2.0·g sodium bicarbonate. Inset presents semilogarithmic plots of urinary excretion rates in the postabsorption phase and shows similar half-life periods of elimination of tetracycline. (From Barr et al., ref. 22, with permission.)

25). Effects of antacids on aspirin are complex. On the one hand, antacids could raise the pH of the gastric contents, reduce lipid solubility of the drug, and decrease gastric absorption, thus favoring absorption in the small bowel. On the other hand, if concurrent alkalinization of the urine is significant, urinary salicylate excretion will be favored. Antacids not only alter gastrointestinal fluid pH but also chelate drugs (tetracycline plus divalent-cation antacids) (26), precipitate drugs (ferrous sulfate plus calcium carbonate), or inhibit gastric emptying (aluminum hydroxide gel and pentobarbital or isoniazid) (23). Examples of the effects of antacids on drug absorption are summarized in Table 3. Most interactions can be avoided by giving the drug and antacid 2 hr apart.

The pH partition hypothesis predicts that weak acids are absorbed more rapidly from the stomach, where the pH is close to 1, than from the intestine, where the pH is closer to 8. Therefore, a delay in gastric emptying could enhance the absorption of acids. However, because of the much greater surface area of the intestine and the greater blood flow, absorption of acids from the intestine is more rapid and more extensive than from the stomach (27). Because of this, the rate of gastric emptying can control the rate of drug absorption by controlling the rate of delivery of drug to the major absorptive surface. Examples include the increased rate and extent of absorption of L-DOPA caused by administration of antacids, which probably increase the rate of gastric emptying (28,29) (and may decrease metabolism

TABLE 3. *Effects of antacids on absorption of some other drugs*

Drug	Antacid type	Effect on absorption	Clinically important
Aminophylline	Mg–Al	↓ Rate (not extent)	No
Atropine and hyoscine	Mg	↓ Extent	Possibly
Chlordiazepoxide	Mg	↓ Rate (not extent)	No
Clorazepate	Mg	↓ Extent[a]	Yes
Cimetidine	Mg	↓ Extent	Possibly[b]
Diazepam	Mg–Al	↓ Rate (not extent)	No
Diflunisal	Al	↓ Extent	Yes
Digoxin	Mg–Al	↓ Extent	Uncertain
Indomethacin	Mg–Al	↓ Extent	?
Levodopa	Mg–Al	↓ Extent	?
Isoniazid	Al	↓ Peak level	?
Nitrofurantoin	Mg	↓ Peak level	?
Oral contraceptives	Mg	Adsorbed *in vitro*	?
Phenothiazines	Mg–Al	Adsorbed *in vitro*	?
Tetracyclines	Al	Adsorbed *in vitro*	Yes
Warfarin	Mg	Adsorbed *in vitro*	Yes

[a]Activity of drug depends on liberation of desmethyldiazepam in the acidic conditions of the gastric contents.
[b]Variable effects from person to person.
From Henry and Langman (24), with permission.

of L-DOPA by gastric mucosa), and the increased rate of absorption of tetracycline when coadministered with metoclopramide (30). Conversely, when a drug is poorly water-soluble, a delay in gastric emptying can increase the rate and extent of absorption by allowing time for the tablet to dissolve. Examples of this interaction include the increased rate and extent of absorption of digoxin when administered with propantheline bromide (see Chapter 2) (31,32) and the decrease with metoclopramide (see Chapter 2, Fig. 1). The bioavailability of dicumarol, which is absorbed poorly, seems to be increased during concurrent ingestion of tricyclic antidepressants (33). The absorption of a drug to nonabsorbable substances is a further mechanism of interaction at the site of absorption. Oral administration of activated charcoal can reduce the rate and extent of absorption of many drugs, including acetaminophen (34), aspirin (35), and phenobarbital, phenylbutazone, and carbamazepine (36). The ion-exchange resin cholestyramine is used to treat certain forms of hyperlipidemia. Cholestyramine adsorbs and reduces absorption of thyroxin (37), loperamide (38), and warfarin (39).

Alteration of the rate of absorption of a drug from the gastrointestinal tract may have more distant effects that could alter the area under the plasma concentration/time curve in the systemic circulation. If a drug undergoes extensive presystemic metabolism in the intestine or liver but demonstrates saturable metabolism in one or both of these organs, the area under the concentration/time curve will depend on the rate of delivery of the drug to the sites of metabolism. For example, the

plasma area under the concentration/time curve of salicylamide is much greater after a dose is administered in solution than when the same dose is administered as a commercial suspension or tablet (40).

Other potential mechanisms for drug-drug interactions during gastrointestinal absorption include alteration in intestinal blood flow, competition for active absorption mechanisms, alteration of metabolism of one drug in the gastrointestinal wall, or alteration in absorption caused by a toxic effect in the gastrointestinal tract. Examples that demonstrate each of these mechanisms will not be discussed here, but the reader is referred to the review of Mayersohn (41) (see also Chapter 2).

Drug Distribution

Drug distribution depends on the partition coefficient of drug between blood and tissue, regional blood flow, binding to plasma proteins and tissue, and active transport to tissue. Theoretically, alteration of these factors can lead to drug interactions (see Chapter 10 for a detailed review).

The most common explanation for altered distribution by drug interaction is displacement of a drug from plasma proteins. Many drugs are bound reversibly to plasma proteins and can compete for common binding sites when administered together. As a result, the free (unbound) plasma concentration of the displaced drug may increase transiently. This has potential importance in that the unbound drug concentration is available for distribution to the drug's sites of action.

Displacement interactions have been studied primarily *in vitro*. Yet, unless drug is bound substantially to and displaced from plasma or tissue binding sites, displacement may be of little therapeutic consequence. Before displacement from plasma proteins can be significant, most of the displaced drug must be bound to plasma proteins, giving a low value for fraction unbound. Second, the displacing drug must have a high affinity for the binding sites and must be present at a concentration that approaches or exceeds the molar concentration of the protein binding sites. Usually, only acidic drugs meet these conditions. Basic drugs, in general, have larger volumes of distribution, are given in smaller doses, and have lower plasma concentrations than acidic drugs, and they do not meet the condition of adequate molar concentration of drug in plasma.

Two general pharmacokinetic situations should be considered: when the displacer is given only once and when the displacer and drug are given together on a multiple-dose regimen. When a drug is displaced from its plasma protein-binding sites by the single dose of a displacer, the increase in unbound concentration is transient because of redistribution of displaced drug into a greater distribution volume. Consequently, the concentration of unbound drug at the site of action may only increase slightly, if at all. Furthermore, if the drug is poorly extracted by the liver, clearance depends on the concentration of unbound drug and increases when this concentration increases. In contrast, for a highly extracted drug, clearance is not dependent on the fraction of unbound drug and does not increase (see Chapter 10). Therefore, in the case of a poorly extracted drug, the elimination half-life of a displaced drug

may show no change or only a slight decrease or increase because of concurrent increases in volume of distribution and clearance. The half-life of a highly extracted drug increases with displacement, parallel to the increase in volume of distribution and lack of change in clearance. Unless clearance of a poorly extracted drug is also impaired by the displacing drug, the potential pharmacologic effect is a temporary increase in intensity of drug action that will decrease as the displacing drug is eliminated.

When a displacing drug is given in a concurrent multiple-dose regimen, the influence of displacement on the unbound concentration at steady state again depends on the extraction ratio of the drug. The total clearance of a low-extraction-ratio drug is influenced by the fraction of unbound drug. After displacement, the unbound fraction increases, which in turn increases the elimination rate, and hence total plasma concentration falls (Fig. 3). When a new steady state is achieved, the concentration of unbound drug in plasma is at the original value, but the total plasma concentration of drug is lower. The pharmacologic response is unaffected. The clearance of a high-extraction-ratio drug is unaffected by the fraction of unbound drug and therefore displacement. Despite displacement, the total plasma concentration of drug at steady state is unaffected. However, in the presence of diminished binding, the unbound concentration is greater, and the response to the drug may also be greater. This may require reduction of the maintenance dosage of the displaced drug.

Despite the large number of *in vitro* studies demonstrating competitive protein-binding displacement between drugs, clinically important examples of interactions due to displacement of drug from plasma proteins are few (43,44). Purported

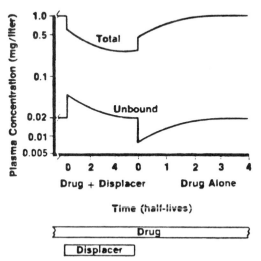

FIG. 3. Effect of administration of a displacing drug on the unbound and total plasma concentrations of a low-extraction-ratio drug being infused constantly. Eventually, the unbound concentration returns to the preexisting value, despite continuous infusion of the displacing drug. (From Rowland and Tozer, ref. 42, with permission.)

examples of displacement interactions include the displacement from plasma proteins of warfarin by phenylbutazone and chloral hydrate and of tolbutamide by phenylbutazone and sulfaphenazole. However, interactions between these drugs may involve other mechanisms as well. For example, phenylbutazone not only displaces warfarin from albumin but also inhibits the biotransformation of the potent S isomer of warfarin (4). In contrast, the elimination of the R isomer, five times less potent, is enhanced. However, the overall result of the drug combination is potentiation of warfarin-induced hypothrombinemia. This is probably related more closely to the inhibition of the metabolism of the S isomer than to displacement from plasma proteins. Sulfaphenazole displaces tolbutamide from serum albumin but also inhibits its hepatic metabolism (45). The combination of decreased clearance of free drug and plasma protein-binding displacement during this interaction potentiates the tolbutamide-induced hypoglycemia. Valproic acid lowers total plasma concentrations of phenytoin by increasing the fraction of drug not bound to plasma proteins and thus increasing metabolism of this fraction over the first 4 weeks of concurrent continuous administration of the two drugs (46). However, the lower total phenytoin concentration persists only for a few weeks, which suggests a subsequent inhibition of phenytoin metabolism by valproic acid.

Data on interactions that alter tissue binding of drugs are meager. However, a probable clinical example of tissue displacement is provided by the observation of increased serum concentration of digoxin even after a single dose of quinidine sulfate (47). Hager et al. (1) demonstrated that the increased serum concentration of digoxin was associated with a decrease in volume of distribution of quinidine. The results may be explained by the displacement of digoxin (by quinidine) from binding sites in tissue. As demonstrated by Schenck-Gustafsson et al. (48) however, the cardiotoxicity of digoxin is enhanced by quinidine, indicating that the displacement of digoxin from tissue stores may be relatively selective, affecting noncardiac tissues but not the heart. Kim et al. (49) demonstrated that in guinea pig and rat heart, quinidine did not modify digoxin Na^+- or K^+-ATPase interactions or the digoxin sensitivity of the myocardium. The adverse effects of the quinidine-digoxin interaction are also mediated by other pharmacokinetic interactions, including the inhibition by quinidine of both renal and nonrenal clearance of digoxin (2,50,51). The levorotatory isomer of quinidine, quinine, also interacts with digoxin primarily by reducing nonrenal clearance of the drug (52,53).

A recent discussion in the literature involved the finding that plasma binding of drugs is reduced in subjects given heparin (54–57). The effect of heparin, however, seems to be indirect. The effect is generally assumed to involve the release of nonesterified fatty acids in blood either before or after its collection. Therefore, the observed decrease in binding in many cases could be an artifact of the test tube, and unbound plasma concentrations of the drug *in vivo* may not be altered. Other blood collection techniques can also affect the measurement of binding. For example, some collection tubes variably decreased quinidine binding when the blood came into contact with the rubber stopper (56). (Further review of this subject is provided in Chapters 21 and 22.)

Enhanced Drug Metabolism

Enhancement of drug metabolism increases metabolic clearance and presumably unbound clearance of drug, decreasing both unbound and total plasma concentrations of drug. The pharmacokinetic consequences of an increased metabolic rate of a drug that is primarily metabolized by the liver, but with a low hepatic extraction ratio, are that clearance increases and half-life decreases, but bioavailability is essentially unaltered. The clearance and half-life of a drug with high hepatic extraction remain essentially unchanged. However, bioavailability is reduced. (The anticipated pharmacokinetics of a drug before and after changes in metabolic clearance after single intravenous and oral doses and intravenous infusions have been discussed in Chapters 3 and 4.)

Drug-induced enhancement of metabolic clearance usually involves enhancement of the hepatic microsomal enzyme hydroxylation system. The enhancement is thought to be mediated by enzyme induction (58) and involves an increase in the number of molecules of cytochrome P-450 or one of its many forms in response to an enzyme-inducing agent (59). The microsomal enzyme hydroxylation systems are unique in that they can be induced by a wide range of biologically and chemically unrelated compounds, including drugs, endogenous steroids, other hormones, and environmental pollutants (60). The molecular biology of the process of induction of P-450 has been reviewed by Bresnick (61). The molecular characteristics of compounds essential for induction have not been defined. Inducers do have several features in common, such as lipophilicity, the ability to bind to cytochrome P-450 enzymes, and relatively long biological half-lives. However, many drugs that have these properties do not induce enzyme synthesis. Chemicals can induce multiple forms of cytochrome P-450, and therefore they have varying effects on a substrate's metabolism, depending on its affinity for the different enzymes.

Inducing drugs include phenobarbital and other barbiturates, glutethimide, phenytoin, carbamazepine, ethanol, rifampin, and griseofulvin. Some clinically important drug interactions associated with induction of the microsomal enzyme hydroxylation systems are listed in Table 4. It is also important to note many chemicals encountered in the environment, such as organochlorine pesticides and polychlorinated biphenyls; charcoal-broiled food, cabbage, and brussels sprouts can also stimulate drug metabolism (85).

The time course of the enhancement of drug metabolism depends on the potency of the inducing agent and enzyme turnover. Rifampin and phenobarbital may produce noticeable changes in the activity of drug-metabolizing enzymes in 48 hr. In contrast, the effects of less potent inducers such as antipyrine may take several days (85,86). Therapeutic doses of inducing drugs may not produce their maximum effects for 1 to 2 weeks (85). Enzyme induction is also dose-dependent, as demonstrated by the response curves constructed for the induction of warfarin metabolism by barbiturates (87) and of antipyrine and cortisone metabolism by rifampin (86). Return to the normal metabolic activity after the inducing drug is withdrawn may take several weeks and depends again on the potency of the inducing drug,

TABLE 4. Some significant drug interactions due to induction of drug metabolism[a]

Interacting drug	Drug affected	Parameter measured	Change Before	Change After	Reference
Phenobarbital	Alprenolol	AUC (ng/ml/hr)	706 ± 77	154 ± 48	63
	Cortisol	Metabolite	↑ in 6-β-hydroxycortisol formation		64
	Dicumarol	Plasma conc. (mg/liter)	21–45	9–14	62
	Digitoxin	Half-life (days)	7.8	4.5	66
	Doxycycline	Half-life (hr)	15.3	11.1	67
	Phenytoin	Plasma conc.	11.4–9.6	7.3–2.7	62
	Warfarin	C_{ss} (µg/ml)	0.73	0.18	68
	Carbamazepine	C_{ss} (µg/ml)	10	7	69
	Nortriptyline	C_{ss} (ng/ml)	28	18	70
	Quinidine	Half-life (hr)	4 hr	1.6 hr	65
Rifampin	Cortisol	Maintenance cortisol dose	↑ requirement		71
	Disopyramide	AUC (µg/ml/hr)	20 ± 9	8 ± 3	72
		Half-life (hr)	5.9 ± 1.6	3.3 ± 0.7	72
	Digitoxin	Half-life (hr)	288	76	73
	Methadone	C_{ss} (µg/ml)	↓ by 33–68%		74
	Warfarin	AUC (µg/ml/hr)	600 ± 54	258 ± 17	75
	Tolbutamide	Half-life (min)	320	195	76
	Metoprolol	AUC (µg/liter/hr)	930 ± 414	624 ± 254	81
	Quinidine	C_{ss} (µg/ml)	4.6	0.6	77
	Oral contraceptives	Half-life (hr)	7.5	3.3	79
Phenytoin	Cortisol	Metabolite	↑ in 6-β-hydroxycortisol formation		78
	Dexamethasone	Low-dose dexamethasone suppression test	No suppression		94
	Dicumarol	C_{ss} (µg/ml)	20	5	80
	Disopyramide	Half-life (hr)	7	4	72
	Carbamazepine	C_{ss} (µg/ml)	6.7	4.4	82
	Methadone	AUC (µg/ml/hr)	4.8	2.3	83
	Quinidine	Half-life (hr)	6.1	2.4	65
	25-Hydroxycholecalciferol	C_{ss} (ng/ml)	20.5 ± 1.0	15.2 ± 1.1	84
	Mianeserin	AUC (nmole/liter/hr)	1453	205	90
		Half-life (hr)	16.9	4.8	90
	Nomifensine	AUC (nmole/liter/hr)	35,456	18,694	90

[a] See Chapter 16 for the effects of smoking on the induction of drug metabolism.

the drug half-life, and the enzyme turnover. Lai et al. (88) studied the time course of interaction between the inducing drug carbamazepine and the affected drug clonazepam. They demonstrated that the new steady-state concentrations of clonazepam were achieved 5 to 15 days after the addition of carbamazepine. The time course of "de-induction" was not studied.

Inhibited Drug Metabolism

Fatalities have resulted from interactions associated with enzyme inhibition. Most of these interactions have involved inhibition of the hepatic microsomal enzyme hydroxylation system, and clinically important combinations are listed in Table 5.

Drugs may inhibit microsomal enzyme drug activity in a variety of ways, including direct competition for substrate binding site, alteration of the conformation of the enzyme and thereby indirect alteration of substrate binding, uncoupling the association between NADPH consumption and drug oxidation, impeding the penetration of substrate through microsomal membranes, and altering the proportions of the various forms of cytochrome P-450 (119). More complex mechanisms than these must no doubt operate.

A problem in assessing whether or not a drug is an inhibitor of metabolism *in vivo*, in contrast to its effects *in vitro*, may arise because chronic administration of some inhibitors, such as SKF 525A, can produce enzyme induction (120,121). This biphasic effect may explain some conflicting data in the literature concerning whether a drug is an inhibitor or an inducer. A further problem in assessing a potential inhibitor of metabolism has been alluded to earlier: Inhibition of drug metabolism may be stereospecific. For example, metronidazole and phenylbutazone inhibit the metabolism of the S enantiomer of warfarin, but they have little effect on or induce the metabolism of the R enantiomer (4,122). Some of the best clinically documented inhibitory interactions involve the oral hypoglycemic agent tolbutamide. Prolonged hypoglycemic crises may ensue from coadministration of chloramphenicol, sulfaphenazole, dicumarol, phenylbutazone, and phenyramidol to patients stabilized on tolbutamide (45,123). Elimination of tolbutamide is particularly sensitive to inhibition because its elimination is dependent on a single route of metabolism, that is, oxidation to hydroxytolbutamide (124). Rowland et al. (125,126) discussed the pharmacokinetics of the effect of an inhibitor on tolbutamide metabolism.

Most compounds that inhibit drug metabolism are assumed to act by direct inhibition of the enzyme system. Thus, inhibition should be dependent on the plasma concentration of the inhibitor and should occur as soon as adequate plasma levels of the inhibiting drug are attained. However, an apparently delayed inhibitory effect of phenylbutazone on the metabolism of tolbutamide has been observed (96) (Fig. 4). Similar blood levels for phenylbutazone, which were achieved by a single 800-mg dose or by 5 days of treatment with the drug, did not produce the same inhibitory effect on the metabolism of tolbutamide. The single large dose of phenylbutazone had no effect on tolbutamide half-life. In contrast, administration of lower doses of phenylbutazone for 7 days, which produced plasma concentrations of phenyl-

TABLE 5. Some clinically significant drug interactions due to inhibition of drug metabolism

Interacting drug	Drug affected	Parameter measured	Change		Reference
			Before	After	
Ethanol	Chloral hydrate	Half-life			89
Sulfaphenazole	Phenytoin	Half-life (hr)	7.8	31.9	91
	Tolbutamide	Half-life (hr)	5.0	21.5	45
Chloramphenicol	Dicumarol	Half-life (hr)	8.7	25	92
	Phenytoin	Half-life (hr)	12	28	92
	Tolbutamide	Half-life (hr)	5.2	14.1	45
Phenylbutazone[a]	Warfarin	Half-life (hr)	44 ± 5	44 ± 4	4,93
	Phenytoin	Half-life (hr)	13.7 ± 5	22 ± 5.5	91,95
	Tolbutamide	Half-life (hr)	8	23	45,96
Cimetidine[b]	Warfarin	CL (ml/min)	3.4	2.5	97–102
	Antipyrine	CL (ml/min)	37.1 ± 6.0	29.7 ± 5.9	172
		Half-life (hr)	12.2 ± 1.8	16.8 ± 2.8	
	Phenindione	↑ prothrombin time			104
	Diazepam	CL (ml/min)	19.9 ± 8.2	11.4 ± 4.2	105–107
	Lidocaine[c]	CL (ml/min)	766 ± 50	576 ± 47	103
	Clorazepate (desmethyldiazepam)	CL (ml/min)	12.0 ± 2.7	8.6 ± 3.2	108
	Chlordiazepoxide	CL (ml/min)	0.38 ± 0.14	0.14 ± 0.03	109,172
	Propranolol	AUC (µg/liter/hr)	450 ± 168	727 ± 126	110,172
	Chlormethiazole	Half-life (hr)	2.33 ± 0.6	3.63 ± 1.3	111,172
	Labetalol	Bioavailability	29.9 ± 2.9%	53.7 ± 14.5%	112
	Theophylline	Half-life (hr)	8.6 ± 2.3	13.9 ± 5.3	113–115
	Indocyanine green	CL (ml/min)	1,192 ± 282	915 ± 328	111
	Caffeine	Half-life (hr)	4.3	6.4	116
	Phenytoin	C_{ss} (µmole/liter)	5.8	9.0	117
	Carbamazepine	C_{ss} (µg/ml)	6–7	10.5	118
Oral contraceptives	Nitrazepam	CL (ml/min)	459 ± 40	323 ± 30	171,173
	Antipyrine	CL (ml/kg/min)	37.7 ± 4.0	26.6 ± 3.1	174

[a] Although the mean half-life remained the same, the half-life for the S isomer of warfarin increased significantly while the half-life for the R isomer decreased (the S isomer is four times as active as the R isomer).
[b] A recent review of cimetidine drug interactions is provided by Sorkin et al. (175).
[c] Knapp et al. (176) recently reported an increase in plasma concentrations of 42–75%.

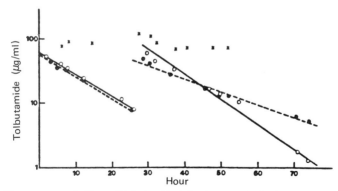

FIG. 4. Plasma concentrations of tolbutamide following two single doses of tolbutamide (500 mg) administered orally on successive days *(open circles)*. Repeat studies were carried out after administration of phenylbutazone, 800 mg, given 4 hr before the first dose of tolbutamide and 200 mg given with the second dose *(filled circles)*. Plasma concentrations of phenylbutazone are also presented (X). Prolongation of tolbutamide half-life was not apparent until 24 hr after the first dose of phenylbutazone. (From Pond et al., ref. 96, with permission.)

butazone that were similar to the concentrations after the large single dose, prolonged the tolbutamide half-life from 8 to 23 hr.

An important recent addition to the list of inhibitors of the microsomal hydroxylation system is the H_2-receptor antagonist cimetidine. As an imidazole derivative, cimetidine is a potent inhibitor of microsomal P-450 enzymes (127). The inhibitory metabolic interactions described with this drug illustrate two important points. First, an inhibiting drug can have differential effects on hepatic drug elimination. Cimetidine inhibits the oxidative metabolism of chlordiazepoxide and diazepam (105,109) but has no effect on the glucuronide conjugation of the benzodiazepines, lorazepam, and oxazepam (128). Second, when the first-pass elimination of a highly extracted drug such as propranolol is inhibited, the area under the curve after an oral dose of the highly extracted drug is increased to a greater extent than the area under the curve after an intravenous dose (111) (see Chapter 3). Cimetidine also may inhibit the metabolism of warfarin (100,101,104), theophylline (115), phenytoin (117), and carbamazepine (118).

Drugs may inhibit nonmicrosomal pathways of metabolism. Clinical examples include the hypertensive reactions that occur in individuals treated with a monoamine oxidase inhibitor who eat cheese or other foods with high tyramine content (129). Inhibition by monoamine oxidase inhibitors of the mitochondrial enzyme impairs the first-pass metabolism of tyramine by the gastrointestinal wall and liver. Disulfiram inhibits acetaldehyde dehydrogenase, which metabolizes ethanol to acetic acid. Concurrent ingestion of alcohol and disulfiram leads to an accumulation of acetaldehyde in the body and accounts for some of the physiologic disturbances of the alcohol-Antabuse® reaction (130). Allopurinol inhibits xanthine oxidase, the enzyme that catalyzes the oxidation of hypoxanthine to xanthine and uric acid (131). Because xanthine oxidase also metabolizes synthetic xanthine analogues such as 6-

mercaptopurine, allopurinol can increase both the toxicity and therapeutic efficacy of 6-mercaptopurine *in vivo*.

Changes in Hepatic Blood Flow

Hepatic blood flow becomes an important determinant of the clearance of drugs that are eliminated extensively and rapidly from the blood by the liver (132–134) (as discussed in Chapters 1, 3, and 10). Perhaps the greatest potential for clinically significant hemodynamic drug interactions occurs in acutely ill patients in whom cardiac output and hepatic blood flow may be changing considerably and rapidly (132). Hepatic blood flow may also be increased or decreased by drugs. For example, phenobarbital increases hepatic blood flow (135), whereas drugs that decrease cardiac output or drugs such as cimetidine and indomethacin, which may decrease splanchnic blood flow (111), decrease hepatic blood flow. Clinical examples of these interactions include the following. By reducing cardiac output and therefore hepatic blood flow, propranolol decreases its own clearance (136) as well as the clearance of lidocaine from plasma (137) (Fig. 5). The recently described interaction between cimetidine and propranolol (111) may provide an example of a similar phenomenon, reduction in propranolol clearance due to reduction of hepatic blood flow. However, more important, cimetidine also inhibits the hepatic metabolism of propranolol.

Interference with Biliary Excretion and Enterohepatic Circulation

Many drugs are secreted actively into bile either unchanged or as conjugates with glucuronide or glutathione. Drugs and their metabolites may compete for biliary excretion or for the preliminary conjugation step. Probenecid decreases the biliary excretion of rifampin and indomethacin (138,139).

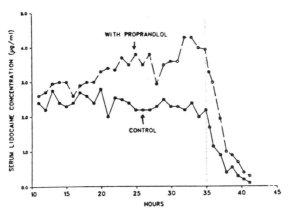

FIG. 5. Serum concentrations of lidocaine in one subject during and after continuous infusion of lidocaine alone and during coadministration of propranolol. (From Ochs et al., ref. 137, with permission.)

Among the various routes of drug elimination, the biliary route is unique in that products excreted have potential access to the large surface area of the intestine and may be reabsorbed with or without intestinal metabolism and returned to the hepatic and/or systemic circulation. Enterohepatic circulation (discussed further in Chapter 5) plays an important role in the delayed excretion of exogenously administered compounds (140–142). Compounds recognized to undergo enterohepatic or enteroenteric circulation in humans include phenobarbital, carbamazepine, phenylbutazone (36,143), dapsone (144), chlordecone (145), methyl mercury (146), digitoxin (147), spironolactone (148), and indomethacin (149). Interruption of the enterohepatic circulation of phenobarbital, carbamazepine, and phenylbutazone has been achieved by repeated oral administration of activated charcoal (36,143). Reduction in the half-life of digitoxin is achieved by administration of ion-exchange resins such as cholestyramine or colestipol (150,151).

Changes in Renal Elimination

During urinary excretion, drugs are eliminated by three mechanisms: glomerular filtration, tubular reabsorption, and active tubular secretion. Theoretically, drug interactions during glomerular filtration could occur if a drug is displaced from its plasma protein-binding sites, enabling the increased amount of free drug in plasma to be filtered by the glomerulus. Clinically significant examples of such an interaction have not been demonstrated. Nonsteroidal antiinflammatory drugs can decrease the glomerular filtration rate and creatinine clearance in patients by inhibiting renal prostaglandin biosynthesis (see Chapter 8). A form of reversible acute renal failure develops, particularly in patients with underlying renal disease (152–154). The effects of the nonsteroidal antiinflammatory drugs on prostaglandin synthesis produce complex changes in renal hemodynamics and tubular function. However, of interest from the point of view of drug interactions is the description by Frölich et al. (155) in 1979 that indomethacin increased plasma concentrations of lithium and decreased renal clearance of lithium in both normal volunteers and psychiatric patients (Fig. 6). The average increase in the plasma concentration of lithium in the psychiatric patients was 59%, whereas in the normal volunteers it was 30%. Renal clearance of lithium was suppressed to the same degree. Interactions affecting renal clearance of lithium are often clinically relevant because lithium is used frequently, has a low therapeutic index and a steep dose–response curve, and has renal excretion as its only route of elimination. The plasma concentration of lithium may increase in relation to decreased renal excretion of sodium. Thus, any cause of sodium loss, for example, excessive sweating, persistent vomiting, or the use of long-term diuretics, can lead to an increased plasma concentration of lithium (156).

The renal tubule can actively secrete or reabsorb a variety of drugs. Active reabsorption is not a major site of drug-drug interactions. However, probenecid, high doses of salicylates, or phenylbutazone probably produce uricosuria by inhibiting the active reabsorption of uric acid in the proximal tubule. The pars recta

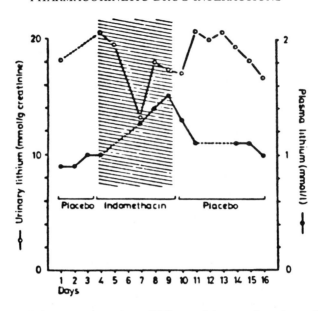

FIG. 6. Increased plasma concentrations of lithium and decreased renal excretion of lithium in a psychiatric patient before, during, and after concurrent administration of indomethacin. (From Frölich et al., ref. 155, with permission.)

(straight segment) of the proximal tubule actively secretes a variety of organic acids and bases into the tubular lumen. (Partial lists of drugs eliminated by these pathways are presented and discussed in Chapter 8.) The transport system for acids is characterized more fully than that for bases. The pathways for acids and bases appear to be separate, but within each pathway there can be competition by substrates for transport and excretion. Many interactions due to this competition have been described, particularly among the various uricosuric agents. Probenecid inhibits renal tubular secretion of sulfinpyrazone (157) and indomethacin (158) and also inhibits the elimination of penicillin and methotrexate. However, coadministration of other organic acids may also lead to similar interactions that could have disastrous clinical consequences if the drug is one such as methotrexate. The combination of penicillin and probenecid is used clinically, but the serum half-life of penicillin is probably also prolonged significantly by phenylbutazone, sulfinpyrazole, indomethacin, sulfaphenazole, and aspirin.

It has been assumed that organic bases can compete with each other for secretion as do acids, but clinically important interactions produced by this mechanism have not been documented.

One drug that is transported by secretion into the tubule but does not follow the organic acid or organic base pathways is digoxin. Its secretion by the distal nephron is reduced by spironolactone (159), leading to decreased renal clearance and increased plasma concentration of digoxin (160). In some individuals, spironolactone also decreases the volume of distribution of digoxin, suggesting that tissue binding of digoxin is also reduced (160).

As in the gastrointestinal tract, the effect of urinary pH on passive reabsorption of weak acids and bases relates to the principles of passive nonionic diffusion (discussed earlier in this chapter and in Chapter 8). Alteration of urinary pH by antacid therapy can alter salicylate (pK_a 3) concentrations significantly in patients taking antirheumatic doses of aspirin (161,162). To increase renal excretion of salicylate, alkalinization of the urine is recommended in salicylate-overdosed patients (163,164). Morgan and Polak (165) demonstrated that renal clearance of salicylate increased fourfold for each one-unit rise in urinary pH. Thus, the renal clearance of salicylate increased from 16 to 164 ml/min as urine pH increased from 6.5 to 7.5. In overdosed patients, forced alkaline diuresis may increase renal clearance of phenobarbital to values as high as 17 ml/min (166). Because the usual renal clearance of phenobarbital under physiologic conditions is 1 to 3 ml/min and the total clearance is 2 to 10 ml/min, forced diuresis can add significantly to total clearance of the drug. Renal elimination of the bases amphetamine and phencyclidine, two drugs that are abused frequently, is sensitive to changes in urinary pH. Approximately 60% of an intravenously administered dose of amphetamine is excreted unchanged in acid urine, whereas less than 20% is excreted in alkaline urine (167). These investigators demonstrated that the plasma half-life of amphetamine in patients with acid urine was shorter (8–10.5 hr) than in patients without an alkaline urine (16–31 hr). Nevertheless, the risks of urine acidification in the presence of amphetamine intoxication may outweigh the benefit of its effect on enhancing renal elimination of amphetamine, as discussed recently by Rosenberg et al. (168). The issue of urinary acidification to increase the renal clearance of phencyclidine is not resolved. Urinary acidification clearly increases the renal clearance of phencyclidine (169,170). However, increased renal clearance may not add significantly to total body clearance of this drug, which is extensively metabolized and has a large volume of distribution.

CONCLUSIONS

It is apparent that drug interactions are potentially hazardous consequences of multiple-drug therapy. One may argue, however, that there has been a pronounced overreaction to their importance. A search through the National Library of Medicine's National Interactive Retrieval Service on the MEDLINE, covering the years 1977 to 1980, retrieved 1,434 references that related only to studies in humans. Reviews of drug interactions abound in the literature. These pertain to interactions between specific drugs used in patients with certain disease states or patients undergoing procedures such as anesthesia. The only practical approach to the problem of identifying clinically important interactions is to follow these lines. The first is identification of the sites of drug interactions and drugs that predictably interact at these sites; thus, some interactions not yet described can be predicted, and steps can be taken to alter therapy to prevent therapeutic failure or drug toxicity. Second, plasma concentrations of drugs with low therapeutic indices or steep dose–response curves should be monitored routinely. Compounds in this list include theophylline,

digoxin, quinidine, lithium, phenytoin, methotrexate, aminoglycoside antibiotics, and lidocaine. Third, a practitioner should become thoroughly familiar with the drugs that are used most frequently and should seek out specific reports on these. Fourth, understanding not only the pathophysiology of the patient's disease but also the pharmacology of the drugs being used will enable the clinician to assess the endpoints of drug efficacy or toxicity and to recognize the interaction(s) when it occurs. Fifth, as few drugs as possible should be prescribed. Finally, one would be wise to remember that interindividual variability in pharmacodynamic and pharmacokinetic responses to drugs can be great and can, in turn, lead to interindividual variability in the pharmacologic consequences of interactions.

REFERENCES

1. Hager, W. D., Fenster, P., Mayersohn, M., Perrier, D., Graves, P., Marcus, F. I., and Goldman, S. (1979): Digoxin-quinidine interaction. Pharmacokinetic evaluation. *N. Engl. J. Med.*, 300:1238–1241.
2. Doering, W., Fichth, B., Hermann, M., and Besenfelder, E. (1982): Quinidine-digoxin interaction: Evidence for involvement of an extrarenal mechanism. *Eur. J. Clin. Pharmacol.*, 21:281–285.
3. Koch-Weser, J., and Sellers, E. M. (1976): Binding of drugs to serum albumin. Parts 1 and 2. *N. Engl. J. Med.*, 294:311–316, 526–530.
4. Lewis, R. J., Trager, W. F., Chan, K. K., Breckenridge, A., Orme, M., Rowland, M., and Schary, W. (1974): Warfarin. Stereochemical aspects of its metabolism and the interaction with phenylbutazone. *J. Clin. Invest.*, 53:1607–1617.
5. Hurwitz, N., and Wade, O. L. (1969): Intensive hospital monitoring of adverse reactions to drugs. *Br. Med. J.*, 1:531–536.
6. Crooks, J., Stevenson, I. H., Shepherd, A. M. M., and Moir, D. C. (1977): The clinical significance and importance of drug interactions. In: *Drug Interactions*, edited by D. G. Grahame-Smith, pp. 3–13. University Park Press, Baltimore.
7. Kellaway, C. S. M., and McCrae, E. (1973): Intensive monitoring for adverse drug effects in patients discharged from acute medical wards. *N. Z. Med. J.*, 78:525–528.
8. Petrie, J. C., Durno, D., and Howie, J. G. R. (1975): Drug interaction in general practice. In: *Clinical Effects of Interactions between Drugs*, edited by L. E. Cluff and J. C. Petrie, p. 237. Excerpta Medica, Amsterdam.
9. May, F. E., Stewart, R. B., and Cluff, L. E. (1977): Drug interactions and multiple drug administration. *Clin. Pharmacol. Ther.*, 22:322–328.
10. Smith, J. W., Seidl, L. G., and Cluff, L. E. (1966): Studies on the epidemiology of adverse drug reactions. V. Clinical factors influencing susceptibility. *Ann. Intern. Med.*, 65:629–640.
11. Talley, R. B., and Laventurier, M. F. (1972): Risk of drug interaction may exist in 1 of 13 prescriptions. *J.A.M.A.*, 220:1287–1288.
12. Stewart, R. B., and Cluff, L. E. (1971): Studies on the epidemiology of adverse drug reactions. VI. Utilization and interactions of prescription and nonprescription drugs in outpatients. *Johns Hopkins Med. J.*, 129:319–331.
13. Mitchell, G. W., Stanaszek, W. F., and Nichols, N. B. (1979): Documenting drug-drug interactions in ambulatory patients. *Am. J. Hosp. Pharm.*, 36:653–657.
14. Robinson, D. S. (1975): The application of basic principles of drug interaction to clinical practice. *J. Urol.*, 113:100–107.
15. Neuvonen, P. J., Gothoni, G., Hackman, R., and Bjorksten, K. (1970): Interference of iron with the absorption of tetracyclines in man. *Br. Med. J.*, 4:532–534.
16. Gothoni, G., Neuvonen, P. J., Mattila, M., and Hackman, R. (1972): Iron-tetracycline interaction: Effect of time interval between the drugs. *Acta Med. Scand.*, 191:409–411.
17. Gibson, T. P., and Nelson, H. A. (1980): Digoxin alters quinidine and quinidine alters digoxin pharmacokinetics in dogs. *J. Lab. Clin. Med.*, 95:417–428.
18. Schwartz, J. B., Keefe, D., Kates, R. E., and Harrison, D. C. (1981): Verapamil and digoxin: Another drug-drug interaction. *Clin. Res.*, 29:501A.

19. Smith, D. E., Gee, W. L., Brater, D. C., Lin, E. T., and Benet, L. Z. (1980): Preliminary evaluation of furosemide-probenecid interaction in humans. *J. Pharm. Sci.*, 69:571–575.
20. Melmon, K. L., and Nierenberg, D. W. (1981): Drug interactions and the prepared observer. *N. Engl. J. Med.*, 304:723–725.
21. Prescott, L. F., Nimmo, W. S., and Heading, R. C. (1977): Drug absorption interactions. In: *Drug Interactions*, edited by D. C. Grahame-Smith, pp. 45–51. University Park Press, Baltimore.
22. Barr, W. H., Adir, J., and Garrettson, L. (1971): Decrease of tetracycline absorption in man by sodium bicarbonate. *Clin. Pharmacol. Ther.*, 12:779–784.
23. Hurwitz, A. (1977): Antacid therapy and drug kinetics. *Clin. Pharmacokinet.*, 2:269–280.
24. Henry, D. A., and Langman, M. J. S. (1981): Adverse effects of anti-ulcer drugs. *Drugs*, 21:444–459.
25. Prescott, L. F. (1974): Gastric emptying and drug absorption. *Br. J. Clin. Pharmacol.*, 1:189–190.
26. Harcourt, R. S., and Hamburger, M. (1957): The effect of magnesium sulfate in lowering tetracycline blood levels. *J. Lab. Clin. Med.*, 50:464–468.
27. Doluisio, J. T., Tan, G. H., Billups, N. F., and Diamond, L. (1969): Drug absorption. II. Effect of fasting on intestinal drug absorption. *J. Pharm. Sci.*, 58:1200–1202.
28. Rivera-Calimlim, L., Dujovne, C. A., Morgan, J. P., Lasagna, L., and Bianchine, J. R. (1970): L-dopa treatment failure: Explanation and correction. *Br. Med. J.*, 4:93–94.
29. Pocelinko, R., Thomas, G. B., and Solomon, H. M. (1972): The effect of an antacid on the absorption and metabolism of levodopa. *Clin. Pharmacol. Ther.*, 13:149.
30. Gothoni, G., Pentikäinen, P., Vapaatalo, H. I., Hackman, R., and Bjorksten, K. A. F. (1972): Absorption of antibiotics: Influence of metoclopramide and atropine on serum levels of pivampicillin and tetracycline. *Ann. Clin. Res.*, 4:228–232.
31. Manninen, V., Apajalahti, A., Melin, J., and Karesoja, M. (1973): Altered absorption of digoxin in patients given propantheline and metoclopramide. *Lancet*, 1:398–399.
32. Medin, S., and Nyberg, L. (1973): Effect of propantheline and metoclopramide on absorption of digoxin. *Lancet*, 1:1393.
33. Pond, S. M., Graham, G. G., Birkett, D. J., and Wade, D. N. (1975): Effect of tricyclic antidepressants on drug metabolism. *Clin. Pharmacol. Ther.*, 18:191–199.
34. Levy, G., and Gwilt, P. R. (1972): Activated charcoal for acute acetaminophen intoxication. *J.A.M.A.*, 219:621.
35. Levy, G., and Tsuchiya, T. (1972): Effect of activated charcoal on aspirin absorption in man. Part I. *Clin. Pharmacol. Ther.*, 13:317–322.
36. Neuvonen, P. J., and Elonen, E. (1980): Effect of activated charcoal on absorption and elimination of phenobarbitone, carbamazepine and phenylbutazone in man. *Eur. J. Clin. Pharmacol.*, 17:51–57.
37. Northcutt, R. C., Stiel, J. N., Hollifield, J. W., and Stant, E. G., Jr. (1969): The influence of cholestyramine on thyroxine absorption. *J.A.M.A.*, 208:1857–1861.
38. Ti, T. Y., Giles, H. G., and Sellers, E. M. (1978): Probable interaction of loperamide and cholestyramine. *Can. Med. Assoc. J.*, 119:607–608.
39. Robinson, D. S., Benjamin, D. M., and McCormack, J. J. (1971): Interaction of warfarin and nonsystemic gastrointestinal drugs. *Clin. Pharmacol. Ther.*, 12:491–495.
40. Barr, W. H., Aceto, T., Chung, M., and Shukar, M. (1978): Dose-dependent drug metabolism during the absorptive phase. *Rev. Can. Biol.*, 32(Suppl.): 31–42.
41. Mayersohn, M. (1979): Physiological factors that modify systemic drug availability and pharmacologic response in clinical practice. In: *Principles and Perspectives in Drug Bioavailability*, edited by J. Blanchard, R. J. Sawchuck, and B. B. Brodie, pp. 211–273. Karger, Basel.
42. Rowland, M., and Tozer, T. N. (1980): *Clinical Pharmacokinetics: Concepts and Applications*. Lea & Febiger, Philadelphia.
43. Wardell, W. M. (1974): Redistributional drug interactions. A critical examination of putative clinical examples. In: *Drug Interactions*, edited by P. L. Morselli, S. Garattini, and S. N. Cohen, pp. 123–134. Raven Press, New York.
44. Sellers, E. M. (1979): Plasma protein displacement interactions are rarely of clinical significance. *Pharmacology*, 18:225–227.
45. Christensen, L. K., Hansen, J. M., and Kristensen, M. (1968): Sulphaphenazole-induced hypoglycemic attacks in tolbutamide-treated diabetics. *Lancet*, 2:1298–1301.

46. Bruni, J., Gallo, J. M., Lee, C. S., Perchalski, R. J., Wilder, B. J. (1980): Interactions of valproic acid with phenytoin. *Neurology (Minneap.)*, 30:1233–1236.
47. Chen, T.-S., and Friedman, H. S. (1980): Alteration of digoxin pharmacokinetics by a single dose of quinidine. *J.A.M.A.*, 244:669–672.
48. Schenck-Gustafsson, K., Jogestrand, T., Nordlander, R., and Dahlqvist, R. (1981): Effect of quinidine on digoxin concentration in skeletal muscle and serum in patients with atrial fibrillation. Evidence for reduced binding of digoxin in muscle. *N. Engl. J. Med.*, 305:209–211.
49. Kim, D.-H., Akera, T., and Brody, T. M. (1981): Effects of quinidine on the cardiac-glycoside sensitivity of guinea-pig and rat heart. *J. Pharmacol. Exp. Ther.*, 217:559–565.
50. Holford, N. H. G. (1980): The quinidine-digoxin interaction. *N. Engl. J. Med.*, 302:864.
51. Dahlqvist, R., Ejvinsson, G., and Schenck-Gustafsson, K. (1980): Effect of quinidine on plasma concentration and renal clearance of digoxin. A clinically important drug interaction. *Br. J. Clin. Pharmacol.*, 9:413–418.
52. Aronson, J. K., and Carver, J. G. (1981): Interaction of digoxin with quinine. *Lancet*, 1:1418.
53. Wandell, M., Powell, J. R., Hager, W. D., Fenster, P. E., Graves, P. E., Conrad, K. A., and Goldman, S. (1980): Effect of quinine on digoxin kinetics. *Clin. Pharmacol. Ther.*, 28:425–430.
54. Routledge, P. A., Kitchell, B. B., Bjornsson, T. D., Skinner, T., Linnoila, M., and Shand, D. G. (1980): Diazepam and *N*-desmethyldiazepam redistribution after heparin. *Clin. Pharmacol. Ther.*, 27:528–532.
55. Wood, M., Shand, D. G., and Wood, A. J. J. (1979): Altered drug binding due to the use of indwelling heparinized cannulas (heparin lock) for sampling. *Clin. Pharmacol. Ther.*, 25:103–107.
56. Kessler, K. M., Leech, R. C., and Spann, J. F. (1979): Blood collection techniques, heparin and quinidine protein binding. *Clin. Pharmacol. Ther.*, 25:204–210.
57. Naranjo, C. A., Sellers, E. M., Khouw, V., Alexander, P., Fan, T., and Shaw, J. (1980): Variability in heparin effect on serum drug binding. *Clin. Pharmacol. Ther.*, 28:545–550.
58. Conney, A. H. (1967): Pharmacological implications of microsomal enzyme induction. *Pharmacol. Rev.*, 19:317–366.
59. Gelehrter, T. D. (1976): Enzyme induction. *N. Engl. J. Med.*, 294:522–526, 589–595, 646–651.
60. Alvares, A. P. (1978): Interactions between environmental chemicals and drug biotransformation in man. *Clin. Pharmacokinet.*, 3:462–477.
61. Bresnick, E. (1978): The molecular biology of the induction of the hepatic mixed function oxidases. *Pharmacol. Ther.*, 2:319–335.
62. Cucinell, S. A., Conney, A. H., Sansur, M., and Burns, J. J. (1965): Drug interactions in man. I. Lowering effect of phenobarbital on plasma levels of bishydroxycoumarin (Dicumarol) and diphenylhydantoin (Dilantin). *Clin. Pharmacol. Ther.*, 6:420–429.
63. Alvan, G., Piafsky, K., Lind, M., and von Bahr, C. (1977): Effect of pentobarbital on the disposition of alprenolol. *Clin. Pharmacol. Ther.*, 22:316–321.
64. Burstein, S., and Klaiber, E. L. (1965): Phenobarbital-induced increase in 6β-hydroxycortisol excretion: Clue to its significance in human urine. *J. Clin. Endocrinol. Metab.*, 25:293–296.
65. Data, J. L., Wilkinson, G. R., and Nies, A. S. (1976): Interaction of quinidine with anticonvulsant drugs. *N. Engl. J. Med.*, 294:699–701.
66. Solomon, H. M., and Abrams, W. B. (1972): Interaction between digitoxin and other drugs in man. *Am. Heart J.*, 83:277–280.
67. Neuvonen, P. J., and Penttilä, O. (1974): Interaction between doxycycline and barbiturates. *Br. Med. J.*, 1:535–536.
68. MacDonald, M. G., Robinson, D. S., Sylwester, D., and Jaffe, J. J. (1969): The effects of phenobarbital, chloral betaine, and glutethimide administration on warfarin plasma levels and hypoprothrombinemic responses in man. *Clin. Pharmacol. Ther.*, 10:480–495.
69. Cereghino, J. J., Brock, J. T., Van Meter, J. C., Penry, J. K., Smith, L. D., and White, B. G. (1975): The efficacy of carbamazepine combinations in epilepsy. *Clin. Pharmacol. Ther.*, 18:733–741.
70. Alexanderson, B., Evans, D. A. P., and Sjöqvist, F. (1969): Steady-state plasma levels of nortriptyline in twins: Influence of genetic factors and drug therapy. *Br. Med. J.*, 4:764–768.
71. Edwards, O. M., Courtenay-Evans, R. J., Galley, J. M., Hunter, J., and Tait, A. D. (1974): Changes in cortisol metabolism following rifampicin therapy. *Lancet*, 2:549–551.
72. Aitio, M. L., Mansury, L., Tala, E., Haataja, M., and Aitio, A. (1981): The effect of enzyme induction on the metabolism of disopyramide in man. *Br. J. Clin. Pharmacol.*, 11:279–285.

73. Peters, U., Hausamen, T. U., and Grosse-Brockhoff, F. (1974): Einfluss von Tuberkulostatika auf die Pharmakokinetik des Digitoxins. *Dtsch. Med. Wochenschr.*, 99:2381–2386.
74. Kreek, M. J., Garfield, J. W., Gutjahr, C. L., and Guisti, L. M. (1976): Rifampin-induced methadone withdrawal. *N. Engl. J. Med.*, 294:1104–1106.
75. O'Reilly, R. A. (1974): Interaction of sodium warfarin and rifampin. Studies in man. *Ann. Intern. Med.*, 81:337–340.
76. Syvälahti, E. K. G., Pihlajamäki, K. K., and Iisalo, E. J. (1974): Rifampicin and drug metabolism. *Lancet*, 2:232–233.
77. Ahmad, D., Mathur, P., Ahuja, S., Henderson, R., and Carruthers, G. (1979): Rifampicin-quinidine interaction. *Br. J. Dis. Chest*, 73:409–411.
78. Choi, Y., Thrasher, K., Werk, E. E., Sholiton, L. J., and Olinger, C. (1971): Effect of diphenylhydantion on cortisol kinetics in humans. *J. Pharmacol. Exp. Ther.*, 176:27–34.
79. Bolt, H. M., and Kappus, N. (1977): Interaction of rifampicin treatment with pharmacokinetics and metabolism of ethinyloestradiol in man. *Acta Endocrinol.*, 85:189–197.
80. Hansen, J. M., Siersbaek-Nielsen, K., Kristensen, M., Skovsted, L., and Christensen, L. K. (1971): Effect of diphenylhydantoin on the metabolism of dicoumarol in man. *Acta Med. Scand.*, 189:15–19.
81. Bennett, P. N., and Whitmarsh, V. B. (1982): Effect of rifampicin on metoprolol and antipyrine kinetics. *Br. J. Clin. Pharmacol.*, 13:387–391.
82. Christiansen, J., and Dam, M. (1973): Influence of phenobarbital and diphenylhydantoin on plasma carbamazepine levels in patients with epilepsy. *Acta Neurol. Scand.*, 49:543–546.
83. Tong, T. G., Pond, S. M., Kreek, M. J., Jaffery, N. F., and Benowitz, N. L. (1981): Phenytoin-induced methadone withdrawal. *Ann. Intern. Med.*, 94:349–351.
84. Hahn, T. J., Hendin, B. A., Scharp, C. R., and Haddad, J. G., Jr. (1972): Effect of chronic anticonvulsant therapy on serum 25-hydroxycalciferol levels in adults. *N. Engl. J. Med.*, 287:900–904.
85. Park, B. K., and Breckenridge, A. M. (1981): Clinical implications of enzyme induction and enzyme inhibition. *Clin. Pharmacokinet.*, 6:1–24.
86. Ohnhaus, E. E., and Park, B. K. (1979): Measurement of urinary 6-β-hydroxycortisol excretion as an *in vivo* parameter in the clinical assessment of the microsomal enzyme-inducing capacity of antipyrine, phenobarbitone and rifampin. *Eur. J. Clin. Pharmacol.*, 15:139–145.
87. Breckenridge, A., Orme, M. E. E., Davies, L., Thorgeirsson, S. S., and Davies, D. S. (1973): Dose-dependent enzyme induction. *Clin. Pharmacol. Ther.*, 14:514–520.
88. Lai, A. A., Levy, R. H., and Cutler, R. E. (1978): Time-course of interaction between carbamazepine and clonazepam in normal man. *Clin. Pharmacol. Ther.*, 24:316–323.
89. Sellers, E. M., Lang, M., Koch-Weser, J., LeBlanc, E., and Kalant, H. (1972): Interaction of chloral hydrate and ethanol in man. I. Metabolism. *Clin. Pharmacol. Ther.*, 13:37–49.
90. Nawisky, S., Hathway, N., and Turner, P. (1981): Interactions of anticonvulsant drugs with mianserin and nomifensine. *Lancet*, 2:871–872.
91. Skovsted, L., Hansen, J. M., Kristensen, M., and Christensen, L. K. (1979): Inhibition of drug metabolism in man. In: *Drug Interactions*, edited by P. L. Morselli, S. Garattini, and S. N. Cohen, pp. 81–90. Raven Press, New York.
92. Christensen, L. K., and Skovsted, L. (1969): Inhibition of drug metabolism by chloramphenicol. *Lancet*, 2:1397–1399.
93. Aggeler, P. M., O'Reilly, R. A., Leong, L., and Kowitz, P. E. (1967): Potentiation of anticoagulant effect of warfarin by phenylbutazone. *N. Engl. J. Med.*, 276:496–501.
94. Jubiz, W., Meikle, A. W., Levinson, R. A., Mizutani, S., West, C. D., and Tyler, F. H. (1970): Effect of diphenylhydantoin on the metabolism of dexamethasone. Mechanism of the abnormal dexamethasone suppression in humans. *N. Engl. J. Med.*, 283:11–14.
95. Andreasen, P. B., Frøland, A., Skovsted, L., Andersen, S. A., and Hauge, M. (1973): Diphenylhydantoin half-life in man and its inhibition by phenylbutazone: The role of genetic factors. *Acta Med. Scand.*, 193:561–564.
96. Pond, S. M., Birkett, D. J., and Wade, D. N. (1977): Mechanisms of inhibition of tolbutamide metabolism: Phenylbutazone, oxyphenbutazone, sulfaphenazole. *Clin. Pharmacol. Ther.*, 22:573–579.
97. Flind, A. C. (1978): Cimetidine and oral anticoagulants. *Br. Med. J.*, 2:1367.
98. Flind, A. C. (1978): Cimetidine and oral anticoagulants. *Lancet*, 2:1054.

99. Breckenridge, A. M., Challiner, M., Mossman, S., Park, B. K., Serlin, M. J., Sibeon, R. G., Williams, J. R. B., and Willoughby, J. M. T. (1979): Cimetidine increases the action of warfarin in man. *Br. J. Clin. Pharmacol.*, 8:392P–393P.

100. Hetzel, D., Birkett, D., and Miners, J. (1979): Cimetidine interaction with warfarin. *Lancet*, 2:639.

101. Serlin, M. J., Challiner, M., Park, B. K., Turcan, P. A., and Breckenridge, A. M. (1980): Cimetidine potentiates the anticoagulant effect of warfarin by inhibition of drug metabolism. *Biochem. Pharmacol.*, 29:1971–1972.

102. Wallin, B. A., Jacknowitz, A., and Raich, P. C. (1979): Cimetidine and effect of warfarin. *Ann. Intern. Med.*, 90:993.

103. Feely, J., McAllister, C. B., Wilkinson, G. R., and Wood, A. J. J. (1982): Reduction in lignocaine clearance by cimetidine. *Br. J. Clin. Pharmacol.*, 13:591P–592P.

104. Serlin, M. J., Sibeon, R. G., Mossman, S., Breckenridge, A. M., Williams, J. R. B., Atwood, J. L., and Willoughby, J. M. T. (1979): Cimetidine: Interaction with oral anticoagulants in man. *Lancet*, 2:317–319.

105. Koltz, U., Anttila, V.-J., and Reimann, I. (1979): Cimetidine/diazepam interaction. *Lancet*, 2:699.

106. Dasta, J., MacKichan, J., Lima, J., and Altman, M. (1980): Diazepam-cimetidine interaction—a preliminary report. *Drug Intell. Clin. Pharm.*, 14:633.

107. Ruffalo, R. L., and Thompson, J. F. (1980): Effect of cimetidine on the clearance of benzodiazepines. *N. Engl. J. Med.*, 303:753.

108. Klotz, U., and Reimann, I. (1980): Influence of cimetidine on the pharmacokinetics of desmethyldiazepam and oxazepam. *Eur. J. Clin. Pharmacol.*, 18:517–520.

109. Desmond, P. V., Patwardhan, R. V., Schenker, S., and Speeg, K. V., Jr. (1980): Cimetidine impairs elimination of chlordiazepoxide (Librium) in man. *Ann. Intern. Med.*, 93:266–268.

110. Donovan, M. A., Heageris, A. M., Patel, L., Castleden, M., and Pohl, J. E. F. (1981): Cimetidine and bioavailability of propranolol. *Lancet*, 1:164.

111. Feely, J., Wilkinson, G. R., and Wood, A. J. J. (1981): Reduction of liver blood flow and propranolol metabolism by cimetidine. *N. Engl. J. Med.*, 304:692–695.

112. Daneshmend, T. K., and Roberts, C. J. C. (1981): Cimetidine and bioavailability of labetalol. *Lancet*, 1:565.

113. Jackson, J. E., Powell, J. R., Mandell, M., Bentley, J., and Dorr, R. (1980): Cimetidine-theophylline interaction. *Pharmacologist*, 22:231.

114. Wood, L., Grice, J., Petroff, V., McGuffie, C., and Roberts, R. K. (1980): Effect of cimetidine on the disposition of theophylline. *Aust. N. Z. J. Med.*, 10:586.

115. Weinberger, M. M., Smith, G., Milavetz, G., and Hendeles, L. (1981): Decreased theophylline clearance due to cimetidine. *N. Engl. J. Med.*, 304:672.

116. Broughton, L. J., and Rogers, H. J. (1981): Decreased systemic clearance of caffeine due to cimetidine. *Br. J. Clin. Pharmacol.*, 12:155–159.

117. Neuvonen, P. J., Tokola, R. A., and Kaste, M. (1981): Cimetidine-phenytoin interaction: Effect of serum phenytoin concentration and antipyrine test. *Eur. J. Clin. Pharmacol.*, 21:215–220.

118. Telerman-Toppet, N., Duret, M. E., and Coërs, C. (1981): Cimetidine interaction with carbamazepine. *Ann. Intern. Med.*, 94:544.

119. Gillette, J., Sasame, H., and Stripp, B. (1973): Mechanisms of inhibition of drug metabolic reactions. *Drug Metab. Disp.*, 1:164–175.

120. Mannering, G. J. (1968): Significance of stimulation and inhibition of drug metabolism in pharmacological testing. In: *Selected Pharmacological Testing Methods*, Vol. 3, edited by A. Burger, pp. 51–119. Marcel Dekker, New York.

121. Kato, R., Chiesara, E., and Vassanelli, P. (1964): Further studies on the inhibition and stimulation of microsomal drug-metabolizing enzymes of rat liver by various compounds. *Biochem. Pharmacol.*, 13:69–83.

122. O'Reilly, R. A. (1976): The stereoselective interaction of warfarin and metronidazole in man. *N. Engl. J. Med.*, 295:354–357.

123. Hansen, J. M., and Christensen, L. K. (1977): Drug interactions with oral sulphonylurea hypoglycemic drugs. *Drugs*, 13:24–34.

124. Thomas, R. C., and Ikeda, C. J. (1966): The metabolic fate of tolbutamide in man and in the rat. *J. Med. Chem.*, 9:507–510.

125. Rowland, M., and Matin, S. B. (1973): Kinetics of drug-drug interactions. *J. Pharmacokinet. Biopharm.*, 1:553–567.

126. Rowland, M., and Tozer, T. N. (1980): *Clinical Pharmacokinetics: Concepts and Applications*, pp. 259–261. Lea & Febiger, Philadelphia.

127. Wilkinson, C. F., Hetnarski, K., and Hicks, L. J. (1974): Substituted imidazoles as inhibitors of microsomal oxidation and insecticide synergists. *Pestic. Biochem. Physiol.*, 4:299–312.

128. Patwardhan, R. V., Yarborough, G., Desmond, P. V., Schenker, S., and Speeg, K. V., Jr. (1980): Differential effect of cimetidine on hepatic drug elimination. *Gastroenterology*, 78:1316.

129. Sjoqvist, F. (1965): Psychotropic drugs. II. Interaction between monoamine oxidase (MAO) inhibitors and other substances. *Proc. R. Soc. Med.* 58(Suppl.):967–978.

130. Raby, K. (1954): Relation of blood acetaldehyde level to clinical symptoms in the disulfiram-alcohol reaction. *Q. J. Stud. Alcohol*, 15:21–32.

131. Elion, G. B., Callahan, S., Nathan, H., Bieber, S., Rundles, R. W., and Hitchings, G. H. (1963): Potentiation by inhibition of drug degradation: 6-substituted purines and xanthine oxidase. *Biochem. Pharmacol.*, 12:85–93.

132. Nies, A. S., Shand, D. G., and Branch, R. A. (1974): Hemodynamic drug interactions. *Cardiovasc. Clin.*, 6:43–53.

133. George, C. F. (1979): Drug kinetics and hepatic blood flow. *Clin. Pharmacokinet.*, 4:433–448.

134. Pirttiaho, H. I., Sotaniemi, E. A., Pelkonen, R. O., Pitkänen, U., Anttila, M., and Sundqvist, H. (1980): Roles of hepatic blood flow and enzyme activity in the kinetics of propranolol and sotalol. *Br. J. Clin. Pharmacol.*, 9:399–405.

135. Branch, R. A., Shand, D. G., Wilkinson, G. R., and Nies, A. S. (1974): Increased clearance of antipyrine and *d*-propranolol after phenobarbital treatment in the monkey. Relative contributions of enzyme induction and increased hepatic blood flow. *J. Clin. Invest.*, 53:1101–1107.

136. Nies, A. S., Evans, G. H., and Shand, D. G. (1973): Regional hemodynamic effects of beta-adrenergic blockade with propranolol in the unanesthetized primate. *Am. Heart J.*, 85:97–102.

137. Ochs, H. R., Carstens, G., and Greenblatt, D. J. (1980): Reduction in lidocaine clearance during continuous infusion and by coadministration of propranolol. *N. Engl. J. Med.*, 303:373–377.

138. Kenwright, S., and Levi, A. J. (1973): Impairment of hepatic uptake of rifamycin antibiotics by probenecid, and its therapeutic implications. *Lancet*, 2:1401–1405.

139. Baber, N., Halliday, L., Sibeon, R., Littler, T., and Orme, M. L. (1978): The interaction between indomethacin and probenecid. A clinical and pharmacokinetic study. *Clin. Pharmacol. Ther.*, 24:298–307.

140. Hanasono, G. K., and Fischer, L. J. (1974): The excretion of tritium-labeled chlormadinone acetate, mestranol, norethindrone, and norethynodrel in rats and the enterohepatic circulation of metabolites. *Drug Metab. Dispos.*, 2:159–168.

141. Katzung, B. G., and Myers, F. H. (1965): Excretion of radioactive digitoxin in the dog. *J. Pharmacol. Exp. Ther.*, 149:257–262.

142. Woods, L. A. (1954): Distribution and fate of morphine in non-tolerant and tolerant dogs and rats. *J. Pharmacol. Exp. Ther.*, 112:158–175.

143. Neuvonen, P. J., and Elonen, E. (1980): Phenobarbitone elimination rate after oral charcoal. *Br. Med. J.*, 1:762.

144. Neuvonen, P. J., Elonen, E., and Mattila, M. J. (1980): Oral activated charcoal and dapsone elimination. *Clin. Pharmacol. Ther.*, 27:823–827.

145. Cohn, W. J., Boylan, J. J., Blanke, R. V., Fariss, M. W., Howell, J. R., and Guzelian, P. S. (1978): Treatment of chlordecone (Kepone) toxicity with cholestyramine. Results of a controlled clinical trial. *N. Engl. J. Med.*, 298:243–248.

146. Bakir, F., Damluji, S. F., Amin-Zaki, L., Murtadha, M., Khalidi, A., Al-Rawi, N. Y., Tikriti, S., Dhahir, H. I., Clarkson, T. W., Smith, J. C., and Doherty, R. A. (1973): Methylmercury poisoning in Iraq. An interuniversity report. *Science*, 181:230–241.

147. Caldwell, J. H., Bush, C. A., and Greenberger, N. J. (1971): Interruption of the enterohepatic circulation of digitoxin by cholestyramine. II. Effect on metabolic disposition of tritium-labeled digitoxin and cardiac systolic intervals in man. *J. Clin. Invest.*, 50:2638–2644.

148. Abshagen, U., von Grodzicki, U., Hirschberger, U., and Rennekamp, H. (1977): Effect of enterohepatic circulation on the pharmacokinetics of spironolactone in man. *Naunyn Schmiedebergs Arch. Pharmacol.*, 300:281–287.

149. Duggan, D. E., and Kwan, K. C. (1979): Enterohepatic recirculation of drugs as a determinant of therapeutic ratio. *Drug Metab. Rev.*, 9:21–41.

150. Bazzano, G., and Bazzano, G. S. (1972): Digitalis intoxication. Treatment with a new steroid-binding resin. *J.A.M.A.*, 220:828–830.

151. Cady, W. J., Rehder, T. L., and Campbell, J. (1979): Use of cholestyramine resin in the treatment of digitoxin toxicity. *Am. J. Hosp. Pharm.*, 36:92–94.
152. Tan, S. Y., Shapiro, R., Kish, M. A. (1979): Reversible acute renal failure induced by indomethacin. *J.A.M.A.*, 241:2732–2733.
153. Brezin, J. H., Katz, S. M., Schwartz, A. B., and Chinitz, J. L. (1979): Reversible renal failure and nephrotic syndrome associated with nonsteroidal anti-inflammatory drugs. *N. Engl. J. Med.*, 301:1271–1272.
154. Mitnick, P. D., Greenberg, A., DeOreo, P. B., Weiner, B. M., Coffman, T. M., Walker, B. R., Agus, Z. S., and Goldfarb, S. (1980): Effects of two nonsteroidal anti-inflammatory drugs, indomethacin and oxaprozin, on the kidney. *Clin. Pharmacol. Ther.*, 28:680–689.
155. Frölich, J. C., Leftwich, R., Ragheb, M., Oates, J. A., Reimann, I., and Buchanan, D. (1979): Indomethacin increases plasma lithium. *Br. Med. J.*, 1:1115–1116.
156. Himmelhoch, J. M., Poust, R. I., Mallinger, A. G., Hanin, I., and Neil, J. F. (1977): Adjustment of lithium dose during lithium-chlorothiazide therapy. *Clin. Pharmacol. Ther.*, 22:225–227.
157. Perel, J. M., Dayton, P. G., Snell, M. M., Yü, T. F., and Gutman, A. B. (1969): Studies of interactions among drugs in man at the renal level: Probenecid and sulfinpyrazone. *Clin. Pharmacol. Ther.*, 10:834–840.
158. Skeith, M. D., Simkin, P. A., and Healey, L. A. (1968): The renal excretion of indomethacin and its inhibition by probenecid. *Clin. Pharmacol. Ther.*, 9:89–93.
159. Steiness, E. (1974): Renal tubular secretion of digoxin. *Circulation*, 50:103–107.
160. Waldorff, S., Andersen, J. D., Heebøll-Nielsen, N., Nielsen, O. G., Moltke, E., Sørensen, U., and Steiness, E. (1978): Spironolactone-induced changes in digoxin kinetics. *Clin. Pharmacol. Ther.*, 24:162–167.
161. Levy, G., and Leonards, J. R. (1971): Urine pH and salicylate therapy. *J.A.M.A.*, 217:81.
162. Levy, G., Lampman, T., Kamath, B. L., and Garrettson, L. K. (1975): Decreased serum salicylate concentrations in children with rheumatic fever treated with antacid. *N. Engl. J. Med.*, 293:323–325.
163. Done, A. K. (1978): Aspirin overdosage: Incidence, diagnosis, and management. *Pediatrics [Suppl.]*, 62:890–897.
164. Temple, A. R. (1978): Pathophysiology of aspirin overdosage toxicity, with implications for management. *Pediatrics* 62(Suppl):873–876.
165. Morgan, A. G., and Polak, A. (1971): The excretion of salicylate in salicylate poisoning. *Clin. Sci.*, 41:475–484.
166. Hadden, J., Johnson, K., Smith, S., Price, L., and Giardina, E. (1969): Acute barbiturate intoxication. Concepts of management. *J.A.M.A.*, 209:93–100.
167. Davies, J. M., Kopin, I. J., Lemberger, L., and Axelrod, J. (1971): Effects of urinary pH on amphetamine metabolism. *Ann. N.Y. Acad. Sci.*, 179:493–501.
168. Rosenberg, J., Benowitz, N. L., and Pond, S. (1981): Pharmacokinetics of drug overdose. *Clin. Pharmacokinet.*, 6:161–192.
169. Aronow, R., Miceli, J. N., and Done, A. K. (1978): Clinical observations during phencyclidine intoxication and treatment based on ion-trapping. *Natl. Inst. Drug Abuse Res. Monogr. Ser.*, 21:218–228.
170. Done, A. K., Aronow, R., and Miceli, J. N. (1978): The pharmacokinetics of phencyclidine in overdosage and its treatment. *Natl. Inst. Drug Abuse Res. Monogr. Ser.*, 21:210–217.
171. Orme, M. L. E. (1982): The clinical pharmacology of oral contraceptive steroids. *Br. J. Clin. Pharmacol.*, 14:31–42.
172. Somogyi, A., and Gugler, R. (1982): Drug interactions with cimetidine. *Clin. Pharmacokinet.*, 7:23–41.
173. Jochemsen, R., Van Der Graaff, M., Boeijinga, J. K., and Breimer, D. D. (1982): Influence of sex, menstrual cycle and oral contraception on the disposition of nitrazepam. *Br. J. Clin. Pharmacol.*, 13:319–324.
174. Chambers, D. M., and Jefferson, G. C. (1982): Antipyrine elimination in saliva after low-dose combined or progestogen-only oral contraceptive steroids. *Br. J. Clin. Pharmacol.*, 13:229–232.
175. Sorkin, E. M., and Darvey, D. L. (1983): Review of cimetidine drug interactions. *Drug Intell. Clin. Pharm.*, 17:110–120.
176. Knapp, A. B., Maguire, W., Keren, G., Karmen, A., Levitt, B., Miura, D. S., and Somberg, J. C. (1983): The cimetidine-lidocaine interaction. *Ann. Intern. Med.*, 98:174–177.

Pharmacokinetic Basis for Drug Treatment,
edited by L. Z. Benet et al., Raven Press,
New York © 1984

Chapter 12

Chronopharmacology and Further Steps Toward Chronotherapy

Franz Halberg and Erna Halberg

Chronobiology Laboratories, Department of Laboratory Medicine and Pathology, University of Minnesota, Minneapolis, Minnesota 55455

ILLUSTRATIVE CHRONOPHARMACOLOGIC EVIDENCE

The right time of administration, just like the right dose, can determine whether the therapy will be of benefit or harm. Timing can (a) influence a desired effect, as in the case of a tumor's response to radiotherapy (1,2), (b) influence carcinostatic chemotherapy (Fig. 1) (3–5), or (c) tip the scale not only between the presence and absence of a response (Figs. 2 and 3) but also between life and death (6–12). In Fig. 3 (effects of bromocriptine on prolactin), timing gains priority over dosing because it determines whether or not a response is produced by a given dose (13). The genetic makeup of an individual may alter the timing of optimal therapy, as seen in Fig. 4 with the use of Nomifensine®.

A caveat is also required for the clinician or investigator applying chronochemotherapy today. As more and more promising results accumulate in chronotherapy (4,11–13), there is the danger that sooner or later enthusiastic chemotherapists will mimic the radiobiologists and give drug therapy ("chronobiologically," as *they* think) under the misapprehension that the body's time structure is invariably tied to environmental time and is related only to a single frequency (1 cycle in 24 hr).

Reference to the fiction of a "steady state" circadian rhythm ignores the extensive, as yet incomplete, evidence documenting a spectrum of rhythms with several frequencies (Table 1), including circannual changes, in most human variables investigated thus far. Failure to take intermodulating rhythms into account may prevent a full exploitation of timing. Just as the search must continue to render screening, diagnosis, and treatment more effective by the application of chronobiological principles, it is necessary in proper studies to secure recent progress that is applicable to the welfare of many patients with cancer and other diseases.

Chronopharmacology

Chronopharmacology is the study of timely and well-timed intervention, accounting for (a) the time dependence of drug effects and (b) the effects of drugs

TABLE 1. *Tentative frequency description and period range for terms describing biologic rhythms[a]*

Domain and region for frequency (*f*)	Range in period ($\tau = 1/f$)
Ultradian	<20 h
Circaduohoran	1.7 ± .1 hr
Circasemidian	12 ± 1hr
Circadian	20–28 hr
Dian	23.8–24.2 hr
Infradian	>28 hr
Circaduodian	2 ± 0.5 days
Circaseptan	7 ± 3 days
Circadiseptan	14 ± 3 days
Circatriseptan (circavigintan)	21 ± 3 days
Circatrigintan	30 ± 5 days
Circannual	1 year ± 2 months

[a]τ = period.

Terms coined by analogy to usage in physics. Just as frequencies higher than those audible or visible are called ultrasonic or ultraviolet, frequencies higher than 1 cycle per 20 hr are designated as ultradian. By the same token, just as frequencies lower than the audible or visible range are called infrasonic or infrared, rhythms with a frequency lower than 1 cycle per 28 hr are designated as infradian.

1. Circadian was intended to indicate the possibility, and thus the need, to search, in the case of several previously synchronized rhythms of an organism, for any consistent desynchronization (a) within the organism and/or (b) from an environmental, e.g., social, schedule. This phenomenon, noted in 1950 in mice after blinding, was of interest since the abrupt change in the temperature rhythm's period after a manipulation (blinding) of the organism indicated that hereditary factors contribute to the period of rhythms that differ from exact environmental counterparts (a precise 24-hr, 7-day, or 1-year period) and among individuals.

2. Equally important in coining circadian was the implication that, in the likely everpresence of biologic noise, a point estimate of a (synchronized or desynchronized) period (or of other rhythm characteristics) should be complemented whenever possible by an inferential statistical interval estimate.

on biologic time structure (i.e., rhythms and age trends). The time dependence of drugs can be drastic, i.e., timing can change the *kind* of response. For example, as a function of timing, the response to the same total dose of the same polysaccharide administered during the same 7-day span to comparable inbred rats subsequently inoculated with the same cancerous growth can be (a) an acceleration of growth and shortening of survival time or (b) a slowing down of growth and lengthening of survival time ($p < 0.05$) (15). Nearly invariably the time dependence of a toxin, a drug, and even of a placebo effect is at least statistically quantitative: as a function of timing, there is less or more of an effect, whether this effect is desired or undesired (16,17).

Chronopharmacology includes, in addition to the study of conventional classic pharmacologic endpoints (and the consequent development of a chronodosimetry for conventional aims), a focus on novel time-dependent drug effects. These effects

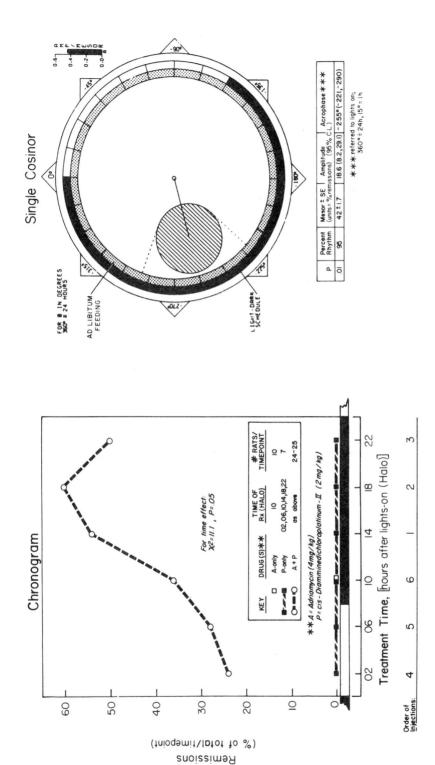

FIG. 1. Circadian-stage dependence of immunocytoma response to *cis*-diamminedichloroplatinum, when adriamycin is given to Louvain rats at optimal circadian intraperitoneal treatment time.

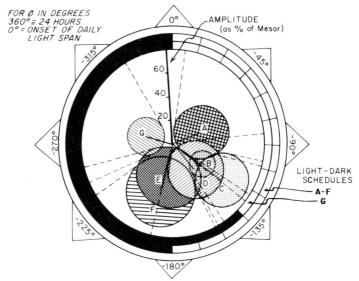

SINGLE COSINOR[1]

Key to Ellipses	Drug Tested[2]	N Studies	Total N Animals	P[3]	% Rhythm[4]	Amplitude[5] (95 % C.L.)	Acrophase, Ø (95 % C.L.)
A	DAUNOMYCIN	4	690	.021	31	29(4,54)	-67°(-8,-127)
B	ADRIAMYCIN	6	1072	<.001	60	33(21,45)	-124°(-103,-146)
C	ARA-C	2	480	<.001	76	56(32,80)	-126°(-100,-151)
D	MELPHALAN	4	456	.015	33	31(18,57)	-138°(- 83,-193)
E	CYCLOPHOSPHAMIDE	6	826	.027	18	32(3,60)	-185°(-123,-255)
F	VINCRISTINE	2	239	.007	67	46(15,76)	-193°(-150,-235)
G	DDPt	11	1503	.002	18	24(8,39)	-289°(-246,-331)

1) Results from least-squares fitting of 24-h cosine curve.
2) i.p.. All drugs, except DDPt, tested in mice kept in LD 12:12; DDPt tested in rats kept in LD: 8:16.
3) P from test of zero-amplitude hypothesis.
4) % Rhythm = % of total variability attributable to fitted cosine.
5) Expressed as % of Mesor.

FIG. 2. Circadian rhythms in murine tolerance of anticancer drugs evaluated from data on survival (%) versus treatment timing. The resistance of nocturnally active mice to toxicity of anticancer drugs varies greatly during a 24-hr span. In studies on the seven drugs summarized here, maximal tolerance occurred in the daily light (rest) span or early in the daily dark (activity) span for six of the drugs and occurred late in the activity span for a seventh drug, cisplatin (DDP). Such results along the 24-hr scale are subject to modulation with lower (infradian) frequency.

include those exerted on parameters of a ubiquitous and important spectrum of rhythms and trends, and they relate to disease prevention as well as therapy.

Chronotherapy

Chronotherapy applies chronopharmacologic and broader chronobiologic facts and principles to the prevention and treatment of disease (17). Chronotherapy, for example, in the case of adrenal corticoids, optimizes known desired effects and/or reduces known undesired effects. Chronotherapy also exploits new pharmacodynamic effects on rhythms, produced by old or new compounds, such as circadian

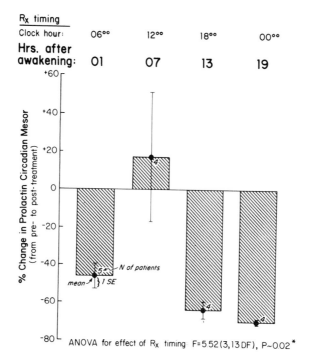

Rx timing

| Clock hour: | 06°° | 12°° | 18°° | 00°° |
| Hrs. after awakening: | 01 | 07 | 13 | 19 |

ANOVA for effect of Rx timing: F=5.52(3,13 DF), P~0.02 *

FIG. 3. Circadian-stage–dependent lowering by bromocriptine mesylate of serum prolactin in patients with prostatic hypertrophy (best effect detected at unconventional rather than conventional times). A bromocriptine mesylate effect on circulating human prolactin was not detected at all times with the conventional dose. Each subject was sampled at 3-hr intervals for 24-hr before and after drug administration; each data series was fitted with 24-hr cosine curve to determine circadian rhythm-adjusted mean (mesor).

*The results from the analysis of variance are questionable for variances are inhomogeneous (Cochran's test ratio = 0.78, $p < 0.05$); a statistically significant effect of treatment timing is indicated separately by the observation that for three of the time points, 95% confidence intervals (approximately three times the indicated SE) do not overlap zero, whereas no response is indicated with treatment at a fourth circadian time.

amplification by Nomifensine (18) and circadian and circaseptan chronization and synchronization by ACTH (19). Prevention by chronobiologic means is the most challenging aim, to be pursued along lines that have proven to be successful in the use of mammary carcinogenesis in certain rodents (1). For example, circadian rhythms in breast surface temperatures have been used to monitor precancerous changes in the human breast (Fig. 5) (20).

Other Definitions

Acrophase (φ)—timing of the highest point in a rhythm defined by a mathematical model (such as a cosine curve) applied to all available data (rather than by the timing of a possibly fortuitous or even informatively influential extreme value).

Amplitude (A)—one-half of the difference between the highest and lowest points in a rhythm defined by a mathematical model (such as a cosine curve) applied to

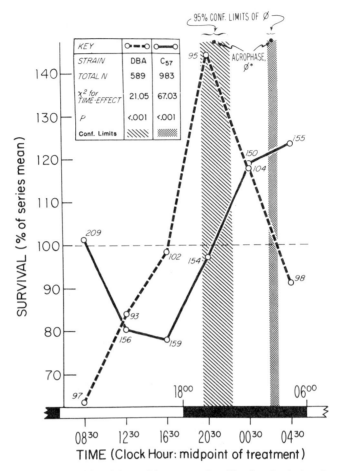

FIG. 4. Overall chronotoxicity of the antidepressant drug Nomifensine in female mice of two inbred strains (differences in timing of murine circadian susceptibility rhythm to Nomifensine evaluated in separate studies). Each point represents the percentage of survivors of overall subtotal of mice injected at a specific time point in three separate studies on DBA mice and four separate studies on C_{57} mice. Evaluation was done at 4 hr after injection in all studies on given strain, irrespective of the dose used. (In any one study, the same dose was used at all time points.) Each dot represents the percentage of survivors of a subtotal at that time, expressed as a percentage of the total series mean (with the latter equated to 100%) in order to eliminate effects of differences among series means.

*ϕ values are from least-squares fit of 24-hr cosine curve.

all available data (rather then by the difference between possibly fortuitous or even informatively influential extreme values).

Amplitude-acrophase test—test of statistical significance for differences in amplitude and acrophase (considered jointly) among different time series (or sets of time series).

Biologic time structure—sum of time-dependent biologic changes, some apparently random, others documentably nonrandom and thus predictable, including a spectrum of rhythms with different frequencies in the context of development, growth, and aging trends.

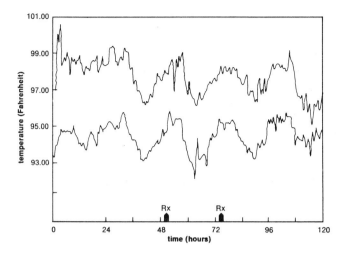

FIG. 5. Comparison of the recorded temperatures for a cancerous left *(top)* and healthy right *(bottom)* breast. Temperatures were obtained from a patient for 52 hr prior to and 62 hr after treatment with estradiol. "High-amplitude" circadian changes in temperature occurred, and the cancerous breast exhibited persistently elevated temperatures prior to treatment. At the end of the study span, less difference in the temperatures of the two breasts is observed, apparently reflecting the effect of treatment. Any interpretation beyond the interbreast difference requires further analysis. The figure shows limitations of exclusive reliance upon inspection of records.

Chronobiology—science of objectively quantifying and investigating biologic time structure and its underlying mechanisms.

Chronodesm—time-specified reference interval.

Chronopharmacokinetics—rhythmic changes in the drug's pharmacokinetics.

Chronoprotopathology—earliest alteration of temporal parameter (e.g., of one or several rhythm characteristics) indicating a progression from a condition of chronorisk toward a potentially or actually harmful state (to be treated in order to prevent overt disease).

Chronopsy—time-specified collection, examination, and interpretation of isolated values or biologic time series for defining health, recognizing risk, screening and diagnosing disease, as a guide to chronotherapy or broadly to assess normality or abnormality against a time-specified reference interval. A time-specified interpretation of body temperature may be referred to as *thermopsy*; the corresponding term for the case of blood pressure is *tensopsy*; for blood, saliva, and urine the terms are *hemopsy, sialopsy,* and *uropsy*, respectively.

Chronorisk—stages of (one or) several rhythms with different frequencies in (one or) several variables placing the individual at enhanced risk of developing chrono-protopathology or disease (21).

Circadian—about 24 hr (20–28 hr).

Circaduodian—about 48 hr.

Circannual—about 1 year.

Merodesm—chronodesm with separate reference intervals computed for a number of time points or time spans throughout a rhythm.

Mesor (M)—mean value of a rhythm defined by a mathematical model (such as a cosine curve).

Mesor-hypertension—transient or lasting elevation of the circadian-rhythm-adjusted mean (mesor) of systolic and/or diastolic blood pressure—validated statistically (e.g., by a mesor test) by comparison with the patient's own mesor at another time and/or against a peer reference standard.

Mesor test—test of statistical significance for differences among mesors of different time series (or sets of time series).

See Table 1 for a description of the period range describing biological rhythms.

CLINOSPECTROMETRY: METHODOLOGIC AND THEORETICAL IMPLICATIONS

Until the early 1950s, the homeostatic dogma of the human body, that is, the belief that all body tissues perform their specific functions in order to maintain constant internal conditions, was not disputed. As rigorous evidence, documenting the ubiquity of rhythms and their critical importance accumulated (see Fig. 6), adherents of the homeostatic cliche started referring in theory to changing set points. The characteristics of these rhythms, vital signs, performance, physiologic responses, and serum and urine variables may change as a function of rhythms. Exploitation of these biological rhythms has great potential value in the therapy of diseases having rhythms to some of their symptoms, such as asthma or seizure disorders. Such chronotherapeutic endeavors must recognize that the effects of many pharmacologic agents depend on the circadian stage at which they are administered. Those who refrain from estimating rhythm parameters use the adjectives "pulsatile" (for regular) and "episodic" (for random) as synonyms in describing a given phenomenon exclusively by "eye-fit" rather than by the often indispensable, inferential statistical complement. By contrast, the chronobiologic concept of the human body recognizes the need for tests and acts on the facts of an inferential statistical time structure. As chronobiology evolved, it began to correlate physiologic results with patient improvement under drug therapy. Most pharmacologists now recognize rhythms but only a few test for them, and even fewer act on them. Chronopharmacologists employing inferential statistical rhythmometry (not to be confused with tests of "time of day" or "seasonal" effects) (22) are scarce in government or in university settings and are virtually absent in industry.

The available evidence shows that rhythms are an indispensable control in most, if not all, drug tests. Figure 2 summarizes pertinent murine data: Circadian rhythms tip the scale between death and survival from a number of agents used in the treatment of human cancer. The rhythm characteristics of such mammalian drug chronotolerance reveal large differences in extent of change and in timing, also apparent in Fig. 2. These differences arise from the resonance between the genetic temporal features of the organism and the environment's cyclic stimuli, and they lead to particularly complex spectral solutions when organismic characteristics are

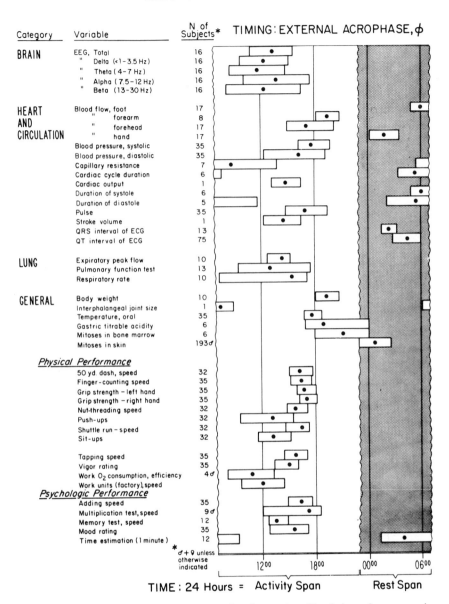

FIG. 6. *(above and following pages)* Human circadian system. The timing values are cosinor approximations of high values in circadian rhythm. Dots = acrophases; bars = 95% confidence limits. Nonoverlapping bars indicate statistically significant differences in timing. **A:** Whole body and organs.

altered by disease. Thus arises the need for self-measurement and for complementary automatic tools, i.e., the polychronor for data collection (see Chapter 19), rapid transfer, transient storage, analysis—and for appropriate data bases. Thereby a

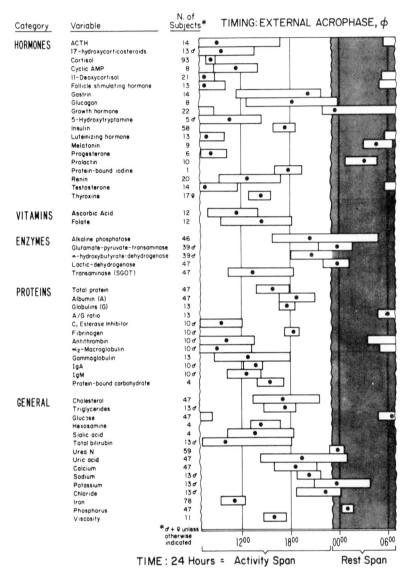

FIG. 6. B. Plasma or serum.

spectrum of rhythms and trends (clinae) can be meaningfully yet cost effectively quantified, in order to predict and exploit timing reliably.

Such clinospectrometry resolves asymmetries in response to schedule shifts and even polarity at the circadian frequency and a host of intermodulations among frequencies within the organism and its environment. The ultimate aim, chronopharmacodynamics, will be to identify pathogenetic time-structure alteration and eventually to prevent it or, if one arrives late, to reverse it. For directions of the

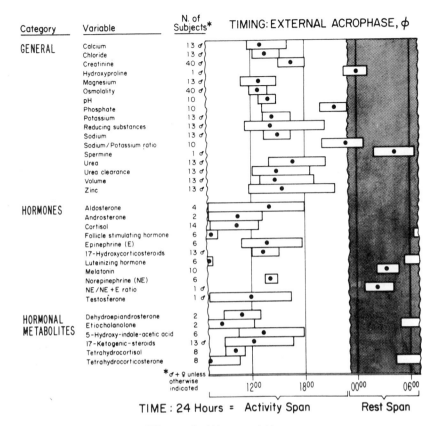

Category	Variable	N. of Subjects*	TIMING: EXTERNAL ACROPHASE, φ
GENERAL	Calcium	13 ♂	
	Chloride	13 ♂	
	Creatinine	40 ♂	
	Hydroxyproline	1 ♂	
	Magnesium	13 ♂	
	Osmolality	40 ♂	
	pH	10	
	Phosphate	10	
	Potassium	13 ♂	
	Reducing substances	13 ♂	
	Sodium	13 ♂	
	Sodium/Potassium ratio	10	
	Spermine	1 ♂	
	Urea	13 ♂	
	Urea clearance	13 ♂	
	Volume	13 ♂	
	Zinc	13 ♂	
HORMONES	Aldosterone	4	
	Androsterone	2	
	Cortisol	14	
	Follicle stimulating hormone	6	
	Epinephrine (E)	6	
	17-Hydroxycorticosteroids	13 ♂	
	Luteinizing hormone	6	
	Melatonin	10	
	Norepinephrine (NE)	6	
	NE/NE+E ratio	1 ♂	
	Testosterone	1 ♂	
HORMONAL METABOLITES	Dehydroepiandrosterone	2	
	Etiocholanolone	2	
	5-Hydroxy-indole-acetic acid	6	
	17-Ketogenic-steroids	13 ♂	
	Tetrahydrocortisol	8	
	Tetrahydrocorticosterone	8	

*♂ + ♀ unless otherwise indicated

TIME: 24 Hours = Activity Span   Rest Span

FIG. 6. C. Urinary variables.

field, the interested reader can refer to the proceedings of international meetings (2,9,10,17,18,23–26).

Individual Variations

Intraindividual differences in the timing of rhythms in different body functions have to be taken into account in specifying, for drug dosing, a circadian and circannual rhythm stage, or at least in attempting to synchronize these stages with known schedules. A specification of the "time of day" or "season" implies standardization as a minimum, preferably chronization or synchronization, and marker rhythmometry as an optimum. It is also desirable to clarify any roles played by interindividual differences in time structure between those who become "active" early or late in the socioecologic day. Such manility or serality, respectively, may have to be assessed not only as such, but also in the light of how it may modify responses to external schedules and/or therapeutic agents.

Furthermore, to whatever "type" (along a manility–serality scale) a given individual may belong, his or her employment schedule may be unusual or irregular, say that of a night guard or a hospital worker on odd shifts, and thus some rhythms

may be shifted largely, if not completely, in relation to local clock time. Similarly, the individual may cross a number of time zones in both directions in the course of working, such as a flight attendant or pilot. Interindividual differences under shifted or shifting conditions may affect various circadian rhythms differently, those associated with the adrenal cortex shifting with the schedule of activity and resting only after a considerable delay (27). Others, such as certain receptor rhythms, may shift at still different speeds after a change in alternation of 24-hr cycles of light and darkness, meal times, and/or other socioecologic schedules. These shift rates may be accelerated or delayed after pinealectomy at certain ages, for the circadian activity rhythm of rats and hamsters (28,29). No case is known, however, for an immediate human circadian adjustment after a 6–12-hr shift in environmental synchronizer. Moreover, reactive as well as spontaneous changes in adrenal cortical and medullary, pineal, and other notably neurohumoral rhythms intermodulate at several frequencies. Drug timing will have to take into account any and all such predictably varying temporal relationships.

For all these reasons, specification of a clock hour or season may not suffice to ensure that a therapy is given at the best time. A comparison of the potential usefulness of chronotherapeutic marker rhythms along several time scales, including that of the menstrual cycle, remains preferable to sole reliance on time of day or time of year. The specification of clock-hour is preferable, however, to total neglect of timing and should involve more than reference to meal times, for mnemotechnical reasons. Moreover, timing should assess variability in disease, as in health, and may prompt us to scrutinize the effects of drugs by rhythm analysis (30).

Penalties for Ignoring Rhythms

Conventional pharmacology and therapy usually ignore biological rhythms and hardly ever rigorously quantify them, with the result that there is real risk of false information being collected and errors committed. By contrast, the recognition and quantification of rhythms can eliminate some of these fallacies and may help us to forestall blunders by action based on erroneous homeostatic concepts, as documented elsewhere (31,32).

Benefits Derived from Assessment of Rhythms

Chronobioassay

A chronobioassay is concerned with testing old and new compounds for (a) any effect on rhythm characteristics and (b) any dependence of effect on the state of rhythms at the time of drug administration.

There are many practicable schemes designed to assess the behavior of circadian rhythm characteristics by the study of responses to environmental changes, with and without drug administration. Data may be collected, for example, on body core temperature by telemetry, on behavioral variables by time-lapse photography, and on biochemical substances by analyses of serial urine, saliva, or blood collections, according to the requirements of a given problem.

Chronobioassays serve to explore rhythm characteristics under such conditions as (a) exposure to one or several (24-hr or other) synchronizers, including the

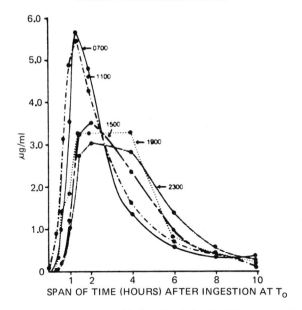

FIG. 7. Mean plasma concentrations of indomethacin in 9 healthy young subjects, each given a single 100-mg dose at different times: T_0 was at 0700, 1100, 1500, 1900, and 2300 hr scheduled at weekly intervals. Samples are missing for 2 subjects at T_0 = 0700 hr and for 4 subjects at T_0 = 1100 hr. (From Clench et al., ref. 34, with permission.)

alternation of light and darkness, alternations of differing environmental temperatures or noise, the availability and nonavailability of food, and of (aggressive, submissive, or neutral) "companions" of the same or different species; (b) institution of one or several changes in the temporal placement along the 24-hr scale of one or more synchronizers, such as the lighting, meal, drug schedules (for rodents), or the living routine, including sleep-wake, work-rest, and meal schedules, as well as other activities and drug regimens; (c) isolation of the subject in a presumably constant environment compatible with a self-selected schedule (and thus with "free running" of one or several rhythms with different frequencies); (d) sampling of blood and/or tissues for a series of special (e.g., biochemical) determinations.

For instance, each of 8 groups of subjects could be dosed at different circadian stages, or with an increase in dose absorbed at certain specified times. The stages chosen for changes in drug dosing schemes could differ by a fixed number of hours (e.g., at 3-hr intervals) on a 24-hr cycle, or more broadly, by a certain number of degrees (e.g., 45°) on any cycle with 360° representing the period length (33). Recently, Clench et al. (34) gave indomethacin at different times and found changes in bioavailability (see Fig. 7). We are clearly dealing in any case with chronodisponibility, as documented originally for erythromycin (17,36). Circadian changes have also been shown with sodium salicylate (35), and theophylline (37). Table 2 lists selected drugs; for these, circadian changes have been shown to alter their pharmacokinetic parameters.

To facilitate the implementation in experimental animals of chronobioassays involving daily drug injections around the clock, including injections at odd hours,

the synchronizers may be manipulated by placing the animals in separate chambers or rooms on different lighting and feeding schedules (33).

For corresponding research on human beings, special drug delivery devices have become available that will program delivery according to some preset time-varying schedule or preferably in a fashion controlled by pertinent marker rhythms of the individual patient, monitored manually or automatically, under computer control.

Chronopharmacokinetics

Of major interest to pharmacologists is the study of temporal aspects of pharmacokinetics, including rhythmic (e.g., circadian) variations of drug bioavailability (Fig. 7) (34); the rate of hepatic drug metabolism; excretion in urine, feces, sweat, saliva, and so on; and variation in the undesired or desired drug effect. The renal excretion of drugs is subject to circadian variations because renal plasma flow, glomerular filtration rate, urine volume, the pH, the content of ions, and so on, fluctuate along the scale of rhythms with several frequencies. A pertinent example is the fluctuations seen in the renal excretion of amphetamine (38). Statistically significant circadian rhythms have been demonstrated for the several parameters used to characterize classical pharmacokinetics (17,34–36,39).

Chronopharmacodynamics

Progress has been made in describing undesired (harmful) or desired effects from physical, chemical, or other agents, including drugs, in relation both to temporal characteristics and to the stage(s) of the test organism at time of dosing (10,40,41). (Much work stems from rodents in the laboratory.) The responsiveness of the human organism to drugs also varies in time. This has been shown with peak expiratory flow in children given methylprednisolone (Fig. 8). Time-dependent drug-induced alterations of physiological functions can therefore influence drug kinetics. Differences in the rhythm spectrum between often diurnally active human beings and largely nocturnal animals, however, should be considered in studies of the dynamic or kinetic effects of drugs.

Chronotherapy: Standardization and Marker Rhythms

Against this background there is a budding interest in chronotherapy—therapeutic action with proper regard for temporal characteristics in the treatment of disease. Chronoprophylaxis for the prevention of disease also must be considered. For such purposes, it hardly suffices to add the prefix "chrono" to a noun. The hard facts of chronotolerance require extensive documentation on appropriate samples obtained under standardized and hence reproducible conditions. Until proof is offered to the contrary, it may not suffice in many clinical cases to specify no more than a pertinent time of day for drug administration. A major task on hand is to investigate further how best to exploit potential "marker rhythms" such as those in host temperature, blood pressure, tumor temperature, urinary Bence Jones protein, polyamine, catecholamine, adrenal corticoid, and electrolyte excretion, to cite but a few examples.

Some markers are gauged in what is presumed to be health for the purposes of detecting constellations of rhythm stages leading to chronorisk, of quantifying and

TABLE 2. *Circadian pharmacokinetic changes of selected drugs[a]*

Drug and dose/24 hr[a]	Time points of administration (clock hours)	Number and type of subjects	Variables investigated	Major circadian changes in pharmacokinetic parameters	Reference
Aspirin (1500 mg) Sd: p.o.	6 a.m. 10 a.m. 6 p.m. 10 p.m.	6 healthy males (20–21 years)	plasma concentration	Peak plasma concentration (C_{max}) and largest area under the curve (AUC) both greatest with admin. at 6 a.m.; smallest C_{max} and AUC with admin. at 11 p.m.	57
Cisplatin (*cis*-diammine dichloroplatinum) 60 mg/m² Sd: i.v.	6 a.m. 6 p.m.	7 women 4 men (25–74 years)	free-platinum urinary excretion	6:00 p.m. infusion resulted in greater urine output, lower peak urinary platinum concentrations, and a lower AUC.	58
Clorazepate dipotassium (50 mg) Sd: p.o.	7 a.m. 7 p.m.	5 healthy adults	plasma concentrations of *N*-desmethyl diazepam	At 7 a.m. time to peak (1 hr) and half-life (3 hr) shortest. At 7 p.m. time to peak (4 hr) and half-life (30 hr) longest.	59
Erythromycin (250 mg × 4) Md: p.o. every 6 hr for 3 days	2 a.m.	24 healthy male adults	plasma erythromycin	Peak concentration greatest at ≈11:30 a.m.; time to peak shortest at ≈8 p.m.; AUC largest at ≈noon.	36
Lithium carbonate	3 types of schedules	5 manic depressive adults	urinary Li, creatinine, and urea	One-third of the daily dose at noon and two-thirds at 8 p.m. reduces both drug nephrotoxicity and large circadian changes in urinary Li compared with 3 equal doses daily or a large dose only in the morning.	60

(continued)

TABLE 2. *(continued)*

Drug and dose/24 hr[a]	Time points of administration (clock hours)	Number and type of subjects	Variables investigated	Major circadian changes in pharmacokinetic parameters	Reference
Midazolam 15 mg, 0.075 mg/kg Sd: p.o., i.v.	morning evening	6 healthy males (24-38 years)	plasma concentration	Clearance differed significantly after both p.o. and i.v. dosing between morning and evening doses.	61
Nortriptyline (100 mg/dose) Sd: p.o.	9 a.m. 9 p.m.	10 healthy adult males	plasma nortriptyline and 10-hydroxynor-triptyline	Mean plasma nortriptyline higher 2 and 3 hr postdrug at 9 a.m. than at 9 p.m. ($p < 0.05$). Mean plasma 10-hydroxynortriptyline (10HP) higher 1, 2, 3, and 4 hr post drug at 9 a.m. than at 9 p.m.; (T_{max}) for 10HP faster after admin. at 9 a.m. than at 9 p.m. ($p < 0.05$).	62
Paracetamol (acetaminophen) (1 g) Sd: p.o.	before sleep and at 8:30 a.m.	4 healthy adult males	paracetamol urinary excretion	The rate of urinary excretion when drug taken before sleep less than when taken at 8:30 a.m.	63
Phenytoin (diphenylhydantoin) (overdose: 5 to 18 mg/kg) Md: p.o.	unknown phenytoin plasma conc. 44–76 mg/liter	4 children; 2M, 2F (6–11 years)	plasma phenytoin, urinary HPPH	Urinary 5-(p-hydroxyphenyl)-5-phenylhydantoin (HPPH) excretion larger during day (up to 75%/24 hr) than during the night.	64

Drug	Times	Subjects	Variable	Comments	Ref.
Propranolol (80 mg) Sd: p.o.	2 a.m. 8 a.m. 2 p.m. 8 p.m.	8 healthy adult males	plasma concentration	Peak concentration of drug lower after admin. at 2 p.m. than after admin. at 8 a.m., 8 p.m. and 2 a.m. ($p < 0.005$; $p \approx 0.1$; $p \approx 0.02$, respectively). AUC after admin. at 2 p.m. lower than after admin. at 8 a.m., 8 p.m. and 2 a.m. ($p < 0.005$, $p < 0.05$; $p < 0.005$, respectively).	65
Synchrodyn Placebo	5 time points (4.8 hr apart)	5 patients with Steinbrocker stage II–III rheumatoid arthritis	urinary cortisol	Circadian change in rhythm-adjusted mean or mesor before and after drug administration. Largest response in summer between 3 and 8 p.m. (95% CL). Percent change in circadian amplitude of urinary free cortisol before and after drug.	50
Theophylline (4.4 mg/kg) Sd: p.o.	1 a.m. 7 a.m. 1 p.m. 7 p.m.	1 healthy adult male	plasma concentration	Time to peak shortest with admin. at 1 a.m. (longest with admin. at 7 p.m.) Peak concentration greatest with admin. at 7 a.m. (smallest with admin. at 7 p.m.).	66
Valproate (50 mg/kg/day)	8 a.m. 8 p.m.	6 healthy patients	plasma concentration Cp_{max}	Time to reach Cp_{max} was longer after 8 p.m. dose due to variation in absorption	67

[a]Sd = single dose, Md = multiple dose, AUC = area under the plasma concentration-time curve, p.o. = oral administration, i.v. = intravenous administration. For comments on indomethacin circadian changes, see Fig. 7. For additional comments concerning theophylline, see Appendix A. Adapted and modified from Reinberg and Smolensky (56), with permission.

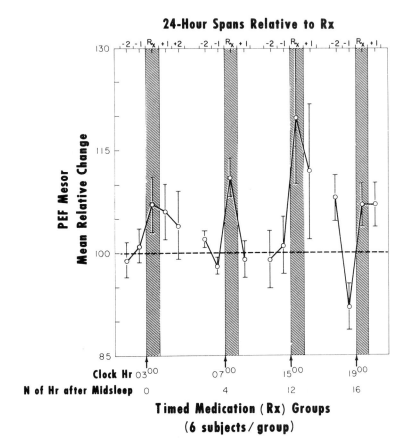

FIG. 8. Peak expiratory flow (PEF) in children. Circadian rhythm-adjusted means (mesors) before and after a single-pulse methylprednisolone sodium succinate injection. For PEF, both mesor and acrophase revealed changes dependent on the timing of the methylprednisolone injection. The circadian mesor of PEF—a measure of airway patency—increased in all instances, but the degree of improvement was greatest when the drug was given at 3 p.m.

testing for statistical significance any alterations in rhythms as harbingers of chronopathology, and thus of signaling the necessity for preventive action. Once the need for action has been identified, perhaps in the form of a deviation from the characteristic rhythm (ecchronism), further research can look for ways of proceeding.

Marker rhythms may also be used once a disease is established, such as mesor-hypertension or cancer (33). Thus, one may endeavor to optimize the treatment of mesor-hypertension with diuretics (Fig. 9) (42–45).

Chronoradiotherapy

Deka and Gupta of Chandigarh, India, have exploited changes in tumor vulnerability by giving radiation to patients with circumoral cancer 5 days each week for weeks, at different times in relation to the peak in tumor temperature assessed "macroscopically" during a 4-day span before treatment was started. In the patients

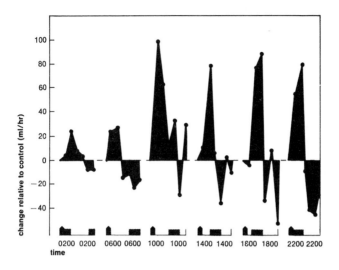

FIG. 9. Chronotherapy for mesor-hypertension: Time and extent of diuresis from chlorothiazide given at different circadian stages in clinically healthy men (positive values are diuresis; negative values are retention). In addition to providing the clinician with personalized standards of blood pressure characteristics, which can reveal abnormalities more precisely, chronobiology may also contribute to therapy. The exact timing of drug administration may be an important consideration in maximizing the therapeutic impact and perhaps in minimizing undesirable side effects. For example, we have studied chlorothiazide and its effect on healthy men depending on the exact time of administration. In this study we administered chlorothiazide to 2 subjects at 2 a.m., to another pair at 6 a.m., and so on at 4-hr intervals. The drug had its most pronounced diuretic effect on subjects who received it at 10 a.m. It then produced a significantly greater urine volume and showed a longer duration of this effect. Obviously, we are not prepared to conclude on the basis of a single study either that chlorothiazide must be administered at 10 a.m. or that this is the optimal timing. The results do suggest, however, that time of administration is potentially an important clinical parameter and that work is needed to specify the optimal time of administration of chlorothiazide and of other drugs used to treat mesor-hypertension. On the basis of our results, it is suggested that the practicing clinician might specify the time of day for administering these therapeutic agents and alter that time of day when necessary to achieve the desired effect by relying on marker rhythms. *Solid obelisk*, chlorothiazide; *solid square*, rest.

investigated, radiotherapy near peak tumor temperature led to a 70% regression of the tumor during the treatment span. By comparison, only a 30% regression occurred when radiotherapy was given either 8 hr before or after the pretreatment peak in tumor temperature (1,2). The (microscopic) acrophase of the rhythm in extent of tumor regression as a function of treatment timing lies near the acrophase of the rhythm in tumor temperature.

Cancer Chronochemotherapy

Figure 10 leads us from chronochemotolerance to chronochemotherapy; it reveals first, in mice free of leukemia, the circadian stages of optimal circadian tolerance for a chemotherapeutic drug, the antimetabolite arabinosyl cytosine (Ara-C). This figure also shows the temporal optimization of the actual cure of leukemic mice by the same drug. Different groups of mice receive so-called sinusoidal treatments

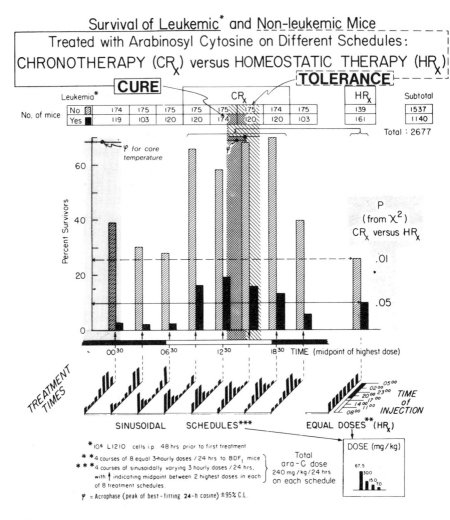

FIG. 10. Treatment of leukemic mice with Ara-C on those sinusoidal schedules to which nonleukemic mice are more tolerant also yields a higher cure rate. As compared with nonsinusoidal (equal dose) schedules, some sinusoidal schedules are much better, in terms of cure as well as tolerance, with others being worse.

(involving gradually increasing and then decreasing doses of the drug) with different temporal placements along the 24-hr scale. Administration of the drug according to certain sinusoidal patterns is associated with favorable cure rates, as compared with equal-dose (or homeostatic) drug administration. Certain other placements of a sinusoidal schedule lead to worse cure rates than the homeostatic treatment and show the need for caution.

Chronopolychemotherapy with cisplatin and doxorubicin has led to apparent cures in a model of a LOU rat plasmacytoma when other treatments had failed in the same rat substrain (although not in others) (46). Individuals concerned with health

care should compare these chronochemotherapeutic lines of evidence with those from currently conventional therapy models, as seen in Figs. 1 and 10.

New Effects

Chronization. Chronization may be defined as the active, practical, and chronobiologically controlled presetting for a predetermined time of a desired organismic state. The presetting of any performance according to the foregoing criteria, including the presetting of a desired state of tolerance for a potentially toxic drug, is a case in point. The presetting of a physiologic performance corresponding to the best one encountered in a spontaneous (e.g., circadian) rhythm may be denoted as relative chronization, whereas a statistically significant further improvement may be denoted as absolute chronization. Chronization may result from a simple or complex treatment. For example, short-chain ACTH-1-17 achieves relative chronization of murine tolerance for doxorubicin (47,48).

Aims. Many agents show effects dependent on the stage of circadian or other rhythms. For example, the tolerance of mice for oncostatic drugs, including doxorubicin, is known to be circadian-stage–dependent. Thus, in many instances, expensive marker rhythmometry may be required to identify optimal treatment time. Hence, to properly specify timing, it is desirable to achieve (by the administration of one or several agents, so-called chronizers) the following:

1. A state corresponding to the best tolerance encountered in the spontaneous circadian tolerance rhythms for a drug, to be denoted as *acrotolerance*

2. Acrotolerance in a logistically convenient way, without the need to identify the best time by marker-rhythm monitoring (which can be costly and complicated)

3. A relative optimization rapidly at any desired time, preferably within 24 hr (of starting any action) and irrespective of (circadian or other) rhythm stage at start

4. For logistic convenience: a staggering of treatment times associated with acrotolerance so that different patients may be scheduled for different clock hours, e.g., for full use of costly radiotherapy or other equipment

5. Documentation of acrotolerance by inferential statistical means, namely by a tolerance associated with the administration of the chronizer and the test substance, comparable to the tolerance associated with the acrophase of the spontaneous tolerance rhythm.

Circadian amplification. A circadian amplitude reduction, if not obliteration, has been found with aging in the SHR-SP rat and also following the experimental lesioning of the two suprachiasmatic nuclei in the inbred Fischer rat (18). Whenever the amplitude reduction can be demonstrated to be undesirable, amplification may constitute a desirable measure. From this viewpoint, further tests are indicated for agents, such as Nomifensine, that have been reported to be potential amplifiers. Great care must be taken, however, to control such studies because amplification may also be unspecific, namely a result of measures involving weighing or injection of a saline solution or placebo in the experimental animal. The same caveat applies to drug-induced (or other) manipulations (49).

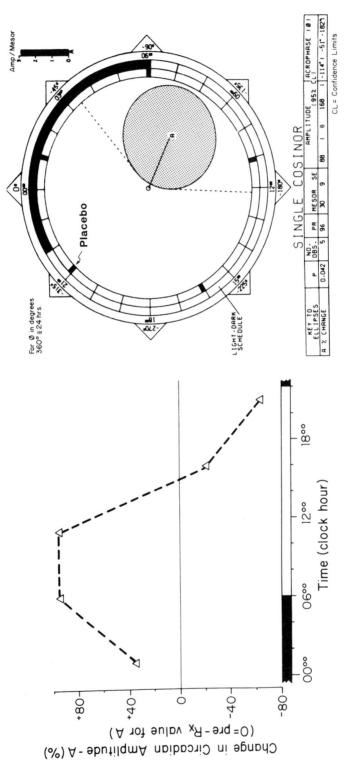

FIG. 11. Circadian rhythmic response to placebo by patients with rheumatoid arthritis. **Left:** Chronogram. **Right:** Single cosinor. Response criterion: Percentage of change in circadian amplitude of urinary free cortisol (μg/hr) from before to after R$_x$. Five men, 45 to 75 years of age, with rheumatoid arthritis provided 6 urine samples in unequal daily fractions (1930–0600 hr, 0600–0830 hr, 0830–1130 hr, 1130–1315 hr, 1315–1730 hr, and 1730–1930 hr) for 24 hr before and after R$_x$. One man was treated at each of 5 different circadian stages. Amplitude determined from fit of 24-hr cosine to each man's data before and after R$_x$.

SINGLE COSINOR

KEY TO ELLIPSES	P	NO. OBS.	PR	MESOR	SE	AMPLITUDE (95% CL)	ACROPHASE (Ø) (CL)
A % CHANGE	0.042	5	96	30 9	88	168 (8	-114°(-51°,-182°)

CL = Confidence Limits

For Ø in degrees 360° ≡ 24 hrs.

Amp./Mesor

Placebo

LIGHT-DARK SCHEDULE

Change in Circadian Amplitude - A (%)
(0= pre-Rx value for A)

Time (clock hour)

Timing the administration of a placebo. Günther et al. (50) demonstrated the circadian-stage–dependent effect of a placebo on urinary free cortisol examined at five different circadian stages in men with Steinbrucker stage II–III rheumatoid arthritis. Population-mean cosinor analysis of urinary cortisol data from the subjects prior to treatment with placebo and during the 24 hr after placebo administration revealed a statistically significant difference in circadian amplitude. Quite clearly, when unspecific circadian amplification is desired or constitutes an unintentional yet beneficial effect, timing may be important to achieve the unspecific benefit (Fig. 11).

STATUS QUO

This chapter primarily illustrates research involving techniques developed in our laboratory and collaborating laboratories. For the broader active field of chrono-biology as it relates to pharmacology and pharmacokinetics, interested readers can refer to references in papers cited herein and to reviews by Halberg et al. (51), Haus and Halberg (23,24), Haus et al. (52), Knapp et al. (53), Scheving et al. (40), Simpson (54), Lemmer (55), and Reinberg and Smolensky (56). Against this background it is surprising that more advantage of the results already obtained in the field of chronobiology has not been taken. One may well anticipate, someday, a label, "Tested and approved for chronotherapeutic administration," on the majority of drugs. Thus, a host of undesirable effects may be minimized, if not avoided, by rhythmometrically guided timing (Table 3). When therapy exploits costly fa-cilities (e.g., for radiation), it will be imperative that timing not only be optimized but also be rendered manipulable for the given patient, i.e., chronized, so that therapeutic desiderata may be combined with logistic realities.

SUMMARY AND CONCLUSION

Whenever tested accurately by chronobiological methods, the responses of living systems to chemical substances (including drugs) have been found to be governed by a spectrum of rhythms characterizing the organism's physiological mechanisms. Among these predictable changes with differing frequencies, circadian rhythms are prominent in the rates of drug absorption, distribution, metabolism, and excretion. They alter human responses to drugs and suggest that timing of drug dosing is an important therapeutic parameter that usually receives too little attention.

The validity of administering potent drugs in equally divided doses almost ran-domly during the day, or at mealtimes, so that compliance is more likely, must be weighed against the advantages of timing according to chronotherapeutic consid-erations, once the latter are proven. Treatment at certain times after awakening, if not at certain times of day (yet to be clarified for the given season), can be suggested. Treatment as to a given spectral stage should become important for administering immunomodulating carcinostatic and antidepressive drugs, to cite a few examples. Drug delivery systems will need to be modified to ensure optimal timing of therapy, e.g., with cyclosporine, according to multifrequency rhythms (67).

TABLE 3. *Introduction of chronobiologic provisions: A choice between alternatives*[a]

Status quo *ad nauseam*	vs.	Toxicology guidelines, good laboratory practices, labeling requirements and funding priorities revised
Ignorance of physiologic timing, e.g., by "the idiocy of three times a day" for everyone and all food and drugs[a]	vs.	Optimization of both food and drug by timing dependent on kind, amount, peer group (or individual) as need be

By making the right choice, literally (above) and figuratively, one not only recognizes but exploits the pertinence of chronobiology to food and drugs:

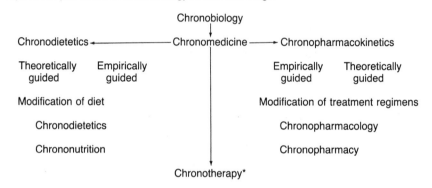

Chronobiology

Chronodietetics ◄─────────── Chronomedicine ───► Chronopharmacokinetics

| Theoretically guided | Empirically guided | | Empirically guided | Theoretically guided |

Modification of diet   Modification of treatment regimens

Chronodietetics   Chronopharmacology

Chrononutrition   Chronopharmacy

Chronotherapy*

*Importance of timing (chronization, synchronization, and development of chronobiotics) documented by:

In rodents

Life or death	Life or death: change of $LD^{30}/_{50}$; improvement of toxic-therapeutic ratio; cure or remission of cancer, unattainable otherwise with same dose

In human beings

Change in relation among metabolic and endocrine rhythm parameters	Amelioration of (a) desired effect, (b) tolerance for undesired effect, (c) novel effects

[a]The evidence is in hand to require that chronobiologic provisions be introduced into the national and international regulation of foods and drugs for a true cooperation between government, industry and university. We continue to confront a choice between alternatives given above.

Education in chronobiology, at as early an age as possible, preferably within the context of secondary education, may achieve not only patient compliance but also the ready implementation of marker rhythmometry. Marker rhythms assessed by self-measurement or automatically can guide the individualized optimization of single- and multiple-drug chronotherapy. Automatic marker rhythm monitoring coupled to automatic drug delivery may eventually adjust therapy according to the characteristics of our time structure.

Even then, the best dose of a drug will be a compromise between the intermodulating stages of maximal and minimal desired activity and greater or lesser susceptibility to side effects. When desired actions and side effects involve different systems, their rhythmical fluctuations may be spontaneously in optimal relation to each other at times that can be predicted by relying on marker rhythms.

Alternatively, best tolerance may be reached by chronization (presetting) or by synchronization and phase shifting with drugs, such as synthetic ACTH 1–17, and in certain cases by timing meals and other aspects of routine (17).

These are just some of the possibilities to be exploited for the time-phased graduation of dosage in practice. Drug therapy that thus succeeds in respecting and exploiting the patient's biological rhythms is both safer and more efficacious. Moreover, new treatment modalities, chronobiotics, can be rationally sought to correct rhythm alteration when it is a determinant of disease.

Rhythmometry in the service of basic and clinical pharmacology is no longer too complex, once its merits are clarified just as the isolation of a chemical compound is not. The usual prescribed timing of a drug may not be optimal; it is often designed merely to assure that the patient is taking the drug, for example, at mealtimes. A schedule of times and doses that takes into account and uses rhythms as a gauge of treatment can be expected to be effective and has been shown to enhance compliance; it immediately reveals the consequences of a failure to comply, notably in the case of a so-called silent disease, such as some illnesses that are associated with an elevated overall blood pressure mean (45).

It is within this broad spectral perspective that the recognition of chronopharmacology as a discipline is becoming realistic. The stream of chronopharmacologic information surely must develop into a mandatory basis of action for the pharmacologist, the physician, the pharmacist, and the remainder of the health care team.

ACKNOWLEDGMENTS

This work was supported by grants from the U. S. National Institute of General Medical Sciences (GM-13981), National Cancer Institute (CA-14445), and National Institute of Occupational Safety and Health (OH-00631) and by the Hoechst Foundation, Milano, Italy. Materials in this chapter were originally prepared for *Chronobiologia* and are here reprinted by kind permission of that journal.

REFERENCES

1. Gupta, B. D., and Deka, A. C. (1975): Application of chronobiology to radiotherapy of tumor of oral cavity. *Chronobiologia*, 2(Suppl. 1):25.
2. Halberg, E., Gupta, B. D., Haus, E., Halberg, E., Deka, A. C., Nelson, W., Sothern, R. B., Cornelissen, G., Lee, J. K., Lakatua, D. J., Scheving, L. E., Burns, E. R. (1977): Steps toward a cancer chronopolytherapy. In: *Proc. XIVth Int. Cong. Therapeutics*, pp. 151–196. L'Expansion Scientifique Francaise, Montpellier, France.
3. Haus, E., Halberg, F., Scheving, L., Cardoso, S., Kühl, J. F. W., Sothern, R., Shiotsuka, R. N., Hwang, D. S., and Pauly, J. E. (1972): Increased tolerance of leukemic mice to arabinosyl cytosine given on schedule adjusted to circadian system. *Science*, 177:80–82.
4. Halberg, F., Haus, E., Cardoso, S. S., Scheving, L. E., Kühl, J. F. W., Shiotsuka, R., Rosene, G., Pauly, J. E., Runge, W., Spalding, J. F., Lee, J. K., and Good, R. A. (1973): Toward a

chronotherapy of neoplasia: Tolerance of treatment depends upon host rhythms. *Experientia*, 29:909–934.

5. Scheving, L. E., Burns, E. R., Pauly, J. E., Halberg, E., and Haus, E. (1977): Survival and cure of leukemic mice after circadian optimization of treatment with cyclophosphamide and arabinosyl cytosine. *Cancer Res.*, 37:3648–3655.

6. Scheving, L. E., Burns, E. R., Pauly, J. E., and Halberg, F. (1980): Circadian bioperiodic response of mice bearing advanced L1210 leukemia to combination therapy with adriamycin and cyclophosphamide. *Cancer Res.*, 40:1151–1515.

7. Sothern, R. B., Halberg, F., and Nelson, W. (1979): Strain-difference in circadian murine chronotolerance to the antidepressant drug nomifensine. *Chronobiologia*, 6:397–404.

8. Scheving, L. E., Haus, E., Kühl, J. F. W., Pauly, J. E., Halberg, F., and Cardoso, S. (1976): Close reproduction by different laboratories of characteristics of circadian rhythm in 1-β-D-arabinofuranosylcytosine tolerance by mice. *Cancer Res.*, 36:1133–1137.

9. Reinberg, A., and Halberg, F. (eds) (1979): *Chronopharmacology*, p. 429. Pergamon, Oxford.

10. Halberg, F. (1962): Physiologic 24-hour rhythms: A determinant of response to environmental agents. In: *Man's Dependence on the Earthly Atomsphere*, edited by Karl. E. Schaefer, pp. 48–98. Macmillan, New York.

11. Reinberg, A., and Halberg, F. (1971): Circadian chronopharmacology. *Ann. Rev. Fharmacol.*, 2:455–492.

12. Levi, F., Halberg, F., Nesbit, M., Haus, E., and Levine, H. (1981): Chrono-oncology. In: *Neoplasms—Comparative Pathology of Growth in Animals, Plants and Man*, edited by H. Kaiser, pp. 267–312. Williams and Wilkins Co., Baltimore.

13. Tarquini, B., Halberg, F., Seal, U. S., Benvenuti, M., and Cagnoni, M. (1981): Circadian aspects of serum prolactin and TSH lowering by bromocriptine in patients with prostatic hypertrophy. *The Prostate*, 2:269–279.

14. Haus, E., Halberg, F., Loken, M. K., and Kim, U. S. (1973): Circadian rhythmometry of mammalian radiosensitivity. In: *Space Radiation Biology*, edited by A. Tobias, and P. Todd, pp. 435–474. Academic Press, New York.

15. Levi, F., and Halberg, F. (1982): Circaseptan (about-7-day) bioperiodicity—spontaneous and reactive—and the search for pacemakers. *La Ricerca Clin. Lab.*, 12:323–370.

16. Halberg, F., Johnson, E. A., Brown, B. W., and Bittner, J. J. (1960): Susceptibility rhythm to *E. coli* endotoxin and bioassay. *Proc. Soc. Exp. Biol.*, 103:142–144.

17. Halberg, F. (1974): Protection by timing treatment according to bodily rhythms—an analogy to protection by scrubbing before surgery. *Chronobiologia*, 1(Suppl. 1):27–68.

18. Halberg, F., Lubanovic, W. A., Sothern, R. B., Brockway, B., Powell, E. W., Pasley, J. N., Scheving, L. E. (1979): Nomifensine chronopharmacology, schedule shifts and circadian temperature rhythms in disuprachiasmatically-lesioned rats—modeling emotional chronopathology and chronotherapy. *Chronobiologia*, 6:405–424.

19. Halberg, F., Günther, R., Herold, M., and Halberg, E. (1981): Circadian and circaseptan (about-7-day) disynchronization of urinary cortisol by synthetic ACTH in arthritics. *Proc. End. Soc. USA*, :331.

20. Halberg, E., Halberg, F., Cornelissen, G., Simpson, H. W., and Taggett-Anderson, M. A. (1979): Toward a chronopsy: Part II. A thermopsy revealing asymmetrical circadian variation in surface temperature of human female breasts and literature review. *Chronobiologia*, 6:231–257.

21. Tarquini, B., Benvenuti, M., Moretti, R., Neri, B., Cagnoni, M., and Halberg, F. (1979): Atherosclerotic chronorisk, recognized by autorhythmometry combined with hemopsies as a step toward chronophylaxis. *Chronobiologia*, 6:162–163.

22. Halberg, F. (1959): Physiologic 24-hour periodicity; general and procedural considerations with reference to the adrenal cycle. *Z. Vitam. Horm. Fermentforsch.*, 10:225–296.

23. Haus, E., and Halberg, F. (1980): Circadian time structure. In: *Chronobiology: Principles and Applications to Shifts in Schedules*, edited by L. E. Scheving, and F. Halberg, pp. 47–94. Sijthoff and Noordhoff, The Netherlands.

24. Haus, E., and Halberg, F. (1980): Endocrine rhythms. In: *Chronobiology: Principles and Applications to Shifts in Schedules*, edited by L. E. Scheving, and F. Halberg, pp. 137–188. Sijthoff and Noordhoff, The Netherlands.

25. Hrushesky, W., Levi, F., Halberg, F., Haus, E., Scheving, L. E., Sanchez, S., Medini, E., Brown, H., and Kennedy, B. J. (1980): Clinical chrono-oncology. In: *Chronobiology: Principles*

and Applications to Shifts in Schedules, edited by L. E. Scheving, and F. Halberg, pp. 513–534. Sijthoff and Noordhoff, Alphen aan den Rijn, The Netherlands.

26. Takahashi, R., Walker, C., and Halberg, F. (eds) (1982): *Toward Chronopharmacology: 8th IUPHAR Congress and Satellite Symposium* (Nagasaki, July 27–28 1981). Pergamon, Oxford.

27. Halberg, F. (1969): Chronobiology. *Ann. Rev. Physiol.*, 31:675–725.

28. Quay, W. B. (1972): Pineal homeostatic regulation of shifts in the circadian activity rhythm during maturation and aging. *Trans. N.Y. Acad. Sci. Ser. II*, 34:239–254.

29. Finkelstein, J. S., Baum, F. R., and Campbell, C. S. (1978): Entrainment of the female hamster to reversed photoperiod: Role of the pineal. *Physiol. Behav.*, 21:105–111.

30. Vukelich, M., Hrushesky, W., Halberg, F., Levi, F., Langevin, T., Levi, F., Kennedy, B. J., Gergen, J., Goetz, F., and Theologides, A. (1981): Elevated circadian mesor of pulse in recumbency predicts doxorubicin-induced congestive heart failure. *Int. J. Chronobiol.*, 7:344.

31. Halberg, F., Kabat, H., and Klein, P. (1980): Chronopharmacology: A therapeutic frontier. *Am. J. Hosp. Pharm.*, 37:101–106.

32. Halberg, F., Klein, P., and Kabat, H. (1980): Circadian rhythms and drug dosing. In: *Biological Rhythms (Documenta Geigy)*, pp. 4–6. Ciba-Geigy Ltd., Basel.

33. Halberg, F., Carandente, F., Cornelissen, G., and Katinas, G. S. (1977): Glossary of chronobiology. *Chronobiologia*, 4(Suppl. 1):189.

34. Clench, J., Reinberg, A. D., Ziewanowska, Z., Ghata, J., and Smolensky, M. (1981): Circadian changes in the bioavailability and effects of indomethacin in healthy subjects. *Eur. J. Clin. Pharmacol.*, 20:359–369.

35. Reinberg, A., Zagula-Mally, Z., Ghata, J., and Halberg, F. (1967): Circadian rhythms in duration of salicylate excretion referred to phase of excretory rhythms and routine. *Proc. Soc. Exp. Biol.*, 124:826–832.

36. DiSanto, A., Chodos, D., and Halberg, F. (1975): Chronobioavailability of three erythromycin test preparations assessed by each of 4 indices, time to peak, peak, nadir, area. *Chronobiol.*, 2(Suppl. 1):17.

37. Maxey, K. G., Smolensky, M. H., and McGovern, J. P. (1979): Circadian variations in the susceptibility of rodents to the toxic effects of theophylline. In: *Chronopharmacology*, edited by A. Reinberg, and F. Halberg, pp. 239–244. Pergamon Press, Oxford.

38. Beckett, A. H., and Rowland, M. (1964): Rhythmic urinary excretion of amphetamine in man. *Nature*, 204:1203–1204.

39. Sturtevant, F. M. (1976): Chronopharmacokinetics of ethanol. *Naunyn-Schmiedebergs Arch. Pharmacol.*, 293:203–208.

40. Scheving, L. E. (1976): The dimension of time in biology and medicine—chronobiology. *Endeavour*, 35:66–72.

41. Haus, E., Halberg, F., Scheving, L. E., and Simpson, H. (1979): Chronotherapy of cancer—a critical evaluation. *Int. J. Chronobiol.*, 6:67–107.

42. Levine, H., and Halberg, F. (1972): Circadian rhythms of the circulatory systems, Literature Review. Computerized case study for transmeridian flight and medication effects on a mildly hypertensive subject. U.S. Airforce Report, SAM-TR-72, p. 64.

43. Bartter, F. C., Delea, C. S., Baker, W., Halberg, F., and Lee, Y. K. (1976): Chronobiology in the diagnosis and treatment of mesorhypertension. *Chronobiol.*, 3:199–213.

44. Scarpelli, P. T., Romano, S., Buricchi, L., Corti, C., Menniti, P., and Gizdulich, P. (1978): Controllo del'effetto antiipertensivo del prazosin mediante autoritmometria della pressione arteriosa. In: *Problemi e Prospettive dell-Ipertensione Arteriosa*, edited by C. Bartorelli, A. Bertelli, A. Giotti, and U. Teodori, pp. 173–190. ESAM.

45. Gullner, H. G., Bartter, F. C., Halberg, F., and Delea, C. (1979): Circadian temperature and blood pressure rhythms guide timed optimization and gauge antimesorhypertensive prazosin effects. *Chronobiologia*, 6:107.

46. Deckers, C., Deckers-Passau, L., and Dubucq-Mace, F. (1977): A transplantable immunocytoma for the rat as a model for the study of immunoglobulin secretion. *Lab. Animal Sci.*, 27:733–736.

47. Halberg, F., Sanchez, S., Brown, H., Haus, E., Lakatua, D., Melby, J., Wilson, T., Sothern, R., Berg, H., and Scheving, L. E. (1980): Pretreatment with time-dependently active short-chain adrenocorticotropin (ACTH-17; HOE 433) for convenient optimization of murine adriamycin chronotolerance. *Proc. AACR/ASCO*, 21:307.

48. Halberg, F., Halberg, E., Herold, M., Vecsei, P., Günther, R., and Reinberg, A. (1982): Toward a clinospectrometry of conventional and novel effects of ACTH 1–17—Synchrodyn®—in rodents

and human beings. In: *Toward Chronopharmacology*. Proc. 8th IUPHAR Cong. and Sat. Symposia, edited by R. Takahashi, C. Walker and F. Halberg, (in press).

49. Baltzer, V., Weiskrantz, L. (1975): Antidepressant agents and reversal of diurnal activity cycles in the rat. *Biol. Psychiat.*, 10:199–209.
50. Günther, R., Herold, M., Halberg, E., Halberg, F. (1980): Circadian placebo and ACTH effects on urinary cortisol in arthritics. *Peptides*, 1:387–390.
51. Halberg, F. (1982): Chronopharmacology and chronotherapy. In: *Cellular Pacemakers*, edited by D. O. Carpenter, pp. 261–297. John Wiley & Sons Inc., New York.
52. Haus, E., Cornelissen, G., Halberg, F. (1980): Introduction to chronobiology. In: *Chronobiology: Principles and Applications to Shifts in Schedules*, edited by L. E. Scheving, and F. Halberg, pp. 1–32. Sijthoff and Noordhoff, The Netherlands.
53. Knapp, M. S., Cove-Smith, J. R., Dugdale, R., Mackenzie, N., and Powell, R. (1979): Possible effect of time on renal allograft rejection. *Br. Med. J.*, 1:75–77.
54. Simpson, H. W. (1980): In: *Chronobiology: Principles and Applications to Shifts in Schedules*, edited by L. E. Scheving, and F. Halberg, pp. 433–446. Sijthoff and Noordhoff, The Netherlands.
55. Lemmer, B. (1981): Chronopharmacokinetics. In: *Topics in Pharmaceutical Sciences*, edited by D. D. Breimer and P. Speiser, pp. 49–68. North Holland Biomedical Press, Amsterdam.
56. Reinberg, A., and Smolensky, M. H. (1982): Circadian changes of drug disposition in man. *Clin. Pharmacokinet.*, 7:401–420.
57. Markiewicz, A., and Semenowicz, K. (1979): Time dependent changes in the pharmacokinetics of aspirin. *Int. J. Clin. Pharmacol. Biopharm.*, 17:409–411.
58. Hrushesky, W. J. M., Borch, R., and Levi, F. (1982): Circadian time dependence in cisplatin urinary kinetics. *Clin. Pharmacol. Ther.*, 32:330–339.
59. Hrushesky, W., Levi, F., and Kennedy, B. J. (1980): Cis-diamine-dichloroplatinium (DDP) toxicity to the human kidney reduced by circadian timing. *Clin. Oncol.*, 21:C45.
60. Lambinet, I., Aymard, N., Soulairac, A., and Reinberg, A. (1981): Chronooptimization of lithium administration in five manic depressive patients: Reduction of nephrotoxicity. *Int. J. Chronobiol.*, 7:274.
61. Klotz, U., and Ziegler, G. (1982): Physiologic and temporal variation in hepatic elimination of midazolam. *Clin. Pharmacol. Ther.*, 32:107–112.
62. Nakano, S., and Hollister, I. E. (1978): No circadian effect on nortriptyline kinetics in man. *Clin. Pharmacol. Ther.*, 23:199–203.
63. Mattok, G. L., and McGilveray, J. (1973): The effect of food intake and sleep on absorption of acetaminophen. *Rev. Can. Biol.*, 32(Suppl. Automne):77–84.
64. Garrettson, L. K., and Jusko, W. J. (1975): Diphenylhydantoin elimination kinetics in overdose children. *Clin. Pharmacol. Ther.*, 17:481–491.
65. Markiewicz, A., Semenowicz, K., Korczynska, J., and Boldys, H. (1980): In: *Recent Advances in the Chronobiology of Allergy and Immunology*, edited by M. H. Smolensky, pp. 185–193. Pergamon, Oxford.
66. Kyle, G. M., Smolensky, M. H., Thorne, L. G., and McGovern, J. P. (1980): In: *Recent Advances in the Chronobiology of Allergy and Immunology*, edited by M. H. Smolensky, pp. 123–128. Pergamon, Oxford.
67. Loiseau, P., Cenraud, B., Levy, R. H., Akbaraly, R., Brachet-Liermain, A., Guyot, M., and Morselli, P. L. (1982): Diurnal variations in steady-state plasma concentrations of valproic acid in epileptic patients. *Clin. Pharmacokinet.*, 7:544–552.

Pharmacokinetic Basis for Drug Treatment,
edited by L. Z. Benet et al., Raven Press,
New York © 1984

Chapter 13

Effects of Pregnancy on Pharmacokinetics

William A. Parker

College of Pharmacy, Dalhousie University, Halifax, Nova Scotia, Canada B3H 3J5

In pregnancy and childbirth (labor), the body becomes a complex, multicompartmental unit consisting of mother, placenta, and fetus. This unit is complicated; not only are the integrated parts of the system interrelated but also considerable physiologic changes occur as pregnancy advances (1,2).

Pharmacokinetic analyses in humans during pregnancy and childbirth are complicated for numerous technical reasons and must be limited for obvious legal and ethical considerations. Such studies are usually isolated cases carried out either in first-trimester pregnancies when abortion is planned or at term shortly before, during, or after delivery. One-point determinations of drug concentrations from maternal, fetal, and neonatal blood samples or arteriovenous (A-V) umbilical vessel drug concentration gradients are often the only available data; this greatly restricts obtaining adequate pharmacokinetic information and leads to confusion and misunderstanding.

COMPARTMENTAL CHARACTERIZATION OF THE MATERNAL–FETAL UNIT

In simple terms, the mother and fetus can be regarded as two separate compartments. However, more complicated models can include further compartments for the amniotic fluid, the placenta, and similar structures (1). Physiologic model representations have also been proposed, as detailed in Fig. 1 (3).

Various computer simulations have been published (2) in which the maternal–fetal unit functions as a one-compartment, two-compartment, or multicompartment system and where mother and/or fetus may possess characteristics of deep and shallow compartments. Most of these models assume all distribution, transfer, and elimination processes to be apparent first-order processes, and they assume that clearances between mother and fetus are equal in both directions, obviously imposing severe limitations.

PHYSIOLOGIC CHANGES OF PREGNANCY/CHILDBIRTH

Physiologic adjustments during pregnancy occur in several different systems, the primary ones being cardiovascular, pulmonary, renal, and gastrointestinal, as well

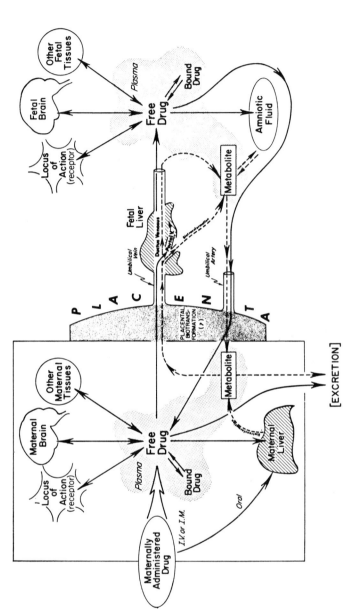

FIG. 1. Relationship between maternal and fetal compartments and distribution of drugs between them. Drug is passed from the maternal compartment via the placenta (a partial barrier) to the fetal compartment where the principles of drug dynamics, i.e., distribution, biotransformation, and excretion, determine the eventual specific organ tissue levels. One purely mechanical barrier exists between the maternal and fetal compartment that attains importance in the late first and second stage of labor, i.e., the umbilical cord, which is susceptible to partial and total occlusion. (From Mirkin, ref. 3, with permission.)

as fat and body water compartments. There is also the development of additional distribution compartments, such as the placenta, amniotic fluid, and fetus (3). Most of these physiologic changes may cause functional changes influencing the pharmacokinetic parameters of drug absorption, distribution, and elimination. As will be seen, these changes develop at different times during gestation and may themselves change over time, especially during childbirth and following parturition.

It is important to delineate key changes during pregnancy and childbirth in order to anticipate either emerging variables needing control for research purposes or patient characteristics necessitating altered therapeutics.

A number of reviews describing drug kinetics in pregnancy (1,2), drug kinetics in childbirth (4), and changing maternal physiology (5) have been published. Table 1 provides pharmacokinetic parameters for a selected list of drugs used in pregnancy, where comparisons of values are made with those values found in nonpregnant women.

DRUG ABSORPTION

Gastrointestinal

As discussed in Chapter 2, gastrointestinal absorption of drugs is influenced by various physiologic factors such as the chemical composition and pH of gastric and intestinal secretions, emptying time, and intestinal blood flow. All of these factors are changing (or are likely to change) during pregnancy.

First, several changes take place in intestinal secretions during pregnancy. There is a 40% reduction in gastric acid secretion, reduced peptic activity, and a significant increase in the secretion of mucus. These alterations result in an increased gastric pH and buffer capacity that may affect dissolution and possibly absorption, as detailed in Chapters 2 and 11.

Second, there is a reduction in intestinal motility, as reflected by a 30 to 50% slowing in gastric and intestinal emptying times, the consequences of which were discussed in Chapter 2 and have been published elsewhere (21).

Third, because of an increased cardiac output *(vide infra)*, one might reasonably expect an increased intestinal blood flow, which might enhance intestinal drug absorption for drugs where membrane transport is the rate-limiting step.

The rate of oral drug absorption in patients in childbirth appears essentially normal, provided that narcotic analgesics have not been administered concurrently. It is clinically important to recognize the possibility of such drug interactions when interpreting and reporting the results of a pharmacokinetic study in order to differentiate between the effects of childbirth per se and the effects of drug interactions.

Pulmonary

Pulmonary absorption and handling of drugs across the alveolar membrane are influenced by various hemodynamic and ventilatory factors (see Chapter 7).

TABLE 1. Pharmacokinetics in pregnancy

Drug (reference)	Number of patients	Route of medication	Vd (liter/kg)	$T_{1/2}$ (hrs)	CL	Comments
Clorazepate (6)	7 7 normals	20-mg i.m. single dose	0.43 (0.26–0.68) 0.33 (0.17–0.67)	1.3 (0.73–2.2) 2 (1.1–3.8)	0.23 (liter/hr/kg) 0.11 (liter/hr/kg)	Pregnant absorption $T_{1/2}$ 0.77 hr, nonpregnant absorption $T_{1/2}$ 0.56 hr, percentage transformed to nordiazepam: 98.1%* in pregnant, 91.3% in nonpregnant
Meperidine (7)	7	50-mg i.v. single dose	2.66 ± 0.66 V_{ss}	3.71 ± 1.69	11.23 ± 4.74 (ml/min/kg)	Normal values for the nonpregnant given from comparisons of other studies
	8 normals 4 normals		4.17 ± 1.33 3.73	3.21 ± 0.80 3.7 ± 1.6	16.5 (ml/min/kg) 14.5 ± 5 (ml/min/kg)	
Meperidine (8)	12 7 normals	50 mg i.v. p.r.n. 50 mg i.v.	187 ± 74 V_{ss} (liters) 209 ± 59 (liters)	2.53 ± 0.6 2.95 ± 1.2	1,010 ± 381 (ml/min) 964 ± 300 (ml/min)	The urinary excretion of meperidine and normeperidine similar in postpartum and nonpregnancy
d-Tubocurarine (10)	10 10 normals	Drug binding determined by equilibrium dialysis				58.9 ± 2.6% free 54.6 ± 1.6% free
Metocurine (10)	3 10 normals	Drug binding determined by equilibrium dialysis				67.1 ± 1.2% free 69.9 ± 1.5% free
Propranolol (10)	15 16 normals	Drug binding determined by equilibrium dialysis				19.9 ± 1.3% free* 14.6 ± 0.8% free
Lidocaine (10,12)	15 16 normals	Drug binding determined by equilibrium dialysis	Increased concentrations of monoethylglycinexylidide throughout labor			47.7 ± 4.7% free* 32.0 ± 1.4% free
Diazepam (10)	11 16 normals	Drug binding determined by equilibrium dialysis				4.5 ± 0.28% free* 2.4 ± 0.07% free*
Dexamethasone (9)	10 6 normals	8-mg i.v. single dose		142 (min)	559 (ml/min) 243 (ml/min)	Plasma binding for pregnant 66.6%, nonpregnant 68.1%, nonpregnant data from other study

Drug	N	Method	Value	$T_{1/2}$ / Clearance	Comments
Salicylic acid and Sulfisoxazole (11)	28 28 normals	Drug binding determined by equilibrium dialysis			↓ Binding of sulfisoxazole and salicylic acid
Carbimazole (methimazole) (13)	7 5 normals	10-mg oral dose 10-mg oral dose		164 ± 16 (ml/min) 110 ± 21 (ml/min)	
Ampicillin (15)	14 6 normals	i.m. dose (10 mg/kg)	0.99 ± 3.1 0.68 ± 0.2*	7.7 ± 3.2 (ml/min/kg) 4.3 ± 1.2 (ml/min/kg)	
Caffeine (16)	62	Weighed amounts of instant coffee	For pregnancy, week of pregnancy	79 (min) 93.5 (min) $T_{1/2}$ (hr)	
			11–14	4.7 ± 0.1	
			15–18	7.9 ± 2.8	
			19–22	7.2 ± 3.3	
			23–26	7.9 ± 2.4	
			27–30	10 ± 3.4	
			31–34	9.8 ± 2.8	
			35–38	10.5 ± 4	
			3–15 post pregnancy	3.9 ± 1.6 3.1 ± 0.9	
Furosemide (17)	14 normals 8	Oral dose 0.66 mg/kg	0.35 ± 0.13	115 ± 37.1 (min)	Single dose study, all gestotic women
	4	i.v. dose 0.6 mg/kg	0.18 ± 0.02	71.8 ± 26.3 (min)	153 ± 48 (ml/min) 152 ± 23 (ml/min)
Atenolol (19)	11	100-mg tablet, single oral dose		8.1 ± 0.5	All in 9th month of gestation, all gestotic, F = 0.5, on other antihypertensives AUC 223 ± 18.2 (µg/hr/ml) AUC 282 ± 75.4 (µg/hr/ml) 10.2 ± 0.2% free
Metronidazole (20)	6 11 normals	1-g oral dose 1-g oral dose		7.73 ± 1.11 7.8 ± 1.3	
Phenytoin (14,18)	4 first trimester 11 third trimester 11 normals				11.2 ± 0.7% free 9.0 ± 1.0% free

*Statistically significant.

Several changes occur in the respiratory system during pregnancy. The respiratory rate remains essentially unchanged throughout pregnancy; however, the tidal volume (that volume of air moved with each normal inspiration and expiration) gradually increases throughout pregnancy so that at term it is 30 to 40% above base-line levels. The increase in respiratory tidal volume associated with the normal respiratory rate necessarily results in increased respiratory minute volume (or hyperventilation), the magnitude of this increase being approximately 40%. This hyperventilation of pregnancy is apparently related, at least in part, to increased levels of progesterone.

Consequently, inhalational drug agents (e.g., anesthetic gases, asthmatic nebulizers) may cross the alveolar membrane at a much higher rate than in nonpregnant patients, especially when one considers the increased cardiac output and higher pulmonary blood flow favoring alveolar drug uptake.

Parenteral

There is generalized peripheral vessel dilatation during pregnancy that results in up to a sixfold increase in peripheral blood flow and peripheral tissue perfusion (22). The mean blood circulation time is not altered. However, late in pregnancy and during childbirth, venous blood flow rates in the lower extremities become markedly decreased due to increased hypostatic pressure in the venous system. Blood flow to the legs is greatly influenced by posture in late pregnancy and during childbirth, being reduced in the supine position but increasing on adoption of a lateral position; this is probably the result of aortocaval compression by the gravid uterus in the supine position.

DRUG DISTRIBUTION

Drug distribution and the intensity and duration of pharmacologic activity are influenced by numerous physiologic factors. These are protein binding, plasma volume, cardiac output and its regional distribution to certain organs, fat and body water compartments, and acid–base equilibrium; there are also unique compartments found in pregnancy that are dependent on placental transfer of drugs. Once again, these are all factors undergoing significant changes during pregnancy, childbirth, and parturition.

PROTEIN BINDING

It has been reported (23) that serum albumin concentrations decrease gradually throughout pregnancy (becoming significantly altered by 15 weeks gestation). They remain at their lowest levels for at least 1 to 5 days after parturition and return to near normal levels within 5 to 7 weeks after parturition. During this time period, serum concentrations of fatty acids, fibrinogen, and various lipoproteins are increasing, while α_1-acid glycoprotein concentrations remain the same as those in nonpregnancy (23,24,64). Fatty acids have been found to be displacers of acidic drug binding to albumin and other proteins. This is caused by direct competitive

inhibition, changes in the electric charge of protein, and/or changes in protein conformations. The end result is an increased free-drug concentration. On the other hand, α_1-acid glycoprotein has been found to bind a number of basic drugs (see Chapter 10), thus resulting in decreased concentrations of free drug. However, as seen in Fig. 2, there is a significant decrease in this protein within the fetus (24). This may result in significantly higher free fractions of drugs (mostly bases) in the developing child. The clinical significance of increased fibrinogen and lipoprotein awaits elucidation.

In general, serum protein binding decreases gradually during pregnancy, following the same temporal pattern as seen with serum albumin. The weakly acidic drugs salicylic acid, sulfisoxazole, and phenytoin and the weakly basic drug diazepam all show significant negative correlations between their free-fraction values in serum and serum albumin concentrations during pregnancy (23).

For drugs that undergo hepatic metabolism and are not rate-limited by blood flow, a decrease in serum protein binding can lower steady state average serum concentrations of total drug while steady state average concentrations of free drug remain unchanged. Because we usually monitor *total* rather than *free* drug levels, unrecognized changes in protein binding during pregnancy may lead to misinterpretation of drug assay results and to inappropriate changes in dosage regimens.

Whereas average steady state free drug concentrations may not always be altered by changes in serum protein binding, the concentration–time profile of free drug during a dosing interval can be modified substantially. Maximum concentrations

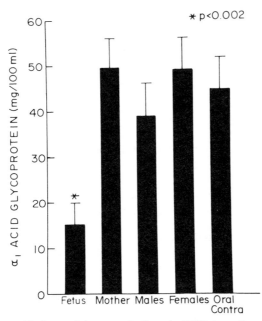

FIG. 2. Mean α_1-acid glycoprotein concentrations ($\pm$ SEM) in mother and fetus, male and nonpregnant female subjects, and women receiving the oral contraceptive pill. (From Wood and Wood, ref. 24, with permission.)

may be higher and minimum concentrations may be lower when serum protein binding is decreased (25).

Considering the maternal–fetal unit, one finds different maternal/fetal albumin concentration ratios at different times during pregnancy. This is most likely due to the fact that maternal serum albumin concentrations are gradually decreasing, while albumin that is produced by the fetus *in utero* and does not cross the placenta increases progressively in the fetal serum. Such differences need to be kept in mind when considering factors influencing the degree of fetal drug exposure (1,2).

PLASMA VOLUME

There is a marked increase in blood volume during pregnancy. The plasma volume is increased by nearly 50%, the maximum being reached between 30 and 34 weeks of gestation. Causes for this hypervolemia most likely include increased aldosterone and estrogenic states. In addition, the intervillous spaces lying between the maternal and fetal placental surfaces may constitute an A-V shunt. Such an effect on plasma volume may have significant effects on drug parameters such as volume of distribution.

CARDIAC OUTPUT/REGIONAL DISTRIBUTION

Cardiac output also increases during pregnancy, averaging about 30% above base line, the maximum being reached between 30 and 34 weeks. The increased cardiac output is a result of the patient's increased heart rate and stroke volume.

Accompanying the increased cardiac output are characteristic changes in the distribution of cardiac output to individual organs:

1. Renal blood flow increases by approximately 50% by the end of the first trimester, with a decrease toward normal as term approaches (as discussed later, this may have significant effects on drug elimination).

2. Pulmonary blood flow increases by approximately 30% (as discussed earlier).

3. Uterine blood flow progressively increases, reaching a maximum of 600 to 700 ml/min at term (80% perfusing the placenta, 20% perfusing the myometrium).

4. Hepatic blood flow does not appear to change significantly during pregnancy. However, the few available studies have not adequately addressed certain variables such as body position (26).

5. Intestinal blood flow has not been adequately assessed, but if increased, it would favor intestinal drug uptake and distribution.

Remarkable changes in cardiac output and its regional distribution have also been shown to occur during childbirth and with changes in body position.

If the patient lies on her back during stage-one labor, the cardiac output increases by approximately 25% with each uterine contraction. If she lies on her side, cardiac output is also increased, but only about 8%. During stage-two labor the mean increase in cardiac output may be between 50% and 100%. It has been estimated that each labor contraction at term injects approximately 400 ml of blood into the

general circulation. This increase in cardiac output with each uterine contraction is fundamentally due to an increased stroke volume because with each contraction there is a slight to moderate decrease in pulse rate as well as an increase in blood pressure.

Pain and anxiety during labor are associated with a cumulative increase of up to 40% in cardiac output, as measured between contractions throughout the first and second stages of labor. The administration of a local anesthetic into the epidural space is therefore likely to modify the cardiac output changes, particularly if the patient is in the supine position. Partial or complete occlusion of the inferior vena cava by the bulky uterus during pregnancy also results in a redirected venous return via collateral channels, such as the vertebral venous system. The resultant engorgement of the internal vertebral venous plexus reduces the size of the epidural space, thereby altering dosage requirements of local anesthetics used for epidural blockade.

Finally, the uteroplacental blood flow mentioned previously is blocked during uterine contractions, thus becoming an important determinant of fetal well-being and placental drug transfer during childbirth.

Therefore, when considering pharmacokinetic drug data during labor, one must consider such things as the stage of labor, the uterine activity phase, and maternal posturing, in addition to things like the mode of drug administration and the interval from maternal drug administration to delivery (4).

FAT AND BODY WATER COMPARTMENTS

The weight gain during pregnancy should be 7 kg or more above the ideal prepregnancy weight. The fetus accounts for approximately 3.25 kg of the increase, amniotic fluid ~ 1 kg, placenta ~ 0.7 to 1 kg, uterine enlargement ~ 1 kg, and breast enlargement ~ 0.5 kg (Fig. 3). The remainder of the weight gain results

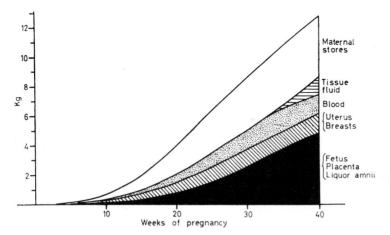

FIG. 3. Components of weight gain in normal pregnancy. (From Hytten and Leitch, ref. 27, with permission.)

TABLE 2. *Estimates of extracellular and intracellular water added during pregnancy*

	Total water (ml)	Extracellular (ml)	Intracellular (ml)
Fetus	2,343	1,360	983
Placenta	540	260	280
Liquor amnii	792	792	0
Uterus	743	490	253
Mammary gland	304	148	156
Plasma	920	920	0
Red cells	163	0	163
Extravascular water	1,195	1,195	0
Total	7,000	5,165	1,835

From Hytten and Leitch (27), with permission.

from an increase in total body water, divided as shown in Table 2 (27). The total increment of body water until term is approximately 7 to 8 liters, of which nearly 80% is extracellular and nearly 20% is intracellular (1,5). Approximately 60% of this increase is from the product of conception and about 40% from the maternal tissues. Where drug distribution and elimination are predominantly perfusion-limited, changes in the circulation velocities will determine the pharmacokinetic consequences.

Fat storage is also a common finding in pregnancy. In studies using serial measurements of skin thickness as a manifestation of body fat, increases of 20% to 40% have been found, depending on the area of skin measured. Such an increase in total body fat may affect certain lipid-soluble drugs (5).

ACID–BASE EQUILIBRIUM

Acid–base changes that occur during pregnancy are primarily the result of the respiratory changes discussed previously. The hyperventilation and consequent blowing off of excess amounts of carbon dioxide result in a mild, compensated respiratory alkalosis. The carbon dioxide tension and standard plasma bicarbonate and base excess concentrations all decrease slightly, resulting in an elevation of blood pH to approximately 7.42 as term approaches (5).

According to the theory of passive nonionic diffusion, nonionized drug molecules with high lipid solubility penetrate biological membranes (like the placenta) more quickly than the less lipid-soluble ionized molecules. Consequently, the transfer of weakly acidic or basic drugs across the placenta will be influenced by the pH of maternal and fetal fluids, especially when the drug's pK_a is close to the plasma's pH. Because the fetal plasma pH is slightly lower than the maternal pH, the concentration of nonionized basic drugs tends to be higher in the maternal circulation, thus leading to a net transfer from mother to fetus of basic drugs (1,2). This

may actually result in fetal drug concentrations higher than maternal drug concentrations once equilibrium has been obtained. The same is true for the situation in the amniotic fluid. The pH of the amniotic fluid being lower than that of the maternal plasma, the accumulation of weakly basic drugs, such as meperidine and diazepam, will be facilitated by ion trapping because the pH gradient will favor the ionization of the basic drug in the more acidic amniotic fluid and, therefore, only a small fraction of nonionized drug molecules will be able to diffuse directly back into the maternal compartment (2). Conversely, ion trapping of acidic drugs may result in higher maternal drug concentrations.

PLACENTAL TRANSFER

The physiochemical properties of drugs and the characteristics of the maternal–placental–fetal unit that modulates the placental transfer of drugs have been reported in detail elsewhere (3,28,63). Table 3 provides the fetal–maternal ratios for a selected list of drugs.

The intervillous spaces that lie between the maternal and fetal placental surfaces are the source of the organ's transport system. The ability of a drug to cross the placenta depends on several major factors:

1. Fick constant, which says that small molecules diffuse more rapidly than larger ones (the desirable molecular weight being less than 500)
2. Transplacental gradient, which is affected by the drug's ability either to bind itself to serum proteins or to remain unbound and in free form for ready diffusion
3. Degree of lipid solubility (not only are lipid-soluble drugs stored for longer periods in the mother than water-soluble drugs, which are metabolized and excreted quickly, but also they often pass unmetabolized into the fetal circulation)
4. Ionization
5. Uterine blood flow
6. Placental age (decreases in thickness and increases in size and surface area as gestation progresses).

BREAST MILK

Drug distribution and elimination in a patient's breast milk are important considerations. Table 4 provides an extensive listing of human milk-to-plasma ratios. The pH partition between breast milk (pH 6.8) and plasma (pH 7.4) favors the accumulation of weak bases in breast milk. Other considerations are degree of ionization, lipid solubility (larger drugs), and water solubility (smaller drugs). Those interested in the topic should consult the extensive review on pharmacokinetic considerations by Wilson and co-workers (42).

DRUG ELIMINATION

Renal Clearance

As discussed earlier, renal plasma flow, glomerular filtration rate (GFR), and consequently creatinine clearance increase early in pregnancy by approximately

TABLE 3. *Placental transfer of drugs*

Drug (reference)[a]	Number of patients studied	Route of administration	Fetal(cord)–maternal ratio	Comments
Ampicillin (33)	30	1 g sodium ampicillin, i.v.	0.16–1.3	Ratio depended on time of sample, at 1 hr approx. 0.43
Atenolol (19)	13	100 mg, oral dose	1.09 ± 0.6	Patients preeclampsic and on other antihypertensives
Atropine (37)	45	i.v. (12.5 µg/kg)	1.2 ± 0.5	Measured 5–15 min postinjection
Bupivacaine (31)	23	Epidural	0.17–0.52	Bound to AAG, which is less in the fetal circulation
(36)	31	Epidural	$49 \pm 27.2/9.3 \pm 6.2$	Single dose, numbers represent % free
Cephalexin (32)	30	1 g, single oral dose	0.25	As measured 2 hr post dose
Cephapirin (32)	30	1 g, single i.m. dose	0.67	As measured 2 hr post dose
Cephradine (41)	24	2 g, i.v. dose	0.13–0.37	
Dexamethasone (9)	6	i.v., single dose	0.32	Also data given for: beta-methasone, 0.37; cortisol, 0.17; prednisolone, 0.1
Lidocaine (12)	25	Epidural	0.66	MEGX ratio 1.45; GX ratio 1.03
Meperidine (38)	4	i.v. (50 mg)	0.72 ± 0.34	
Morphine (34)	20	4–6 mg, epidural	0.69–1.4	Ratio depended on time of sample, at 1 hr approx. 0.95
Normeperidine (38)	4	i.v. (50 mg)	0.68 ± 0.28	
Pivampicillin (as ampicillin) (40)	7	350 mg four times daily, oral doses	0.8	As measured 3 hr post dose
Propranolol (35)	1	Chronic oral dosing, 40–60 mg every 6 hr	1.09–1.27	
Theophylline (39)	12	Oral doses	0.95	35% bound in neonate, 56% bound in adult; metabolite, 3-keto ratio 1.5 ± 0.4
Valproic acid (30)	6	7.7–31 mg/kg/day, oral doses	1.7 ± 0.6	Neonatal half-life found to be 47 ± 15 hr

[a]For a recent review on the transplacental transfer of anticonvulsants during pregnancy, see Nau et al. (65).

TABLE 4. *Drug excretion in human breast milk*

Drug (reference)[a]	M/P[b]	Drug (reference)[a]	M/P[b]
Aspirin	0.6–1	Iodine 131	65
Acenocoumarol (48)	Not detected	Isoniazid	1.0
Alcohol (ethanol) (55)	0.9–0.95	Kanamycin sulfate	0.05–0.4
Amoxacillin (50)	0.014–0.043[c]	Lincomycin	0.13–0.17
Antipyrine (49)	<0.01	Lithium carbonate	0.25–0.77
Atenolol (46)	1.5–6.8	Lormetazepam (52)	0.06
Bishydroxycoumarin	0.01–0.02	Meprobamate	2–4
(dicoumarol)		Methadone (55)	0.83
Bis-3:3-4-oxycoumarinyl-	0.6–0.8	Methotrexate	0.1
ethylacetate		Methotrexate (55)	0.08
Captopril (45)	<0.01	Metoprolol (46)	2.6–3.7
Carbamazepine	0.6–0.7	Metronidazole	0.6–1.4
Cefadroxil (50)	0.009–0.019[c]	Metronidazole (55)	0.45–1.6
Cefotaxime (50)	0.029–0.160[c]	Nadolol (44)	2.7–4.6
Cephalexin (50)	0.008–0.140[c]	Nalidixic acid	0.08–0.13
Cephalothin (50)	0.073–0.500[c]	Nitrofurantoin (55)	0.3
Cephapirin (50)	0.068–0.480[c]	*d*–Norgestrel	0.2
Chloral hydrate	0–0.5	Novobiocin	0.1–0.25
Chloral hydrate	0.27	Penicillin	0.02–0.2
(and metabolite	0.5–1	Phenobarbital	0.21–0.71
trichloroethanol) (55)		Pentothal	1.0
Chloramphenicol	0.5–0.6	Phenytoin	0.12–0.24
Chlorotetracycline (54)	0.12–1	Phenylbutazone	0.1–0.3
Chlorpromazine	0.3, 0.5	Propoxyphene (55)	0.5
Chlorthalidone	0.03	Propranolol (55)	0.5
Colistin sulfate	0.17–0.18	Propylthiouracil	12
Cycloserine	0.67–0.75	Propylthiouracil (47)	0.1
Cycloserine (55)	0.31–1.18	Pyrazolone	1.0
Demeclocycline (54)	0.70	Pyrimethamine	0.2–0.43
Desmethyldiazepam	0.1	Quinine sulfate	0.14
Diazepam (55)	0.08–0.13	Rifampicin (rifampin)	0.2–0.6
Digoxin	0.6–0.8	Streptomycin sulfate	0.5–1
Dihydroxystreptomycin	0.021–0.1	Sulfathiazole (55)	0.33–0.5
Doxycycline (54)	0.3–0.4	Sulphanilamide	1.0
Epoxycarbamazepine	0.6–1	Sulphapyridine	1.0
Erythromycin	2.5–3	Sulphatrone	6.4
Ethanol	0.9–1.0	Tetracycline	0.62–0.81
Ether	1.0	hydrochloride	
Ethosuximide (43)	0.8	Theophylline (51)	0.57 ± 0.07
Ethyl biscoumacetate	0.6–0.8	(55)	0.7
(55)		Thiopental	1.0
Flufenamic acid	<0.01	Thiouracil	3.0
Heparin	<0.01	Tolbutamide	0.25
Hydralazine (53)	1.4	Tolbutamide (55)	0.09–0.4
Imipramine hydrochloride	0.08–0.5	Warfarin	<0.01

[a]Drugs not referenced are from Wilson et al. (42).
[b]The M/P ratio is shown for milk to maternal plasma.
[c]Smaller numbers as measured 1 hr post dose, and larger numbers as 3 hr post dose.
Adapted from Wilson et al. (42) and from Anderson (55).

50%. Therefore, the elimination of drugs that are primarily excreted by the kidneys will be increased, provided such factors as the drug's tubular reabsorption remain unchanged. In women in spontaneous labor, the creatinine clearance appears to remain essentially constant throughout the course of labor. However, creatinine clearance has been shown to be lower in those parturients whose labor is induced by administration of oxytocin (5).

Another factor that may modify the renal clearance of drugs during pregnancy is the extent of plasma binding, as discussed earlier.

Hepatic Clearance

The clearance rates of drugs primarily eliminated by the liver may also be different in pregnant patients, although comprehensive studies are lacking.

As discussed in Chapters 3 and 4, the major biological determinants of hepatic clearance of total drug are (a) the extent of drug binding in plasma, (b) the intrinsic hepatic clearance, and (c) the hepatic blood flow. As mentioned earlier, protein binding is altered, and hepatic blood flow is minimally affected. In normal pregnancy, steroid production is significantly increased, offering several considerations for clearance:

1. High progesterone levels appear to stimulate hepatic microsomal enzyme activity, resulting in increased hepatic intrinsic clearance.

2. Progesterone and estradiol have also been shown to be competitive inhibitors of microsomal oxidases for drugs such as ethylmorphine, therefore reducing the elimination rate of such compounds.

3. Finally, estrogens have a cholestatic effect that when coupled with decreased gallbladder emptying during pregnancy could impair the hepatic elimination of some drugs, such as rifampin (1,2).

PLACENTAL/FETAL METABOLISM

Drug metabolism by the human fetus has recently been reviewed (56). Drug-metabolizing activity has been detected in human placental tissue and in fetal tissues, including the liver.

From the data available, it would appear that in most instances the biotransformation of drugs in the human embryo and fetus does not affect maternal serum concentrations significantly.

Unless the fetal tissues are capable of metabolizing a drug more rapidly than the maternal tissues, fetal drug metabolism usually will exert little effect on the steady-state concentrations of drugs and their metabolites in the fetus. The mass and the activity of the maternal drug biotransforming tissues render it improbable that fetal drug metabolism will ever occur at more rapid rates than maternal drug metabolism (56).

A fetal enzyme will have a greater effect on the concentration of a drug in fetal blood (assuming steady state concentrations) when the drug diffuses slowly across

the placental membrane than when it diffuses rapidly (as with lipid-soluble drugs). In terms of single or widely spaced drug exposures, steady state concentrations are not reached, and fetal/placental drug metabolism could then play a more significant role in drug clearance from the fetal serum.

PLASMA DRUG LEVEL MONITORING DURING PREGNANCY

Because of the progressively changing maternal physiology during pregnancy and the rather more rapid return to the normal state after parturition, monitoring of plasma drug concentrations needs to be carried out at frequent intervals during pregnancy, and even more frequently in the puerperium (57). These recommendations hold primarily for chronic maintenance medications used throughout pregnancy, such as anticonvulsants.

In the majority of cases, prospective plasma level monitoring for a given patient in childbirth is not appropriate or advantageous, primarily because (a) most medications administered in childbirth are given acutely, usually as a single dose, (b) the relative magnitudes of assay time and length of labor make plasma level monitoring impractical, and (c) rapidly changing physiology in childbirth may also render useless such monitoring for prospective adjustments (4). Eadie and coworkers (57) have reviewed available data on plasma level monitoring during pregnancy (see Chapter 21).

ANTICONVULSANTS

There appears to be good evidence that plasma phenytoin levels fall during pregnancy and rise again during the puerperium, unless dosage increases and decreases are made, respectively (58), which corresponds with the changes in free fraction noted in Table 1. There is reasonable evidence that similar blood level changes occur in plasma phenobarbital levels during pregnancy, and there is a suspicion that such changes may also occur with other anticonvulsants, such as ethosuximide and carbamazepine (57), although possibly because of different mechanisms.

The major causative factor is believed to be an increased rate of biotransformation and clearance, with an increased extracellular fluid and tissue volume of the maternal-fetal unit playing a minor secondary role. Higher serum folate levels observed during pregnancy have been linked to lower serum phenytoin levels; similarly, lower serum folate levels following parturition have corresponded to higher serum phenytoin levels (59). However, the clinical relevance of this interaction is debatable (60).

Because plasma anticonvulsant levels may fall early in pregnancy (first trimester) and may be associated with increased seizure frequency, it is desirable to measure drug levels every 4 weeks from the onset of pregnancy, adjusting drug dosage accordingly. Because anticonvulsant requirements may change within a few days of parturition, or not for several weeks, it is recommended to monitor plasma drug

levels weekly after birth for 2 to 3 weeks, and then every 2 weeks, making dosage adjustments as necessary until drug levels stabilize at prepregnancy levels.

LITHIUM

There is also good evidence that plasma lithium levels fall during pregnancy and rise again sharply during the puerperium. The major causative factor is believed to be increased renal clearance of lithium secondary to the increased GFR and creatinine clearance of pregnancy.

Plasma lithium levels should be monitored at regular intervals during pregnancy, especially every 2 weeks during the final trimester, and every few days after birth until levels stabilize at prepregnancy concentrations.

Also, should toxemia of pregnancy develop and require treatment with salt restriction and diuretics, there will be a particular need to monitor plasma lithium levels more closely.

DIGOXIN

Like lithium, digoxin is eliminated by the kidneys predominantly unchanged. Therefore, one might reasonably expect that maternal drug dose requirements would increase during pregnancy and fall again in the puerperium.

ANTIBIOTICS

Philipson (61) has recently reviewed the pharmacokinetics of antibiotics in pregnancy and childbirth. Significantly lower antibiotic serum or plasma concentrations have been well documented during pregnancy for ampicillin (see Table 1), and other studies suggest the same for cephalexin, cefazolin, pivampicillin, aminoglycosides, erythromycin, and nitrofurantoin (61). In general, levels of antibiotics in urine seem to be unchanged in pregnancy. Studies of metronidazole pharmacokinetics in pregnant women indicate no need for dosage adjustment of this drug (20) (see Table 1).

FETAL DRUG CONCENTRATIONS

Recently, Anderson and co-workers (62) have reported on a model for predicting fetal drug concentrations. Equations are derived for the fetal concentrations of a drug during and after the slow release of the drug into the maternal circulation. To use the model, it is necessary to know the placental drug clearance, the clearance of the drug from the fetal circulation by the fetal tissues, and the volume of distribution of the drug in the fetal compartment. Their theoretical approach demonstrates the importance of determining maternal and fetal drug concentrations over an extended period of time and emphasizes that it is not sufficient to take samples of maternal and fetal blood at a single point in time (as has usually been done in the past) and make generalizations with regard to the mechanism of transfer.

TABLE 5. *Summary of measurable pregnancy changes*

Parameter	Percent increase	Percent decrease	Unchanged
Respiratory system			
Tidal volume	30–40		
Respiratory rate			x
Resistance of tracheobronchial tree		36	
Expiratory reserve		40	
Residual volume		40	
Functional residual capacity		25	
Vital capacity			x
Respiratory minute volume	40		
Cardiovascular system			
Heart			
Rate	0–20		
Stroke volume	x		
Cardiac output	20–30		
Blood pressure			x
Peripheral blood flow	600		
Blood volume	48		
Blood constituents			
Leukocytes	70–100		
Fibrinogen	50		
Platelets	33		
Carbon dioxide		25	
Standard bicarbonate		10	
Proteins		15	
Lipids	33		
Phospholipids	30–40		
Cholesterol	100		
Clotting factors I, VII, VIII, IX, X,	x		
XIII		x	
Gastrointestinal system			
Cardiac sphincter tone		x	
Acid secretion		x	
Motility		x	
Gallbladder emptying		x	
Urinary tract			
Renal plasma flow	25–50		
Glomerular filtration rate	50		
Ureter tone		x	
Ureteral motility			x
Metabolism			
Nitrogen stores	x		
General stores of			
Sodium	x		
Potassium	x		
Calcium	x		
Oxygen consumption	14		

CONCLUSION

In conclusion, a number of physiologic changes occurring during pregnancy and childbirth (Table 5) have been summarized, some with proven effects on pharmacokinetic parameters, others with a theoretical basis for potential alterations. It is hoped that future studies on pharmacokinetics during pregnancy and childbirth will be improved by considering the physiologic adjustments reviewed here.

REFERENCES

1. Krauer, B., and Krauer, F. (1977): Drug kinetics in pregnancy. *Clin. Pharmacokinet.*, 2:167–181.
2. Krauer, B., Krauer, F., and Hytten, F. E. (1980): Drug disposition and pharmacokinetics in the maternal-placental-fetal unit. *Pharmacol. Ther.*, 10:301–326.
3. Mirkin, B. L. (1973): Drug distribution in pregnancy. In: *Fetal Pharmacology*, edited by L. O. Boreus, Raven Press, New York.
4. Nation, R. L. (1980): Drug kinetics in childbirth. *Clin. Pharmacokinet.*, 5:340–364.
5. Quilligan, E. J., and Kaiser, I. H. (1982): Maternal physiology. In: *Obstetrics and Gynecology*, 3rd Ed., edited by D. N. Danforth, pp. 326–341. Harper & Row, New York.
6. Rey, E., Giraux, P., de Lauture, D., Turquais, J. M., Chavinie, J., and Olive, G. (1979): Pharmacokinetics of clorazepate in pregnant and non-pregnant women. *Eur. J. Clin. Pharmacol.*, 15:175–180.
7. Morgan, D., Moore, G., Thomas, J., and Triggs, E. (1978): Disposition of meperidine in pregnancy. *Clin. Pharmacol. Ther.*, 23:288–295.
8. Kuhnert, B. R., Kuhnert, P. M., Prochaska, A. L., and Sokol, R. J. (1980): Meperidine disposition in mother, neonate, and nonpregnant females. *Clin. Pharmacol. Ther.*, 27:486–490.
9. Tsuei, S. E., Petersen, M. C., Ashley, J. J., McBride, W. G., and Moore, R. G. (1980): Disposition of synthetic glucocorticoids. II. Dexamethasone in parturient women. *Clin. Pharmacol. Ther.*, 28:88–97.
10. Wood, M., and Wood, A. J. J. (1981): Changes in plasma drug binding and α_1-acid glycoprotein in mother and newborn infant. *Clin. Pharmacol. Ther.*, 29:522–526.
11. Dean, M., Stock, B., Patterson, R. J., and Levy, G. (1980): Serum protein binding of drugs during and after pregnancy in humans. *Clin. Pharmacol. Ther.*, 28:253–260.
12. Kuhnert, B. R., Knapp, D. R., Kuhnert, P. M., and Prochaska, A. L. (1979): Maternal, fetal, and neonatal metabolism of lidocaine. *Clin. Pharmacol. Ther.*, 26:213–219.
13. Kampmann, J., and Hansen, J. M. (1980): The metabolism of methimazole in pregnancy. *Br. J. Clin. Pharmacol.*, 10:314.
14. Perucca, E., Richens, A., and Ruprah, M. (1981): Serum protein binding of phenytoin in pregnant women. *Proc. Br. Pharmacol. Soc.*, 11:409P–410P.
15. Assael, B. M., Como, M. L., Miraglia, M., Pardi, G., and Sereni, F. (1979): Ampicillin kinetics in pregnancy. *Br. J. Clin. Pharmacol.*, 8:286–288.
16. Knutti, R., Rothweiler, H., and Schlatter, C. (1981): Effect of pregnancy on the pharmacokinetics of caffeine. *Eur. J. Clin. Pharmacol.*, 21:121–126.
17. Riva, E., Farina, ?., Tognoni, G., Bottino, S., Orrico, C., and Pardi, G. (1978): Pharmacokinetics of furosemide in gestosis of pregnancy. *Eur. J. Clin. Pharmacol.*, 14:361–366.
18. Chen, S. S., Perucca, E., Lee, J. N., and Richens, A. (1982): Serum protein binding and free concentrations of phenytoin and phenobarbitone in pregnancy. *Br. J. Clin. Pharmacol.*, 13:547–552.
19. Thorley, K. J., McAinsh, J., and Cruickshank, J. M. (1981): Atenolol in the treatment of pregnancy-induced hypertension. *Br. J. Clin. Pharmacol.*, 12:725–730.
20. Amon, I., Amon, K., Franke, G., and Mohr, C. (1981): Pharmacokinetics of metronidazole in pregnant women. *Chemotherapy*, 27:73–79.
21. Nimmo, W. S. (1976): Drugs, diseases and altered gastric emptying. *Clin. Pharmacokinet.*, 1:189–203.
22. Katz, M., and Sahal, M. M. (1980): Skin perfusion in pregnancy. *Am. J. Obstet. Gynecol.*, 137:30–33.

23. Dean, M., Stock, B., Patterson, R. J., and Levy, G. (1980): Serum protein binding of drugs during and after pregnancy in humans. *Clin. Pharmacol. Ther.*, 28:253–261.
24. Wood, M., and Wood, A. J. J. (1981): Changes in plasma binding and α_1-acid glycoprotein in mother and newborn infant. *Clin. Pharmacol. Ther.*, 29:522–526.
25. Levy, G. (1976): Effect of plasma protein binding of drugs on duration and intensity of pharmacological activity. *J. Pharm. Sci.*, 65:1264–1265.
26. Munnell, E. W., and Taylor, H. C. (1947): Liver blood flow in pregnancy—hepatic vein catheterization. *J. Clin. Invest.*, 26:952–956.
27. Hytten, F. E., and Leitch, I. (1964): *The Physiology of Human Pregnancy*. Blackwell, Oxford.
28. Mirkin, B. L., and Singh, S. (1976): Placental transfer of pharmacologically active molecules. In: *Perinatal Pharmacology and Therapeutics*, edited by B. L. Mirkin, pp. 1–69. Academic Press, New York.
29. Morselli, P. L. (1976): Clinical pharmacokinetics in neonates. *Clin. Pharmacokinet.*, 1:81–98.
30. Nau, H., Pating, D., Koch, S., Hauser, I., and Helge, H. (1981): Valproic acid and its metabolites: Placental transfer, neonatal pharmacokinetics, transfer via mother's milk and clinical status in neonates of epileptic mothers. *J. Pharmacol. Exp. Ther.*, 219:768–776.
31. Petersen, M. C., Moore, R. G., Nation, R. L., and W. McMenima (1981): Relationship between the transplacental gradients of bupivacaine and α_1-acid glycoprotein. *Br. J. Clin. Pharmacol.*, 12:859–862.
32. Creatsas, G., Pavlatos, M., Lolis, D., and Kaskarelis, D. (1980): A study of the kinetics of cephapirin and cephalexin in pregnancy. *Curr. Med. Res. Opin.*, 7:43–46.
33. Kraybill, E. N., Chaney, N. E., and McCarthy, L. R. (1980): Transplacental ampicillin: Inhibitory concentrations in neonatal serum. *Am. J. Obstet. Gynecol.*, 138:793–796.
34. Nybell-Lindahl, G., Carisson, C., Ingemarsson, I., Westgren, M., and Paalzow, L. (1981): Maternal and fetal concentrations of morphine after epidural administration during labor. *Am. J. Obstet. Gynecol.*, 139:20–21.
35. Cottrill, C. M., McAllister, R. G., Jr., Gettes, L., and Noonan, J. A. (1977): Propranolol therapy during pregnancy, labor, and delivery: Evidence for transplacental drug transfer and impaired neonatal drug disposition. *J. Pediatr.*, 91:812–814.
36. Thomas, J., Long, G., Moore, G., and Morgan, D. (1975): Plasma protein binding and placental transfer of bupivacaine. *Clin. Pharmacol. Ther.*, 19:426–433.
37. Onnen, I., Barrier, G., d'Athis, P., Sureau, C., and Olive, G. (1979): Placental transfer of atropine at the end of pregnancy. *Eur. J. Clin. Pharmacol.*, 15:443–446.
38. Morrison, J. C., Tood, E. L., Lipshitz, J., Anderson, G. D., Schneider, J. M., and Dilts, P. V., Jr. (1982): Meperidine metabolism in the parturient. *Obstet. Gynecol.*, 59:359–364.
39. Labovitz, E., and Spector, S. (1982): Placental theophylline transfer in pregnant asthmatics. *J.A.M.A.*, 247:786–788.
40. Jordheim, O., and Hagen, A. G. (1980): Study of ampicillin levels in maternal serum, umbilical cord serum and amniotic fluid following administration of pivampicillin. *Acta Obstet. Gynecol. Scand.*, 59:315–317.
41. Craft, I., and Forster, T. C. (1978): Materno-fetal cephradine transfer in pregnancy. *Antimicrob. Agents Chemother.*, 14:924–926.
42. Wilson, J. T., Brown, R. D., Cherek, D. R., Dailey, J. W., Hilman, B., Jose, P. C., Manno, B. R., Manno, J. E., Redetzki, H. M., and Stewart, J. J. (1980): Drug excretion in human breast milk: Principles, pharmacokinetics and projected consequences. *Clin. Pharmacokinet.*, 5:1–66.
43. Rane, A., and Tunell, R. (1981): Ethosuximide in human milk and in plasma of a mother and her nursed infant. *Br. J. Clin. Pharmacol.*, 12:855–858.
44. Devlin, R. G., and Duchin, K. L. (1981): Nadolol in human serum and breast milk. *Br. J. Clin. Pharmacol.*, 12:393–396.
45. Devlin, R. G., and Fleiss, P. M. (1981): Captopril in human blood and breast milk. *J. Clin. Pharmacol.*, 21:110–113.
46. Liedholm, H., Melander, A., Bitzen, O.-O., Helm, G., Lonnerholm, G., Mattiasson, I., Nilsson, B., and Wahlin-Boll, E. (1981): Accumulation of atenolol and metoprolol in human breast milk. *Eur. J. Clin. Pharmacol.*, 20:229–231.
47. Kampmann, J. P., Hansen, J. M., Hohansen, K., and Helweg, J. (1980): Propylthiouracil in human milk. Revision of a dogma. *Lancet*, 1:736–737.
48. Houwert-de Jong, M., Gerards, L. J., Tetteroo-Tempelman, C. A. M., and de Wolff, F. A. (1981): May mothers taking acenocoumarol breast feed their infants? *Eur. J. Clin. Pharmacol.*, 21:61–64.

49. Berlin, C. M., and Vesell, E. S. (1982): Antipyrine disposition in milk and saliva of lactating women. *Clin. Pharmacol. Ther.*, 31:38–43.

50. Kafetzis, D. A., Siafas, C. A., Georgakopoulos, P. A., and Papadatos, C. J. (1981): Passage of cephalosporins and amoxicillin into the breast milk. *Acta Paediatr. Scand.*, 70:285–288.

51. Stec, G. P., Greenberger, P., Ruo, T. I., Henthorn, T., Morita, Y., Atkinson, A. J., Jr., and Patterson, R. (1980): Kinetics of theophylline transfer to breast milk. *Clin. Pharmacol. Ther.*, 28:404–408.

52. Humpel, M., Stoppelli, I., Milia, S., and Rainer, E. (1982): Pharmacokinetics and biotransformation of the new benzodiazepine, lormetazepam, in man. *Eur. J. Clin. Pharmacol.*, 21:421–425.

53. Liedholm, H., Wahlin-Boll, E., Hanson, A., Ingemarsson, I., and Melander, A. (1982): Transplacental passage and breast milk concentrations of hydralazine. *Eur. J. Clin. Pharmacol.*, 21:417–419.

54. Vorherr, H. (1974): Drug excretion in breast milk. *Postgrad. Med.*, 56:97–101.

55. Anderson, P. O. (1977): Drugs and breast feeding, a review. *Drug Intell. Clin. Pharm.*, 11:208–223.

56. Juchau, M. R., Chao, S. T., and Omiecinski, C. J. (1980): Drug metabolism by the human fetus. *Clin. Pharmacokinet.*, 5:320–339.

57. Eadie, M. J., Lander, C. M., and Tyrer, J. H. (1977): Plasma drug level monitoring in pregnancy. *Clin. Pharmacokinet.*, 2:427–436.

58. Puprah, M., Perucca, E., and Richens, A. (1981): Phenytoin binding in pregnancy. *Lancet*, 1:97.

59. Strauss, R. G., Ramsey, R. E., Willmore, L. J., and Wilder, B. J. (1978): Hematologic effects of phenytoin therapy during pregnancy. *Obstet. Gynecol.*, 51:682–685.

60. Gibberd, F. B., Nicholls, A., and Wright, M. G. (1981): The influence of folic acid on the frequency of epileptic attacks. *Eur. J. Clin. Pharmacol.*, 19:57–60.

61. Philipson, A. (1979): Pharmacokinetics of antibiotics in pregnancy and labour. *Clin. Pharmacokinet.*, 4:297–309.

62. Anderson, D. F., Phernetton, T. M., and Rankin, J. H. G. (1980): Prediction of fetal drug concentrations. *Am. J. Obstet. Gynecol.*, 137:735–738.

63. Levy, G., and Hayton, W. L. (1973): Pharmacokinetic aspects of placental transfer. In: *Fetal Pharmacology*, edited by L. O. Boreus, pp. 29–39. Raven Press, New York.

64. Morgan, D. J., Koay, B. B., and Paull, J. D. (1982): Plasma protein binding of etidocaine during pregnancy and labour. *Eur. J. Clin. Pharmacol.*, 22:451–457.

65. Nau, H., Kuhnz, W., Egger, H. J., Rating, D., and Helge, H. (1982): Anticonvulsants during pregnancy and lactation: Transplacental, maternal and neonatal pharmacokinetics. *Clin. Pharmacokinet.*, 7:508–543.

Pharmacokinetic Basis for Drug Treatment,
edited by L. Z. Benet et al., Raven Press,
New York © 1984

Chapter 14

Clinical Pharmacokinetics: Pediatric Considerations

Thomas P. Green and Bernard L. Mirkin

*Division of Clinical Pharmacology, University of Minnesota,
Minneapolis, Minnesota 55455*

The physiologic processes that determine drug disposition undergo radical changes during biological maturation. Correspondingly, the processes of drug absorption, distribution, metabolism, and elimination are modified throughout infancy and childhood. These changes give rise to two characteristics of pediatric therapeutics: (a) Drug disposition both changes throughout biological maturation and differs from adult norms. (b) A large interpatient variability in drug disposition is observed for most drugs in this patient population.

The utility of pharmacokinetics in pediatric drug therapy is therefore obvious. Studies with individual drugs can be designed to delinate the modifications in disposition that occur with maturation and establish scientifically based dosage regimens for pediatric patients of various ages. Therapeutic drug monitoring strategies for individual patients can be devised that will compensate for the expected interindividual variation. Regretfully, most drugs are marketed with little or no information regarding their pharmacology in children. Poorly constructed regulatory statutes of the Food and Drug Administration have perpetuated this situation in the past (1–3), but major changes in the premarketing drug testing procedure may help in the future.

This chapter discusses the potential for pharmacokinetic analyses to improve drug therapy in pediatric patients. Examples of the effects of biological maturation on drug disposition will be presented as they influence the practitioner's ability to apply the pharmacokinetic methods elaborated in this and other chapters. For those readers desiring tabulations of pharmacokinetic values in children, several excellent recent reviews are available (3–6). The difficulties in applying standard pharmacokinetic analyses in pediatric subjects will be discussed, and approaches that may be particularly well suited to this patient population will be highlighted.

BIOLOGICAL MATURATION AND DRUG DISPOSITION

Each of the classic subdivisions of drug disposition, i.e., absorption, distribution, metabolism, and elimination, will be considered separately. Some of the difficulty

in drawing general conclusions from the data in the literature derives from the nonuniform age ranges of patient populations in the various studies. We have attempted to maintain a consistent nomenclature here: premature infant, a child born before 36 weeks gestation and still less than 1 month old; newborn, a child less than 1 month of age; infant, 1 month to about 12 months; child, 1 to 11 years; adolescent, 12 to 18 years; adult, older than 18 years. A general summary of the physiologic changes that occur during development and that affect drug disposition is given in Table 1.

Absorption

Enteral absorption is influenced by many factors that change during development, including gastric pH, gastric emptying time, intestinal motility, and intestinal blood flow. Gastric pH is neutral at birth and decreases to values between 1 and 3 by 24 hr of age (3). Infants after the newborn period have a relative achlorhydria; gastric acid secretion increases with the development of gastric mucosa and reaches adult values by 3 years of age (3). This relative achlorhydria apparently accounts for the increased bioavailability of the acid-labile penicillins in newborns (7,8). Increased gastric pH might also decrease the absorption of weak acids from the stomach. However, the surface area of gastric mucosa is small relative to that of the small intestine, and most drugs are absorbed from the intestine rather than the stomach, regardless of their ionization (9) (see Chapter 2). The speculation that the higher gastric pH of young infants accounts for the delayed absorption of phenobarbital, phenytoin, and nalidixic acid (3) in this population requires verification before this explanation can be accepted.

In general, drugs that are not acid-labile, show equivalent bioavailability in infants, children, and adults. Acetaminophen (10), digoxin (11), and sulfonamides (12) are well absorbed in children of all ages. Some exceptions do exist: The bioavailability of enterally administered iron continues to increase from birth until adolescence (13).

However, for all drugs, the rate at which enteral absorption occurs varies strikingly with age. Newborns clearly absorb drugs at slower rates than older children or adults. This may be due to the delayed gastric emptying time and irregular intestinal peristalsis characteristic of this age group. Heimann (12), however, has suggested that the intestinal mucosa may be a more important factor in limiting the rate of absorption. Studies in which the saturation kinetics of L-(+)-arabinose were analyzed demonstrated a lower V_{max} of absorption for neonates, as well as a decreased affinity constant, as compared with older children. Some reports suggest that preadolescent children may absorb drugs at faster rates than either neonates or adults (14,15).

Because of the slow rate of enteral absorption and the differences in distribution, metabolism, and elimination in newborns (vide infra), overall bioavailability of drugs must be assessed by carefully designed studies that account for these factors. Some of the literature that suggests a decreased bioavailability for many drugs in

TABLE 1. *Maturation of physiologic variables that determine drug disposition*

Aspect of drug disposition	Physiologic variable	Representative values[a]				Examples (references)
		Premature	Newborn	One-year-old	Adult	
Absorption, oral	Gastric acid secretion (mEq/kg/hr)		0.015		0.2	Penicillin G: increased bioavailability in newborns (7)
	Gastric emptying time (min)		87		65	Phenobarbital: slower rate of absorption in newborns (12)
	Intestinal peristalsis	↓[b]	↓[b]	↔		Phenobarbital: slow rate of absorption in newborns (12)
Absorption, intramuscular	Regional muscular blood flow	c	c	↔		Digoxin, gentamicin: erratic absorption in newborns (3,18)
Distribution	Total body water (% of total body weight)	87	79	67	60	
	Extracellular water (% of total body weight)	62	45	27	20	Amikacin, ticarcillin: increased distribution volumes in young subjects (19,22)
	Adipose tissue (% of total body weight)	3	12	23	12–25	
	Total serum proteins (g/dl)	5.9	6.0	6.4	7.2	Sulfadiazine: decreased serum drug protein binding in newborns (31)
	Serum albumin (g/dl)	3.7	4.5	4.9	4.9	
Metabolism	Sulfation[a]		↔	↔		Acetaminophen: predominantly sulfated in infants (10)
	Glucuronidation[a]	→	→			Chloramphenicol: delayed elimination in prematures and newborns (35)
	Mixed-function oxidase	→	→	↔		Theophylline: possible decreased rate of metabolism in newborns (41,61)
Elimination	Glomerular filtration (ml/min/m²)	5	15	50	70	Gentamicin: delayed elimination in newborns (40)
	Tubular anion secretion (PAH clearance: ml/min/1.73 m²)	50	50	245	380	Furosemide: delayed elimination in newborns (41)

[a] For physiologic variables for which no quantitation in children is available, the values are qualitatively expressed relative to the adult (5,20,62,63).
[b] Peristalsis tends to be slow and irregular in premature and newborn infants.
[c] Muscular blood flow appears to be more labile in very young subjects.

newborns must be questioned on methodologic grounds. For example, Evans et al. (15) have reported that plasma drug concentrations following oral administration of indomethacin are lower in premature infants than in adults. These authors concluded that the bioavailability of this drug was lower in these patients than the bioavailability of similar preparations in adults. However, drug distribution volumes and the rate (not the total amount) of drug absorption were probably more important determinants of the values of peak drug concentrations in this study.

Very few studies of the first-pass phenomenon (hepatic extraction during oral absorption, as described in Chapters 1 and 3) have been conducted in children. Wilson et al. (16) examined the serum levels achieved after oral administration of propoxyphene and propranolol to children from 2 to 13 years of age. The large intersubject differences and low serum concentrations achieved were consistent with the extensive first-pass effect seen for these drugs in adult subjects. A developmental difference in hepatic extraction would be more likely to occur in a younger patient population, but such studies have not been performed.

Absorption from intramuscular sites depends strongly on regional blood flow (17), which can vary depending on the site of injection and coexisting disease states. These variables cloud the interpretation of studies in newborns that show decreased absorption of digoxin (3) and gentamicin (18) from intramuscular sites. Other studies, by contrast, have shown rapid absorption of amikacin (19).

Distribution

The apparent volume of distribution of drugs is influenced by many factors, including the actual volume of tissue compartments, the binding of drugs to serum proteins, and the binding of drugs in tissue. In general, distribution volumes expressed per mass of body weight tend to be larger in neonates than in adults and decrease toward adult values during childhood.

The relative mass of various tissues changes throughout maturation (4). Total body water, as a fraction of body weight, decreases throughout the first year of life, and during this time there is a shift from predominantly extracellular to intracellular fluid (2). Correspondingly, drugs that are normally confined to extracellular fluids are found to have larger distribution volumes in this age group when compared with those of adults. Examples of this phenomenon from recent studies include ampicillin (21), ticarcillin (22) and amikacin (19).

A larger volume of distribution for more lipid-soluble drugs has also been documented. This is somewhat surprising, because neonates have a relatively low percentage of adipose tissue. The local anesthetics lidocaine (23) and mepivacaine (24) have been shown to have volumes of distribution in the neonate that are significantly larger than those in adults; these authors speculated that the high blood flow to lipid-rich organs, such as liver and brain, might account for this difference.

For most drugs that have been studied, a large interpatient variability in volume of distribution has been found. The likely explanation for such variability would seem to be that the rate of maturation varies greatly among individual patients.

Such variability undoubtedly accounts for the failure of several studies to demonstrate a relationship between distribution volume and age in studies where patients of limited age range have been examined (21,25–27).

In general, drugs bind less extensively to serum proteins of newborn infants than to those of older children and adults; this appears to be true for acidic drugs, which bind primarily to albumin, as well as for basic drugs, which are more avidly bound to globulins, primarily α_1-acid glycoprotein (28). Although albumin concentrations are not signficantly lower in neonates than in the adult population, α_1-acid glycoprotein concentrations tend to be lower (29) (see Chapter 13, Fig. 2). Factors deemed responsible for this observation include the persistence of fetal serum proteins (28,30), hypoproteinemia (especially in premature infants), the presence of competing ligands such as bilirubin (28,31), and developmentally unique albumin-globulin interactions (28).

Tissue binding of drugs is difficult to quantitate and therefore is seldom studied. Investigations of the tissue binding of digoxin have revealed that the myocardial concentrations achieved are higher in infants than in adults (32,33). These differences are apparently not explainable by differences in serum drug concentration or regional blood flow. Although these findings are in conflict with the results of other investigations, more avid tissue binding would explain the larger distribution volume of digoxin found in newborn patients.

Metabolism

The various pathways of drug metabolism mature at different rates, and therefore the ability of the newborn to metabolize drugs differs both quantitatively and qualitatively from that of older subjects. No general rule concerning the metabolic competence of immature subjects relative to adults can be stated. Several examples will illustrate the diverse nature of this area.

Newborns are relatively slow metabolizers of caffeine (34). During the first months of life, little metabolism occurs, and the drug is eliminated primarily by renal excretion of the unchanged drug. A very long $T_{1/2}$ (4 days) thereby results. Between 3 and 7 months of age, this drug is metabolized to urates and demethylated xanthines as in adults, and correspondingly the elimination rate increases to adult values during this period.

A similar situation exists for lidocaine in patients of this same age group (23). Neonates excrete a considerable portion of the unchanged drug in the urine, but with maturation more extensive metabolism occurs. In this case, however, metabolism does not occur at a rate appreciably faster than renal elimination in the newborn, and therefore the change in route of elimination is not associated with a change in the overall elimination rate.

Many investigations have demonstrated that the various drug-metabolizing systems mature at differing rates (13). The very inefficient state of the hepatic microsomal glucuronidation system at birth has been well described. For drugs with no major alternate metabolic pathway, such as chloramphenicol, this produces a slower

overall rate of elimination in newborns than is found in older subjects (35). However, other drugs, normally glucuronidated in the adult, may become substrates for alternate metabolic pathways when glucuronidation is less well developed. Acetaminophen is an example of this phenomenon: Sulfate conjugation is the predominant route of metabolism in infants, and the overall elimination rate is not different from that in adults (10). The adult pattern of metabolism is not reached until about 12 years of age.

Whenever enzyme saturation kinetics can be achieved, further information concerning drug metabolism can be obtained. Chiba et al. (36) have examined the Michaelis-Menten kinetics of phenytoin in children of various ages. (Nonlinear kinetics are discussed in Chapters 17 and 21.) The K_m for phenytoin metabolism remained unchanged in patients ranging in age from 6 months to 16 years. V_{max} (expressed on a weight basis), however, progressively fell during development. These authors correlated this fall to the decrease in liver size relative to total body mass that occurs at the same time in development.

Most available evidence indicates that even the youngest subjects can undergo induction of hepatic microsomal metabolism (27,37). This characteristic has been used therapeutically to increase the endogenous detoxification of bilirubin in infants at risk for hemolytic disease of the newborn by pretreating the mother (and the fetus *in utero*) with phenobarbital (38).

The maturation of the various metabolic pathways is mediated by processes that are not understood at present. Postnatal enzyme induction may be one mechanism. Redmond et al. (39) have advanced the interesting hypothesis that hormonal influences may be an important part of this process. They found an increase in amobarbital elimination rate after growth-hormone-deficient children received replacement therapy with growth hormone.

Elimination

The immature state of glomerular filtration and renal tubular function in premature infants and newborns is familiar to most practitioners. The glomerular filtration rate (GFR) normalized for surface area increases gradually, reaching adult values at about 6 months of life; renal tubular capacity, measured by renal clearance of *p*-aminohippurate, achieves adult values 1 to 2 months later (4). (For a further discussion of GFR and a method for prediction of creatinine clearance in pediatrics, see Chapter 8.) Drugs that depend primarily on the renal route of elimination, such as gentamicin (40), ampicillin (21), and furosemide (41), therefore have prolonged elimination time courses in neonates and young infants. The maturation of renal clearance of these drugs closely corresponds to the development of the corresponding renal function (40). In spite of this close relationship between organ function and drug excretion, wide interpatient variability is quite prominent for these drugs (21). This variability is not improved by normalizing doses on the basis of either body weight or surface area (25).

PHARMACOKINETICS AND PEDIATRIC THERAPEUTICS

The changes in drug disposition that occur during biological maturation and the interpatient variability that is characteristic of the pediatric population pose therapeutic problems that are potentially soluble by pharmacokinetic techniques. Investigations by pharmacokineticists will further delineate the influence of development for each therapeutic agent and define appropriate strategies for therapeutic drug monitoring. However, in these processes some problems arise that are unique to this population and demand special considerations.

Technical Problems in Applying Pharmacokinetics in Pediatric Patients

The most obvious obstacles in performing kinetic studies in pediatric patients are accessibility to blood samples and specimen volume. Venipuncture in newborns and infants can be difficult, even for skilled personnel. When repeated samples are necessary, this problem can multiply in difficulty as satisfactory access to a vein decreases after repeated venipuncture. Although the volume of blood that can be safely obtained from an infant varies, physicians recognize the need to limit the volume of blood drawn from very small infants. A 5-ml blood sample from a 1,000-g premature infant represents about 6% of his blood volume, and the need for such a large sample must be clearly established. Repeated sampling of this sort would be out of the question.

Another technical problem probably unique to the pediatric population has been pointed out by Gould and Roberts (42). After observing grossly inconsistent serum drug concentrations in infants receiving intravenous medications, they investigated the influence of infusion rates and the sites of injection into the intravenous system on the time course of the drug concentration. When the rate of fluid administration was at the lower limit of what is commonly used clinically in small infants, the drug remained in the intravenous tubing for 4 hr or more. Because of drug diffusion in the fluid in the tubing, the time over which drug was actually infused was also considerably prolonged beyond what was anticipated. Taking into account that the intravenous tubing was routinely changed in their nursery every 24 hr, these workers determined that 36% of the daily doses of the various intravenous medications were inadvertently discarded. Clearly, the dynamics of drug administration demand special care when flow rates for intravenous solutions are less than 25 ml/hr.

Techniques for Determination of Serum Drug Concentration

The development of analytical methods for measuring serum drug concentrations with microliter quantities of serum has been extremely valuable in allowing the application of pharmacokinetic principles to pediatric patients. Radioimmunoassay, high-pressure liquid chromatography, and gas chromatography/mass spectroscopy have been the principal techniques involved. An additional benefit has been the improved sensitivity and specificity characteristic of these techniques. The fact that specimens of smaller volume will suffice has also eased the various access problems, because capillary samples obtained by heel prick are now feasible.

The development of pharmacokinetic methods that use body fluids other than serum is particularly attractive for pediatric patients. The monitoring of salivary drug concentrations has been favored by some because it spares patients the trauma and difficulty of venipuncture. The limitations and advantages of this technique are summarized in Chapter 21, as well as by Mucklow et al. (43) and Danhof and Breimer (44). The utility of this technique depends greatly on the particular drug in question, its protein binding, its ionization potential, and perhaps its active secretion into saliva. In general, this technique has not found widespread applicability in pediatrics for any drug. Further testing may establish selected circumstances favorable to the application of salivary drug concentrations. For example, Khanna et al. (45) have recently reported that salivary concentrations of theophylline and caffeine can be used to monitor therapy with these drugs. Their findings suggest that salivary drug concentrations are valid as a drug-monitoring index if they remain less than 8 μg/ml (see Chapter 21, Table 1). Above that level, the correlation of salivary and serum concentrations was poor, except for selected drugs, and thus serum level monitoring was required.

Methods of Pharmacokinetic Analysis in Pediatric Patients

All pharmacokinetic principles used in adult patients could, in theory, be applied to pediatric patients. However, the limitations described earlier, particularly those dealing with numbers of serum samples, make some methods of analysis more attractive than others. Two areas of application of pharmacokinetics will be addressed: (a) pharmacokinetics as a research tool used to understand the changes in drug disposition that occur during biological maturation, and (b) pharmacokinetics as a clinical technique to improve therapeutics in individual patients.

Pharmacokinetics and research. The foregoing review of pharmacokinetic information in pediatric patients, while not exhaustive, should serve to demonstrate that large gaps exist in our knowledge of drug disposition at varying stages of development. The generation of rational dosage regimens for patients of various ages depends on the aquisition of additional information. Some of the problems that have hindered this research have now been overcome, as detailed earlier. The recognition of the importance of this information has overcome the previous reluctance to conduct investigations in children. Nonetheless, absolute limitations on plasma sample sizes and numbers make some methods of experimental design more attractive in children.

The observation that the time course of drug urinary excretion rate parallels the decline in serum drug concentration can be used to study drug elimination or to enhance the interpretation from a limited number of serum samples. Two treatments of urinary excretion data are commonly employed (46). By one method, the "amount remaining to be excreted" for a drug following one-compartment-model kinetics is given by

$$\ln (Ae_\infty - Ae) = \ln \frac{k_e}{k} D - kt$$

where Ae is the cumulative amount of unchanged drug excreted in the urine at time t, Ae_∞ is the amount of unchanged drug eventually excreted, D is the total dose given, k_e is the rate constant governing urinary drug elimination, and k is the overall elimination-rate constant. The second method, the "excretion-rate" plot, is represented by the following equation:

$$\ln \frac{dAe}{dt} = \ln k_e D - kt$$

Note that both equations represent linear plots with slope k, the same slope found when the natural logarithm of serum concentration is plotted against time. Urinary data can therefore be used to augment a few serum points. Evans et al. (47), studying the elimination of gentamicin in children, used urinary excretion data to define the terminal elimination phase for this drug. Their data support the importance of this phase in determining steady state gentamicin levels. Clearly, this study would have been impossible using serum samples alone.

Other workers have used urinary data alone in other circumstances. Miller et al. (10) studied the urinary excretion of acetaminophen and its conjugates and analyzed the data using plots of the amount remaining to be excreted. Because relatively complete excretion of drug was assured, the rate constants could then be obtained for unchanged drug and both glucuronide and sulfate conjugate, and then the overall elimination constant computed. Morgan et al. (48) used urinary data to determine the half-life of elimination for etidocaine in newborns whose mothers had received the drug during labor. Because the quantity of drug delivered to the infant could not be assessed, no information concerning volume of distribution and clearance could have been obtained. However, urinary monitoring did offer information about the elimination rate without the necessity of drawing blood.

Pharmacokinetics and clinical therapeutics. Regardless of how and when additional pharmacokinetic information for pediatric therapy becomes available, the large interpatient variability previously noted will remain a problem complicating the application of population-derived pharmacokinetic parameters to individual patients. Appropriate strategies for therapeutic drug monitoring and subsequent adjustments in dosage schedules for most drugs have not been clearly devised in a form useful to the pediatrician. Some exceptions, however, exist and warrant further examination.

The strategy that is most commonly used in therapeutic drug monitoring has had little systematic evaluation. It is the hit-or-miss method of choosing a dose, waiting a while, getting a level, then incrementing the dose on the basis of the result. This derisive description is not to say that the determination of single serum drug concentrations is without value. Indeed, a dosage increase in this circumstance will produce a proportional increase in the serum drug concentration, assuming the

sample was taken at steady state and first-order elimination was obtained. The difficulty with this approach is that these conditions are seldom met; in addition, no account is taken of the change in drug concentration during the dosage interval. However, investigation will undoubtedly define the role for this type of monitoring because of the relatively few blood samples involved and therefore its ease of applicability and, perhaps, its cost-effectiveness (49). It is likely to be useful in circumstances where (a) the drug does not reach saturation kinetics, (b) there is little urgency to reach steady state concentration, and (c) the elimination rate is slow or relatively constant between patients. Single-point determinations might still be useful if elimination occurred rapidly if there was no need to maintain therapeutic levels throughout the dosage interval. (The method of single-point determination is discussed in Chapter 21.)

A second method of applying pharmacokinetics to individual patients is exemplified by the study of Koup et al. (50). These workers designed nomograms relating a single steady state concentration obtained at a fixed time after the initial dose to the maintenance dose required to maintain an average steady state drug concentration. A good correlation for chloramphenicol and theophylline was found for this method. The potential for application of this type of analysis to pediatric patients seems limited, however. These nomograms compensate for differences in drug clearance, and the wide variability in distribution volume would render this method inaccurate. This is particularly exemplified with theophylline variability in infancy (51).

In theory, the most accurate method of overcoming a large interindividual variation in pharmacokinetics would be a measurement in each patient of a pharmacokinetic profile. Naturally, the limitations discussed earlier may make this method impractical for pediatric patients. For example, the definition of two compartments may require 10 or more sampling points (52). Nevertheless, even for the many drugs for which two compartments define more accurately the disposition pattern, conclusions reached using a one-compartment model can prove satisfactory for clinical application (53). Therefore, several methods of assessing first-order kinetic constants have been developed and applied to pediatric patients.

In one study, individual kinetic parameters for gentamicin have been calculated by collecting as few as three points after a single intravenous injection (54). A satisfactory agreement was noted between the predicted and achieved steady state levels, although trough concentrations were slightly but significantly greater than predicted.

Alternate methods are available to calculate first-order kinetic constants. Bjornsson and Shand (55) have proposed obtaining an interdose minimum concentration after the first dose and at steady state. As their calculations show, kinetic constants can be calculated from these two values. This method, however, seems to have no advantages over the determination of kinetic parameters from a single dose, at least as far as individual therapeutics are concerned. There is no savings on the number of samples needed, and there are additional requirements of knowing the time the

steady state is reached and of maintaining a constant dose and consistent dosage interval.

However, an analogous method may be useful for determining individual kinetic constants of drugs that achieve saturation kinetics. The method was elaborated by Ludden et al. (56) and applied to pediatric patients by Chiba et al. (36). It is based on the concept that when the steady state is reached, the rate of drug administration, D/τ, is equal to elimination, and the Michaelis-Menten constants V_{max} and K_m can be calculated:

$$\frac{D}{\tau} = \frac{V_{max} \cdot C}{K_m + C}$$

Therefore, the determination of steady state concentration at two or more dosage rates allows calculation of V_{max}, K_m, and, by extrapolation, the anticipated concentrations at other doses.

Some workers have argued that although first-order kinetics are not an accurate approximation, they can be applied if the departure from first-order kinetics is systematic so that a corresponding systematic adjustment can be made. Two such proposals have been made for gentamicin, which shows a slow terminal elimination phase. One method suggests obtaining first-order elimination constants after the fourth or fifth dose (57). A second method was proposed that uses the first-order constants calculated for individual patients together with a nomogram that includes the contribution of the second compartment from population-derived values (47).

Clearly, there is a need for more pharmacokinetic studies in pediatric patients. It is important, however, to emphasize a crucial and ultimate limitation of pharmacokinetics; i.e., pharmacokinetic data must be collected in conjunction with pharmacodynamic data if the former are to prove useful in clinical practice. Said another way, biological maturation, in addition to the influences enumerated earlier, appears to affect the relationship between serum concentration and drug effect as well. Several examples will serve to illustrate this problem.

The response to nondepolarizing curare-type muscle relaxants is accentuated in neonates and small infants, resembling that seen in adult myasthenic patients (58). Infants seem to demonstrate enhanced responsiveness to vagal stimulation, and atropine doses are correspondingly higher in these patients (58). Finally, this phenomenon for some drugs may represent itself not as a shift in the concentration–response relationship but as a difference in the effect. Imipramine, used to treat enuresis in children, induces an increase in circulating norepinephrine and increases in systolic and diastolic blood pressures (59). This contrasts strikingly with the postural hypotension seen in adults treated with this agent (60). Whether the direct actions of imipramine or compensatory cardiovascular reflexes account for these differences is unknown.

CONCLUSION

Abundant data support the conclusion that the maturation of physiologic processes accounts for the changes in drug disposition that occur during childhood. Because

these processes are independent, drug disposition in young children is not predictable from the known disposition as determined in adult patients. More thorough study of selected populations of pediatric patients should better define the changes in drug disposition that occur with age and allow better estimations of initial drug dosages. However, a wide interindividual variation in drug disposition seems to be characteristic of this patient population, and monitoring of serum drug concentrations along with determination of individual pharmacokinetic parameters in selected patients are often necessary to assure safe yet effective therapy.

REFERENCES

1. Finkel, M. J. (1978): Proposed regulations for the study of new drugs in children. In: *Clinical Pharmacology and Therapeutics: A Pediatric Perspective*, edited by B. L. Mirkin, pp. 299–304. Year Book, Chicago.
2. Wilson, J. T. (1975): Pragmatic assessments of medicines available for young children and pregnant or breast-feeding women. In: *Basic and Therapeutic Aspects of Perinatal Pharmacology*, edited by P. L. Morselli, S. Garattini, and F. Sereni, pp. 411–421. Raven Press, New York.
3. Morselli, P. L. (1976): Clinical pharmacokinetics in neonates. *Clin. Pharmacokinet.*, 1:81–98.
4. Rane, A., and Wilson, J. T. (1976): Clinical pharmacokinetics in infants and children. *Clin. Pharmacokinet.*, 1:2–24.
5. Hilligoss, D. M. (1980): Neonatal pharmacokinetics. In: *Applied Pharmacokinetics*, edited by W. E. Evan, J. J. Schentag, and W. J. Jusko, pp. 76–94. Applied Therapeutics Inc., San Francisco.
6. Morselli, P. L., Franco-Morselli, R., and Bossi, L. (1980): Clinical pharmacokinetics in newborns and infants. *Clin. Pharmacokinet.*, 5:485–527.
7. Huang, N. N., and High, R. H. (1953): Comparison of serum levels following the administration of oral and parenteral preparations of penicillin to infants and children of various age groups. *J. Pediatr.*, 42:657–668.
8. Silverio, J., and Poole, J. W. (1973): Serum concentrations of ampicillin in newborn infants after oral administration. *Pediatrics*, 51:578–580.
9. Rowland, M. (1978): Drug administration and regimens. In: *Clinical Pharmacology*, 2nd Ed., edited by K. L. Melmon, and H. F. Morrelli, pp. 25–70. Macmillan, New York.
10. Miller, R. P., Robert, R. J., and Fischer, L. J. (1970): Acetaminophen elimination kinetics in neonates, children and adults. *Clin. Pharmacol. Ther.*, 19:284–294.
11. Larese, R. J., and Mirkin, B. L. (1974): Kinetics of digoxin: Absorption and relation of serum levels to cardiac arrhythmias. *Clin. Pharmacol. Ther.*, 15:387–396.
12. Heimann, G. (1980): Enteral absorption and bioavailability in children in relation to age. *Eur. J. Clin. Pharmacol.*, 18:43–50.
13. Gladtke, E., and Heimann, G. (1975): The rate of development of elimination functions in kidney and liver of young infants. In: *Basic and Therapeutic Aspects of Perinatal Pharamcology*, edited by P. L. Morselli, S. Garattini, and F. Sereni, pp. 393–403. Raven Press, New York.
14. Morselli, P. L. (1977): Drug absorption. In: *Drug Disposition during Development*, edited by P. L. Morselli, pp. 51–60. Spectrum, New York.
15. Evans, M. A., Bhat, R., Vidyasagar, D., Vadapulli, M., Fisher, E., and Hastreiter, A. (1979): Gestational age and indomethacin elimination in the neonate. *Clin. Pharmacol. Ther.*, 26:746–751.
16. Wilson, J. T., Atwood, G. F., and Shand, D. G. (1976): Disposition of propoxyphene and propranolol in children. *Clin. Pharmacol. Ther.*, 19:264–270.
17. Evans, E. F., Proctor, J. D., Fratkin, M. J., Velandia, J., and Wasserman, A. J. (1975): Blood flow in muscle groups and drug absorption. *Clin. Pharmacol. Ther.*, 17:44–47.
18. Assael, B. M., Gianni, V., Marnin, A., Peneff, P., and Sereni, F. (1977): Gentamicin dosage in preterm and term neonates. *Arch. Dis. Child.*, 52:883.
19. Sardemann, H., Colding, H., Hendel, J., Kampmann, J. P., Hvidberg, E. F., and Vejlsgaard, R. (1976): Kinetics and dose calculations of amikacin in the newborn. *Clin. Pharmacol. Ther.*, 20:59–66.
20. Winters, R. W. (1973): Regulation of normal water and electrolyte metabolism. In: *The Body Fluids in Pediatrics*, edited by R. W. Winters, pp. 95–112. Little, Brown, Boston.

21. Dreissen, O. M., Sargedrager, N., Michel, M. F., Kerrebijn, K. J., and Hermans, J. (1979): Variability and predictability of plasma concentrations of ampicillin and kanamycin in newborn infants. *Eur. J. Clin. Pharmacol.*, 15:133–137.
22. Nelson, J. D., Kusmiesz, H., Shelton, S., and Woodman, E. (1978): Clinical pharmacology and efficacy of ticarcillin in infants and children. *Pediatrics*, 61:858–863.
23. Mihaly, G. W., Moore, R. G., Thomas, J., Triggs, E. J., Thomas, D., and Shauks, C. A. (1978): The pharmacokinetics and metabolism of the anilide local anesthetics in neonates. *Eur. J. Clin. Pharmacol.*, 13:143–152.
24. Moore, R. G., Thomas, J., Triggs, E. J., Thomas, D. B., Burnard, E. D., and Shauks, C. A. (1978): The pharmacokinetics and metabolism of the anilide local anesthetics in neonates. III. Mepivacaine. *Eur. J. Clin. Pharmacol.*, 14:203–213.
25. Evans, W. E., Feldman, S., Ossi, M., Taylor, R. H., Chaudhary, W., Melton, E. T., and Baker, L. F. (1980): Gentamicin dosage in children: A randomized prospective comparison of body weight and body surface area as dose determinants. *J. Pediatr.*, 96:479–484.
26. Hilligoss, D. M., Jusko, W. J., Koup, J. R., and Gracola, G. (1980): Factors affecting theophylline pharmacokinetics in premature infants with apnea. *Dev. Pharmacol. Ther.*, 1:6–15.
27. Pitlick, W., Painter, M., and Pippenger, C. (1978): Phenobarbital kinetics in neonates. *Clin. Pharmacol. Ther.*, 23:346–350.
28. Kurz, H., Mauser-Ganshorn, A., and Stickel, H. H. (1977): Differences in the binding of drugs to plasma proteins from newborn and adult man. *Eur. J. Clin. Pharmacol.*, 2:463–467, 469–472.
29. Piafsky, M. D., and Mpamugo, L. (1981): Dependence on neonatal drug binding of α_1-acid glycoprotein concentrations. *Clin. Pharmacol. Ther.*, 29:272.
30. Wallace, S. (1977): Altered plasma albumin in the newborn infant. *Br. J. Clin. Pharmacol.*, 4:82–85.
31. Wallace, S. (1976): Factors affecting drug protein binding in the plasma of newborn infants. *Br. J. Clin. Pharmacol.*, 3:510–512.
32. Gorodischer, R., Jusko, W. J., and Yaffe, S. J. (1976): Tissue and erythrocyte distribution of digoxin in infants. *Clin. Pharmacol. Ther.*, 19:256–263.
33. Wettrell, G., and Andersson, K. E. (1977): Clinical pharmacokinetics of digoxin in infants. *Clin. Pharmacokinet.*, 2:17–31.
34. Aldridge, A., Aranda, J. F., and Neims, A. A. (1979): Caffeine metabolism in the newborn. *Clin. Pharmacol. Ther.*, 25:447–453.
35. Friedman, C. A., Lovejoy, F. C., and Smith, A. L. (1979): Chloramphenicol disposition in infants and children. *J. Pediatr.*, 95:1071–1077.
36. Chiba, K., Ishizaki, T., Munra, H., and Minagawa, K. (1980): Michaelis-Menten pharmacokinetics of diphenylhydantoin and application in the pediatric age patient. *J. Pediatr.*, 96:479–484.
37. Painter, M. J., Pippenger, C., MacDonald, H., and Pitlick, W. (1978): Phenobarbital and diphenylhydantoin levels in neonates with seizures. *J. Pediatr.*, 92:315–319.
38. Thomas, C. R. (1976): Routine phenobarbital for prevention of neonatal hyperbilirubinemia. *Obstet. Gynecol.*, 47:304.
39. Redmond, G. P., Bell, J. J., and Perel, J. M. (1978): Effect of human growth hormone on amobarbital metabolism in children. *Clin. Pharmacol. Ther.*, 24:213–218.
40. Haugey, D. B., Hilligoss, D. M., Grassi, A., and Schentag, J. J. (1980): Two compartment gentamicin pharmacokinetics in premature infants: A comparison to adults with decreased glomerular filtration rates. *J. Pediatr.*, 96:325–330.
41. Aranda, J. V., Turmen, T., and Sasynuik, B. I. (1980): Pharmacokinetics of diuretics and methylxanthines in the neonate. *Eur. J. Clin. Pharmacol.*, 18:55–63.
42. Gould, T., and Roberts, R. F. (1979): Therapeutic problems arising from the use of the intravenous route for drug administration. *J. Pediatr.*, 95:465–471.
43. Mucklow, J. C., Bending, M. R., Kahn, G. C., and Dollery, C. T. (1978): Drug concentration in saliva. *Clin. Pharmacol. Ther.*, 24:563–570.
44. Danhof, M., and Breimer, D. D. (1978): Therapeutic drug monitoring in saliva. *Clin. Pharmacokinet.*, 3:39–57.
45. Khanna, N. N., Bada, H. S., and Somani, S. M. (1980): Use of salivary concentrations in the prediction of serum caffeine and theophylline concentrations in premature infants. *J. Pediatr.*, 96:494–499.
46. Martin, B. K. (1967): Treatment of data from drug urinary excretion. *Nature*, 214:247–249.

47. Evans, W. E., Taylor, R. H., Feldman, S., Crom, W. R., Rivera, G., and Yee, G. C. (1980): A model for dosing gentamicin in children and adolescents that adjusts for tissue accumulation with continuous dosing. *Clin. Pharmacokinet.*, 5:295–306.
48. Morgan, D., McQuillan, D., and Thomas, J. (1978): Pharmacokinetics and metabolism of the anilide local anesthetics in neonates. II. Etidocaine. *Eur. J. Clin. Pharmacol.*, 13:365–371.
49. Sheiner, L. B., Beal, S., Rosenberg, B., and Marathe, V. V. (1979): Forecasting individual pharmacokinetics. *Clin. Pharmacol. Ther.*, 26:294–305.
50. Koup, J. R., Sack, C. M., Smith, A. L., and Gibaldi, M. (1979): Hypothesis for the individualization of drug dosage. *Clin. Pharmacokinet.*, 4:460–469.
51. Nassif, E. G., Weinberger, M. M., Shanon, D., Guiany, S. F., Hendeles, L., Jimenez, D., and Ekivo, E. (1981): Theophylline disposition in infancy. *J. Pediatr.*, 98:158–160.
52. Fell, P. J., and Stevens, M. T. (1975): Pharmacokinetics—uses and abuses. *Eur. J. Clin. Pharmacol.*, 8:241–248.
53. Dvorchik, B. H., and Vessell, E. S. (1978): Significance of error associated with use of the one-compartment formula to calculate clearance of thirty-eight drugs. *Clin. Pharmacol. Ther.*, 23:617–623.
54. Sawchuck, R. J., Zaske, D. E., Apolle, R. J., Wargin, W. A., and Strate, R. G. (1977): Kinetic model for gentamicin dosing with the use of individual patient parameters. *Clin. Pharmacol. Ther.*, 21:362–369.
55. Bjornsson, T. D., and Shand, D. G. (1979): Estimation of kinetic parameters from a two-point determination of the drug cumulation factor. *Clin. Pharmacol. Ther.*, 26:540–547.
56. Ludden, T. M., Allen, J. P., Valutsky, W. A., Vicuna, A. V., Nappi, J. M., Hoffman, S. F., Wallace, J. E., Lalka, D., and McNay, J. L. (1977): Individualization of phenytoin dosage regimens. *Clin. Pharmacol. Ther.*, 21:287–293.
57. Evans, W. E., Feldman, S., Barber, L. F., Ossi, M., and Chaudhary, S. (1978): Use of gentamicin serum levels to individualize therapy in children. *J. Pediatr.*, 93:133–137.
58. Nugent, S. K., Laravuso, R., and Rogers, M. C. (1979): Pharmacology and use of muscle relaxants in infants and children. *J. Pediatr.*, 94:481–487.
59. Lake, C. R., Mikkelsen, E. J., Rapoport, J. L., Zavadil, A. P., and Kopin, I. J. (1979): Effect of imipramine on norepinephrine and blood pressure in enuretic boys. *Clin. Pharmacol. Ther.*, 26:647–653.
60. Glassman, A. H., Bigger, J. T., Giardina, E., Kantor, S., Perel, J., and Davies, M. (1979): The clinical characteristics of imipramine induced orthostatic hypotension. *Lancet*, 1:468–472.
61. Tserng, K. Yi, King, K. C., and Takieddine, F. N. (1981): Theophylline metabolism in premature infants. *Clin. Pharmacol. Ther.*, 29:594–600.
62. Foman, S. J. (1974): *Infant Nutrition*, p. 575. W. B. Saunders, Philadelphia.
63. Vaughn, V. C., McKay, J. R., and Nelson, W. E. (1975): *Textbook of Pediatrics*, p. 1876. W. B. Saunders, Philadelphia.

Pharmacokinetic Basis for Drug Treatment,
edited by L. Z. Benet et al., Raven Press,
New York © 1984

Chapter 15

Pharmacokinetic Considerations in Geriatric Patients

Neil Massoud

*Division of Clinical Pharmacology, University of California, San Francisco,
San Francisco, California 94143*

Aging is a biological process difficult for us to understand and accept. Yet, in the future, we as clinicians can expect to spend much more of our time catering to the health needs of the geriatric population (i.e., persons 65 years of age and older). These patients freqently present with perplexing multiple disorders and complaints. In deciding whether or not treatment is required, it is often difficult to differentiate between those symptoms due to disease and those due to aging (1). As one ages, the total number of cells in the human body decreases 25% to 30% between adolescence and old age. However, cellular mass may be larger and structure increasingly irregular. The cell loss is particularly of the postmiotic type (cells not capable of reproducing), and obscure changes occur in compositional distribution (2). Many of these physiologic changes and pathologic disorders are irreversible, inevitable, and additive (Table 1 and Fig. 1). There may also be behavioral changes prompted by emotional adjustments to loneliness, changes in financial status, insomnia, senility, depression, and anxiety, resulting in deterioration of the individual's health. As a result, aging is often regarded with negativism by both the public and health care professionals (2). This attitude is often exacerbated by the complexity of the treatment for ailments in geriatric patients.

Although geriatric patients constitute only 11% of the population in North America, they incur 30% of the total costs of drugs (3). Within the next 30 years, these figures are expected to reach 16% to 18% and 40%, respectively (4). Considering that about one-half of all drugs will be used in geriatric patients, and the fact that the majority of therapeutic, pharmacologic, and pharmacokinetic studies have been done in individuals less than 55 years of age, it is important that special attention be given to geriatric patients who have variable diseases (e.g., cardiac disease, osteoarthritis, osteoporosis, diabetes, cerebrovascular disease, emphysema, paralysis, malignancies, renal infection, influenza, pneumonia) and use multiple drugs (5). Seventy-eight percent of hospitalized geriatric patients have at least four major diseases; 38% have six or more, and approximately 13% have eight or more diseases (3). Clinicians are finding more drug-related toxicities in the elderly, possibly

TABLE 1. *Changes in regional perfusion with aging[a]*

	Rate of change (% per year)	
	Approximate[b]	Average[c]
Cardiac output	−0.75	−1.01
Cerebral flow	−0.35	−0.5
Coronary flow	−0.5	
Visceral flow (liver)	−1.1	−0.3
		(−0.36[d])
Renal flow	−1.1	−1.9
Remainder (by difference)		−1.3

[a]For an excellent review, see Danon et al. (123).
[b]Data from Bender (120).
[c]Data from Landowne and Stanley (121).
[d]Data from Flood et al. (122).

because of the increased numbers of drugs used to treat multiple disease states, in addition to overresponses to certain drugs. There is a sevenfold increase in drug toxicities as one ages from 20 to 79 years (3% at 20–29 years of age, 21% at 70–79 years of age) (1,6). Perhaps this is related to altered pharmacokinetic parameters (i.e., absorption, distribution, metabolism, and/or excretion) (ADME) involved in the handling of the drug and/or in response to the drug with aging (7). Table 2 is a summary of the factors affecting drug disposition and response in geriatric patients. It is important to distinguish between those elderly persons who are long-term bedridden patients and those who are ambulatory and living independently within the community (8). Totally bedridden patients may have impaired circulation, altering the pharmacokinetic profiles of drugs. It is possible, therefore, that the immobility of the elderly, their multiple disease states, and multiple medications contribute to the pharmacokinetic differences that distinguish them from the younger population. The clinician who is aware of these altered pharmacokinetic parameters will be able to make therapeutic recommendations aimed at lowering the incidence of toxicity while optimizing therapy and compliance in the elderly (3).

ABSORPTION

There are a number of associated physiologic changes occurring in the elderly that are expected to alter drug absorption from the gastrointestinal tract or parenteral sites (intramuscular, subcutaneous, intradermal). However, there has been little evidence to suggest that this is of any major significance. On the other hand, there have been few systematic studies of this aspect (5).

From youth to old age, there are a number of physiologic changes that occur within the gastrointestinal (GI) tract that influence absorption. As one ages, the pH rises slightly in the stomach, gastric acid secretion decreases (to 25–35% of that of a 20-year-old), and possibly the production of pancreatic trypsin is lowered.

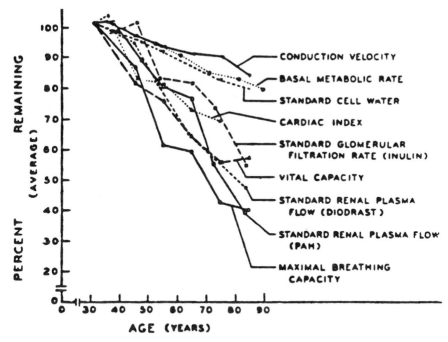

FIG. 1. Loss of efficiency with age for several human physiologic functions. (From Ritschel, ref. 11, with permission.)

There are also decreases in blood flow, gastric emptying time, tissue surface area, and the numbers of Peyer's patches and the follicles within them, and there is a thickening of the muscularis of the colon (2,9). In the geriatric population, the incidence of duodenal diverticula disease is greater than in the young. This may allow for bacterial colonization of the small intestine, resulting in absorption changes in the elderly. Defects occur in deglutition (swallowing) due to the combination of dilatation of the esophagus, relaxation of the lower esophageal sphincter, delay of esophageal emptying, and an increase in the nonpropulsive contractions (2). This should be kept in mind particularly when designing dosage forms. Once-daily dosing, based on pharmacokinetic parameters (i.e., long half-life) and an effort to increase compliance, can lead to the use of abnormally large capsules and tablets that are difficult to swallow.

Salivary drug concentrations of many orally administered drugs correlate with concurrent free serum drug concentrations (see Chapter 21). When using saliva as a means to measure drug concentrations and perhaps further correlate this with therapeutic effect, it is important to remember that different age groups produce varying amounts of saliva. It has been found that in both stimulated and unstimulated geriatric patients there is only about one-third the amount of saliva produced by a young person. Just the physical process of collection may be difficult in the geriatric age group.

TABLE 2. *Summary of factors affecting drug disposition and responses in the elderly*

Effect	Altered physiology[a]	Clinical considerations
Absorption	↓ Gastric acid secretion ↑ Gastric pH ↓ GI blood flow ↓ Pancreatic trypsin ↓ Number of absorbing cells ↓ GI motility	Altered dissolution rate, possible decreased absorption rate, "longer time" for onset of effect
Distribution Body composition	↓ Total body water ↓ Lean body weight (mass/kg body weight) ↑ Body fat (females ≥ males)	Polar drugs tend to have ↓ Vd, lipid-soluble drugs tend to have ↑ Vd, "hangover phenomenon," delayed onset, followed by accumulation and "overdosing" in multiple dosing
Protein binding	↓ Serum albumin ↔↑ AGP[b] ↔↑ Gammaglobulin ↔↓ RBC binding	↑ Free fraction of highly bound acidic drugs ↔ ↓ free fraction of highly bound basic drugs
Metabolism (hepatic)	↔↓ Enzyme inducibility ↓ Hepatic blood flow ↓ Hepatic mass ↔ Acetylation ↔ Alcohol dehydrogenase metabolism ↔↓ Glucuronidation ↔↓ Mixed-function oxidase system	Apparently decreased metabolism and clearance of certain drugs; influenced by environmental factors (e.g., smoking and/or nutritional)
Excretion (renal)	↓ GFR ↓ Renal plasma flow ↓ Active secretion	Decreased renal clearance; ↑ half-life of drugs significantly excreted via the kidney (see Chapter 8)
Response (Multiple disease states; multiple drug use)	↔↓ Altered receptor number ? Altered receptor sensitivity Organ-specific age changes Changes in CNS enzyme activity Possible altered second-messenger function Baroreceptor reflex sensitivity	↑ Variation in dose response; ↑ adverse drug reactions; ↑ paradoxic drug reactions

[a] ↓ decrease; ↑ increase; ↔ no change; ? questionable change.
[b] Alpha-glycoprotein.
Adapted from Vestal (3), with permission.

Passive absorption, as measured by xylose uptake, is reduced, but this is of clinical significance only in the older geriatric group (i.e., 80–85 years of age and above). For the majority of drugs, neither the rate nor the extent of absorption by passive diffusion processes will be altered as a result of physiologic alterations in

the aging GI tract. However, this is still a matter of dispute (10,11). With advancing age, active absorption processes are thought to be more significantly decreased, based on the limited absorption found for galactose, 3-methylglucose, calcium, thiamine, vitamin B_{12}, and iron (5,12).

Recently, there have been a few studies concerning GI absorption of drugs in the geriatric population. Evans et al. (13) demonstrated in 5 elderly (71–86 years) parkinsonian outpatients and 6 young (22–34 years) healthy controls that when 300 mg of L-DOPA was given, the rates of absorption did not differ (13). However, there was an increase in the area under the serum concentration curve *(AUC)* in the geriatric group ($p < 0.01$) (Fig. 2) (13). In a further follow-up of this study, Evans et al. (14) also demonstrated significant increases in both Cp_{max} (1.9 $\pm$ 0.39 vs. 0.88 $\pm$ 0.29 µg/ml) and $Cp_{6\text{-}hr}$ (0.25 $\pm$ 0.22 vs. 0.05 $\pm$ 0.04 µg/ml) for the old and young, respectively (14). These authors suggested that the increase in *AUC* may be due to an age-related alteration in the disposition of the orally administered L-DOPA or that this enhancement may be a consequence of an age-related decrease in the activity of DOPA decarboxylase in the gastric mucosa (13,14). Sartor et al. (15) demonstrated the effects of age on the absorption of tolbutamide (500 mg) and chlorpropamide (250 mg) in 12 elderly (74–75 years) and 12 young (23–28 years) healthy community volunteers (15). In the measurements of peak concentration (Cp_{max}), time to peak concentration (T_{max}), elimination half-life ($T_{1/2}$), and *AUC*,

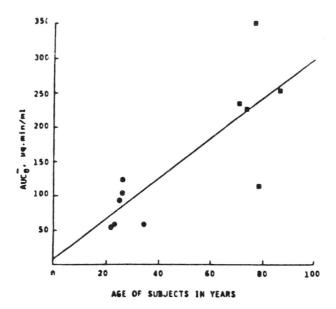

FIG. 2. Relationship for elderly Parkinsonian patients *(squares)* and young healthy volunteers *(circles)* between the area under the plasma L-DOPA curve to infinite time *(AUC_0^∞)* and age [$N = 11$; $r = 0.7970$ ($p < 0.01$)]. (From Evans et al., ref. 13, with permission.)

only the T_{max} concentration of tolbutamide differed. In the elderly patients, the T_{max} was significantly greater ($p < 0.05$) (15). Kendal et al. (16) demonstrated the effects of age on the absorption of metoprolol (100 mg) in 8 young (21–26 years) and old (62–72 years) otherwise healthy hypertensive patients. Both the mean plasma metoprolol concentrations and AUC did not differ significantly, although there was a tendency for the older subjects to have later and higher peaks, as well as a greater 24-hr plasma metoprolol concentration. In 1980, Schneider et al. (8) evaluated another beta blocker, propranolol, with respect to age. After giving single 40-mg and 80-mg doses to both young (19–25 years) and old (63–81 years) otherwise healthy nonsmoking individuals with sedimentation rates less than 30 mm/hr, differences in the AUC were not significant at the 5% level (8). Sedimentation rates below 20 to 30 mm/hr tend to indicate the absence of both inflammatory disease activity and elevation in α_1-acid glycoprotein. Redolfi et al. (17) found the Cp_{max} (3,667 ± 297 ng/ml in the young vs. 6,390 ± 366 ng/ml in the elderly) for a single 200-mg tablet of cimetidine to be greater in the elderly (66–84 years) than in the young (22–57 years). Cusack et al. (18) found a similar (although not as significant) pattern with digoxin bioavailability. In both the latter studies, both oral and intravenous doses were given. This allowed for a greater number of possibilities for considering the demonstrated changes of bioavailability, because it is incorrect to equate plasma drug concentrations or areas under the serum concentration/time curves with the completeness of absorption (or changes in metabolism) unless intravenous data are also available. Conversely, equal absorption in no way implies that the systemic bioavailability (i.e., rate and/or amount) of certain drugs may not differ in old age (19). For example, as with cimetidine, it is not that the drug is absorbed better in the elderly but rather that clearance decreases with age, providing higher plasma drug concentrations (17). Raised steady state plasma drug concentrations in the elderly, therefore, may be a function of reduced plasma clearance, rather than a change in passive or active absorption. Thus, when considering a few of the most recent studies, there are increases, decreases, and even no changes in both the rate and extent of GI absorption with aging.

There are very few data on the relationship between the effect of age and the rate and completeness of drug absorption from extravascular sites (20). Recently, however, Greenblatt et al. (20) demonstrated that the intramuscular systemic bioavailability of lorazepam did not vary between the young and old. In both age groups, the absorption half-life averaged 15.6 min, and peak plasma concentrations occurred no later than 2 hr after injection. In both groups, lorazepam absorption was essentially 95% to 100%. Although many physiologic changes occur within the GI tract with aging, only few major alterations in the absorption of drugs occur. In most cases, any change in passive or active absorption is balanced by an alteration in binding, metabolism, excretion, or distribution (10,11).

DISTRIBUTION

Great changes occur in body composition as the patient ages (Fig. 3). Much of the metabolically active tissue is slowly replaced by fat as one ages from 15 years

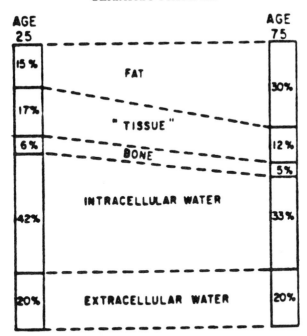

FIG. 3. Distribution of major body components with age. (From Rossman, ref. 2, with permission.)

to 60 years; body fat increases by 18 to 36% in males and in females by 33 to 48% (5). As a result, there is a reduction of lean body mass in proportion to total body weight. Drugs that are more highly lipid-soluble should have an increase in the volume of distribution (this may be more dramatic in females), whereas those that are highly water-soluble should result in greater plasma concentrations due to a decreased volume of distribution. For example, Wilkinson (21) and Shull et al. (22) demonstrated that volume of distribution for diazepam and chlordiazepoxide increased with age, whereas for the closely related derivatives, lorazepam and oxazepam, the volume of distribution remained relatively unaltered. The lipid solubilities of diazepam and chlordiazepoxide are much greater than the values reported for lorazepam and oxazepam (21,22). For other drugs, such as propicillin or digoxin, the volume of distribution has been stated to diminish with age, and for digoxin the effects have been explained largely by the decrease in body mass (23). There is a slight tendency to convert body fat back to a "normal" body composition after the age of 80 to 85 years (5). Total body water, unlike fat, decreases approximately 10 to 15% between the ages of 20 and 80 years (3). The extracellular fluid (Fig. 3) remains unchanged, but constitutes a greater portion of the total body water in the elderly. The reductions in total body water in males and females are approximately 0.37 and 0.27% per year, respectively (11). Because of these changes in water distribution, Ritschel (11) has suggested the following correction factor for the volume of distribution coefficient of a drug in elderly patients, for drugs that

have a higher degree of water solubility: Distribution coefficient of drug corrected for age, in males:

$$V \text{ in elderly} \approx \frac{V_{25}(54.25 - 0.199(\text{age} - 25))}{54.25}$$

Distribution coefficient of drug corrected for aged, in females:

$$V \text{ in elderly} \approx \frac{V_{25}(49.25 - 0.130(\text{age} - 25))}{49.25}$$

where V_{25} is the volume of distribution determined in healthy young individuals (i.e., 25 years old).

In addition to body fluids and lipid solubility, carrier proteins (depending on the degree of binding) are important when one considers the distribution of drugs. Although total protein concentrations remain relatively constant, albumin concentrations fall in the elderly by approximately 0.4–0.6 g/dl whereas a rise in gammaglobulin concentration occurs (5,24,25). These changes are partially explained by the relative inactivity of most elderly patients (24). There are also differences in albumin between geriatric outpatients and their hospitalized counterparts, as depicted in Fig. 4. In the elderly, a drop in the serum albumin can be an indication of the severity of systemic illnesses. In the hospitalized, an immediate fall in serum albumin has been noted after acute myocardial infarction, inflammatory disease (e.g., ulcerative colitis), burns, large pressure sores, and/or severe infection. On recovery, the serum albumin returns to the patient's normal values within a few weeks (26,27). Wallace and Whiting (24) demonstrated the effects of decreased albumin concentration on the percentage of drug unbound for salicylate, sulphadiazine, and phenylbutazone in four groups (two young, with mean ages 27 and 30 years; two old, with mean ages 79 and 84 years). In the elderly, the percentage unbound for all three drugs increased significantly (at least $p < 0.05$), as shown in Fig. 5. Triggs and Nation (6) reviewed the studies concerning albumin binding of phenytoin in the elderly. Affinity did not appear to change with age, but the

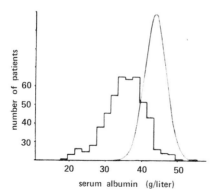

FIG. 4. Serum albumin results for 605 elderly Northwick Park Hospital patients (histogram) compared with those of healthy old subjects (normal curve). (From Hodkinson, ref. 27, with permission.)

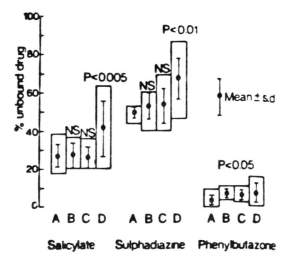

FIG. 5. Binding of salicylate, sulphadiazine, and phenylbutazone in groups A, B, C, and D. The mean ages of the groups were 27, 30, 79, and 84 years, respectively. Group A: normal young volunteers receiving no drugs. Group B: young surgical and gynecological patients receiving drug therapy. Group C: elderly patients receiving no drugs. Group D: elderly patients receiving drug therapy. Groups B, C, and D are compared to group A. (From Wallace and Whiting, ref. 24, with permission.)

maximum albumin binding of phenytoin or binding capacity correlated directly with albumin concentration (727 $\pm$ 22 μmole/liter for the young; 595 $\pm$ 21 μmole/liter for the old) (5). This 25 to 40% increase of unbound drug (i.e., fraction unbound 0.099 at 17 years vs. 0.127 at 53 years) could conceivably result in toxic levels for phenytoin, a drug with a narrow therapeutic concentration range. However, as will be noted subsequently, changes in albumin concentrations, which result in more unbound phenytoin, also result in an increased phenytoin clearance in the older age group. Perhaps this increase in clearance is enough to balance the increased unbound drug, thus requiring no dosage modification. However, this is only speculative and still very much debatable (6,28). Recently, Greenblatt et al. (29) demonstrated the influence of binding on diazepam. Here it was found that the percentage of unbound diazepam was positively correlated with increasing age, but only in females ($p < 0.001$) (29). For lipid-soluble drugs, the change in fraction of drug unbound may be accentuated in the female more than the male, because of the increase in fat stores with aging. Considering that the average geriatric hospitalized patient is receiving six or more drugs, competition for similar binding sites may cause increased displacement from plasma proteins, resulting in definite changes in drug distribution. With the concomitant average drop of 0.6 g/dl in serum albumin from 17 years of age to 80 years, one would expect binding interactions to be of clinical significance. Wallace and Whiting (24) demonstrated the effects of a number of drugs being taken simultaneously on the binding of salicylate in patients over 69 years of age (24). Patients receiving two or more additional drugs exhibited a significant increase in the percentage of free salicylate ($p < 0.001$). In patients aged

60 to 92 years regularly receiving salicylates, the free salicylate changed from 28% ($\pm 6\%$) to 48% ($\pm 8\%$) when there was an increase from no drug or one drug to two or more drugs taken simultaneously with their salicylate. Interesting studies have also suggested that red blood cell (RBC) binding of medications may decrease as one ages. This has been shown with meperidine, pentazocine, diazepam, and chlormethiazole (29,30). However, to what degree the buffering capacity of the blood cells and nontarget tissues will be decreased and more free drug (active) will become systemically available needs further investigation. Theoretically, higher concentrations should occur at both metabolic and effector sites, resulting in changes in both metabolism and activity (19).

Recently, there has been increased interest in the binding of drugs to plasma proteins other than albumin and red cells (see Chapter 10). Interest has centered around α_1-acid glycoprotein (AGP) with relation to basic (cationic) drugs. AGP increases are associated with a number of pathologic findings, including local inflammation, acute myocardial infarction, neoplastic growths, renal failure, erythrocyte sedimentation rate (ESR) greater than 30, Crohn's disease, celiac disease, surgery, trauma, and aging (31). Braithwaite et al. (31) found the AGP differences to be significant between the young (20–32 years) and the old (74–95 years). The mean AGP concentrations for the young and the old were approximately 0.70 and 1.30 g/liter, respectively. This may be of particular importance with highly bound basic drugs such as alprenolol, lidocaine, propranolol, quinidine, chlorpromazine, and disopyramide and antidepressants (e.g., amitriptyline, mianserin, viloxazine), where measurements of plasma drug concentrations are now more available. It is important to consider the AGP levels when measuring such drugs in the elderly. Norman et al. (32) reviewed the literature and noted increased plasma concentrations of imipramine, desipramine, and amitriptyline, but no mention of AGP was made. As a result, one is unable to differentiate between total changes in plasma antidepressant concentrations and unbound concentrations (active drug). It would appear, therefore, that the combination of decreased albumin, decreased RBC binding, and increased AGP, along with multiple drug therapy, is responsible for the increases in free concentrations of drugs, with their resulting increased toxicities.

When considering binding changes in the elderly, it would therefore be appropriate to consider albumin, RBC binding, AGP concentration, numbers and types of binding sites, sex, underlying disease processes, and renal function. Because only the free fraction is available for diffusion from the vascular system to sites of activity and biotransformation, it is the unbound rather than the total drug concentration that will reflect more accurately changes in distribution. Drugs that are considered highly bound (greater than 90%) and/or have a low volume of distribution (less than 0.20 liter/kg) are more likely to be affected through these changes with aging.

The variations in rate and/or extent of blood flow to different organs can alter the distribution of drugs. As one ages, the primary organs involved with distribution, such as the heart and blood vessels, undergo extensive changes. In the aging heart there is a decrease in the speed of contraction, and an increase in the refractory

interval between stimuli (2,33); the heart valves become stiffer; the left ventricular wall thickens (approximately 25% from ages 30 to 80), but the resting heart rate remains essentially unchanged. With a fatter, "stiffer," slower heart, cardiac output decreases, as would be expected (approximately 0.9% per year after the age of 20). As a result, when a maximal load is presented, both the rate and stroke volume are unable to compensate. Cardiac output consequently decreases 40% by the eighth decade (2). In an attempt to compensate, there is an increase in sympathetic tone (34), allowing vital organs (heart, skeletal muscle, and brain) to receive preference for circulation, with a concomitant decrease in peripheral and renal blood flow, although circulation to the brain may be countered by arterial and atherosclerotic changes. In the elderly, other mechanisms may also be involved in decreasing blood flow to the kidneys, because this appears to be reduced more than would be expected from a decrease in cardiac output (6). There is a decrease in hepatic blood flow of approximately 0.3 to 1.5% per year after the age of 20 that is partially explained by the decrease in cardiac output. The reduction in hepatic blood flow may result in decreased metabolic clearance for flow-dependent drugs with high extraction ratios (6). (For further discussion of high ER drugs, see Chapters 1 and 3.)

As one ages, there is a consistent decrease of elastin within the blood vessels. There is also an increase in the thickness of the basement membrane, from 700 Å in youth to 1,100 Å in old age. With atherosclerosis, aggregates of fatty substances are deposited in blood vessel linings. Plaques are apt to form about these deposits, thus decreasing or altering the distribution of blood flow. This decreased elasticity, narrowing of the artery, and changes in both the permeability of various tissues and barriers contribute to an abnormal distribution profile, as compared with that seen in the young (2). For example, considering the decrease of total body water, increase in fat composition, and decrease in peripheral blood flow, certain drugs could possibly remain localized longer after intramuscular, subcutaneous, or intradermal injection in the elderly.

METABOLISM

The liver is the major organ involved in metabolism. Hepatic drug metabolism can activate a drug, terminate its pharmacologic action, and/or generate a more polar ionized metabolite, allowing for renal excretion. In the elderly, hepatic metabolism is generally reduced; however, there is a great deal of variation (2–5,28,35,36). The aging liver undergoes cellular changes, a loss in weight (a decrease from 2.5% of body weight to 1.6% occurring from the sixth decade to the tenth decade), and a reduction in hepatic flow (0.3–1.5% per year after the age of 30 or approximately a 40% reduction by 65 years of age), but metabolism does not decrease as significantly (2,3). Clearance of bilirubin is not changed with age, and there are no significant differences in SGOT, SGPT, and alkaline phosphatase. Total protein decreases insignificantly, but there are significant decreases in serum albumin and the production of clotting factors (2). Thus, two of the three determinants of hepatic drug clearance are decreased: liver blood flow and the degree of binding of certain

drugs (average decrease in albumin from age 20 to 80 is 0.4–0.8 g/liter). The third factor, intrinsic hepatic clearance, is highly variable (Fig. 6). The latter is a measure of the efficiency with which an unbound drug is irreversibly removed from blood perfusing the hepatic sinusoids, and it reflects a rate-limiting process (18). As depicted in Fig. 6, only in 5% of the individuals studied can the decline in intrinsic hepatic clearance be explained as a function of aging. With cardiac output (as discussed earlier) decreasing 30% to 40% by 65 years of age, there is an approximate 12% to 40% decrease in hepatic blood flow. If liver metabolism is maintained, this reduction in hepatic flow could result in decreased extraction of highly cleared drugs (i.e., hepatic extraction ratio > 0.70).

Acetylation seems to be undisturbed with aging (as measured with isoniazid), but there is a generalized decrease in microsomal oxidation with aging (3,35,36). Although there has not been a large series of biopsies performed on the aging liver, it appears that the activity of the genetically controlled polymorphic N-acetyltransferase responsible for hepatic acetylation is preserved to even the advanced age of 90 to 95 years (37). Reynolds et al. (38) measured the metabolism of a single 25-mg oral dose of methaqualone and the excretion of its five C-hydroxy metabolites excreted in the urine, and the pattern of C-oxidation metabolites indicated that the C and N oxidative metabolic pathways do not change with age (at least as far as methaqualone is concerned) (38). However, this study provided evidence for a delay

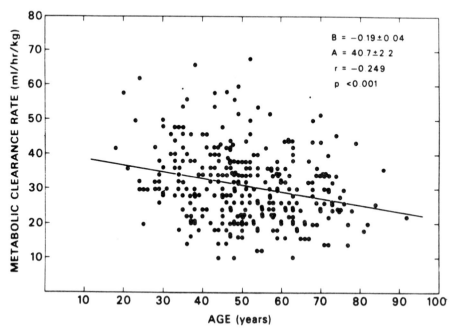

FIG. 6. Decline of metabolic clearance rate for antipyrine with age. (From Vestal et al., ref. 36, with permission.)

in the formation of oxidative metabolites and a greater interindividual variation in the elderly.

Unlike many other drugs metabolized within the liver, ethanol is primarily oxidized by alcohol dehydrogenase (ADH). Vestal et al. (39) demonstrated that the mean rate of hepatic ADH metabolism was not affected by age. The greater ethanol peak blood concentrations found in the elderly ($p < 0.01$) were related to a smaller volume of body water, a decrease in lean body mass, and a smaller volume of distribution, not a change in metabolism (39).

There are some who believe that a "decline" in certain other aspects of the mixed-function oxidative system is a mere reflection of the decreased use of common enzyme "inducers" (cigarettes, alcohol, certain foods) in the elderly (40). In a letter to the editor, Smithhard et al. (41) stressed that in the elderly, poor nutrition is at least partly responsible for the decline in microsomal enzyme function. They noted that both vitamin C and folate often are below therapeutic concentrations in the elderly admitted to geriatric wards. A deficiency in humans of either of these vitamins has shown impairment in the hepatic metabolism of certain drugs (41). In the rat, as perhaps in humans, the induction of the P-450 and P-448 mixed-function oxidase pathways by cigarette smoking requires prolonged exposure. Salem et al. (42) demonstrated, in the elderly, that after a 2-week course of dichloralphenazone (a drug used to evaluate the hepatic induction capabilities of cigarette smoking), hepatic induction was reduced in the elderly. However, Cusack et al. (43) recently demonstrated a 40% higher clearance of theophylline in geriatric smokers versus nonsmokers. This may be compared to the 55% higher clearance of theophylline in smoking versus nonsmoking young volunteers. Pfeifer and Greenblatt (44) have also reported a reduction in the incidence of theophylline adverse reactions in geriatric smokers versus nonsmokers. Perhaps an age-related effect of smoking may reflect a reduced capacity for enzyme induction and may require more time than the usual 2 to 3 weeks for induction. It is therefore important to consider smoking, in elderly patients, when assessing drug metabolism involving particular pathways (45). In humans, the effect of aging on glucuronide conjugation is not well understood, partly because of the limited number of drugs involved that can be given by both oral and intravenous routes. However, Greenblatt et al. (20) recently demonstrated, with lorazepam, that although glucuronidation appeared to decline with age, this decline was not statistically significant when cigarette smokers were omitted from the data analysis. Only negligible or slight alterations in oxazepam and acetaminophen glucuronidation have been found with age (20). Clearly, the various enzymes involved in drug metabolism show considerable differential sensitivity to the aging process, and as a result it is likely that each drug of interest will require individual investigation to define the magnitude of any change in hepatic clearance (46).

The activity of nonmicrosomal enzymes may also change with age. For example, Shanor et al. (47) reported a decline in plasma cholinesterase activity with age in men when acetylcholine or succinylcholine was used as substrate, whereas no such

change was noted in women. The effect of age on biliary excretion is still relatively unexplored. With diminished hepatic function and hepatic blood flow in the elderly, reduced biliary clearance would be anticipated, but results have been extremely variable (48). For digoxin, as the rate of renal excretion diminishes with age, the relative excretion by biliary route becomes more pronounced, suggesting that for this drug, renal clearance is altered more by aging than by extrarenal excretion.

The half-lifes for drugs in the elderly, similar to hepatic metabolism, are highly variable. However, changes in metabolism are more appropriately reflected by clearance, as emphasized in Chapter 1. This is exemplified with the drug diazepam, where half-life increases in proportion to a change in volume of distribution (with age) and is not a reflection of decreased metabolism (49). During chronic therapy, plasma drug concentrations accumulate at a rate dependent on half-life, but the steady state concentration is dependent on clearance (46). In situations such as this, where the half-life is increased and clearance maintained, the steady state will be reached more slowly, and fluctuations between peak and trough drug concentrations will be blunted, although the "average" plasma drug concentration will remain the same. Nation and Triggs (50) described a similar pattern for lidocaine with respect to steady state plasma concentrations in the elderly. In geriatric patients, it is important to remember that although plasma drug concentrations may be similar to those found in younger populations, the amount of drug at the receptor site could be quite different. Table 3 provides clearance values (as well as volume of distribution and half-life) for some commonly used drugs in both the young and old.

EXCRETION

The kidney is the major route of excretion for most drugs, either as the unchanged species or as the metabolic products. Like other organs, the kidney will undergo physiologic and anatomic changes with aging. Some changes reflect a consistent decrease in cardiac output, whereas others reflect internal renal changes. Drugs and their metabolites appear in the urine as a consequence of glomerular filtration, tubular reabsorption, and secretion, or a combination of processes (1) (see Chapter 8).

Any drug that is unbound within the plasma will be filtered. With advancing age, this glomerular filtering process is reduced as a result of a 20% weight reduction in kidney size, partly due to a loss of 35% of the number of nephrons (whose function is partially compensated for by the residual nephrons), a 30% loss in the number of functional glomeruli, and a decrease in the renal blood flow by 45% to 53% (2,5). As expected, there is an increase in serum creatinine, because the majority of creatinine is excreted via glomerular filtration and 10% via tubular secretion. However, this increase in serum creatinine is countered by a decrease in the production of creatinine as the proportion of muscle mass to body weight is decreased in the elderly. This decrease in glomerular filtration rate (GFR) after the age of 20 is approximately 6% per 10 years (2). This reduction is not exactly linear, because there is a greater fall in GFR after the fifth and sixth decades (76). However,

TABLE 3. Pharmacokinetic data in the elderly and the young[a]

Drug	Geriatrics			Young			Age and comments
	V_d (liter/kg)	$T_{1/2}$ (hr)	CL	V_d (liter/kg)	$T_{1/2}$ (hr)	CL	
N-acetylprocainamide (NAPA) (51,52)	1.75 (based on mean weight of 72 kg)	8.8	2.46 (ml/min/kg)	1.4 ± 0.2	6 ± 0.2	3.1 ± 0.4 (ml/min/kg)	Mean age 69 years, range 49–80 years; mean CL_{cr} 57.6 ± 5.53 ml/min (range 35–100 ml/min); 4 patients had pacemakers
Acetaminophen (3,5,55)	1.05 ± 0.08	2.1 ± 0.02	379 ± 35 (ml/min/1.73 m²)	1.03 ± 0.08	1.6 ± 0.2	477 ± 36 (ml/min/ 1.73 m²)	Young, 25 years mean; old, 60 years mean; absorbed: young, 98 ± 3%; old, 95 ± 11%
Alprazolam (124)		19.0	0.64 (ml/min/kg)		11.1	1.33 (ml/min/ kg)	
Ampicillin (500 mg i.v.) (53)	0.30 ± 0.04	6.7 ± 5.85	0.08 (liter/hr/kg)	0.29 ± 0.04	1.7 ± 0.54	0.18 (liter/hr/kg)	Young, 22–36 years; old, 67–84 years
Amitriptyline (54)	16.7 ± 0.03	37.3 ± 2.4	0.29 ± 0.05 (liter/kg/hr)				Study involved 6 females, ages 72–83 years, with single 125-mg dose
Antipyrine (5,45,55)	0.58 ± 0.04	12.6 ± 1.40	32.8 ± 3.50 (ml/hr/kg)	0.67 ± 0.03	13.7 ± 1.40	35.8 ± 5.23 (ml/hr/kg)	Represents a capacity-limited binding-insensitive drug; young, 21–37 years; old, 46–68 years
Antipyrine (28)	29.5 ± 8.6 (liters)	12.3 ± 6.2	29.6 ± 9.5 (ml/min)	40 ± 9.1 (liter)	7.65 ± 2	61.9 ± 13.9 (ml/min)	Smoking may alter CL_{cr} in geriatrics
Atenolol (115)	0.75	3.5 (i.v.)	163 (ml/min)	0.55	3.3 hr (i.v.)	203 (ml/min)	Bioavailability for both groups 0.55
Cefoxitin (15 mg/kg i.v.) (56)	0.29	1.3	5.7 (liters/hr)	0.148	0.64		Young, 15–55; CL_{cr} = 75–184; old, 66–94; CL_{cr} = 31.5–174
Cefuroxime (150 mg i.v.) (58,59)	18.9 ± 6.4 (liters)	2.3 ± 1.3	5.7 (liters/hr)	19.1 (liters)	1.4	9.4 (liters/hr)	
Chlordiazepoxide (46)	0.38	40	10 (ml/min)	0.26	7	30 (ml/min)	Age ranges 20–80
Cimetidine (17)	1.37 ± 0.17	2.6 ± 0.2	0.37 ± 0.04 (ml/min/kg)	1.63 ± 0.13	2.0 ± 0.15	0.55 ± 0.04 (ml/min/kg)	Young, 22–57 years; old, 66–84 years
Clobazam (57) Males	1.4	47.7	0.36 (ml/min/kg)	0.87	16.6	0.63 (ml/min/kg)	
Females	1.83	48.6	0.48 (ml/min/kg)	1.37	30.7	0.56 (ml/min/kg)	
Diazepam (5,29) Males	1.8 ± 0.9	98.5 ± 45	0.24 ± 0.1 (ml/min/kg)	1.1 ± 0.4	36 ± 16	0.39 ± 0.1 (ml/min/kg)	Young, 27.5 years mean; old, 68.5 years mean
Females	2.6 ± 1.4	71.8 ± 30	0.48 ± 0.2 (ml/min/kg)	1.7 ± 0.4	42 ± 14	0.51 ± 0.15 (ml/min/kg)	% Unbound: males, 1.34 (young), 1.66 (old); females, 1.23 (young), 1.72 (old)

(continued)

TABLE 3. (continued)

Drug	Geriatrics			Young			Age and comments
	Vd (liter/kg)	$T_{1/2}$ (hr)	CL	Vd (liter/kg)	$T_{1/2}$ (hr)	CL	
Digitoxin (60)	0.62 ± 0.02	8.3 ± 0.8 (days)	0.054 ± 0.006 (liter/kg/day)	0.64 ± 0.03	10.0 ± 0.5 (days)	0.045 ± 0.002 (liter/kg/day)	Young, 25–30 years; old, 69–79 years; 5 females + 1 male in each age group; based on single i.v. injection
Digoxin (18,23)[b]	4.1 ± 0.9	69.6 ± 13	0.8 ± 0.2 (ml/min/kg)	5.3 ± 0.6	36.8 ± 4.5	1.7 ± 0.2 (ml/min/kg)	% Absorbed: young, 84 ± 6%; old, 76 ± 10%; young, 34–61 years; old, 72–91 years
Indocyanine green (45)	41.1 ± 5.3	4.7 ± 0.57 (min)	6.1 ± 0.6 (ml/min/kg)	41.6 ± 6.4	3.1 ± 0.3 (min)	7.1 ± 1.2 (ml/min/kg)	Representing a drug whose clearance is dependent on hepatic blood flow
Isoniazid (37) Fast acetylators	0.39 ± 0.2	1.3 ± 0.65	8.36 ± 3.6 (ml/min/kg)	0.34 ± 0.2	1.1 ± 0.1	7.4 ± 2 (ml/min/kg)	Young, 39 ± 13 years; old, 80 ± 10 years
Slow acetylators	0.59 ± 0.3	3.1 ± 0.5	3.63 ± 1.8 (ml/min/kg)	0.37 ± 0.5	3.1 ± 1	3.7 ± 1 (ml/min/kg)	
Lidocaine (61)	0.85 ± 0.17	2.1 ± 0.14	5.0 ± 1.2 (ml/min/kg)	0.7 ± 0.2	1.5 ± 0.18	5.3 ± 1.5 (ml/min/kg)	% Bound: young, 48 ± 5.4%; old, 69.5 ± 4.8%; % absorbed (p.o.): young, 13 ± 2%; old, 27 ± 5.5%; young, 24–34 years; old, 73–87 years
Lorazepam (20)	0.99 ± 0.03	13.13	0.78 (ml/min/kg)	1.11 ± 0.03	14.14	0.96 (ml/min/kg)	Intramuscular absorption = 88%, p.o. = 98%; young, 27 years mean; old, 69 years mean
Midazolam (119)	2.46 ± 0.63	4.3	0.43 ± 0.16 (liter/hr/kg)	1.71 ± 0.3	2.77	0.45 ± 0.11 (liter/hr/kg)	
Morphine (62)	4.7 ± 0.2	4.4 ± 0.25	12.4 ± 1.2 (ml/min/kg)	3.2 ± 0.3	2.95 ± 0.5	14.7 ± 0.9 (ml/min/kg)	Four geriatric patients, all had some degree of cardiac disease; young, 28 years mean; old, 66 years mean
Netilmicin (63) (1 mg/kg) (2 mg/kg)	0.25 ± 0.07 0.22 ± 0.03	5 ± 2.6 6.2 ± 2.3	54 ± 27 (ml/min) 34 ± 15 (ml/min)	0.2 ± 0.02 0.16 ± 0.03	2.3 ± 0.7 2.1 ± 0.5	64 ± 14 (ml/min) 77 ± 32 (ml/min)	Geriatrics had CL_{cr} = 50–100 ml/min; Young group CL_{cr} = 100–130 ml/min; young, 48–58 years; old, 61–83 years
Nitrazepam (64)	4.8 ± 1.7	40.4 ± 16.2	4.7 ± 1.5 (liter/hr)	2.4 ± 0.8	28.9 ± 7.4	4.1 ± 2 (liter/hr)	Young, 18–38 years; old, 66–89 years

							Comments
Nortriptyline (65-67)	61 (liters)	45 hr (23.5-79)	18.8 (liter/hr) (8.3-38.4)	48 (liters)	26.8	54 ± 24 (liter/hr)	Single-dose determinations; geriatric group had a number of diseases; young, 22-38 years; old, 69-100 years; no mention of AGP binding; no mention of hepatic or renal function
Oxazepam (68)		5.6	136 (ml/min)		5.1	114 (ml/min)	Mostly males; young, 14-30 years; old, 45-84 years
Pancuronium (69)	0.32 ± 0.1	3.5 ± 1.1	1.1 ± 0.4 (ml/min/kg)	0.28 ± 0.06	1.7 ± 0.4	1.9 ± 0.4 (ml/min/kg)	Young, 25-55 years; old, 75-86 years
Phenylbutazone (5,6)	0.1 ± 0.02	87 ± 11	2.75 (ml/min/kg)	0.16 ± 0.02	110 ± 13	2.9 (ml/min/kg)	Young, 26 years mean; old, 81 years
Phenytoin (28,104)	44.4 ± 18.1 (liters)	10.6 ± 3.65	50.5 ± 36.9 (ml/min)	40.9 ± 8.5 (liters)	11.96 ± 3.65	48.4 ± 16.6 (ml/min)	In elderly (62-87), percent unbound 12.8 ± 1.8%; in young (18-33), percent unbound 11.1 ± 2.5%
Prazepam (70)[c]	2.56	128 (males) 75 (females)	0.36 (ml/min/kg)	1.6	62 (males) 84 (females)	0.37 (ml/min/kg)	Young, 22-42 years; old, 62-85 years
Prazosin (71)	0.89 ± 0.26	3.2 ± 0.6	3.53 ± 1.0 (ml/min/kg)	0.63 ± 0.14	2.05 ± 0.3	3.94 ± 0.73 (ml/min/kg)	
Propranolol (42)	4.2 ± 0.5	5.6 ± 0.6	9.0 ± 0.9 (ml/min/kg)	3.8 ± 0.3	4.5 ± 0.4	10.6 ± 1.3 (ml/min/kg)	Representing a drug whose clearance is relatively insensitive, but both flow- and capacity-limited; young, 21-37 years; old, 46-73 years
Salicylate (72)		3.7 ± 0.4	1.7 ± 0.2 (ml/hr)		2.4 ± 0.11	1.61 ± 0.09 (ml/hr)	Only males studied; used 1-g dose
Temazepam (108) Males	1.32 (0.9-2)	11.9 (8.3-14.2)	1.35 (0.7-2.5)	1.53 (0.7-2.8)	12.8 (9.4-23.3)	1.36 (0.8-1.7)	Clearance expressed in ml/min/kg
Females	1.39 (0.7-2.3)	17.2 (8.9-37.9)	0.97 (0.7-1.5)	1.4 (1.2-1.8)	16.2 (10.1-25.3)	1.10 (0.6-1.5)	
Theophylline (9,43,73)							Young, 21-30 years; old 67-81 years
Smokers	0.36 ± 0.15	5.9 ± 0.8	0.71 ± 0.06 (liter/kg/hr)	0.30 ± 0.06	5.9 ± 0.3	0.72 ± 0.06 (liter/hr/kg)	Young < 50; old > 50, smoked 15-23 cigarettes/day
Non-smokers	0.36 ± 0.06	8 ± 0.5	0.5 ± 0.2 (liter/kg/hr)	0.30 ± 0.03	7.6 ± 0.6	0.46 ± 0.05 (liter/kg/hr)	Young, 20-39 years; old, 60-79 years; all patients had $CL_{cr} \geq 85$ ml/min
Tobramycin (102)	0.25 ± 0.04	2.4 ± 0.5	1.25 ± 0.4 (ml/min/kg)	0.25 ± 0.04	2.3 ± 0.5	1.34 ± 0.48	
Warfarin (74,75)	0.2 ± 0.01	44 ± 9.9	3.26 ± 0.5 (ml/min/kg)	0.19 ± 0.26	37 ± 2	3.8 ± 0.55 (ml/min/kg)	Young, 20-40 years; old, 65-94 years

[a] Mean ± SD, except where noted.
[b] Tsujimoto et al. (125) provides a recent comparison of proposed digoxin nomograms.
[c] Measured as desmethyldiazepam.

a general formula can be applied to represent GFR with aging; it depicts the decrease in GFR in the creatinine clearance formulas provided in Chapter 8. On the average, there is a decrease of 0.5 to 1.0 ml/min/1.73 m² (Fig. 7) "beginning" after the age of 25 to 30. In other words, there is a drop from 120 to 60 ml/min/1.73 m² as one ages from 20 to 90 (6,9).

Once filtered, a drug may be reabsorbed back into the plasma across the renal tubules (depending on such variables as lipid solubility, pH, concentration gradient, and molecular size) (1). As one ages, there are decreases in both the cell mass and the numbers of tubules. The former is reflected in the following table:

Age	Proximal tubule length	Proximal volume	Glomerular surface
20–39 years	19.36 mm	0.076 mm³	0.254 mm²
60–69 years	17.38 mm	0.067 mm³	0.222 mm²
80–101 years	12.50 mm	0.052 mm³	0.155 mm²

When the glomerular filtrate enters the proximal tubule, there is neither a pH gradient nor a concentration gradient with respect to plasma. However, as urine progresses through the renal tubules, water is reabsorbed, and the pH changes, initiating both a concentration gradient and a pH gradient. As one ages, there is a decrease in the capacity to concentrate this water. As a result, the mean maximum urine specific gravity decreases from 1.030 to 1.021 (2,3,76). There is also a reduction in the ability to conserve sodium and reabsorb phosphate with aging (76). The pH gradient, which is usually in the direction of acidity, is hampered with aging (46). This decrease in the ability to acidify the urine could affect the rate and extent of reabsorption of drugs that are weakly acidic (i.e., pK_a 3–7.5) or basic (i.e., pK_a 7.5–10) (1) (see Chapter 8).

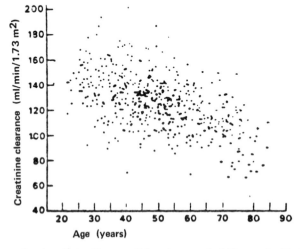

FIG. 7. Cross-sectional analysis of true creatinine clearance in 548 normal subjects ($r = -0.54$, slope $= -0.80$ and intercept at age zero $= 165.6$). These values are equivalent to values by the automated total chromogen method when multiplied by 0.80. (From Vestal, ref. 3, with permission.)

Tubular secretion plays a major role in the excretion of many drugs. The transport mechanisms that are responsible for organic acids or bases involve active transport processes that are carrier-mediated and are not affected by protein binding (e.g., methotrexate, choline, procainamide, chlorothiazide) (1). Once transported into the kidney, the drug will respond according to the principles described in Chapters 8 and 9.

In the geriatric patient who has had a nephrectomy, the ability to compensate is blunted, whereas in youth, the maturing residual kidney will demonstrate a 60% to 80% increase in function. The aging single kidney can compensate only to a maximim increase of 30% (2). The greatest increase in size and function in the remaining kidney occurs within the first week, with slower increases occurring within the month. Only relatively minor increases occur thereafter.

In geriatric patients receiving drugs, reduced renal function will assume greater importance. Drugs metabolized to active compounds that might accumulate due to impaired renal excretion in the elderly include methyldopa, oxyphenbutazone, triamterene, spironolactone, levodopa, acetohexamide, acetylated sulfonamides and oxypurinal. Chapter 9 provides a more detailed listing of drugs with active metabolites excreted by the kidney. However, at this time, there is little information available on the renal excretion of these drug metabolites in the elderly.

PHARMACOLOGIC RESPONSE

Clinical experience has often shown the elderly to be more responsive to drugs than younger adults. There are two possible explanations for this increased response. First, the target cell or organ could have an increase in sensitivity, resulting in an increased response with a given drug concentration (pharmacodynamics). Second, and the most common, is that the amount of drug within the body is modified (pharmacokinetic changes) (19). This modification may be due to the redistribution (as compared with the younger population) of drug or the size or weight changes of specific organs. For example, from 20 to 80 years of age, the brain decreases 20% in weight. With this weight reduction there is a gradual loss of neurons from the cerebral cortex, accumulation of lipofuscin pigments, a decline in cerebral blood flow that is aggravated by atherosclerosis, a change in catecholamine ratio, and endocrine changes possibly affecting the central nervous system (CNS). Reichlmier et al. (77) demonstrated age-dependent changes in human brain enzyme activity. His study evaluated the influence of aging on 14 glycolytic enzymes and some enzymes related to neurotransmitter function from the frontal cortex and putamen homogenates. The activities of five enzymes decreased (fructose-6-phosphate kinase, phosphoglycerate mutase, carbonic anhydrase, acetylcholinesterase, protein kinase), whereas hexokinase activity increased (77). Because biological responses usually are a direct function of tissue concentrations to these hormone receptors, sensitivity to many such substrate drugs has been shown to decrease with age. Specifically, responsiveness to the beta-adrenoceptor agonist isoproterenol has been shown to decrease in old age (111). This has been reported by Dillon et al. (78)

and others using lymphocytes as an index of beta-adrenoceptor responsiveness. However, recently an investigation by Abrass et al. (79) has shown that beta-adrenoceptors on human lymphocytes are unaltered in the elderly. It has also been demonstrated in rats that the characteristics of the blood-brain barrier are altered, allowing more drug to enter the brain (19). The role of age in the sensitivity of adrenergic, serotonin, acetylcholine, and histamine receptors is still unclear. Thus, in the elderly, the increased response to drugs acting within the CNS is a combination of organ weight losses, pharmacodynamics, and pharmacokinetic changes. These interrelated factors and the relationship that exists among them can be described mathematically:

$$\text{Effect} \propto fC_T \propto C_P \propto \frac{(FD)(T_{1/2})}{(V_{ss})(\tau)}$$

where f is sensitivity, C_T is the concentration at the site of action, C_p is plasma concentration, FD is bioavailability, $T_{1/2}$ is metabolism, V_{ss} is distribution, and τ is dosing interval. This relationship attempts to describe the pharmacokinetic parameters (absorption, distribution, metabolism, and excretion) and the observed response at any given time within the usual linear range.

In certain cases the response is considered proportional to the plasma concentration and the level of drug at its site of action (e.g., anticonvulsants, certain cardiac and antidepressant drugs) and the sensitivity of the target tissue. Because it is not practical at this time to sample tissue drug concentrations, one uses the closest and most easily accessible tissue (blood, plasma, or saliva), making the assumption that drug levels at the sampling site reflect tissue drug concentrations (19,80,81). Our knowledge of pharmacokinetics of drugs in the elderly is, at present, rudimentary. However, one can quickly see that associated changes in binding (decreased albumin and RBC binding, increased concentrations of AGP), bioavailability (the rate and extent of absorption), and distribution (increased fat content, decreased total body water, decreased organ function, arteriosclerosis and atherosclerosis) in old age could easily alter the concentration of drug at the site of action, and ultimately, the response. This would especially be true if doses were based on weights extrapolated from the average 70-kg, 30- to 50-year-old individual.

Clinicians have noticed (and studies have verified) that their geriatric patients are generally more sensitive to the effects of various drugs. Such alterations in pharmacologic reponses are usually due to age-related changes in drug disposition and elimination. In 1977, Castleden et al. reported increased sensitivity to nitrazepam in the elderly after a 10-mg nightly dose (64). It was demonstrated that in 36 partly immobilized geriatric patients (66–94 years) and 41 young healthy volunteers (18–38 years) given 5 mg of nitrazepam daily that the geriatric group had a larger volume of distribution at steady state. They concluded that in aged subjects there is a greater amount of the administered dose within the tissue compartment, and presumably at the receptor sites in the CNS (64). This increased incidence of nitrazepam toxicity could be due to the increased volume of distribution and slower

CNS elimination. Triggs and Nation (6) reviewed a number of studies involving meperidine (pethidine) in older age groups. They found a direct correlation between the age of the patient and the fraction of unbound drug in the plasma ($p < 0.001$). One of the studies concluded that unless this increase in unbound meperidine is buffered by erythrocytes, which would seem likely in the elderly (decreased RBC buffering capacity with increasing age), the increase in absolute free drug concentration would account for the increased sensitivity to meperidine's respiratory depressant effects (6). Husted and Andersen (74) and Shepard et al. (75) examined the response and sensitivity, respectively, of anticoagulants in the aged. The average individual daily doses for phenprocoumon, bishydroxycoumarin, and warfarin decreased significantly with advancing age. There was a significant correlation between the maintenance dosage of phenprocoumon and the albumin concentration in the aged. Only with bishyroxycoumarin was there a correlation between the daily maintenance dose and weight of the patient (74). Warfarin, one of the most studied anticoagulants, did not show any major age-related differences in the measured pharmacokinetic parameters (75). The possibilities for the increased response in the elderly to anticoagulants include a decreased affinity of the system for vitamin K_1, an increased affinity for anticoagulants, a dietary deficiency of vitamin K, a significantly lower level of vitamin-K-dependent clotting factor ($p < 0.001$), defective absorption or alterations in the pharmacokinetics of vitamin K, altered affinity for the receptor site in the liver, and, in a select group of acute myocardial infarction patients, an increase in the degradation rate of coagulation factors (74,75). The three examples (nitrazepam, meperidine, warfarin) show that we are beginning to understand why the elderly respond to certain drugs differently. In most cases these changes in response are a result of pharmacokinetic alterations with age, but as with the anticoagulants or beta blockers, there are still some unresolved reasons for the changes in response. Table 4 is a summary of responses to commonly used drugs in the geriatric population. Of those changes in response, only those of anticoagulants, beta blockers, and possibly alpha agonists (118), are not explainable by pharmacokinetic changes.

CONCLUSION

The effects of age on drug disposition depend on the particular compound in question and the characteristics of the population being studied. When evaluating geriatric studies, it is important to differentiate between those who are long-term-care patients not considered healthy or active and those who are old (>65 years) but living in the community and in some cases working independently in the community (7). It is important to remember that the changes in the pharmacokinetic parameters in the elderly can reflect the immobility of the patients, their numbers or types of diseases, and/or their number of medications, rather than an actual change due to aging alone. Because of the changes in body composition between males and females (with aging), it is important to differentiate these groups when evaluating data. If the half-life of a drug is thought to increase, the time to reach

TABLE 4. Summary of response changes in the geriatric population for commonly used drugs and the mechanisms involved[a]

Drug or class	Response	Pharmacokinetic mechanism & comments
Acetaminophen (3,5,82–84)	↔ ↑	↔ Bioavailability (oral 0.95 ± 0.11); ↔ ↑ $T_{1/2}$ (2.1 hr); ↔ ↑ Vd (0.99 liter/kg males, 0.86 liter/kg females); ↓ CL (0.335 liter/kg/hr);
ACTH (3)	↓ →	↓ Sensitivity of adrenal gland
Antihypertensives (31,83)	↑	Propensity to orthostatic hypotension, impaired baroreceptor
Anticoagulants (3,74,75,100)	↑	Warfarin ↔ PPB (98.5 ± 0.1%); ↔ V_{ss} (200 ± 12 ml/kg); ↔ CL (3.26 ± 0.49 ml/hr/kg); ↔ $T_{1/2}$ (44 ± 3.9 hr); ↓ binding baroreceptors; ↓ dietary vitamin K; phenprocoumon ↑ free drug with aging
Amitriptyline (3,31,54)	↑ ↑	↔ ↑ $T_{1/2}$; ↓ CL; ↑ bioavailability; ↓ Vd
Atenolol (116)	NR	↔ Effective renal blood flow, ↔ glomerular filtration rate ↔ renal vascular conductance
Barbiturates (3)	↑	↑ Sensitivity; increase in paradoxical responses
Carbenoxolone (85)	↔ ↑	↑ $T_{1/2}$ (22.9 hr); ↔ PPB; ↓ CL (3.3 ml/hr/kg)
Chlordiazepoxide (46,83)	↔ ↑	↑ $T_{1/2}$ (40 hr); ↓ CL (10 ml/min); ↑ Vd (0.38 liter/kg)
Clomipramine (86)	NR	PPB N.R.; Cp_{ss} with equivalent dose given to younger group
Desipramine (31,128)	↑ ↑	↔ ↑ $T_{1/2}$ (76 hr); ↓ CL; ↑ C_{ss}; studies as a metabolite of imipramine, ↑ metabolite formation
Digoxin (3,23,83,87)	↔ ↑	↑ $T_{1/2}$ (69.6 ± 13); ↓ CL (0.8 ± 0.2 ml/min/kg); ↔ ↓ Vd (4.1 ± 0.9 liter/kg); ↓ rate of absorption; often used with diuretics and low serum potassium; oral maintenance dose is 1.4 times higher than those of metildigoxin; this is not different from the ratio in younger age groups
Diazepam (3,29,49,88,107,113)	↑	↔ ↑ $T_{1/2}$ (72 hr females, 98.5 hr males); ↔ ↑ V_{ss} (males 1.83 liter/kg, females 2.64 liter/kg); ↔ ↓ CL (males 0.24, females 0.48 ml/min/kg)
Chlormethiazole (3,19)	↑ ↔	↓ (Vd, CL, PPB, RBC binding); ↑ $T_{1/2}$
Chlorpropamide (3,15)	↔ →	Impairment of endogenous insulin release
Cimetidine (17,89,101)	NR	↑ Cp_{max}; ↔ ↑ $T_{1/2}$ (156 ± 12.8 min); ↑ AUC_0^∞ ↓ Vd (1.37 ± 0.17 liter/kg); ↓ CL (0.37 ± 0.04 liter/hr/kg)
Clobazam (57,126)	NR	↑ $T_{1/2}$ in males (62.3 hr); ↓ CL in males (0.32 ml/min/kg).
Ethanol (39)	↑	↔ $T_{1/2B}$; ↑ Cp_{max}; ↓ Vd_{ss} (0.6 ± 0.07 liter/kg-LBM); ↔ V_{max} (76.4 mg/kg/hr ± 2.55); ↔ CL
Flunitrazepam (90)	↑	↔ $T_{1/2B}$; ↔ CL (total); ↔ V_{ss} (increased in elderly with serious disease only)
Flurazepam (3,83)	↑	↑ $T_{1/2}$; ↔ CL (total); ↔ V_{ss} (in elderly with serious disease only)
Imipramine (3,31)	↑	↑ $T_{1/2}$; ↑ C_{ss}
L-DOPA (3,13,14,83)	↔ ↑	↑ AUC_0^∞ ↔ $T_{1/2}$ (66 ± 11.1 min); ↑ Cp_{max}
Lidocaine (12,50,61)	NR	↑ $T_{1/2}$ (2.1 ± 0.14 hr); ↑ C_{ssi}; ↔ ↑ Vd (0.85 ± 0.17 liter/kg); oral bioavailability (26.6 ± 5.6%)
Lithium (91)	NR	↑ $T_{1/2}$

Drug (references)		Effects
Lorazepam (3,20)	↔↑	↓ Vd (0.99 liter/kg); ↔↑ $T_{1/2}$ (15.9 hr); ↔↓ CL (0.77 ml/min/kg)
Lorcainide (112)	↔↓↑	↓ $T_{1/2}$ (7.7 hr); ↑ Vd (7.8 liter/kg); ↔↓ CL
Morphine (3,62,92,100)	↑	↑ Vd (4.7 ± 0.2 liter/kg); ↔↑ $T_{1/2}$ (4.5 ± 0.3 hr); ↓ CL (12.4 ± 1.2 ml/min/kg); progressive age-related pain relief, duration of pain relief
Metoprolol (93,94,100)	↔↓	↔ $T_{1/2}$ ↔↓ CL; ↔ AUC (↑ if metabolites are involved)
Nadolol (116)	NR	↓ Effective renal blood flow, ↔ glomerular filtration rate; ↔ renal vascular conductance
Oxazepam (15)	↔↓	↔ Increased plasma nortriptyline concentrations ($p < 0.001$); ↔↑ $T_{1/2}$; ↔↑ CL; ↑ Vd
Nitrazepam (64,65,95,114)	↑	↔ $T_{1/2}$ (40.4 ± 16.2 hr); ↑ Vd (4.8 ± 1.7 liter/kg)
Nortriptyline (96)	↔↑	↔↑ $T_{1/2}$ (23–79 hr); ↔↓ CL (8–38.5 liter/hr)
Pancuronium (110)	↓↑	↓ $T_{1/2}$ (201 min)
Pethidine (3,83)	↓↑	↓ Albumin binding; ↑ $T_{1/2}$; ↔ CL; ↑ Vd_{ss}
Phenytoin (3,5,28,83,97,105)	↔↑	↓ V_{max} (6.0 ± 1.9 mg/day/kg); ↔ K_m (5.4–5.8 µg/ml); V_{ss} (44 ± 18 liters); albumin binding;
Pindolol (127)	NR	↑ T_{max} (2.3 ± 0.4); ↓ ke (0.257 ± 0.039); ↔ Cp_{max}
Propranolol (111)	↓ ↓	Response also demonstrated for isoproterenol
Quinidine (3,83)	↔↓↑	↓ CL related to renal function; ↑ in cardiac abnormalities
Ranitidine (117)	NR	↑ $T_{1/2}$ (243 ± 7 min); ↔ V (142 ± 29 liter); ↓ CL (322 ± 31, ml/min); ± 45 bioavailability
Salicylates (72,106)	NR	↑ $T_{1/2}$ (3.7 hr); ↔ CL (1.7 ± 0.2 ml/hr); ↑ gentisic to salicylic acid ratio over age 60 (renal data not given)
Sulfamethiazole (85)	↔↓	↑ $T_{1/2}$ (3 hr); ↓ CL (90 ml/min/1.73 m²)
Tolbutamide (3,15)	↔↓	Cp_{max}, impairment of endogenous insulin release with aging
Theophylline (3,43,103)	↔↓	↔↑ $T_{1/2}$ (8.0 ± 0.5 hr); ↔↓ CL (0.51 ± 0.20 ml/min/kg)
Thiopental (109)	↑	70% of dose required when compared with younger groups; ↑ $T_{1/2}$; ↑ Vd; ↓ CL (50%)
Triazolam (124)	NR	↑ $T_{1/2}$ (4 hr); ↓ CL (3.66 ml/min/kg)
Phenylbutazone (3,5)	NR	↑ $T_{1/2}$ (104.6 hr); ↔ Vd (9.2 liter/kg); ↓ CL (0.065 liter/hr)
Procainamide (98)	↑	↑ Serum drug concentrations; ↓ renal tubular secretion
Zimelidine (99)	NR	↑ $T_{1/2}$ (10.1 ± 2.6 hr); metabolite (norzimelidine $T_{1/2}$ 35.5 ± 10.9 hr); ↑ AUC; ↓ PPB

[a] Data in parentheses are actual values for elderly.

Symbols: ↑ increased; ↓ decreased; ↔ no difference; ↔↓ possible decrease or no change; ↔↑ possible increase or no change; CL, clearance; V_{ss}, volume of distribution at steady state; $T_{1/2}$, half-life in terminal phase; PPB, plasma protein binding; parentheses indicate value of kinetic parameter in the elderly; NR, not reported or suggested; AUC_0^∞, area under the plasma concentration curve from zero to infinite time; RBC, red blood cell; Cp_{max}, Serum or plasma drug maximum as reported at steady state; LBM, lean body mass; V_{max}, maximum rate of metabolism by an enzymatically mediated reaction; K_m, Michaelis-Menten constant.

a steady state drug concentration will be longer; thus, the timing of blood sampling for drug concentrations must take this into consideration. It is the active and objectively disease-free geriatric patient who would be appropriate for investigation involving the effects of age on pharmacokinetic parameters (8).

REFERENCES

1. Kenny, A. D. (1979): Designing therapy for the elderly. *Drug Ther.*, July:49–64.
2. Rossman, I. (1979): *Clinical Geriatrics*, 2nd Ed., pp. 23–52, 132–137, 224–229. J. B. Lippincott, Philadelphia.
3. Vestal, R. E. (1978): Drug use in the elderly. A review of problems and special considerations. *Drugs*, 16:358–382.
4. Ouslander, J. G. (1981): Drug therapy in the elderly. *Ann. Intern. Med.*, 95:711–722.
5. Crooks, J., O'Malley, K., and Stevenson, I. H. (1976): Pharmacokinetics in the elderly. *Clin. Pharmacokinet.*, 1:280–296.
6. Triggs, E. J., and Nation, R. L. (1975): Pharmacokinetics in the aged: A review. *J. Pharmacokinet. Biopharm.*, 3:387–417.
7. Hurwitz, N. (1969): Predisposing factors in adverse reactions to drugs. *Br. Med. J.*, 1:536–539.
8. Schneider, R. E., Bishop, H., Yates, R. A., Auarterman, C. P., and Kendal, M. J. (1980): Effects of age on plasma propranolol levels. *Br. J. Clin. Pharmacol.*, 10:169–170.
9. Schumacher, G. E. (1980): Pharmacokinetic factors influencing drug therapy in the aged. *Am. J. Hosp. Pharm.*, 37:559–562.
10. Castleden, C. M., Volans, C. N., and Raymond, K. (1977): The effect of aging on drug absorption from the gut. *Age Ageing*, 6:138–142.
11. Ritschel, W. A. (1976): Pharmacokinetic approach to drug dosing in the aged. *J. Am. Geriatr. Soc.*, 24:344–354.
12. Holloway, D. A. (1974): Drug problems in the geriatric patient. *Drug Intell. Clin. Pharm.*, 8:632–642.
13. Evans, M. A., Triggs, E. J., Broe, G. A., and Saines, N. (1980): Systemic availability of orally administered L-dopa in the elderly parkinsonian patient. *Eur. J. Clin. Pharmacol.*, 17:215–221.
14. Evans, M. A., Broe, G. A., Triggs, E. J., Cheung, M., Creasy, H., and Paull, P. D. (1981): Gastric emptying rate and the systemic availability of levodopa in the elderly parkinsonian patient. *Neurology (Minneap.)*, 31:1288–1294.
15. Sartor, G., Melander, A., Schersten, G., and Wahlin, B. E. (1980): Influence of food and age on the single-dose kinetics and effects of tolbutamide and chlorpropamide. *Eur. J. Clin. Pharmacol.*, 17:285–293.
16. Kendal, M. J., Brown, D., and Yates, R. A. (1977): Plasma metoprolol concentrations in young, old, and hypertensive patients. *Br. J. Clin. Pharmacol.*, 4:497–499.
17. Redolfi, A., Borgogelli, E., and Lodola, E. (1979): Blood level of cimetidine in relation to age. *Eur. J. Clin. Pharmacol.*, 15:257–261.
18. Cusack, B., Horgan, J., Kelly, J. G., Lowan, J., Noel, J., and O'Malley, K. (1978): Pharmacokinetics of digoxin in the elderly. *Br. J. Clin. Pharmacol.*, 6:439–440.
19. Witts, D. J., Bowkay, A. A., Garland, M., McLean, A. E. M., and Exton-Smith, A. (1979): Studies in the elderly: Pharmacokinetic aspects. *Age Ageing*, 8:271–281.
20. Greenblatt, D. J., Allen, M. C., Locniskar, A., Harmatz, J. S., and Shader, R. I. (1979): Lorazepam kinetics in the elderly. *Clin. Pharmacol. Ther.*, 26:103–113.
21. Wilkinson, G. R. (1978): Effects of aging and liver disease on disposition of lorazepam. *Clin. Pharmacol. Ther.*, 24:411–419.
22. Shull, H. J., Wilkinson, G. R., Johnson, R., and Schenker, S. (1976): Normal disposition of oxazepam in acute viral hepatitis and cirrhosis. *Ann. Intern. Med.*, 84:420–425.
23. Cusack, B., Kelly, J., and O'Malley, K. (1979): Digoxin in the elderly: Pharmacokinetic consequences of old age. *Clin. Pharmacol. Ther.*, 25:772–776.
24. Wallace, S., and Whiting, B. (1976): Factors affecting drug binding in plasma of elderly patients. *Br. J. Clin. Pharmacol.*, 3:327–330.
25. Greenblatt, D. J. (1979): Reduced serum albumin concentration in the elderly: A report from the Boston Collaborative Drug Surveillance Program. *J. Am. Ger. Soc.*, 28:20–22.

26. Keating, F. R., Jones, J. D., and Elveback, L. R. (1969): The relation of age and sex to distribution of values in healthy adults of serum calcium, inorganic phosphorus, magnesium, alkaline phosphatase, total protein, albumin, and blood urea. *J. Lab. Clin. Med.*, 73:825–834.

27. Hodkinson, H. (1977): *Biochemical Diagnosis of the Elderly*, pp. 234–268. Wiley, New York.

28. Bach, B., Hansen, J. M., Kampmann, J. P., Rasmussen, S. N., and Skovsted, L. (1981): Disposition of antipyrine and phenytoin correlated with age and liver volume in man. *Clin. Pharmacokinet.*, 6:389–396.

29. Greenblatt, D. J., Allen, M. D., Hartmatz, J. S., and Shader, R. I. (1980): Diazepam disposition determinants. *Clin. Pharmacol. Ther.*, 27:301–311.

30. Hayes, M. J., Langman, M. J. S., and Short, A. H. (1975): Changes in drug metabolism with increasing age: Phenytoin clearance and protein binding. *Br. J. Clin. Pharmacol.*, 2:73–79.

31. Braithwaite, R. A., Heard, R., and Snape, A. (1978): Plasma protein binding of maprotiline in geriatric patients—influence of α_1-acid-glycoprotein. *Br. J. Clin. Pharmacol.*, 6:448–449.

32. Norman, T. R., Burrows, G. D., Scoggins, B. A., and Davies, B. (1979): Pharmacokinetic and plasma levels of antidepressants in the elderly. *Med. J. Aust.*, 1:273–274.

33. Urthaler, F., Walker, A. A., and James, T. N. (1978): The effect of aging on ventricular contractile performance. *Am. Heart J.*, 6:381–483.

34. Sato, I., Hasegawa, Y., Tahahashi, N., Hiruta, Y., Shimoiaura, K., and Hotta, K. (1981): Age related changes in cardiac control function in man. *J. Gerontol.*, 36:564–572.

35. Farah, F., Taylor, W., Rawlins, M. D., and James, D. (1977): Hepatic drug acetylation and oxidation: Effects of aging in man. *Br. Med. J.*, 2:155–156.

36. Vestal, R. E., Norris, P. K., Tobin, J. D., Cohen, B. H., Shock, N. W., and Andres, R. (1975): Antipyrine metabolism in man: Influence of age, alcohol, caffeine and smoking. *Clin. Pharmacol. Ther.*, 18:425–432.

37. Advenier, C., Saint-Aubin, A., Gobert, C., Houin, G., Albengres, E., and Tillement, J. R. (1980): Pharmacokinetics of isoniazid in the elderly. *Br. J. Clin. Pharmacol.*, 10:167–168.

38. Reynolds, C. N., Wilson, K., and Burnett, D. (1978): Metabolism of methaqualone in geriatric patients. *Eur. J. Clin. Pharmacol.*, 13:285–289.

39. Vestal, R. E., McGuire, E. A., Tobin, J. D., Andres, R., Norris, A., and Mezey, E. (1977): Aging and ethanol metabolism. *Clin. Pharmacol. Ther.*, 21:343–354.

40. Anon (1978): Drugs in the elderly. *Br. Med. J.*, 1:1168.

41. Smithhard, D. J., and Langman, M. J. S. (1977): Drug metabolism in the elderly. *Br. Med. J.*, 2:520–521.

42. Salem, S. A. M., Rajgayabun, P., Shepard, A. M. M., and Stevenson, L. H. (1978): Reduced induction of drug metabolism in the elderly. *Age Ageing*, 7:68–73.

43. Cusack, B., Kelly, J. G., Lavan, J., Noel, J., and O'Malley, K. (1980): Theophylline kinetics in relation to age: The importance of smoking. *Br. J. Clin. Pharmacol.*, 10:109–114.

44. Pfeifer, H. J., and Greenblatt, D. J. (1978): Clinical toxicity of theophylline in relation to cigarette smoking. *Chest*, 73:455–459.

45. Vestal, R. E., and Wood, A. J. J. (1980): Influence of age and smoking on drug kinetics in man. *Clin. Pharmacokinet.*, 5:309–319.

46. Roberts, R. K., Wilkinson, G. P., Branch, R. A., and Schender, S. (1978): Effect of age and parenchymal liver disease on the disposition and elimination of chlordiazepoxide. *Gastroenterology*, 75:479–485.

47. Shanor, S. P., Van Hees, G. R., Baart, N., Erdos, E. G., and Foldes, F. F. (1961): The influence of age and sex on human plasma and red cell cholinesterase. *Am. J. Med. Sci.*, 242:357–361.

48. Whiting, B., and Lawrence, J. R. (1979): Digoxin in pharmacokinetics in the elderly. In: *Drugs and the Elderly*, edited by J. Crooks and I. H. Stevenson, pp. 89–101. University Park Press, Baltimore.

49. Klotz, U., Avant, G. R., and Hayumpa, A. (1975): The effects of age and liver disease on the disposition and elimination of diazepam in adult man. *J. Clin. Invest.*, 55:347–359.

50. Nation, R. L., and Triggs, E. J. (1977): Lignocaine kinetics in cardiac patients and aged subjects. *Br. J. Clin. Pharmacol.*, 4:439–448.

51. Galeazzi, R. L., Omar-Amberg, C., and Karlaganis, G. (1981): *N*-acetyl-procainamide kinetics in the elderly. *Clin. Pharmacol. Ther.*, 29:440–446.

52. Benet, L. Z., and Sheiner, L. B. (1980): Design and optimization of dosage regimens; pharmacokinetic data. In: *The Pharmacological Basis of Therapeutics*, 6th Ed., edited by A. G. Gilman, L. S. Goodman, and A. Gilman, p. 1686. Macmillan, New York.

53. Triggs, E. J., Johnson, J. M., and Learoyd, B. (1980): Absorption and disposition of ampicillin in elderly. *Eur. J. Clin. Pharmacol.*, 18:195–198.
54. Henry, J. F., Altamura, C., Gomerri, R., Hervy, M. P., Forette, F., and Morselli, P. L. (1981): Pharmacokinetics of amitriptyline in the elderly. *Int. J. Clin. Pharmacol.*, 19:1–5.
55. Mucklow, J. C., and Fraser, H. S. (1980): The effects of age and smoking upon antibyrine metabolism. *Br. J. Clin. Pharmacol.*, 9:613–614.
56. Garcia, M. J., Garcia, A., Nieto, M. J., Dominguez-Gil, A., Alonso, G., and Mellado, L. (1980): Disposition of cefoxitin in the elderly. *Int. J. Clin. Pharmacol.*, 18:503–509.
57. Greenblatt, D. J., Divoll, M., Puri, S. K., Ho, I., Zinny, M. A., and Shader, R. I. (1981): Clobazam kinetics in the elderly. *Br. J. Clin. Pharmacol.*, 12:631–636.
58. Douglas, J. G., Box, R. P., and Munro, J. F. (1980): The pharmacokinetics of cefuroxime in the elderly. *J. Antimicrob. Chemother.*, 6:543–549.
59. Broekhuysen, J., Deger, F., Douchamps, J., Freschi, E., Mal, N., Neve, P. Parfait, R., Siska, G., and Winand, M. (1981): Pharmacokinetic study of cefuroxime in the elderly. *Br. J. Clin. Pharmacol.*, 12:801–805.
60. Donovan, M. A., Castleden, C. M., Pohl, J. E. F., and Kraft, C. A. (1981): The effect of age on digitoxin pharmacokinetics. *Br. J. Clin. Pharmacol.*, 2:401–402.
61. Cusack, B., Kelly, J. G., Lavan, J., Noel, J., and O'Malley, K. (1980): Pharmacokinetics of lignocaine in the elderly. *Br. J. Clin. Pharmacol.*, 9:293–294.
62. Stanski, D. R., Greenblatt, D. J., and Lowenstein, E. (1978): Kinetics of intravenous and intramuscular morphine. *Clin. Pharmacol. Ther.*, 24:52–58.
63. Welling, P. G., Baumueller, A., and Lau, C. C. (1977): Netilmicin pharmacokinetics after single intravenous doses to elderly male patients. *Antimicrob. Agents Chemother.*, 12:328–334.
64. Kangas, L., Iisalo, E., Kanto, J., Lehtinen, V., Pynnonen, S., Ruikha, I., Salminen, J., and Syvalahte, E. (1979): Human pharmacokinetics of nitrazepam. Effect of age and disease. *Eur. J. Clin. Pharmacol.*, 15:163–170.
65. Braithwaite, R. A., Crome, P., and Dawling, S. (1980): Pharmacokinetics of nortriptyline in elderly depressed patients and prediction of optimal dosage regimens. *Br. J. Clin. Pharmacol.*, 9:306–307.
66. Dawling, S., Crome, P., and Braithwaite, R. (1980): Pharmacokinetics of single oral doses of nortriptyline in depressed elderly hospital patients and young healthy volunteers. *Clin. Pharmacokinet.*, 5:394–401.
67. Dawling, S., Crome, P., Braithwaite, R. A., and Lewis, R. R. (1980): Nortriptyline therapy in elderly patients; dosage prediction after single dose pharmacokinetic study. *Eur. J. Clin. Pharmacol.*, 18:147–150.
68. Greenblatt, D. J. (1981): Clinical pharmacokinetics of oxazepam and lorazepam. *Clin. Pharmacokinet.*, 6:89–105.
69. Duvaldestin, P., Berger, J. L., Saada, J., and Demonts, J. M. (1980): Pancuronium, pharmacokinetics and pharmacodynamics in the elderly. *Anesthesiology*, 53:5284 (abstract).
70. Allen, M. D., and Greenblatt, D. J. (1980): Desmethyldiazepam kinetics following oral prazepam in the elderly. *Clin. Pharmacol. Ther.*, 27:244.
71. Rubin, P. C., Scott, P. J. W., and Reid, J. L. (1981): Prazosin disposition in young and elderly. *Br. J. Clin. Pharmacol.*, 12:401–404.
72. Cuny, G., Roger, R. J., Mur, J. M., Serot, J. M., Netter, F. P., Maillard, A., and Penin, F. (1979): Pharmacokinetics of salicylates in elderly. *Gerontology*, 25:49–55.
73. Bauer, L. A., and Blouin, R. A. (1981): Influence of age on theophylline clearance in patients with chronic obstructive pulmonary disease. *Clin. Pharmacokinet.*, 6:469–474.
74. Husted, S., and Andersen, F. (1977): The influence of age on the response to anticoagulants. *Br. J. Clin. Pharmacol.*, 4:559–565.
75. Shepard, A. M. M., Hewick, D. S., Moreland, T. A., and Stevenson, I. H. (1977): Age as a determinant of sensitivity to warfarin. *Br. J. Clin. Pharmacol.*, 4:315–320.
76. McLachlan, M. S. F. (1978): The aging kidney. *Lancet*, 2:143–146.
77. Reichlmier, K., Eng, A., Ivangoff, P., and Meier-Ruge, W. (1978): Age related changes in human brain enzymes: Basis for pharmacological intervention. In: *Pharmacological Intervention in the Aging Process*, edited by J. Roberts, R. C. Addman, and V. J. Cristofalo, pp. 251–252. Plenum Press, New York.
78. Dillon, N., Chung, S., Kelly, J., and O'Malley, K. (1980): Age and beta-adrenoceptor-mediated function. *Clin. Pharmacol. Ther.*, 27:769–772.

79. Abrass, I. B., and Scarpace, P. J. (1981): Human lymphocyte beta-adrenergic receptors are unaltered with age. *J. Gerontol.*, 36:298–301.
80. Fleisch, J. G. (1980): Age-related changes in the sensitivity of blood vessels to drugs. *Pharmacol. Ther.*, 8:477–487.
81. Poe, W. D., and Holloway, D. A. (1980): *Drugs and the Aged*, p. 48. McGraw-Hill, New York.
82. Fulton, B., James, O., and Rawlins, M. D. (1979): The influence of age on the pharmacokinetics of paracetamol. *Br. J. Clin. Pharmacol.*, 7:418.
83. Wallace, D. E., and Watanabe, A. S. (1977): Drug effects of geriatric patients. *Drug Intell. Clin. Pharm.*, 11:597–602.
84. Divoll, M., Abernethy, D. R., Ameer, B., and Greenblatt, D. J. (1982): Acetaminophen kinetics in the elderly. *Clin. Pharmacol. Ther.*, 31:151–155.
85. Avery, G. S. (1980): *Drug Treatment*, ed. 2, pp. 158–181. Adis Press, Sydney.
86. John, V. A., Lus Combe, D. K., and Kemp, H. (1980): Effects of age, cigarette smoking and the oral contraceptive on the pharmacokinetics of clomipramine and its desmethyl metabolite during chronic dosing. *J. Intern. Med. Res., [Suppl. 3]*, 8:88–95.
87. Kaufmann, B., Olcay, A., Schaumann, W., Teufel, W., and Weib, W. (1981): Pharmacokinetics of methyldigoxin and digoxin in geriatric patients with normal and elevated serum creatinine levels. *Clin. Pharmacokinet.*, 6:463–468.
88. Reidenberg, M. M., Levy, M., Warner, H., Coutinho, C. B., Schwartz, M. A., Yu, G., and Cheripko, J. (1978): Relationship between diazepam dose, plasma level, age, and central nervous system depression. *Clin. Pharmacol. Ther.*, 23:371–374.
89. Schentag, J. J., Cerra, F. B., Calleri, G. M., Leising, M. E., French, M. A., and Bernhard, H. (1981): Age, disease, and cimetidine in healthy subjects and chronically ill patients. *Clin. Pharmacol. Ther.*, 29:737–743.
90. Kanto, J., Kangos, L., Aaltonen, L., and Hilke, H. (1981): Effect of age on the pharmacokinetics and sedative effect of flunitrazepam. *Acta Psychiatr. Scand.*, 63(Suppl. 290):400–403.
91. Hicks, R., Dysken, M. W., Davis, J. M., Lesser, J., Ripeckyl, A., and Lazarus, L. (1981): The pharmacokinetics of psychotropic medication in the elderly: A review. *J. Clin. Psychiatry*, 42:374–385.
92. Kaiko, R. F. (1980): Age and morphine analgesia in cancer patients with postoperative pain. *Clin. Pharmacol. Ther.*, 28:823–826.
93. Regardh, C. G., and Hohnson, G. (1980): Clinical pharmacokinetics of metoprolol. *Clin. Pharmacokinet.*, 5:557–569.
94. Quaterman, C. P., Kendall, M. J., and Jack, D. B. (1981): The effect of age on the pharmacokinetics of metoprolol and its metabolites. *Br. J. Clin. Pharmacol.*, 2:287–294.
95. Kangos, L., and Breimer, D. D. (1981): Clinical pharmacokinetics of nitrazepam. *Clin. Pharmacokinet.*, 6:346–366.
96. Sorensen, P., and Laresen, N. E. (1980): Factors influencing nortriptyline steady-state kinetics: Plasma and saliva levels. *Clin. Pharmacol. Ther.*, 28:796–803.
97. Lambie, D. C., and Caird, F. I. (1977): Phenytoin dosage in the elderly. *Age Ageing*, 6:133–136.
98. Reidenberg, M. M., Camacho, M., and Kluger, J. (1980): Aging and renal clearance of procainamide and acetylprocainamide. *Clin. Pharmacol. Ther.*, 28:732–735.
99. Dehlin, O., Bjornsson, G., and Lundstrom, J. (1981): Zimelidine to geriatric patients: A pharmacokinetic and clinical study. *Int. J. Clin. Pharmacol.*, 19:410–424.
100. Ramsay, L. E., and Tucker, G. T. (1981): Clinical pharmacology; drugs in the elderly. *Br. Med. J.*, 1:125S–127S.
101. Drayer, D. E., Romankiewicz, J., Lorenzo, B., and Reidenberg, M. M. (1982): Age and renal clearance of cimetidine. *Clin. Pharmacol. Ther.*, 31:45–50.
102. Bauer, L. A., and Blouin, K. A. (1981): Influence of age on tobramycin pharmacokinetics in patients with normal renal function. *Antimicrob. Agents Chemother.*, 20:587–589.
103. Talseth, T., Kornstad, S., Boye, N. P., and Bredesen, J. E. (1981): Individualization of oral theophylline dosage in elderly patients. *Acta Med. Scand.*, 210:489–492.
104. Patterson, M., Heazelwood, R., Smithurst, B., and Eadie, M. J. (1982): Plasma protein binding of phenytoin in the aged: In vivo studies. *Br. J. Clin. Pharmacol.*, 13:423–425.
105. Bauer, L. A., and Blouin, R. A. (1982): Age and phenytoin kinetics in adult epileptics. *Clin. Pharmacol. Ther.*, 31:301–304.
106. Montgomery, P. R., and Sitar, D. S. (1981): Increased serum salicylate metabolites with age in patients receiving chronic acetylsalicylic acid therapy. *Gerontology*, 27:329–333.

107. Ochs, H. R., Greenblatt, D. J., Divoll, M., Abernethy, D. R., Feyerabend, H., and Dengler, H. J. (1981): Diazepam kinetics in relation to age and sex. *Pharmacology*, 23:24–30.
108. Divoll, M., Greenblatt, D. J., Harmatz, J. S., and Shader, R. I. (1981): Effect of age and gender on disposition of temazepam. *J. Pharm. Sci.*, 70:1104–1107.
109. Christensen, J. H., Andreasen, F., and Jansen, J. A. (1981): Influence of age and sex on the pharmacokinetics of thiopentone. *Br. J. Anaesth.*, 53:1189–1195.
110. Duvaldestin, P., Saada, J., Berger, J. L., Hollander, A. D., and Desmonts, J. M. (1982): Pharmacokinetics, pharmacodynamics, and dose-response relationship of pancuronium in control and elderly subjects. *Anesthesiology*, 56:36–40.
111. Vestal, R. E., Wood, A. J. J., and Shand, D. G. (1979): Reduced β-adrenoceptor sensitivity in the elderly. *Clin. Pharmacol. Ther.*, 26:181–186.
112. Klotz, U., and Wilkinson, G. R. (1978): Hepatic elimination of drugs in the elderly. In: *Liver and Aging*, edited by K. Kitani, pp. 367–380. North-Holland, Amsterdam.
113. Tsang, C. C., Speeg, K. V., and Wilkinson, G. R. (1982): Aging and benzodiazepine binding in the rat cerebral cortex. *Life Sci.*, 30:343–346.
114. Morgon, K. (1982): Effect of low-dose nitrazepam on performance in the elderly. *Lancet*, 1:516.
115. Rubin, P. C., Scott, P. J. W., McLean, K., Pearson, A., Ross, D., and Reid, J. L. (1982): Atenolol disposition in young and elderly subjects. *Br. J. Clin. Pharmacol.*, 13:235–237.
116. O'Callaghan, W. G., Laker, M. S., McGarry, K., O'Brien, E. T., and O'Malley, K. (1982): Antihypertensive and renal haemodynamic effects of atenolol and nadolol in elderly hypertensive patients. *Br. J. Clin. Pharmacol.*, 14:135P–136P.
117. Young, C. J., Daneshmend, T. K., and Roberts, C. J. C. (1982): Pharmacokinetics of ranitidine in hepatic cirrhosis and in the elderly. *Br. J. Clin. Pharmacol.*, 14:152P.
118. Elliott, H. L., Sumner, D. J., McLean, K., and Reid, J. L. (1982): Effect of age on the responsiveness of vascular alpha-adrenoceptors in man. *J. Cardiovasc. Pharmacol.*, 4:388–392.
119. Collier, P. S., Kawar, P., Gamble, J. A. S., and Dundee, J. W. (1982): Influence of age on pharmacokinetics of midazolam. *Br. J. Clin. Pharmacol.*, 13:602P.
120. Bender, A. D. (1965): The effect of increasing age on the distribution of peripheral blood flow in man. *J. Am. Geriatr. Soc.*, 13:192.
121. Landowne, M., and Stanley, J. (1960): Aging of the cardiovascular system. In: *Aging: Some Social and Biological Aspects*, edited by N. W. Shock. American Association for the Advancement of Science, Washington, D.C.
122. Flood, C., Gherondache, C., Pincus, G., Tait, S. A. S., and Willoughby, S. (1967): The metabolism and secretion of aldosterone in elderly subjects. *J. Clin. Invest.*, 46:960.
123. Danon, D., Shock, N. W., and Marois, M. (eds.) (1982): *Aging: A Challenge to Science and Society*. Oxford University Press, Oxford.
124. Greenblatt, D. J., Abernethy, D. R., Divoll, M., Smith, R. B., and Shader, R. I. (1983): Old age, cimetidine, and disposition of alprazolam and triazolam. *Clin. Pharmacol. Ther.*, 33:61.
125. Tsujimoto, G., Sasaki, T., Ishizaki, T., Suganuma, T., and Hirayama, H. (1982): Reexamination of digoxin dosage regimen: Comparison of the proposed nomograms or formulae in elderly patients. *Br. J. Clin. Pharmacol.*, 13:493–500.
126. Greenblatt, D. J., Divoll, M., Puri, S. K., Ho, I., Zinny, M. A., and Shader, R. I. (1983): Reduced single dose clearance of clobazam in elderly men predicts increased multiple dose accumulation. *Clin. Pharmacokinet.*, 8:83–94.
127. Hitzenberger, G., Fitscha, P., Beveridge, T., Nuesch, E., and Pacha, W. (1982): Effects of age and smoking on the pharmacokinetics of pindolol and propranolol. *Br. J. Clin. Pharmacol.*, 13:217S–222S.
128. Kitanaka, I., Ross, R. J., Cutler, N. R., Zavadil, A. P., and Potter, W. Z. (1982): Altered hydroxydesipramine concentrations in elderly depressed patients. *Clin. Pharmacol. Ther.*, 31:51–55.

Pharmacokinetic Basis for Drug Treatment,
edited by L. Z. Benet et al., Raven Press,
New York © 1984

Chapter 16

Smoking Effects in Pharmacokinetics

William J. Jusko

*Department of Pharmaceutics, School of Pharmacy, State University of New York
at Buffalo, Amherst, New York 14260*

Depending on one's point of view, the changes in pharmacokinetics induced by tobacco smoking can be considered to be the results of a habit, a disease, use of a social drug, or environmentally induced alterations of drug disposition. Approximately one of three adults uses tobacco regularly, and smoking thus offers extensive possibilities of modifying clinical effects and drug dosage needs in patients.

The literature related to smoking effects in pharmacokinetics was reviewed in 1978–1979 (1,2) and assessed as part of the most recent Surgeon General's Report on Smoking and Health (3). The purpose of this chapter will be to (a) update the topic, including itemization of those drugs whose pharmacokinetics have been examined in relation to smoking, (b) consider interactions of smoking with other drug, disease, and physiological factors affecting pharmacokinetics, and (c) attempt to detail further the mechanisms of tobacco-induced changes in drug elimination.

ARRAY OF DRUG STUDIES

A listing of drugs that have been examined with respect to total clearance or elimination rate in relation to smoking is provided in Table 1. The number of drugs examined has nearly doubled since 1978, indicating the rapid growth of interest in the topic and the observance of an earlier recommendation that all studies should report and consider the smoking status of their subjects or patients.

As indicated in Table 1, the array of compounds evaluated in relation to smoking ranges from such common social stimulants as nicotine, ethanol, and caffeine to numerous important and frequently used therapeutic agents. Increased coffee drinking is associated with smoking, and the disposition of caffeine is thus of interest. Plasma clearances of caffeine determined in smokers and nonsmokers by Parsons and Neims (5) are shown in Fig. 1. The mean clearance of caffeine was 155 ml/hr/kg in smokers, compared with 94 ml/hr/kg in nonsmokers.

Theophylline and caffeine, both methylxanthines, share pharmacologic properties, biotransformation mechanisms, and the effects of smoking. These compounds have been evaluated extensively by numerous investigators in relation to smoking (8–12). We found that use of both tobacco and marijuana causes an increased rate

TABLE 1. *Summary of drugs examined in relation to*
tobacco smoking in humans[a]

Compounds with increased clearance or
   elimination
  Antipyrine (15–17,57)
  Caffeine (5–7)
  Clorazepate (desmethyldiazepam) (54)
  Imipramine (23)
  Clomipramine (58)
  Lidocaine (18)
  Nicotine (4)
  Nortriptyline (25)
  Oxazepam (24)
  Pentazocine (22)
  Phenacetin (19–21)
  Propranolol (14)
  Theophylline (8–13)
Compounds with slight or uncertain
   changes
  Diazepam (32)
  Ethanol (26,27)

  Indocyanine green (17,30)
  Lorazepam (31)
  Warfarin (28,29)
  Chlorpromazine (56)
Compounds not affected
  Chlordiazepoxide (38)
  Codeine (60)
  Dexamethasone (39)
  Diazepam (33)
  Epoprostenol (61)
  Meperidine (36)
  Nortriptyline (37)
  Oral contraceptives (40)
  Phenytoin (34,35)
  Pindolol (62)
  Prednisolone (39)
  Prednisone (39)
  Glucaric acid (59)

[a]Reference numbers in parentheses.

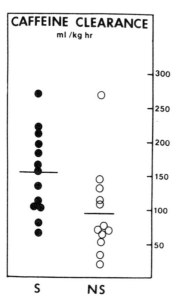

FIG. 1. Plasma clearances of caffeine in adult (20–45 years) smokers (S) and nonsmokers (NS). Horizontal lines indicate mean values. (Data from Parsons and Neims, ref. 5.)

of metabolism of theophylline. As shown in Fig. 2, the dual smoking of both plants seems to result in an additive increase in plasma clearance of theophylline. A similar finding has recently been reported for antipyrine (57).

The drug exhibiting the most striking change in disposition in relation to smoking is propranolol. Figure 3 represents propranolol intrinsic clearances (uncorrected for protein binding) obtained by Vestal et al. (14,41) in young and old smokers. The

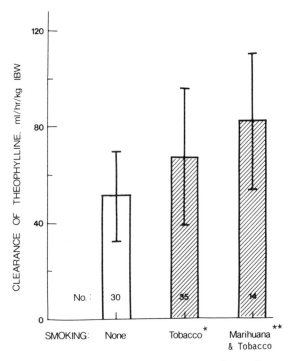

FIG. 2. Effect of smoking tobacco or marijuana plus tobacco on plasma clearances (mean ± SD) of theophylline in adult subjects (20–40 years). Numbers in bars indicate numbers of subjects per group. *Individuals in this group smoked a mean of 25 (± 9.6) cigarettes per day. **Individuals smoked 21 (±7.3) cigarettes per day, plus marijuana at least twice a week (mean of four times a week). (From Jusko et al., ref. 11, with permission.)

younger smokers exhibited a 2.7-fold greater clearance than did the nonsmokers. As will be discussed later, this difference was largely dissipated in old age. The interaction of smoking with beta blockers is of further interest in view of the pharmacologic effects of nicotine from smoking. The beta blockers have been shown to unmask the vasoconstrictor effect of smoking mediated by vascular alpha receptors (42). This results in decreased peripheral blood flow and increased diastolic blood pressure caused by the marked increase in plasma adrenaline concentrations induced by cigarette smoking.

Tobacco use may have a slight effect on ethanol clearance. As depicted in Fig. 4 (27), somewhat greater rates of metabolism of ethanol were found in persons who were either smokers or drinkers or both. Several other compounds, namely warfarin (28,29), indocyanine green (17), and lorazepam (31), may be affected slightly by smoking, but the effects are either marginal or unresolvable from the information reported.

The disposition of an appreciable number of important therapeutic drugs is not modified by smoking. Whereas imipramine disposition is markedly altered in smokers (23), nortriptyline metabolism is not changed (37). Both compounds undergo hydroxylation and demethylation as elimination pathways. The plasma clearances

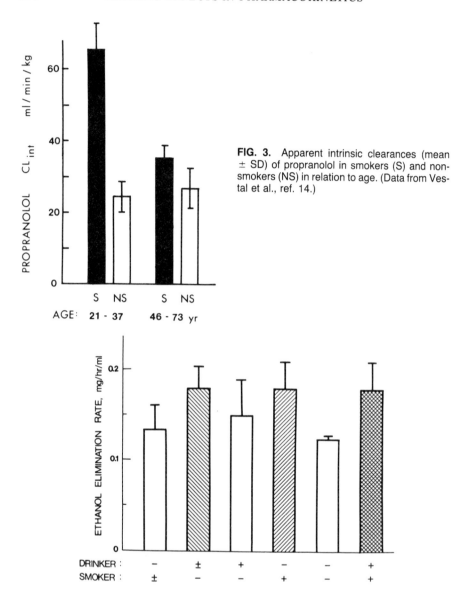

FIG. 3. Apparent intrinsic clearances (mean ± SD) of propranolol in smokers (S) and non-smokers (NS) in relation to age. (Data from Vestal et al., ref. 14.)

FIG. 4. Elimination rates of ethanol (mean ± SD) in persons who were either smokers or drinkers or both or neither. Drinkers: minimum 60 g ethanol/day. Smokers: more than 25 cigarettes/day. (Data from Kopun and Propping, ref. 27.)

of two benzodiazepines, diazepam (33) and chlordiazepoxide (38), are not increased in smokers. This is intriguing because the Boston Collaborative Drug Surveillance Program (43) found a markedly lower incidence of CNS depression in heavy smokers (about 3%) using these drugs than in nonsmokers and light smokers (6%–10%). The differences in side effects must therefore be related to pharmacologic rather than pharmacokinetic differences.

We evaluated the apparent intrinsic clearances of several corticosteroids in relation to smoking (39). These compounds are of interest because their biotransformation mechanism probably differs from the P-448 and P-450 pathways accounting for most (except for ethanol and lorazepam) of the other drugs in Table 1. The clearances of prednisone and dexamethasone were examined in the same group of smokers and nonsmokers (Fig. 5). There is covariance in metabolism of these steroids, but the data from the smokers and nonsmokers are mingled in the graph and show no differences.

INTERACTIONS WITH SECONDARY FACTORS

More complicated questions to be resolved include assessing the effects of smoking when other factors, such as physiologic, occupational, disease, or drug interactions, are also present. Generally, it becomes more difficult to maintain proper control in prospective assessment of multiple factors that may affect the pharmacokinetics of various drugs.

Most clearly evaluated is the role of age. Vestal et al. examined antipyrine (15), propranolol (14), and indocyanine green (17) in relation to both age and smoking. When the smoking effect was present, it occurred only in young to middle-aged adults, as shown in Fig. 3 for propranolol (perhaps those smokers most sensitive to the enzyme inductive and other effects of tobacco did not survive long enough to be assessed in old age). We noted a similar phenomenon in evaluating factors affecting theophylline plasma clearances (12). The smoking effect was found primarily in 20- to 40-year-old persons.

Attempts have been made to evaluate drug disposition in relation to smoking and one or more additional factors. A summary of such studies is provided in Table 2. Generally, if a disease is present causing major organ dysfunction, such as liver

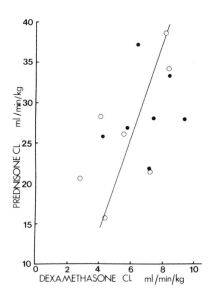

FIG. 5. Oral dose clearances of prednisone and dexamethasone in smokers *(filled circles)* and nonsmokers *(open circles)*. The correlation ($r = 0.55$) is statistically significant ($p < 0.05$). (From Rose et al., ref. 39, with permission.)

TABLE 2. *Interactions of tobacco smoking and other drug, disease,*
or physiologic factors

Drug	Second factor	Observation	References
Antipyrine	Age	No effect of smoking on clearance in older persons[a]	17
Antipyrine	Liver disease	No smoking effect when cirrhosis or hepatitis present	45
Antipyrine	Glutethimide	Drug enhances metabolism in both smokers and nonsmokers	46
Antipyrine	Cannabis	Additive effect of cannabis on clearance	57
Insulin	Diabetes mellitus	Insulin absorption is decreased by 113%; $T_{1/2}$ nonsmoking, 158 min; during smoking, 336 min	47
Propranolol	Age	No effect of smoking on clearance in older persons	14
Propranolol	Angina	Effective treatment of angina with propranolol is limited by cigarette smoking	55
Theophylline	Obesity	No difference in clearance in obese persons	44
Theophylline	Oral contraceptives	OCs reduced clearance in smokers	12
Theophylline	CHF	Increased clearance found in patients with moderate and severe CHF	12
Theophylline	Marijuana	Possible additive effects of tobacco and marijuana on clearance	11

[a]Clearance refers to total plasma clearance of the principal drug.

impairment or congestive heart failure, the altered capability for clearance of the drug predominates over the potential for enzyme induction caused by smoking.

Genetic considerations may be involved in determining the degree to which tobacco smoking enhances the biotransformation rate of drugs. Kellerman and Luyten-Kellerman (48) found a correlation between antipyrine and theophylline clearances and the inducibility of aryl hydrocarbon hydroxylase in mitogen-stimulated lymphocytes. Betlach and Tozer (49) examined the effects of polycyclic aromatic hydrocarbons on theophylline clearance in six inbred mice strains. Two strains were nonresponsive to such treatment. When examining theophylline clearances in large numbers of young adult subjects, we found considerable variability in disposition of the drug, with numerous persons showing relatively low clearance. The possibility thus exists that the degree of sensitivity to changes in drug metabolism related to smoking is genetically determined.

MECHANISMS OF SMOKING EFFECTS

The predominant mechanism of tobacco-increased clearance of drugs is probably the induction of the microsomal P-448 mixed-function oxidase system. This was proposed (1) based on the analogies between the selective effects of polycyclic

aromatic hydrocarbons in animal systems and the limited array of drugs that are affected by smoking in humans. Most of the drugs in Table 1 that exhibit marked increases in clearance are metabolized by hydroxylation and demethylation. On the other hand, many drugs that undergo similar metabolic routes are not affected by smoking. Corticosteroids are biotransformed by another pathway involving 11-β-hydroxydehydrogenase enzymes and other metabolic routes that are not affected by smoking. There are multiple forms of inducible drug-metabolizing enzymes (50), and it appears that only the P-448 type of mechanism is affected by smoking in humans.

Vestal et al. (14,41) evaluated hepatic blood flow in smokers and nonsmokers using oral and intravenous doses of propranolol and suitable pharmacokinetic methods. No effect of smoking was found. In contrast, Huet and Lelorier (18), using lidocaine with similar pharmacokinetic methods, observed lower hepatic blood flows in smokers. Unlike phenobarbital, which causes multiple physiologic changes in liver function, the polycyclic aromatic hydrocarbons do not affect hepatic blood flow in animals (51). We found no difference in liver sizes in autopsy studies of smokers and nonsmokers (52).

McNamara et al. (53) found an interesting difference in plasma protein binding of lidocaine between smokers and nonsmokers. Increased binding of the drug was found in smokers (increased 19%). They suggested that smokers may have increased plasma concentration of α_1-acid glycoprotein (for further comments on α_1-acid glycoprotein, see Chapters 10, 13, and 15). Possible changes in binding should be assessed further with other drugs in relation to smoking.

ACKNOWLEDGMENT

This work was supported in part by Grant 20852 from the National Institute of General Medical Sciences, National Institutes of Health, Bethesda, Maryland.

REFERENCES

1. Jusko, W. J. (1978): Role of tobacco smoking in pharmacokinetics. *J. Pharmacokinet. Biopharm.*, 6:7–39.
2. Jusko, W. J. (1979): Influence of cigarette smoking on drug metabolism in man. *Drug Metab. Rev.*, 9:221–236.
3. Smoking and Health: A Report of the Surgeon General. DHEW Publication No. (PHS)79–50066. Superintendent of Documents, U.S. Government Printing Office, Washington, D.C., 1979.
4. Beckett, A. H., and Triggs, E. J. (1967): Enzyme induction in man caused by smoking. *Nature*, 216:587.
5. Parsons, W. D., and Neims, A. H. (1978): Effect of smoking on caffeine clearance. *Clin. Pharmacol. Ther.*, 24:40–45.
6. Christensen, H. D., and Whitsett, T. L. (1979): Measurements of xanthines and their metabolites by means of high pressure liquid chromatography. In: *Biological/Biomedical Applications of Liquid Chromatography*, edited by G. L. Hawk, pp. 507–537. Marcel Dekker, New York.
7. Descotes, J., Brazier, J. L., Ollagnier, M., and Evreaux, J. C. (1979): Influence de la consommation de tabac sur la pharmacocinetique de la caféine. *Thérapie*, 34:619–624.
8. Jenne, J., Nagasawa, H., McHugh, R., MacDonald, F., and Wyse, E. (1975): Decreased theophylline half-life in cigarette smokers. *Life Sci.*, 17:195–198.
9. Hunt, S. N., Jusko, W. J., and Yurchak, A. M. (1976): Effect of smoking on theophylline disposition. *Clin. Pharmacol. Ther.*, 19:546–551.

10. Powell, J. R., Thiercelin, J.-F., Vozeh, S., Sansom, L., and Riegelman, S. (1977): The influence of cigarette smoking and sex on theophylline disposition. *Am. Rev. Respir. Dis.*, 116:17–24.

11. Jusko, W. J., Schentag, J. J., Clark, J. H., Gardner, M., and Yurchak, A. M. (1978): Enhanced biotransformation of theophylline in marijuana and tobacco smokers. *Clin. Pharmacol. Ther.*, 24:406–410.

12. Jusko, W. J., Gardner, M. J., Mangione, A., Schentag, J. J., Koup, J. R., and Vance, J. W. (1979): Factors affecting theophylline clearances: Age, tobacco, marijuana, cirrhosis, congestive heart failure, obesity, oral contraceptives, benzodiazepines, barbiturates and ethanol. *J. Pharm. Sci.*, 68:1358–1366.

13. Grygiel, J. J., Birkett, D. J., and Phil, D. (1981): Cigarette smoking and theophylline clearance and metabolism. *Clin. Pharmacol. Ther.*, 30:491–495.

14. Vestal, R. E., Wood, A. J. J., Branch, R. A., Shand, D. G., and Wilkinson, G. R. (1979): Effects of age and cigarette smoking on propranolol disposition. *Clin. Pharmacol. Ther.*, 26:8–15.

15. Vestal, R. E., Norris, A. H., Tobin, J. D., Cohen, B. H., Shock, M. W., and Andres, R. (1975): Antipyrine metabolism in man: Influence of age, alcohol, caffeine, and smoking. *Clin. Pharmacol. Ther.*, 18:425–432.

16. Hart, P., Farrell, G. C., Cooksley, W. G. E., and Powell, L. W. (1976): Enhanced drug metabolism in cigarette smokers. *Br. Med. J.*, 2:147–149.

17. Wood, A. J. J., Vestal, R. E., Wilkinson, G. R., Branch, R. A., and Shand, D. G. (1979): Effect of aging and cigarette smoking on antipyrine and indocyanine green elimination. *Clin. Pharmacol. Ther.*, 26:16–20.

18. Huet, P.-M., and Lelorier, J. (1980): Effects of smoking and chronic hepatitis B on lidocaine and indocyanine green kinetics. *Clin. Pharmacol. Ther.*, 28:208–215.

19. Pantuck, E. J., Kuntzman, R., and Conney, A. H. (1972): Decreased concentration of phenacetin in plasma of cigarette smokers. *Science*, 175:1248–1250.

20. Pantuck, E. J., Hsiao, K.-C., Maggio, A., Nakamura, K., Kuntzman, R., and Conney, A. H. (1973): Effect of cigarette smoking on phenacetin metabolism. *Clin. Pharmacol. Ther.*, 15:9–17.

21. Murdock, J. R., and Robilard, N. F. (1979): Use of smokers in bioavailability studies. *Clin. Pharmacol. Ther.*, 25–238 (Abstr.).

22. Vaughan, D. P., Beckett, A. H., and Robbie, D. S. (1976): The influence of smoking on the intersubject variation in pentazocine elimination. *Br. J. Clin. Pharmacol.*, 3:279–283.

23. Perel, J. N., Hurvic, M. J., and Kanzler, M. B. (1975): Pharmacodynamics of imipramine in depressed patients. *Psychopharmacol. Bull.*, 11:16–18.

24. Ochs, H. R., Greenblatt, D. J., and Otten, H. (1981): Disposition of oxazepam in relation to age, sex, and cigarette smoking. *Klin. Wochenschr.*, 59:899–903.

25. Linnoila, M., George, L., Guthrie, S., and Leventhal, B. (1981): Effect of alcohol consumption and cigarette smoking on antidepressant levels of depressed patients. *Am. J. Psychiatry*, 138:841–842.

26. Vestal, R. E., McGuire, E. A., Tobin, J. D., Andres, R., Norris, A. H., and Mezey, E. (1977): Aging and ethanol metabolism. *Clin. Pharmacol. Ther.*, 21:343–354.

27. Kopun, M., and Propping, P. (1977): The kinetics of ethanol absorption and elimination in twins and supplementary repetitive experiments in singleton subjects. *Eur. J. Clin. Pharmacol.*, 11:337–344.

28. Yacobi, A., Udall, J. A., and Levy, G. (1976): Serum protein binding as a determinant of warfarin body clearance and anticoagulant effect. *Clin. Pharmacol. Ther.*, 19:552–558.

29. Bachman, K., Shapiro, R., Fulton, R., Carroll, F. T., and Sullivan, T. J. (1979): Smoking and warfarin disposition. *Clin. Pharmacol. Ther.*, 25:309–315.

30. Blain, P. G., Mucklow, J. C., Wood, P., Roberts, D. F., and Rawlins, M. D. (1982): Family study of antipyrine clearance. *Br. Med. J.*, 1:150–152.

31. Greenblatt, D. J., Allen, M. D., Locniskar, A., Harmatz, J. S., and Shader, R. I. (1979): Lorazepam kinetics in the elderly. *Clin. Pharmacol. Ther.*, 26:103–113.

32. Greenblatt, D. J., Allen, M. D., Harmatz, J. S., and Shader, R. I. (1980): Diazepam disposition determinants. *Clin. Pharmacol. Ther.*, 27:301–312.

33. Klotz, U., Avant, G. R., Hoyumpa, A., Schenker, S., and Wilkinson, G. R. (1975): The effects of age and liver disease on the disposition and elimination of diazepam in adult man. *J. Clin. Invest.*, 55:347–359.

34. Rose, J. Q., Barron, S. A., and Jusko, W. J. (1978): Phenytoin disposition in smokers and nonsmokers. *Int. J. Clin. Pharmacol.*, 16:547–550.

35. DeLeary, E. G., McLeay, C. D., Eadie, M. J., and Tyrer, J. H. (1979): Effects of subjects' sex, and intake of tobacco, alcohol and oral contraceptives on plasma phenytoin levels. *Br. J. Clin. Pharmacol.*, 8:33–36.

36. Mather, L. E., Tucker, G. T., Pflug, A. E., Lindop, M. J., and Wilkerson, C. (1975): Meperidine kinetics in man, intravenous injection in surgical patients and volunteers. *Clin. Pharmacol. Ther.*, 17:21–30.

37. Norman, T. R., Burrows, G. D., Maguire, K. P., Rubinstein, G., Scoggins, B. A., and Davies, B. (1977): Cigarette smoking and plasma nortriptyline levels. *Clin. Pharmacol. Ther.*, 21:453–456.

38. Desmond, P. V., Roberts, R. K., Wilkinson, G. R., and Schenker, S. (1979): No effect of smoking on metabolism of chlordiazepoxide. *N. Engl. J. Med.*, 300:199–200.

39. Rose, J. Q., Yurchak, A. M., Meikle, A. W., and Jusko, W. J. (1981): Effect of smoking on prednisone, prednisolone, and dexamethasone pharmacokinetics. *J. Pharmacokinet. Biopharm.*, 9:389–417.

40. Crawford, F. E., Back, D. J., Orme, M. L. E., and Breckenridge, A. M. (1981): Oral contraceptive steroid plasma concentrations in smokers and non-smokers. *Br. Med. J.*, 2:1829–1830.

41. Vestal, R. E., and Wood, A. J. J. (1980): Influence of age and smoking on drug kinetics in man. Studies using model compounds. *Clin. Pharmacokinet.*, 5:309–319.

42. Trap-Jensen, J., Carlsen, J. E., Svendsen, T. L., and Christensen, N. J. (1979): Cardiovascular and adrenergic effects of cigarette smoking during immediate non-selective and selective beta adrenoceptor blockade in humans. *Eur. J. Clin. Invest.*, 9:181–183.

43. Jick, H. (1974): Smoking and clinical drug effects. *Med. Clin. North Am.*, 58:1143–1149.

44. Gal, P., Jusko, W. J., Yurchak, A. M., and Franklin, B. A. (1978): Theophylline disposition in obesity. *Clin. Pharmacol. Ther.*, 23:438–444.

45. Farrell, G. C., Cooksley, W. G. E., Hart, P., and Powell, L. W. (1978): Drug metabolism in liver disease. Identification of patients with impaired hepatic drug metabolism. *Gastroenterology*, 75:580–588.

46. Cooksley, W. G. E., Farrell, G. C., Cash, G. A., and Powell, L. W. (1979): The interaction of cigarette smoking and chronic drug ingestion on human drug metabolism. *Clin. Exp. Pharmacol. Physiol.*, 6:527–533.

47. Klemp, P., and Staberg, B. (1982): Smoking reduces insulin absorption from subcutaneous tissue. *Br. Med. J.*, 1:237.

48. Kellerman, G., and Luyten-Kellerman, M. (1978): Benzo(a)pyrene metabolism and plasma elimination rates of phenacetin, acetanilide and theophylline in man. *Pharmacology*, 17:191–200.

49. Betlach, C. J., and Tozer, T. N. (1980): Biodisposition of theophylline. II. Effect of aromatic hydrocarbon treatment in mice. *Drug Metab. Dispos.*, 1:271–273.

50. Nebert, D. W. (1979): Mutliple forms of inducible drug-metabolizing enzymes: A reasonable mechanism by which any organism can cope with adversity. *Mol. Cell. Biochem.*, 27:27–46.

51. Nies, A. S., Wilkinson, G. R., Rush, B. D., Strother, J. T., and McDevitt, D. G. (1976): Effects of alteration of hepatic microsomal enzyme activity on liver blood flow in the rat. *Biochem. Pharmacol.*, 25:1991–1993.

52. Lewis, G. P., Jusko, W. J., Coughlin, L. L., and Hartz, S. (1972): Cadmium accumulation in man: Influence of smoking, occupation, alcoholic habit and disease. *J. Chronic Dis.*, 25:717–726.

53. McNamara, P. J., Slaughter, R. L., Visco, J. P., Elwood, C. M., Siegel, J. H., and Lalka, D. (1980): Effect of smoking on binding of lidocaine to human serum proteins. *J. Pharm. Sci.*, 69:749–751.

54. Norman, T. R., Fulton, A., Burrows, G. D., and Maguire, K. P. (1981): Pharmacokinetics of *N*-desmethyldiazepam after a single oral dose of clorazepate: The effect of smoking. *Eur. J. Clin. Pharmacol.*, 21:229–233.

55. Deanfield, J., Jonathan, A., Selwyn, A., and Fox, K. M. (1981): Treatment of angina pectoris with propranolol: The harmful effects of cigarette smoking. *Cardiology*, 68(Suppl. 2):186–189.

56. Pantuck, E. J., Pantuck, C. B., Anderson, K. E., Conney, A. H., and Kappas, A. (1982): Cigarette smoking and chlorpromazine disposition and actions. *Clin. Pharmacol. Ther.*, 31:533–537.

57. Uppal, R., Garg, S. K., Sharma, P. R., Varma, V. K., and Chaudhury, R. R. (1981): Antipyrine kinetics in cannabis smokers. *Br. J. Clin. Pharmacol.*, 11:522–523.

58. John, V. A., Luscombe, D. K., and Kemp, H. (1980): Effects of age, cigarette smoking, and the oral contraceptive on the pharmacokinetics of clomipramine and its desmethyl metabolite during chronic dosing. *J. Int. Med. Res.*, 8:88–95.

59. Fiedler, K., Schröter, E., and Cramer, H. (1980): Glucaric acid excretion. Analysis of the enzymatic assay and findings in smokers and nonsmokers. *Eur. J. Clin. Pharmacol.*, 18:429–432.
60. Rogers, J. F., Findlay, J. W. A., Hull, J. H., Butz, R. F., Jones, E. C., Bustrack, J. A., and Welch, R. M. (1982): Codeine disposition in smokers and non-smokers. *Clin. Pharmacol. Ther.*, 32:218–227.
61. Hassen, S., MacDougall, I. C., O'Grady, J., and Pickles, H. (1982): Cigarette smoking does not attenuate the cardiovascular effects of epoprostenol (Prostacyclin) in humans. *Br. J. Clin. Pharmacol.*, 14:97–98.
62. Hitzenberger, G., Fitscha, P., Beveridge, T., Nüesch, E., and Pachaw, W. (1982): Effects of age and smoking on the pharmacokinetics of Pindolol and Propranolol. *Br. J. Clin. Pharmacol.*, 13:217(S)–222(S).

Pharmacokinetic Basis for Drug Treatment,
edited by L. Z. Benet et al., Raven Press,
New York © 1984

Chapter 17

Nonlinear Kinetics and Theophylline Elimination

Lawrence J. Lesko

Clinical Pharmacokinetics Laboratory, School of Pharmacy, University of Maryland, Baltimore, Maryland 21201

Theophylline (1,3-dimethylxanthine) is an effective bronchodilator for the treatment and prevention of bronchospasms. Because of its narrow therapeutic index and the wide interpatient variability in its pharmacokinetics, serum theophylline concentrations are a useful guide to dosage titration. Target serum concentrations for optimal bronchodilation are 5 to 20 mg/liter (see Appendix A and Chapters 19 and 22). There are many physiological and environmental factors that significantly influence the plasma clearance of theophylline and may lead to an unpredictable relationship between maintenance dosages and serum concentrations. Smoking (Chapter 16), obesity (Appendix D), interactions (Chapter 11), hepatic disease (Chapters 3 and 4), and cardiovascular diseases (Appendix A) are just a few of these factors. More recently, there has been an increasing awareness that the elimination kinetics of theophylline are dose-dependent or nonlinear in some patients. This adds yet another complication to the predictability of serum theophylline concentrations from the daily dose.

The purpose of this chapter is to discuss nonlinear kinetics as they pertain to theophylline and to evaluate the clinical significance of this phenomenon.

BACKGROUND

In a clinical setting, the pharmacokinetics of a drug are generally assumed to be log linear or first order, unless there is a change with dose in the value of any one or more of the pharmacokinetic parameters listed in Table 1 (1). When the kinetics of a drug are log linear, the clearance of that drug is independent of dose, and serum drug concentrations are proportional to the dose. When nonlinear kinetics occur, the clearance of the drug decreases with increasing doses and serum drug concentrations. Serum drug concentrations increase or decrease disproportionally with a change in dose. Typically, the time course of the serum concentration following a dose would not be superimposable following any other dose if the serum concentration were normalized to the dose administered. This lack of superposition

TABLE 1. *Recognition of nonlinear kinetics: changes in parameter values[a]*

Pharmacokinetic parameter			
Absorption	Distribution	Elimination	Observation
Availability	Volume of distribution	Renal clearance	Blood (plasma) concentration
Absorption rate constant	(Fraction unbound in plasma)	Extrarenal clearance	Unbound concentration
		(Fraction excreted unchanged)	Amount excreted unchanged

[a]Route, method of administration, and dosage form held constant.
From Tozer et al. (1), with permission.

is indicative of dose-dependent kinetics (see Chapter 21, Fig. 3). Relative to the total number of drugs used in therapeutics, the incidence of nonlinear kinetics is an exception rather than the rule at therapeutic doses and concentrations. The following drugs are considered to follow nonlinear kinetics in drug therapy: acetaminophen (hepatotoxic at higher doses), alcohol (enzyme saturation, diuretic effect), diazepam (metabolite inhibition), disopyramide (plasma protein binding changes), griseofulvin (gastrointestinal insolubility), propranolol (saturable first-pass metabolism, altered hepatic blood flow), phenytoin (capacity-limited metabolism), salicylamide (saturable first-pass metabolism), salicylic acid (saturable protein binding, capacity-limited metabolism), and theophylline (diuretic effect, capacity-limited metabolism) (1).

In the case of theophylline pharmacokinetics, evidence of nonlinearity has taken several forms. In therapeutic drug monitoring, by comparing steady state serum theophylline concentrations obtained at two different doses, one may observe that the ratio of percent change in serum level to percent change in dose (dose ratio) is greater than unity. For example, it was reported that the dose ratio was 1.5 in 13 of 83 (16%) adults with obstructive lung disease (2). These patients did not have any evidence of significant impairment of hepatic or renal function that might contribute to nonlinear kinetics. In 42 pediatric patients with chronic asthma, where two dose/serum concentration pairs were available, 30 patients (71%) had dose ratios of at least 1.5 (3). Similar evidence of nonlinearity has been observed in 4 of 23 (17%) pediatric asthmatics (4) and 21 of 44 (48%) patients with chronic airway obstruction (5). Dose ratios significantly greater than unity strongly suggest that the clearance of theophylline is dose-dependent. It was reported that the mean clearance of theophylline in 20 pediatric patients was 1.37 ml/min/kg at a low mean infusion rate of 0.74 mg/kg/hr and only 1.20 ml/min/kg at a higher mean infusion rate of 1.42 mg/kg/hr (6).

In acute theophylline overdoses where serum theophylline concentrations are measured, one may observe nonlinear pharmacokinetics in the form of an initial slow rate of decline in serum concentrations, followed by a faster rate of decline

at lower concentrations. This type of "biphasic" convex log serum-level/time curve was observed in an infant accidentally administered a theophylline dose of 192 mg/kg. Beginning with an initial serum theophylline concentration of 182 mg/liter, the first phase of elimination had an apparent elimination half-life of 15.2 hr, and the second phase showed 8.5 hr (7). Similar biphasic mixed-order patterns of theophylline elimination have been reported for other pediatric patients (8,9). However, one must consider that the pharmacokinetics in a drug overdose may drastically differ from the pharmacokinetics of therapeutic doses with many drugs, as with theophylline (10).

Another form of nonlinearity that has been observed is an increase in the elimination half-life of theophylline after chronic dosing, compared with the single-dose elimination half-life in the same subject or patient. In one study, the single-dose average elimination half-life in 12 volunteers was 4.6 hr, and after chronic dosing the average terminal elimination half-life increased to 6.3 hr (11). This increase in half-life differs from the well-known intrasubject variability in half-life in that the increase was greater than expected if due to interday variability alone; it occurred over a relatively short time period, and the increase was observed in a majority of individuals.

A classic test for detecting nonlinearity in a pharmacokinetic system is to administer a drug at two or more dose levels to the same subject, measure serum drug concentrations over time, calculate the areas under the serum concentration/time curves, and divide each area by the dose. If the quotients for each area–dose pair are different, nonlinearity is highly probable. This test was applied to data obtained after administration of 100- and 200-mg doses of theophylline to 17 normal volunteers; indeed, the two area–dose quotients were unequal, indicative of dose-dependent kinetics (12).

These examples, and others, are representative of nonlinear pharmacokinetic data for theophylline. There are also many pharmacokinetic studies of theophylline and case reports of accidental theophylline ingestion in which the elimination kinetics appear to be log linear over a wide range of serum theophylline concentrations (13–16). However, not all of these studies included enough serum theophylline concentration/time data to exclude the possibility that nonlinear kinetics had occurred but were not detected.

METABOLISM OF THEOPHYLLINE

Theophylline is eliminated primarily by demethylation and oxidation by the liver. The major metabolites found in the urine are 3-methylxanthine (MX), 1,3-dimethyluric acid (DMU), and 1-methyluric acid (MU) (17,18). The relative average amounts (as percentage of dose) of theophylline and its major metabolites recovered in 24-hr urines collected after acute or chronic dosing of theophylline in adults are as follows: unchanged theophylline, 7–13%; MX, 13–36%; DMU, 29–39%; MU, 15–35% (17,19,20,31–34). The range of recovery percentages for theophylline and its metabolites is apparently due in part to differences in sensitivity and specificity of assay methods.

The most probable cause of nonlinear theophylline pharmacokinetics is the operation of Michaelis-Menten kinetics. Current evidence suggests that the formation of MX is a potentially saturable metabolic pathway. One study presented evidence that the urine MX fraction is inversely related to serum theophylline concentrations at steady state (19). In another study of urinary excretion patterns of theophylline and its metabolites, the data for each metabolite were plotted according to a linearized form of the Michaelis-Menten equation (20) as follows:

$$S/v = K_m/V_{max} + 1/V_{max} \times S \qquad (1)$$

where S is the amount of unmetabolized theophylline in the body, v is the elimination rate of metabolite, reflecting its rate of formation, K_m is the apparent Michaelis constant, and V_{max} is the theoretical maximum rate of metabolite formation (21). With respect to theophylline disposition, the use of Eq. 1 makes the following assumptions: (a) the major metabolites are eliminated solely by renal excretion, (b) the rate-limiting step in the elimination of metabolites is the formation step, (c) the recovery of theophylline and its metabolites after a dose is quantitatively complete, and (d) the body represents a constant "volume." If the data follow Michaelis-Menten kinetics, a plot of S/v versus S is linear, with a y-axis intercept of K_m/V_{max} and a slope of $1/V_{max}$. The data for MX yielded a plot describable by Michaelis-Menten kinetics. If the data follow first-order kinetics, a plot of S/v versus S will have a slope of zero. Plots for theophylline, DMU, and MU all had slopes of zero.

Thus, the concept of enzyme saturation may be used to explain the nonlinear kinetics of theophylline. However, there are insufficient data to eliminate the possibility that dose-dependent kinetics may occur as a result of feedback inhibition of demethylation of theophylline by MX.

INFLUENCE OF DIET ON THEOPHYLLINE METABOLISM

Dietary factors have been shown to influence theophylline metabolism (see Appendix A). A low-carbohydrate high-protein diet ingested by normal volunteers for 2 weeks resulted in a decrease in theophylline elimination half-life from 8.1 hr (baseline) to 5.2 hr. Subsequently, a low-protein high-carbohydrate diet produced an increase in half-life from 5.2 to 7.6 hr (22). A diet containing charcoal-broiled beef ingested by normal volunteers for 5 days resulted in a 22% decrease in the elimination half-life of theophylline as compared with control diet (23). Presumably, dietary constituents alter the capacity of the microsomal system in the liver to oxidize theophylline although the mechanisms for these effects are unclear.

Perhaps more closely related to nonlinear theophylline kinetics, it has been shown that the presence or absence of dietary methylxanthines can significantly alter the rate of metabolism of ^{14}C-theophylline (20). The absence of dietary methylxanthines for 1 week resulted in a decrease in the urinary elimination half-life of radioactivity, as compared with base line (9.8 to 7.0 hr). The recovery of MX in the urine was also greater in the absence of dietary methylxanthines. It is hypothesized that dietary methylxanthines (caffeine, theobromine, theophylline) compete with exogenously

administered theophylline for metabolizing enzymes in the liver. The N-demethylation pathway responsible for the formation of MX from theophylline is apparently saturable, and Michaelis-Menten kinetics occur when methylxanthines compete with theophylline for oxidizing enzyme sites. Similarly, the plasma elimination half-life of another methylxanthine, theobromine, was decreased by 33% when dietary methylxanthines were restricted (24).

PHARMACOKINETIC ANALYSIS OF THEOPHYLLINE NONLINEARITY

The overall elimination rate of theophylline may be represented by a model with simultaneous supply- and capacity-limited elimination from a single compartment:

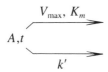

where A is the amount of theophylline in the body at time t; V_{max} and K_m are the maximal metabolic rate and Michaelis constant, respectively, for the formation of MX; and k' is a pooled first-order rate constant representing the sum of the individual rate constants describing the first-order elimination of unchanged theophylline via the urine and first-order metabolism of theophylline to DMU and MU. It is assumed that the formation of MX is characterized by relatively low K_m and V_{max} values, that clearance via this pathway is highly dependent on low serum theophylline concentrations, and that the metabolic pathway becomes saturated quickly as serum theophylline concentrations increase. Furthermore, it is assumed that renal elimination of theophylline is concentration-independent, as it is likely to be after chronic dosing or after acute intoxication, and that the formation of DMU and MU is apparent first order. Conceptually, all saturable elimination processes with similar K_m values have been hybridized in the model through single K_m and V_{max} values, and the renal and remaining pseudolinear metabolic processes have been hybridized through a single first-order rate constant k'.

Mathematically, using concentration terms rather than amount terms, the change in serum concentration, dC/dt, may be described by Eq. 2:

$$dC/dt = -k[(1 - f) + fK_m/(K_m + C)]C \tag{2}$$

where k is the overall observed first-order rate constant at low serum concentrations, f is the fraction of the plasma clearance that occurs by the capacity-limited metabolic pathway, and C is the serum concentration of theophylline. The implicit solution of this model for C as a function of time t is as follows (25):

$$\ln C = \ln C(0) + f/1 - f \ln \left[\frac{1 + (1 - f) C(0)/K_m}{1 + (1 - f) C/K_m} \right] - kt \tag{3}$$

where $C(0)$ is the extrapolated intercept of the initial plasma concentrations.

In the clinical setting, a graphic method for calculation of K_m and V_{max} from a limited amount of serum drug concentration/time data has been described for phenytoin (26). From a linear plot of daily dose (D) steady state serum concentrations (C_{av}) versus daily dose, a straight line is obtained whose slope provides an estimate of K_m and whose x intercept yields an estimate of V_{max}. There have been attempts to apply this method to theophylline data in order to approximate K_m and V_{max} (6). Values of K_m and V_{max} using mean C_{av} data obtained at two different infusion rates of theophylline were 70 mg/liter and 6.6 mg/kg/hr, respectively. However, as these authors pointed out, this graphic method is an oversimplification because a significant fraction of theophylline, unlike phenytoin, is eliminated by multiple apparent first-order pathways in parallel with the Michaelis-Menten pathways, and the first-order component cannot be ignored. In practice, if this method were used to obtain estimates of K_m and V_{max}, the serum theophylline concentrations predicted from a daily dose would be overestimated. Furthermore, a plot of D/C_{av} versus D using several D,C_{av} pairs would most likely not be linear, but concave and asymptotic, with the abscissa at higher doses (27). This trend was beginning to emerge in a plot of the D,C_{av} data obtained for one patient who was reported to exhibit dose-dependent kinetics of theophylline (3). This trend supports the use of a model for theophylline that incorporates the first-order elimination processes, and it suggests that the clearance (expressed as D/C_{av}) decreases as doses are increased. However, at the asymptote achieved at higher doses, the contribution of the nonlinear component of elimination becomes negligible, and the clearance becomes dose-independent.

There is a graphic method that may be used to obtain initial estimates of the apparent Michaelis-Menten constants describing the dose-dependent metabolism $(K_m$ and $V_{max})$ of theophylline and the apparent rate constant describing the dose-independent component of theophylline elimination (k) (25). This method is most precise when a large number of experimental serum drug concentration/time data points are available after administration of a large single bolus dose. Figure 1 is a plot of data obtained after accidental administration of 750 mg of aminophylline over 30 min to a 4-week-old 3.9-kg infant (7).

K_m can be estimated from the time shift, Δt, between the straight line describing the terminal linear phase of the serum concentration/time curve and a parallel straight line originating at the real intercept of the initial serum concentration, $C(0)$ (see Fig. 1):

$$K_m = (1 - f) \, C(0)/\text{antilog} \, [0.434k\Delta t(1 - f)/f] - 1 \qquad (4)$$

where f is the fraction of theophylline clearance occurring via the capacity-limited pathway, determined from the ratio of the slopes of the two straight-line segments in Fig. 1, and k is determined from the slope of the extrapolated terminal linear line segment. V_{max} can be calculated by

$$V_{max} = fkVK_m \qquad (5)$$

where V, the apparent volume of distribution, is determined from $D/C(0)$.

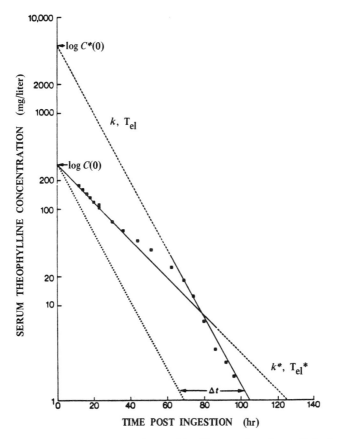

FIG. 1. Serum concentration curve showing combined linear and nonlinear elimination kinetics of theophylline and the procedure for estimating K_m and V_{max}: $C(0)$ is the extrapolated intercept of the initial plasma concentrations; k is the first-order rate constant; T_{el} = time constant $1/k$. *Asterisk* refers to extrapolated line at high concentrations. (Data from Simons et al., ref. 7, and Van Ginneken et al., ref. 25.)

Using this method, the estimated values of the parameters describing supply- and capacity-limited elimination of theophylline are shown in Table 2 for the patient of Simons et al. (7). In addition, serum concentration/time data obtained from two other reports of acute theophylline overdoses were analyzed in a similar way, and the estimated parameters are also shown in Table 2 (8,9).

Under conditions of high serum drug levels ($C \gg K_m$), Eq. 2 becomes

$$dC/dt = -(1 - f) kC - fk K_m \tag{6}$$

Integration of Eq. 6 with the boundary conditions $t = 0$, $C = C(0)$ leads to

$$C = C(0)^{-k^*t} - f/[1 - f K_m(1 - e^{-k^*t})] \tag{7}$$

where $k^* = (1 - f)k$. This equation can be used to predict the serum theophylline concentration curve in the region where $C \gg K_m$.

TABLE 2. *Estimated parameters for simultaneous supply-
and capacity-limited elimination kinetics of theophylline[a]*

	Estimated dose		
	Simons et al. (7) 163.5 mg/ kg	Buchanan et al. (9) 55.6 mg/ kg	Kadlec et al. (8) 97.5 mg/ kg[b]
$C^*(0)$ (mg/liter)[c]	5000	450	1900
$C(0)$ (mg/liter)[c]	300	165	195
V (liter/kg)	0.54	0.34	0.50[d]
k^* (hr^{-1})[c]	0.0456	0.0578	0.0555
k^* (hr^{-1})[c]	0.0815	0.0866	0.128
f	0.44	0.33	0.57
K_m (mg/liter)	4.13	15.3	18.3
V_{max} (mg/kg/hr)	0.095	0.16	0.67

[a]Procedure according to Van Ginneken et al. (25).
[b]Estimated from $D = C(0)V_d$, where V_d is assumed to be 0.5
liter/kg.
[c]Obtained from plot of log C vs. t.
[d]Assumed value.
Asterisk refers to rate constant of initial extrapolated line.

At low serum theophylline levels ($C << K_m$), Eq. 3 becomes

$$\ln C = \ln C(0) + f/1 - f \ln [1 + (1 - f) C(0)/K_m] - kt \qquad (8)$$

This equation can be used to predict the plasma concentration curve along the
terminal linear segment.

Using Eqs. 3 and 7 and the estimated parameters for the patient of Simons et al.
(7) shown in Table 2, the serum theophylline concentrations at selected times were
predicted and compared to the actual serum levels measured in the patient. These
data are shown in Table 3, and it is apparent that there is good agreement between
the actual and predicted levels.

DISCUSSION

The major factors, other than dose or serum concentration, that determine if the
pharmacokinetics of theophylline will be dose-dependent in a given patient are the
following: f, the fraction of clearance that occurs via the saturable metabolic pathway; V_{max}, the metabolic capacity of the liver enzymes involved; and K_m, the
Michaelis-Menten constant. It appears that f is widely variable from patient to
patient, based on 24-hr urine recovery studies of MX. The fraction of theophylline
dose recovered as MX ranges from 0.13 (20) to 0.36 (19). As f increases, the
probability of nonlinear kinetics also increases. From Eq. 5 it can be observed that
for a given V_{max} and constant clearance, K_m is inversely proportional to f. Therefore,
as f increases, K_m decreases, leading to the appearance of dose-dependent kinetics

TABLE 3. *Observed and predicted serum theophylline concentrations at selected times after administration of 750 mg aminophylline to a 3.9-kg 4-week-old infant*

Time after dose (hr)	Serum theophylline concentration (mg/liter)	
	Observed	Predicted
12	177	173[a]
14	158	157[a]
16	143	142[a]
18	131	130[a]
20	119	118[a]
23	106	103[a]
30	74	73[a]
36	59	54[a]
44	47	36[a]
51	38	26[b]
62	25	15[b]
69	18	10[b]
74	12.3	7.7[b]
80	6.8	5.4[b]
86	3.4	3.5[b]
92	2.5	2.5[b]
98	1.8	1.6[b]
107	1.0	0.9[b]

[a]Calculated from Eq. 7 (where observed $C \gg K_m$).
[b]Calculated from Eq. 3.
Data from Simons et al. (7).

at low serum theophylline concentrations. In addition, f is highly dependent on the dietary methylxanthine intake, decreasing as methylxanthine in the diet increases (20). Age does not appear to influence the value of f, based on one study where the patterns of urinary metabolite excretion were found to be the same in children and adults (28) (see Appendix A). Values for K_m and V_{max} are likely to show wide interpatient variability; based on the parameter values in Table 2, V_{max} for the MX pathway is relatively small. In addition, K_m is also small relative to the therapeutic range of theophylline, suggesting that as serum concentrations increase into the therapeutic range above K_m, the process metabolizing theophylline to MX quickly approaches saturation. The contribution of the MX pathway to the overall clearance of theophylline becomes less important as serum levels increase. At high serum levels of theophylline, the elimination half-life will be related to k^* (see Fig. 1), and the kinetics of theophylline will appear to be log linear. At low serum concentrations of theophylline (relative to K_m), the elimination half-life will be determined by k (see Fig. 1) and will again appear to be log linear or first order.

In a clinical setting it seems impossible to correctly estimate f, K_m, and V_{max}. It is likely that doses that would produce the high serum levels needed to define k^*

would lead to toxicity in most patients. A large number of data points would also be required to define both k^* and k.

Several nomograms and methods for individualizing theophylline doses based on single-dose pharmacokinetic data have been described and reported to work well (29,30). However, these approaches to dosing theophylline assume first-order kinetics throughout the range of serum theophylline levels and must therefore be used cautiously. These methods should be considered experimental and should not be accepted routinely until they are proved experimentally to be accurate in a large percentage of patients.

CONCLUSIONS AND THERAPEUTIC IMPLICATIONS

The elimination kinetics of theophylline appear to be nonlinear in a significant percentage of patients receiving the drug. Evidence of nonlinear kinetics include disproportionate changes in serum theophylline concentrations with changes in dosage, biphasic log-linear decay of serum theophylline concentrations following acute administration of high doses, and increases in serum elimination half-life with chronic theophylline dosing. Elimination of theophylline occurs via parallel apparent first-order and Michaelis-Menten pathways, and the nonlinearity arises primarily from the saturation of the 3-methylxanthine metabolic pathway. Dietary intake of methylxanthines appears to influence the rate of formation of 3-methylxanthine. Graphic estimates of K_m and V_{max} in overdosed pediatric patients suggest that nonlinear kinetics are likely to occur in the therapeutic range. Interpatient variability in K_m and V_{max} will be related to the fraction of theophylline cleared via the 3-methylxanthine pathway.

It is clear that adjustments of maintenance theophylline dosages designed to achieve serum concentrations of theophylline in the therapeutic range should be made cautiously and in small increments. There is no proven graphic or mathematical procedure for estimating K_m and V_{max} using a limited number of serum theophylline concentrations obtained in therapeutic drug monitoring. Additional pharmacokinetic studies are needed to define a mathematic model for predicting dose/serum concentration relationships in patients and for defining more clearly the mechanism(s) that account for nonlinear elimination of theophylline.

There is a definite need to conduct additional studies of theophylline elimination kinetics to expand our knowledge of the mechanisms of nonlinearity. Because the majority of reports of nonlinear theophylline kinetics have been in children, this population needs to be included in subsequent studies. The effects of chronic multiple doses on the distribution equilibrium and accumulation of theophylline metabolites, the effects of various dietary methylxanthine regimens, and the effects of high (toxic) serum theophylline concentrations all need to be evaluated with respect to their influence on the appearance of nonlinear elimination kinetics of theophylline.

REFERENCES

1. Tozer, T. N., Tang, D. S., and Riegelman, S. (1981): Linear vs nonlinear kinetics. In: *Topics in Pharmaceutical Sciences*, edited by D. D. Breimer and P. Speiser, pp. 3–17. North-Holland, Amsterdam.
2. Jenne, J. W., Wyze, E., Rood, F. S., and McDonald, F. M. (1972): Pharmacokinetics of theophylline; application to adjustment of the clinical dose of aminophylline. *Clin. Pharmacol. Ther.*, 13:349–360.
3. Sarrazin, E., Hendeles, L., Weinberger, M., Muir, K., and Riegelman, S. (1980): Dose-dependent kinetics for theophylline: Observations among ambulatory asthmatic children. *J. Pediatr.*, 97:825–828.
4. Ginchansky, E., and Weinberger, M. (1977): Relationship of theophylline clearance to oral dosage in children with chronic asthma. *J. Pediatr.*, 91:655–660.
5. Marlin, G. E., Butcher, M. A., Klumpp, J. A., and Thompson, P. J. (1981): Pharmacokinetics of a single evening dose of slow-release theophylline in patients with chronic lung disease. *Br. J. Clin. Pharmacol.*, 12:443–445.
6. Weinberger, M., and Ginchansky, E. (1977): Dose-dependent kinetics of theophylline disposition in asthmatic children. *J. Pediatr.*, 91:820–824.
7. Simons, F. E. R., Friesen, F. R., and Simons, K. J. (1980): Theophylline toxicity in term infants. *Am. J. Dis. Child.*, 134:39–41.
8. Kadlec, G. J., Jarboe, C. H., Pollard, S. J., and Sublett, J. L. (1978): Acute theophylline intoxication. Biphasic first order elimination kinetics in a child. *Ann. Allergy*, 41:337–339.
9. Buchanan, N., Wainwright, L., and DeVilliers, F. (1979): Theophylline poisoning in an infant. *S. Afr. Med. J.*, 56:811–812.
10. Rosenberg, J., Benowitz, N. L., and Pond, S. (1981): Pharmacokinetics of drug overdose. *Clin. Pharmacokinet.*, 6:161–192.
11. Shen, D. D., Fixley, M., and Azarnoff, D. L. (1978): Theophylline bioavailability following chronic dosing of an elixir and two solid dosage forms. *J. Pharm. Sci.*, 67:916–919.
12. Sved, S., McGilveray, I. J., and Wilson, D. L. (1978): Dose-dependent pharmacokinetics of theophylline and the contribution to estimation of bioavailability studies. *Acad. Pharm. Sci.*, 8:77(abstr.).
13. Gotz, V. P., Drayer, D. E., Schned, E. S., and Reidenberg, M. M. (1979): Unusual case of theophylline toxicity. *N. Y. State J. Med.*, 7:1232–1234.
14. Vaucher, Y., Lighter, E. S., and Walson, P. D. (1977): Theophylline poisoning. *J. Pediatr.*, 90:827–830.
15. Weinberger, M., and Bronsky, E. A. (1974): Evaluation of oral bronchodilator therapy in asthmatic children. *J. Pediatr.*, 84:421–427.
16. Nielsen-Kudsk, R., Magnussen, I., Staehelin-Jenson, T., and Naser, K. (1980): Bioavailability and pharmacokinetics in man of orally administered theophylline. *Acta Pharmacol. Toxicol.*, 46:205–212.
17. Cornish, H. H., and Christman, A. A. (1957): A study of the metabolism of theobromine, theophylline, and caffeine in man. *J. Biol. Chem.*, 228:315–323.
18. Thompson, R. D., Nagasawa, H. T., and Jenne, J. W. (1974): Determination of theophylline and its metabolites in human urine and serum by high-pressure liquid chromatography. *J. Lab. Clin. Med.*, 84:584–594.
19. Jenne, J. W., Nagasawa, H. T., and Thompson, R. D. (1976): Relationship of urinary metabolites of theophylline to serum theophylline levels. *Clin. Pharmacol. Ther.*, 19:375–381.
20. Monks, T. J., Caldwell, J., and Smith, R. L. (1979): Influence of methylxanthine-containing foods on theophylline metabolism and kinetics. *Clin. Pharmacol. Ther.*, 26:513–524.
21. Levy, G., Tsuchiya, T., and Amsel, L. P. (1972): Limited capacity for salicyl phenolic glucuronide formation and its effect on the kinetics of salicylate elimination in man. *Clin. Pharmacol. Ther.*, 13:258–268.
22. Kappas, A., Anderson, K. E., Conney, A. H., and Alvares, A. P. (1976): Influence of dietary protein and carbohydrate on antipyrine and theophylline metabolism. *Clin. Pharmacol. Ther.*, 20:643–653.
23. Kappas, A., Alvares, A. P., Anderson, K. E., Pantuck, E. J., Pantuck, C. B., Chang, R., and Conney, A. H. (1978): Effect of charcoal-broiled beef on antipyrine and theophylline metabolism. *Clin. Pharmacol. Ther.*, 23:445–450.

24. Drouillard, D. D., Vesell, E. S., and Dvorchick, B. H. (1978): Studies on theobromine disposition in normal subjects. *Clin. Pharmacol. Ther.*, 23:296–302.
25. Van Ginneken, C. A. M., Van Rossum, J. M., and Fleuren, H. L. J. M. (1974): Linear and non-linear kinetics of drug elimination with or without simultaneous supply-limited elimination. *J. Pharmacokinet. Bipharm.*, 2:395–415.
26. Ludden, T. M., Allen, J. P., Valutsky, W. A., Vincuna, A. V., Nappi, J. M., Hoffman, S. F., Wallace, J. E., Lalka, D., and McNay, J. L. (1977): Individualization of phenytoin dosage regimens. *Clin. Pharmacol. Ther.*, 21:287–292.
27. Martin, E., Tozer, T. N., Sheiner, L. B., and Riegelman, S. (1977): The clinical pharmacokinetics of phenytoin in man. *J. Pharmacokinet. Biopharm.*, 5:579–596.
28. Verbesselt, R., Tjandramaga, T. B., and DeSchepper, P. J. (1980): A simple method for simultaneous determination of theophylline and its metabolites in urine. World Conference on Clinical Pharmacology and Therapy (Abstr.).
29. Koup, J. R., Sack, C. M., Smith, A. L., and Gibaldi, M. (1979): Hypothesis for the individualization of drug dosage. *Clin. Pharmacokinet.*, 4:460–469.
30. Pancorbo, S., Sawchuk, R. J., Zaske, C. H., and Schallock, M. (1979): Use of pharmacokinetic model for individualizing intravenous doses of aminophylline. *Eur. J. Clin. Pharmacol.*, 16:251–254.
31. Bonati, M., and Latini, R. (1980): Theophylline and 3-methylxanthine kinetics in man. World Conference on Clinical Pharmacology and Therapy (Abstr.).
32. Jonkman, J. H. G., Tang, D., Upton, R. A., and Riegelman, S. (1981): Measurement of excretion characteristics of theophylline and its major metabolites. *Eur. J. Clin. Pharmacol.*, 20:435–441.
33. Tang-Liu, D., Williams, R. L., and Riegelman, S. (1982): Nonlinear theophylline elimination. *Clin. Pharmacol. Ther.*, 31:358–369.
34. Remy-Gundert, U., Hildebrandt, R., Hengen, N., and Weber, E. (1983): Nonlinear elimination processes of theophylline. *Eur. J. Clin. Pharmacol.*, 24:71–78.

Pharmacokinetic Basis for Drug Treatment,
edited by L. Z. Benet et al., Raven Press,
New York © 1984

Chapter 18

Drug Absorption and Disposition in Burn Patients

Ronald J. Sawchuk

*Department of Pharmaceutics, College of Pharmacy, University of Minnesota,
Minneapolis, Minnesota 55455*

The absorption, distribution, metabolism, and renal excretion of a therapeutic agent are related to its physicochemical properties and the pathophysiologic state of the patient. Thermal injury produces a wide variety of intricate physiologic alterations that often involve cardiovascular, hepatic, renal, and dermatological functions. Individual responses to varying degrees of burns and secondary complications may produce unpredictable changes in the pharmacokinetics of drugs.

This chapter briefly reviews pathophysiologic changes that occur following burns and summarizes the results of studies that have investigated the pharmacokinetics of systemic and topical agents in burn patients.

PATHOPHYSIOLOGIC CONSIDERATIONS IN BURN PATIENTS

Following extensive thermal injury, an inflammatory reaction occurs, rapidly resulting in edema formation owing to increased microvascular permeability, vasodilation, and increased extravascular osmotic activity. This reaction results from the direct effect of heat on capillary beds and, in remote tissues, from the effect of histamine and other mediators of inflammation. Such changes are accompanied by increased prostaglandin synthesis from arachidonic acid. Prostaglandins inhibit the release of norepinephrine and are thus believed to be important in altering the responsiveness of the adrenergic nervous system.

Interstitial tissue changes also occur following burn injury. Fluid loss from the vasculature in the injured area results in a rapid decrease in plasma volume and a rise in hematocrit, with decreased cardiac output and tissue hypoperfusion. Unless fluid loss is corrected, burn shock will develop. The word *shock* denotes a clinical entity in which there is inadequate cardiac output and deficient perfusion of organs and tissues. In addition, the burn patient is dangerously exposed to surface infection with a great risk of septic shock. Pathophysiologic changes and the principles of management of the burn patient have been reviewed (1).

333

Cardiovascular Alterations

Abnormal cardiac output can theoretically alter the pharmacokinetic profiles of certain agents by altering perfusion to sites of absorption, distribution, elimination, and the biophase. Ten patients with burns averaging 64.5% of the body had cardiac outputs determined by an indocyanine green dilution technique (2). Within 6 hr of burn injury, cardiac outputs decreased as much as 50%. Concurrent fluid and colloid resuscitation offset the circulatory deficiency and produced supranormal cardiac outputs within 1 to 4 days.

Cardiac output and splanchnic blood flow were measured simultaneously in 3 patients using indocyanine green by Gump et al. (3). Extent of burns ranged from 25% to 60% of body surface. Seven to 26 days after trauma a smaller than normal fraction of the cardiac output was delivered to the right hepatic vein. However, the hepatic flow rate was greater than normal because of elevated cardiac output.

In a study by Aulick et al. (4), the effect of thermal injury on visceral blood flow was examined by measuring paraaminohippuric acid (PAH) clearance and indocyanine green (ICG) clearance. From an analysis of 13 nonbacteremic patients with burns averaging 50% of body surface area (BSA) studied 6 to 25 days post injury these authors found that the effective renal blood flow (ERBF), as measured by PAH clearance, was not different from that in controls ($N = 5$). They concluded that ERBF does not always rise after burn injury, but rather is dependent on sodium load and/or vascular volume. However, in a matched group of 10 burn patients, they found significant increases in splanchnic blood flow (SBF) and cardiac output using ICG clearance and dilution techniques, respectively. SBF was found to be twice normal and to be 19% of the cardiac output. The effect of increased cardiac output on peripheral perfusion remains open to speculation.

Variations in plasma volume determined by administering labeled albumin correspond to changes in cardiac output. Destruction of red blood cell mass further reduces blood volume in burn patients (5).

A recent report (6) has described the existence of cardiotoxic substances in the sera of severely burned patients. One of these appears to be a small protein (molecular weight 12,000–14,000). A purified preparation of this material has yielded a lower-molecular-weight substance capable of altering ECG patterns, indicating decreased cardiac output and other disturbances. These authors suggested that this toxic factor may explain, in part, the cardiovascular complications observed in some burn patients.

Factors Affecting Fluid Balance and Drug Distribution

Burn-induced alterations in transcapillary transport have been reviewed (7). Following a burn, an inflammatory reaction results in edema because of (a) dilatation of resistance vessels, with an increased filtration pressure across the capillary, (b) increased osmotic activity in burned tissue, and (c) increased permeability of the microvasculature to macromolecules. In extensive burn injury, the latter has also

been observed in nonburned tissues, presumably because of the release of histamine and other mediators of inflammation.

It has been shown that the normal circadian pattern of serum aldosterone and cortisol levels, as well as renin activity, is altered in patients immediately following thermal injury (8). The circadian rhythm was not evident during the 5 consecutive days post burn; instead, the hormone levels were found to be very elevated, and 4 of the 10 patients studied developed hypertensive crisis.

Intravascular albumin concentrations in burn patients may fluctuate because of increased catabolism, altered capillary permeability, and transfusion of albumin-containing fluids, but they tend to be depressed to 1.0 to 3.0 g/dl for several weeks (9–12).

The volume of distribution for some drugs may be increased by extravascular movement of fluids and albumin. Also, a substantially faster rate of insensible water loss attributed to damaged stratum corneum and hyperventilation (13), combined with fluid resuscitation, may result in a fluctuating distribution volume for some drugs in burn patients.

In addition, an albumin deficit decreases the number of drug binding sites, allowing more free drug to distribute into greater volumes. Furthermore, hyperbilirubinemia (14) and elevated free fatty acid concentrations associated with burns (15,16) may reduce the bound fraction for certain drug agents.

Lipoprotein changes were examined in a study of 16 burn-injured patients (17). It was observed that high-density lipoprotein (HDL) serum levels fell drastically in these patients, and it was suggested that because HDL is required in the conversion of very-low-density lipoprotein to low-density lipoprotein, this loss in HDL may account in part for the hypertriglyceridemia, hypocholesterolemia, and hypophospholipidemia noted after burn injury.

In a study (18) of 30 patients with burned body surface area averaging 60%, it was observed that the essential fatty acid composition of total plasma lipids was decreased. The ratio of free fatty acids to albumin in plasma, however, was greatly increased. It is conceivable that the protein binding for a number of basic drugs can be altered significantly in burn patients, because the level of α_1-acid glycoprotein, which appears to be responsible for the binding of some bases (19,20), is increased by inflammatory reactions. In addition to the changes in distribution patterns induced by binding alterations, it is clear that a disturbance of plasma protein drug binding can alter the metabolic or renal clearance of certain drugs.

Alterations in Metabolic Function

Hypercatabolism is often a consequence of major burns and has been related to evaporative heat loss (21) and excessive catecholamine secretion (22–24).

Metabolic studies on 23 burned children studied sequentially were performed to examine the effect of occlusive dressings on energy requirements (25). The investigators used a heat-balance equation, employing measurements of oxygen consumption and carbon dioxide production rates, rectal temperature, average surface

temperature, rate of body weight loss, and body heat content. It was found that occlusive dressings substantially reduced the energy requirements to manageable levels and that increased heat production in burn patients is a response to an increased rate of heat loss, not vice versa. This is confirmed by the findings of Crabtree et al. (26), who examined heat production and loss in anesthetized children with burns. Heat production increased significantly, although not enough to offset increased heat loss, reflecting a block in central thermoregulation induced by methoxyflurane anesthesia.

Systemic metabolic and circulatory alterations induced by thermal injury as they relate to energy production and utilization have been reviewed (27); however, the mechanisms responsible for these alterations are not known.

In a recent study (28) on burn patients it was demonstrated that the iron-binding glycoprotein in transferrin was more rapidly synthesized and degraded during burn injury than following recovery.

The effects of severe burns on the activity of drug-metabolizing enzymes have not been extensively investigated. A prospective monitoring of 81 burn patients provided clinical and/or laboratory evidence of hepatic injury in 58% of the subjects (14). Enzyme patterns and histological findings were consistent with acute hemolysis and anoxic hepatocellular damage.

One report has compared 24-hr urinary D-glucaric acid measurements in 5 treated burn patients and 6 healthy controls (29). Burns ranged from 6% to 53%, and sample collection varied from the first days following injury to 3 months. Urinary D-glucaric acid output was 14.4 ± 5.4 (mean ± SE) μmoles/day versus 28.7 ± 6.5 for controls ($p < 0.002$). Although it has not been proved that a decrease in urinary glucaric acid results from a decrease in drug-metabolizing enzyme activity, there is a strong correlation between increased urinary output of glucaric acid and increased drug metabolism. It is conceivable, therefore, that drug-metabolizing activity is decreased in some burn patients. This may have implications for therapy with drugs that, although extensively metabolized, exhibit low intrinsic clearances. The clearance of such agents may be affected more by changes in enzyme activity than by alterations in the perfusion of metabolizing organs.

Additional evidence suggesting decreases in enzyme activity associated with burn injury comes from animal studies. *In vitro* investigations using rat liver homogenates demonstrated a significant decrease in the metabolism of benzopyrene to 3-hydroxybenzopyrene after 15% third-degree burns (30).

Alterations in Renal Function

Varying degrees of renal dysfunction may occur secondary to burn trauma. The renal clearance of a drug following a burn injury may be affected by tubular necrosis, altered renal plasma flow, and altered protein binding in an unpredictable manner. Glomerular filtration rate is a function of the mean transcapillary hydraulic pressure, the ultrafiltration coefficient, the renal plasma flow rate, and the protein concentration in afferent plasma (31). Twelve-hour creatinine clearances were calculated

from total creatinine excreted in urine and the midpoint plasma creatinine concentration in 110 patients with greater than 15% burns (32). Although actual data were not presented, the clearances were reported to be depressed in all severely burned patients. Maximum reductions occurred 2 to 4 days after injury and usually normalized within 2 to 3 weeks. Some patients became oliguric or anuric either immediately or several days following the burn. Oliguria did not always correlate with reduced creatinine clearances, nor was oliguria related to fluid therapy.

A second study determined serial creatinine clearances in burn patients (33). Values fluctuated, but a downward trend was evident in most of the 13 subjects. Several patients with reduced creatinine clearance had normal urine output. The excretion of filtered water was inversely related to the glomerular filtration rate. Kidney specimens from 7 patients were examined and found to be histologically consistent with tubular casts and necrosis. These authors postulated that oliguria occurs only when there is a substantial reduction in functional tubular mass and when decreased glomerular filtration cannot be countered by the increased excretion of filtered water. Other data suggest that urine output in burn patients correlates with impaired osmolal regulation (34).

Some investigators have detected elevated glomerular filtration rates after burn trauma (35). Creatinine clearances in 20 patients with burns averaging $33 \pm 21.3\%$ of total body surface were 172.1 ± 48 ml/min/1.73 m^2. Eight normal subjects had clearance values of 125.4 ± 10.4 ml/min/1.73 m^2 ($p < 0.02$). These studies were performed from 4 to 35 days post burn, but those patients who exhibited "higher" creatinine clearance were evaluated within the first 2 weeks.

Percutaneous Absorption

Percutaneous absorption, the process of diffusive penetration through the skin, may be substantially increased through burned tissue. Normally, a drug must diffuse from a topically administered dosage form into the stratum corneum and pilosebaceous gland ducts. Further movement transcending the epidermal strata is required before the drug becomes available to the systemic circulation (36). Burn injury can destroy these normal barriers, and depending on the degree of burn and surface area involved, the systemic absorption of topical medications may be clinically significantly enhanced if the local vasculature remains intact.

Research involving humans to investigate the net effects of these pathophysiologic changes on the pharmacokinetics of drugs and the clinical consequences of such changes is generally lacking. A review of specific drug studies follow.

PHARMACOKINETIC STUDIES AND OBSERVATIONS IN BURN PATIENTS

Systemic Therapy

Tobramycin

Ciarpella and Lombardi (37) reported treating 10 burn patients with infections. Intramuscular tobramycin at doses ranging from 2.3 to 5.8 mg/kg/day for 1 to 4

weeks resulted in recovery for 9 patients. Although tobramycin levels were determined after the first dose and on the third, sixth, and ninth days of therapy, the concentrations were not reported; however, these authors observed no accumulation of antibiotic.

In a more recent study by Loirat et al. (35), glomerular filtration rates were found to rise significantly in 13 of 20 burned patients. Creatinine clearances were more than 2 standard deviations above the normal mean. No correlation was found between these elevated creatinine clearances and fluid intake, urinary output, temperature, or burned surface area. However, patients with high creatinine clearances were significantly younger than patients with normal clearances. The increased values were confirmed by measuring inulin or iothalamate clearance in 9 of these patients. The pharmacokinetic profile of tobramycin, which is eliminated primarily as unchanged drug by the kidneys, was characterized in 11 of the 20 burned patients and in 8 normal individuals. The calculated volumes of distribution were not significantly different between normals (0.23 liter/kg) and the burn patients exhibiting a high creatinine clearance (0.28 liter/kg), but a significant difference ($p < 0.01$) in mean tobramycin serum half-life was found between the former (1.13 hr) and the latter (0.85 hr) group. Hypoproteinemia was observed in the burned patients in this study when plasma protein concentrations were determined. Although renal plasma flow was not measured, these authors postulated that an increase in this parameter may result from supranormal cardiac output. These authors concluded that the reduced half-life of tobramycin in these patients was related to increased renal clearance, but factors other than glomerular filtration rate may be involved.

Two other investigators have suggested possible mechanisms explaining increased glomerular filtration rates in burned patients. Harrison (38) has suggested that prostaglandins, which significantly increase the glomerular filtration rate (39), are formed in the skin after burn injury (40) and can be present in sufficient concentration to produce glomerular filtration rate changes at the time Loirat et al. (35) would have observed these alterations. The second hypothesis (41) to explain these observations is based on increased glucagon secretion in patients with severe burn trauma (16,42). Glucagon has been reported to enhance glomerular filtration (43).

Gentamicin

Eleven burn patients, ranging in age from 1.5 to 64 years, received much higher than recommended doses of gentamicin to maintain therapeutic peak serum concentrations (44). One 4-year-old patient who exhibited a gentamicin half-life of 0.7 hr needed 16.7 mg/kg body wt per day. Two other children required doses in excess of 10 mg/kg daily for optimal therapy, and they showed gentamicin half-lives of 1.2 and 1.6 hr. Others (45–47) have reported gentamicin half-life in unburned children as 2.5 to 3.5 hr. Because none of these 3 patients demonstrated abnormal creatinine clearances or gentamicin distribution volumes, the relatively short half-life periods may be due, in part, to loss of drug via burn wounds.

Glew et al. (48) calculated that 20% of the daily dose of gentamicin was lost into burn-wound dressings when a 15-year-old boy with 45% body surface area

burns was treated. However, negligible amounts of gentamicin were recovered in the dressings of a 9-year-old with 30% body surface area burns. In their study of 18 burned children, larger doses at more frequent intervals than normally utilized were often necessary. They surmised that the increased dosage requirements resulted from either loss of drug across burn wounds or increased renal excretion. In small children and infants, wound losses may be more significant because of their relatively high surface area/volume ratio.

Similarly, an additional study of 14 burn patients demonstrated that the recommended daily dose of gentamicin (5 mg/kg/day) yielded low serum gentamicin concentrations (49). Patients ranged in age from 1.5 to 64 years, and surface area burns from 25% to 85%. All patients were at least 5 days post burn. Gentamicin half-life periods were unusually short, especially in patients under 20 years of age (1.1 ± 0.44 hr). To maintain peak serum gentamicin levels in the range of 7 to 8 µg/ml, the average dose required in the group of older patients was 7.2 mg/kg/day, and in the younger patients 12.8 mg/kg/day. For patients with relatively short half-life periods, it was necessary to decrease the dosing interval to 4 hr to prevent prolonged periods of subtherapeutic serum concentrations. These authors strongly recommended individualization of gentamicin dosing regimens for burned patients with life-threatening infections.

In a report (50) describing the successful treatment of 4 burn patients with ecthyma gangrenosum, the authors individualized gentamicin therapy using daily doses (15–30 mg/kg) that were three to six times those recommended. A fifth patient who received much lower daily doses did not survive. No nephrotoxic or ototoxic reactions were noted in any of the patients.

In a comparative study of the efficacy of tobramycin and gentamicin in treating surgical infections, 20 burn patients were among those evaluated (51). Patients received 1 mg/kg of aminoglycoside intramuscularly every 8 hr for 7 to 10 days. Burn patients also received topical therapy using a neomycin-polymyxin aerosol. Serum aminoglycoside concentrations were determined by a microagar punch technique at 2 and 6 hr following administration. The average aminoglycoside serum concentration achieved at 2 hr in nonburn patients was less than 2 µg/ml, compared with a mean level exceeding 10 µg/ml in the burn patients. These authors believed that the topical neomycin-polymyxin therapy augmented these values, but they did not speculate as to the reason. Assay interference, relatively small distribution volumes for the aminoglycoside (< 0.10 liter/kg), or more rapid intramuscular absorption rates in burn patients may have been contributing factors.

Amikacin

Zaske et al. (52) investigated extended periods of subtherapeutic serum levels of amikacin initially observed in 5 burn patients receiving the recommended intravenous dose of 7.5 mg/kg every 12 hr. For the 10 patients subsequently studied, the mean amikacin half-life was unusually short (1.4 ± 0.54 hr). An intravenous dosage regimen of 7.5 mg/kg every 6 hr produced therapeutic peak concentrations

of amikacin and shortened periods of subtherapeutic concentrations. Although a transient episode of tinnitus occurred in 1 subject, no other signs of ototoxicity or nephrotoxicity were evident in any patient. Because of the wide interpatient variability of amikacin elimination, even in patients with normal renal function, these authors recommend individualization of amikacin dosage to provide optimal serum concentrations.

The pharmacokinetics of amikacin have been studied in an additional 30 burn patients (53). An intravenous dose of 2 mg/kg was administered, and four serum levels were determined over the next 2 hr. Because of the short sampling period, their results are difficult to evaluate. A more rapid decline of serum concentrations was seen in patients who were more than 8 days post burn, as compared with patients within 3 days of burn trauma. Unfortunately, renal function could not be assessed in these patients.

Another study of amikacin in patients with 20% to 60% body surface area burns was reported by Palayret et al. (54). Dosages of 7 to 10 mg/kg infused over 60 to 90 min provided efficacious serum concentrations in most patients. Average peak levels of 20.6 mg/liter ($N = 14$) were obtained after the initial dose, decreasing to 5.4 mg/liter within 6 hr. These authors observed no drug accumulation after three doses; however, a mean value of 5.4 mg/liter 6 hr after infusion of the initial dose suggests that some degree of accumulation could be expected on a regimen of dosing every 6 hr. The adoption of a standard dose of amikacin for burn patients may result in inappropriate therapy for some; thus, these authors suggested that monitoring serum amikacin levels is desirable in burn patients.

d-*Tubocurarine*

A recent study on the plasma protein binding of *d*-tubocurarine in the plasma of burn patients has shown a 1.7-fold increase in *d*-tubocurarine binding over that in normal plasma in 1 to 2 weeks following burn injury (55). This timing corresponds to the onset of hyposensitivity of burn patients to this drug observed here and in an earlier report (56). Calculations based on the results of their equilibrium dialysis experiments using radiolabeled drug accounted for only a fraction of the observed hyposensitivity. Despite lower total plasma protein, burn patients ($N = 16$) exhibited 71% binding, compared with 51% binding in control plasma at equivalent free concentrations of 0.34 μg/ml. In an additional study of 7 burn patients discussed in the same report, these authors similarly examined the binding of labeled metocurine (tubocurarine dimethyl ether) and found that, despite lower total plasma protein concentrations, the binding of this skeletal muscle relaxant was increased ($p < 0.005$) over that in control plasma.

Interestingly, these investigators noted that because all plasma proteins (including α_1- and γ-globulin) except for albumin were within normal limits in the plasma of these patients, there must be a qualitative change in a subfraction responsible for the binding alterations observed. They suggested that α_1- and γ-globulin may be involved. It has been demonstrated that increased levels of α_1-acid glycoprotein

induced by inflammation are associated with increased binding of cationic drugs (57). These authors suggested that other factors, such as alterations involving synaptic membranes in the target tissue, also contribute to the decreased sensitivity of burn patients to these agents.

Phenytoin

The observation of unexpectedly low serum phenytoin concentrations in burned epileptic patients maintained on their normal regimen prompted Bowdle et al. (58) to examine phenytoin plasma binding in 4 burned patients. These investigators found that the plasma protein binding of this drug was significantly decreased, with 25.8% unbound (normal, approximately 10%). Serum albumin was decreased (2.68 vs 3.5 g/dl in normals) as expected. These authors pointed out that although it has been reported that the free fraction of phenytoin is inversely proportional to albumin concentration, and that the increase in phenytoin free fraction may be due to the decrease in plasma albumin, other factors may be involved for other drugs. They reported that their preliminary studies showed a fivefold increase in free fraction of valproic acid in the plasma of burn patients, with only a 50% decrease in albumin, and they suggested that displacers may also be present in the plasma of these patients.

Topical Therapy

Nitrates

Although the use of topical silver nitrate is no longer common in therapy for burn patients, it was often applied to burn wounds using a thick dressing of coarse mesh gauze kept continuously wet with 0.5% silver nitrate solution. However, its use gradually declined because of a number of objections and apparent problems, not the least of which were argyria (59,60) and methemoglobinemia (61).

Three workers sprayed with molten chemicals, including potassium nitrate, in an industrial accident suffered body burns encrusted with these chemicals (62). All three rapidly developed methemoglobinemia from nitrate absorption via their burns. Following a brief delay in diagnosis, appropriate therapy (high-flow oxygen and methylene blue) resulted in favorable outcomes for two of the burn patients.

Mafenide

Mafenide acetate is a sulfonamide derivative active against *Pseudomonas* organisms when applied as a cream to burn wounds. The effectiveness against bacterial colonization has been related to good penetration of the eschar (63,64). Systemic effects on the acid–base balance and ventilatory patterns in burn patients have been observed following topical administration (63,65,66).

Drug absorption and metabolism were studied in 10 burn patients receiving topical mafenide acetate applications within 48 hr of injury (67). Peak blood levels of mafenide and its metabolite, *p*-carboxybenzene sulfonamide, occurred 2 and 4 hr, respectively, after application to the burn tissue. The maximum concentrations

ranged from 0.05 to 1.7 μmoles/liter and were higher in patients with evidence of reduced glomerular filtration rate. Blood levels of both parent drug and metabolite were undetectable 24 hr after application of the cream. Because the data reported were incomplete, quantitation of the absorption and elimination kinetics of mafenide was not possible.

Harrison et al. (68) investigated the absorption of ^{14}C-mafenide acetate through burned human and rat skin. The penetration studies demonstrated that the drug reached the subeschar tissue within 30 min in both species. Analysis of drug depletion from the cream showed that only 10% of the inital concentration remained after 4 to 6 hr of application under their experimental conditions. Factors controlling the rate of absorption of mafenide acetate were identified as (a) the nature of the layer between the cream and the wound tissue, (b) the nature of hydration of the cream, (c) the thickness of the cream layer, and (d) the concentration of drug in the cream. Delivery of mafenide acetate from gauze dressings saturated with a 5% aqueous solution to excised human and burned rat skin was also investigated (69). Peak tissue concentrations observed at 4 hr were similar to those previously observed using 11.2% mafenide acetate in a cream base. The favorable concentration gradient from the application vehicle to the wound tissue may be attributable to the appreciable amount of water absorbed by the wound. The rate of drug delivery was calculated to range from 0.24 to 0.40 g/kg/hr for each square meter of burn treated.

Povidone Iodine

Povidone iodine has been used as an effective nonabsorbable antimicrobial agent for many patients. Current marketed preparations provide approximately 1% free iodine. When povidone iodine is applied to burn wounds, evidence suggests that the traumatized areas allow substantial systemic absorption of iodine.

In a study of 5 patients suffering 23% to 86% second- and third-degree burns, serum iodide levels ranged from 1.4 to 41.3 mg/dl subsequent to treatment with povidone iodine ointment (70). The most elevated serum iodide concentrations were observed in the subjects with varying degrees of renal dysfunction. One patient with an initial serum iodide of 41.3 mg/dl underwent peritoneal dialysis, resulting in the collection of 17 g of free iodide during a 48-hr period. The peritoneal dialysis clearance was estimated to be 50 to 70 ml/min.

Two other patients with 35% and 75% burns had serum iodide concentrations of 17.6 and 48 mg/dl after povidone iodine ointment therapy (71). Both patients concentrated free iodine in the urine to approximately 50 mg/dl.

Another 17 burn patients treated with povidone iodine ointment within 24 hr of injury had peak serum iodide levels ranging from 0.6 to 4.9 mg/dl (72). Systemic iodine accumulated as treatment continued and remained elevated for as long as 1 week following discontinuation. Reduced urine outputs were coincidental with lower urinary iodine concentrations. The amount of iodine absorbed from the wound appeared to correlate with the size of the burn injury.

The potential for nephrotoxicity and metabolic acidosis resulting from excessive iodine levels in burn patients treated with topical iodine preparations requires further study.

Silver Sulfadiazine

Twelve hospitalized patients with variable extent and depth of burns were treated daily for a period of 5 to 15 days with 1% silver sulfadiazine cream (73). Plasma concentrations and daily urinary output of unconjugated and total sulfonamide were determined. In 3 patients with 17% to 46% burned surface area, approximately 20% to 25% of the daily topical dose could be accounted for in the urine as conjugated sulfonamide. Unconjugated drug represented from 35% to 95% of the total output. Total plasma sulfonamide concentrations did not exceed 10 μg/ml.

A more recent study (74) examined the attachment of ^{110}Ag-labeled silver sulfadiazine to burned human skin, as well as full- and partial-thickness scald burns of rats. Less than 8% of the topical dose was localized in the rat skin after 24 hr, and only 1.4% was localized in human full-thickness burns. Over 80% of the silver was associated with the epidermal layer. Only background radioactivity was detected in the blood and visceral organs of the rats studied. The surface attachment of silver observed was in agreement with the results of Lazare et al. (75), who examined pig scald burns, and it also confirms the findings of Catania and King (76), who concluded, based on data from burned guinea pigs, that silver sulfadiazine would not be the agent of choice when treating subeschar infections.

Propylene Glycol

In a recent report, serum hyperosmolality was noted in a group of hospitalized burn patients (77). Further analysis of the patients' serum by gas chromatography revealed propylene glycol as the compound responsible for most of the osmolal discrepancy. The only exposure to this glycol was from a topical cream containing silver sulfadiazine.

These authors did not try to determine the extent of absorption of propylene glycol via the burn wounds. This report confirmed the earlier observations of others (78), who found propylene glycol in the serum of 2 patients treated with a similar preparation.

Lidocaine

The absorption of lidocaine from a topically applied dosage form was examined in patients undergoing treatment of skin graft donor sites and treatment of burns (79). These authors found a significant degree of absorption of lidocaine from the jelly only in patients with thermal burns, with the extent of absorption dependent on the surface area of the wound. These authors recommend caution in using this jelly in burn patients, although no systemic toxicity was noted in their study.

Gentamicin

Stone et al. (80) reported on the systemic absorption of topical gentamicin in burn patients using either a water-miscible cream or a petrolatum ointment. Patients (N = 22) with 22% to 88% third-degree burns were studied. Based on urinary gentamicin output, greater systemic absorption occurred from the cream, but absorbed amounts were negligible. Increased absorption from the cream was thought to be related to the extent of hydration; this appeared to be maximal immediately post injury or during profuse exudation.

A preliminary report evaluating the efficacy of topical gentamicin described systemic absorption from a 0.1% cream (81). Fourteen patients with burns ranging from 11% to 75% were treated by covering all burned areas with gentamicin cream. Occlusive gauze dressings were changed daily. Periodic serum gentamicin assays revealed concentrations ranging from 0.6 to 2.5 μg/ml. Serum levels were not correlated with percentage of body surface area burned. The extent of absorption could not be calculated from the data. The appearance of a gentamicin-resistant strain of *Pseudomonas* was alluded to by these authors. This problem has been documented elsewhere, and the use of topical aminoglycoside preparations has been seriously questioned (82,83).

Two patients suffering extensive thermal trauma were treated with topical gentamicin for 10 and 22 days (84). Although details of the amount of drug applied and time of serum sampling are lacking, both patients, who had normal renal function, developed progressive hearing loss. Serum levels measured were 1.0 to 3.0 μg/ml and 3.3 to 4.3 μg/ml, respectively.

CONCLUSIONS

Many of the reports concerning the absorption and elimination of drugs in burn patients do not provide sufficient information for proper interpretation of the study results. In some cases, available data were not included in the reports. In other instances, it is likely that required data could not be collected during the study. It is clear that prospective controlled studies in a population of burn patients are difficult to perform. In addition, the marked variability in the nature of the injury (the extent and degree of burn) suggests that comparisons between burn and nonburn patients would be unlikely to demonstrate significant differences in pharmacokinetic parameters.

Although there has been some research in the area of urinary excretion of drugs in burn patients, the results are contradictory. Again, the nature of the injury and the timing of the study relative to the burn probably account, at least in part, for these discrepancies.

There is a need for well-controlled studies to further investigate pathophysiologic changes secondary to burn injury and the effects of changes on drug disposition. Additional research using animal models will assist in defining the mechanisms responsible for alterations in drug absorption, distribution, and elimination in burn patients.

REFERENCES

1. Arturson, G. (1980): Pathophysiology of the burn wound. *Ann. Chir. Gynaecol.*, 69:178–190.
2. Pruitt, B. A., Mason, A. D., and Moncrief, J. A. (1971): Hemodynamic changes in the early postburn patient: The influence of fluid administration and of a vasodilator (hydralazine). *J. Trauma*, 11:36–46.
3. Gump, F. E., Price, J. B., and Kinney, J. M. (1970): Blood flow and oxygen consumption in patients with severe burns. *Surg. Gynecol. Obstet.*, 130:23–28.
4. Aulick, L. H., Goodwin, C. W., Jr., Becker, R. A., and Wilmore, D. W. (1981): Visceral blood flow following thermal injury. *Ann. Surg.*, 193:112–116.
5. Davies, J. W. L. (1964): Blood volume changes in patients with burns treated with either colloid or saline solutions. *Clin. Sci.*, 26:429–443.
6. Moati, F., Sepulchre, C., Miskulin, M., Huisman, O., Moczar, E., Robert, A. M., Monteil, R., and Guilbaud, J. (1979): Biochemical and pharmacological properties of a cardiotoxic factor isolated from the blood serum of burned patients. *J. Pathol.*, 127:147–156.
7. Arturson, G., and Jonsson, C. E. (1979): Transcapillary transport after thermal injury. *Scand. J. Plast. Reconstr. Surg.*, 13:29–38.
8. Molteni, A., Warpeha, R. L., Brizio-Molteni, L., Albertson, D. F., and Kaurs, R. (1979): Circadian rhythms of serum aldosterone, cortisol and plasma renin activity in burn injuries. *Ann. Clin. Lab. Sci.*, 9:518–523.
9. Alexander, J. W., Brown, W., Mason, A. D., and Moncrief, J. A. (1966): The influence of infection upon serum protein changes in severe burns. *J. Trauma*, 6:780–789.
10. Alexander, J. W., Ogle, C. K., Stinnett, J. D., White, M., MacMillan, B. G., and Edwards, B. K. (1979): Fresh-frozen plasma vs plasma protein derivative as adjunctive therapy for patients with massive burns. *J. Trauma*, 19:502–511.
11. Birke, G., Liljedahl, S.-O., Plantin, L.-O., and Wetterfors, J. (1959–60): Albumin catabolism in burns and following surgical procedures. *Acta Chirurg. Scand.*, 118:353–366.
12. Davies, J. W. L., Ricketts, C. R., and Bull, J. P. (1962): Studies of plasma protein metabolism. Part I. Albumin in burned and injured patients. *Clin. Sci.*, 23:411–423.
13. Fallon, R. H., and Moyer, C. A. (1963): Rates of insensible perspiration through normal, burned, tape stripped, and epidermally denuded living human skin. *Ann. Surg.*, 158:915–923.
14. Czaja, A. J., Rizzo, T. A., Smith, W. R., and Pruitt, B. A. (1975): Acute liver disease after cutaneous thermal injury. *J. Trauma*, 15:887–894.
15. Carlson, I. A. (1970): Mobilization and utilization of lipids after trauma: Relation to caloric homeostasis. In: *Energy Metabolism in Trauma*, edited by R. Porter and J. Knight, pp. 155–163. Churchill, London.
16. Shuck, J. M., Eaton, R. P., Shuck, L. W., Wachtel, T. L., and Schade, D. S. (1977): Dynamics of insulin and glucagon secretions in severely burned patients. *J. Trauma*, 17:706–713.
17. Coombes, E. J., Shakespeare, P. G., and Batstone, G. F. (1980): Lipoprotein changes after burn injury in man. *J. Trauma*, 20:971–975.
18. Harris, R. L., Cottam, G. L., Johnston, J. M., and Baxter, C. R. (1981): The pathogenesis of abnormal erythrocyte morphology in burns. *J. Trauma*, 21:13–21.
19. Borga, O., Piafsky, K. M., and Nilsen, O. G. (1977): Plasma protein binding of basic drugs. I. Selective displacement from α_1-acid glycoprotein by tris (2-butoxyethyl) phosphate. *Clin. Pharmacol. Ther.*, 22:539–544.
20. Piafsky, K. M., and Borga, O. (1977): Plasma protein binding of basic drugs. II. Importance of α_1-acid glycoprotein for interindividual variation. *Clin. Pharmacol. Ther.*, 22:545–549.
21. Harrison, H. N., Moncrief, J. A., Duckett, J. W., and Mason, A. D. (1964): The relationship between energy metabolism and water loss from vaporization in severely burned patients. *Surgery*, 56:203–211.
22. Harrison, T. S., Seaton, J. F., and Feller, I. (1967): Relationship of increased oxygen consumption to catecholamine excretion in thermal burns. *Ann. Surg.*, 165:169–172.
23. Wilmore, D. W., Long, J. M., Mason, A. D., Skreen, R. W., and Pruitt, B. A. (1974): Catecholamines: Mediator of the hypermetabolic response to thermal injury. *Ann. Surg.*, 180:653–669.
24. Zawacki, B. E., Spitzer, K. W., Mason, A. D., and Johns, L. A. (1970): Does increased evaporative water loss cause hypermetabolism in burned patients? *Ann. Surg.*, 171:236–240.
25. Caldwell, F. T., Jr., Bowser, B. H., and Crabtree, J. H. (1981): The effect of occlusive dressings on the energy metabolism of severely burned children. *Ann. Surg.*, 193:579–591.

26. Crabtree, J. H., Bowser, B. H., Campbell, J. W., Guinee, W. S., and Caldwell, F. T. (1980): Energy metabolism in anesthetized children with burns. *Am. J. Surg.*, 140:832–835.
27. Wilmore, D. W., and Aulick, L. H. (1978): Metabolic changes in burned patients. *Surg. Clin. North Am.*, 58:1173–1187.
28. Zeineh, R. A. (1979): The metabolism of transferrin in burned patients. *Res. Commun. Chem. Pathol. Pharmacol.*, 26:347–356.
29. Ciaccio, E. I., and Fruncillo, R. J. (1979): Urinary excretion of D-glucaric acid by severely burned patients. *Clin. Pharmacol. Ther.*, 25:340–344.
30. Ciaccio, E. I., and Fruncillo, R. J. (1979): Decreased aryl hydrocarbon hydroxylase after 15% burn injury. *Biochem. Pharmacol.*, 28:3151–3152.
31. Brenner, B. M., and Humes, H. D. (1975): Mechanics of glomerular ultrafiltration. *N. Engl. J. Med.*, 297:148–154.
32. Cameron, J. S., and Miller-Jones, C. M. H. (1967): Renal function and renal failure in badly burned children. *Br. J. Surg.*, 54:132–141.
33. Graber, I. G., and Sevitt, S. (1959): Renal function in burned patients and its relationship to morphological changes. *J. Clin. Pathol.*, 12:25–44.
34. Eklund, J., Granberg, P.-O., and Liljedahl, S.-O. (1970): Studies on renal function in burns. *Act. Chirurg. Scand.*, 136:627–640.
35. Loirat, P., Rohan, J., Baillet, A., Beaufils, F., David, R., and Chapman, A. (1978): Increased glomerular filtration rate in patients with major burns and its effect on the pharmacokinetics of tobramycin. *N. Engl. J. Med.*, 299:915–919.
36. Flynn, G. (1979): Topical drug absorption and topical pharmaceutical systems. In: *Modern Pharmaceutics*, edited by G. S. Banker and C. T. Rhodes, pp. 263–327. Marcel Dekker, New York.
37. Ciarpella, E., and Lombardi, P. (1976): Preliminary research on the activity of a new aminoglycoside antibiotic, tobramycin, in patients with gram-negative infected burns. In: *Treatment of Burns*, edited by L. Donati, J. Burke, and A. Bertelli, pp. 181–184. Piccin Medical Books, Padua.
38. Harrison, S. D., Jr. (1979): Increased glomerular filtration in burned patients. *N. Engl. J. Med.*, 300:680.
39. Lee, J. B., Patak, R. V., and Mookerjee, B. K. (1976): Renal prostaglandins and the regulation of blood pressure and sodium and water homeostatis. *Am. J. Med.*, 60:798–816.
40. Anggard, E., and Jonsson, C. E. (1972): Formation of prostaglandins in the skin following a burn injury. In: *Prostaglandins in Cellular Biology*, edited by P. W. Ramwell and B. P. Pharriss, pp. 269–284. Plenum Press, New York.
41. Golper, T. A. (1979): Increased glomerular filtration in burned patients. *N. Engl. J. Med.*, 300:680.
42. Orton, C. I., Segal, A. W., Bloom, S. R., and Clarke, J. (1975): Hypersecretion of glucagon and gastrin in severely burnt patients. *Br. Med. J.*, 2:170–172.
43. Johannesen, J., Lie, M., and Kiil, F. (1977): Effect of glycine and glucagon on glomerular filtration and renal metabolic rates. *Am. J. Physiol.*, 233:F61–F66.
44. Sawchuk, R. J., and Zaske, D. E. (1976): Pharmacokinetics of dosing regimens which utilize multiple intravenous infusions: Gentamicin in burn patients. *J. Pharmacokinet. Biopharm.*, 4:183–195.
45. McCracken, G. H., Jr. (1972): Clinical pharmacology of gentamicin in infants 2 to 24 months of age. *Am. J. Dis. Child.*, 124:884–887.
46. Paisley, J. W., Smith, A. L., and Smith, D. H. (1973): Gentamicin in newborn infants. *Am. J. Dis. Child.*, 126:473–477.
47. Riley, H. D., Jr., Rubio, T., Hinz, W., Nunnery, A. W., and Englund, J. (1971): Clinical and laboratory evaluation of gentamicin in infants and children. *J. Infect. Dis.*, 124(Suppl.):S236–S246.
48. Glew, R. H., Moellering, R. C., Jr., and Burke, J. F. (1976): Gentamicin dosage in children with extensive burns. *J. Trauma*, 16:819–823.
49. Zaske, D. E., Sawchuk, R. J., Gerding, D. N., and Strate, R. G. (1976): Increased dosage requirements of gentamicin in burn patients. *J. Trauma*, 16:824–828.
50. Solem, L. D., Zaske, D., and Strate, R. G. (1979): Ecthyma gangrenosum: Survival with individualized antibiotic therapy. *Arch. Surg.*, 114:580–583.
51. Stone, H. H., Kolb, L. D., Geheber, C. E., and Currie, C. A. (1975): Treatment of surgical infections with tobramycin. *Am. Surg.*, 41:301–308.
52. Zaske, D. E., Sawchuk, R. J., and Strate, R. G. (1978): The necessity of increased doses of amikacin in burn patients. *Surgery*, 84:603–608.

53. Flandrois, J. P., Marichy, J., and Ceyrat, J. (1979): Pharmacocinétique de l'amikacine chez le brûlé. *Nouv. Presse Méd.*, 8:3501–3502.
54. Palayret, D., Manelli, J. C., Perez-Cappellano, R., Garabedian, M., Lombard, C., Kiegel, P., and Caniggia, M. (1979): Étude clinique et pharmacocinétique de l'amikacine au cours des septicémies compliquant des brûlures étendues. *Nouv. Presse Méd.*, 8:3503–3506.
55. Leibel, W. S., Martyn, J. A., Szyfelbein, S. K., and Miller, K. W. (1981): Elevated plasma binding cannot account for the burn-related *d*-tubocurarine hyposensitivity. *Anesthesiology*, 54:378–382.
56. Martyn, J. A., Szyfelbein, S. K., Ali, H. H., Matteo, R. S., and Savarese, J. J. (1980): Increased *d*-tubocurarine requirement following major thermal injury. *Anesthesiology*, 52:352–355.
57. Piafsky, K. M., Borga, O., and Odar-Cedelof, I. (1978): Increased plasma binding of α-propranolol and chlorpromazine mediated by disease induced elevation of plasma α_1-acid glycoprotein. *N. Engl. J. Med.*, 299:1435–1439.
58. Bowdle, T. A., Neal, G. D., Levy, R. H., and Heimbach, D. M. (1980): Phenytoin pharmacokinetics in burned rats and plasma protein binding of phenytoin in burned patients. *J. Pharmacol. Exp. Ther.*, 213:97–99.
59. Bader, J. E. (1966): Organ deposition of silver following silver nitrate therapy of burns. *Plast. Reconstr. Surg.*, 37:550–551.
60. Marshall, J. P., and Schnieder, R. P. (1977): Systemic argyria secondary to topical silver nitrate. *Arch. Dermatol.*, 113:1077–1079.
61. Ternberg, J. L., and Luce, E. (1968): Methemoglobinemia: A complication of the silver nitrate treatment of burns. *Surgery*, 63:328–330.
62. Harris, J. C., Rumack, B. H., Peterson, R. G., and McGuire, B. M. (1979): Methemoglobinemia resulting from absorption of nitrates. *J.A.M.A.*, 242:2869–2871.
63. Lindberg, R. B., Moncrief, J. A., Switzer, W. E., Order, S. E., and Mills, W., Jr. (1965): The successful control of burn wound sepsis. *J. Trauma*, 5:601–612.
64. Muir, I. F. K., Owen, D., and Murphy, J. (1969): Sulfamylon acetate in the treatment of *Pseudomonas pyocyanea* infection of burns. *Br. J. Plast. Surg.*, 22:201–206.
65. Haynes, B. W., Jr. (1971): Mafenide acetate in burn treatment. *N. Engl. J. Med.*, 284:1324.
66. Petroff, P. A., Hander, E. W., and Mason, A. D. (1975): Ventilatory patterns following burn injury and effect of sulfamylon. *J. Trauma*, 15:650–656.
67. White, M. G., and Asch, M. J. (1971): Acid-base effects of topical mafenide acetate in the burned patient. *N. Engl. J. Med.*, 284:1281–1286.
68. Harrison, H. N., Blackmore, W. P., Bales, H. W., and Reeder, W. (1972): The absorption of C^{14}-labeled sulfamylon acetate through burned skin. I. Experimental methods and initial observations. *J. Trauma*, 12:986–993.
69. Harrison, H. N., Bales, H. W., and Jacoby, F. (1972): The absorption into burned skin of sulfamylon acetate from 5 percent aqueous solution. *J. Trauma*, 12:994–998.
70. Lavelle, K. J., Doedens, D. J., Kleit, S. A., and Forney, R. B. (1975): Iodine absorption in burn patients treated topically with povidone-iodine. *Clin. Pharmacol. Ther.*, 17:355–362.
71. Pietsch, J., and Meakins, J. L. (1976): Complications of povidone-iodine absorption in topically treated burn patients. *Lancet*, 1:280–282.
72. Hunt, J. L., Sato, R., Heck, E. L., and Baxter, C. R. (1980): A critical evaluation of povidone-iodine absorption in thermally injured patients. *J. Trauma*, 20:127–129.
73. Delaveau, P., and Friedrich-Noue, P. (1977): Absorption cutanée et elimination urinaire d'une combinasion sulfadiazine-argent utilisée dans le traitement des brûlures. *Therapie*, 32:563–572.
74. Harrison, H. N. (1979): Pharmacology of sulfadiazine silver. *Arch. Surg.*, 114:281–285.
75. Lazare, R., Watson, P. A., and Winter, G. D. (1974): Distribution and excretion of silver sulfadiazine applied to scalds in the pig. *Burns*, 1:57–64.
76. Catania, P. N., and King, J. C. (1975): Inhibition of supraeschar and subeschar *Pseudomonas* infection by silver sulfadiazine dry foam. *J. Pharmaceut. Sci.*, 64:457–458.
77. Kulick, M. I., Lewis, N. S., Bansal, V., and Warpeha, R. (1980): Hyperosmolality in the burn patient: Analysis of an osmolal discrepancy. *J. Trauma*, 20:223–228.
78. Bekeris, L., Baker, C., Fenton, J., Kimball, D., and Bermes, E. (1979): Propylene glycol as a cause of an elevated serum osmolality. *Am. J. Clin. Pathol.*, 72:633–636.
79. Read, J. M., and Bach, P. H. (1980): Sterile topical lignocaine jelly in plastic surgery: An assessment of its systemic toxicity. *S. Afr. Med. J.*, 57:704–706.

80. Stone, H. H., Kolb, L. D., Pettit, J., and Smith, R. B., III (1968): The systemic absorption of an antibiotic from the burn wound surface. *Am. Surg.*, 34:639–643.

81. Snelling, C. F. T., Ronald, A. R., and Johnson, G. E. (1970): Topical gentamicin therapy on the burn wound. *Plast. Reconstr. Surg.*, 46:158–163.

82. Holder, I. A. (1976): Gentamicin resistant *Pseudomonas aeruginosa* in a burns unit. *J. Antimicrob. Chemother.*, 2:309–311.

83. Keighley, M. R. B., and Burdon, D. W. (1979): Burns. In: *Antimicrobial Prophylaxis in Surgery*, edited by M. R. B. Keighley and D. W. Burdon, pp. 213–224. Pitman Medical, Tunbridge Wells.

84. Dayal, V. S., Whitehead, G. L., and Smith, E. L. (1975): Gentamicin—progressive cochlear toxicity. *Can. J. Otolaryngol.*, 4:348–351.

Pharmacokinetic Basis for Drug Treatment,
edited by L. Z. Benet et al., Raven Press,
New York 1984

Chapter 19

Computer-assisted Clinical Pharmacokinetics

Carl C. Peck*

*Division of Clinical Pharmacology, Departments of Medicine and Pharmacology,
Uniformed Services University of the Health Sciences, Bethesda, Maryland 20814*

Optimal therapy with a number of drugs requires achieving a blood concentration range that exceeds a minimal effective concentration (MEC) but remains below a maximal safe concentration (MSC) (see Chapters 1, 21, and 22). Dosing decisions aimed at achieving such a target concentration range are particularly critical when exceeding the MSC may cause potentially lethal toxicity. Commonly used drugs that fall into the latter category are theophylline, digitalis glycosides, aminoglycosides, and phenytoin. Large interpatient variability in pharmacokinetic disposition of these drugs owing to individual variability and disease factors confound the physician's ability to make optimal dosing decisions (see Appendix A).

Throughout the last decade, computer programs have been developed for the purpose of assisting physicians in individualizing drug dosing regimens for patients. The most elementary programs simply calculate the dosage for a given patient from the patient's body weight or body surface area using an algorithm that relates dosage to body size parameters. Although such algorithms may be modified for use in particular disease states, a more comprehensive approach is to ascertain the patient's extent of disease and the resultant influence on drug pharmacokinetics. Once the individual patient's pharmacokinetics [e.g., drug clearance (CL) and distribution volume *(Vd)*] are known for a particular drug, a dosage regimen may be determined that is consistent with the goals and constraints of therapy. The essential element of this approach is the determination of the relationship between measurable disease-state parameters (such as creatinine clearance as a measure of extent of renal disease) and pharmacokinetic parameters (*Vd*, CL). This relationship is usually determined by careful study of drug disposition in a population of diseased individuals from whom the average disease/pharmacokinetic relationship is derived. Several computer programs based on this approach have been proposed and evaluated (1–4).

Unfortunately, estimation of individual patient pharmacokinetics from the average disease/pharmacokinetic relationship has been found to be of limited accuracy be-

---

*For those interested in recent computer programs, Dr. Peck can be reached by mail or telephone at the above address.

cause individual effects vary significantly from the average effects of disease states on drug disposition. Hence, it has become evident that fine-tuning of dosage regimens in diseased individuals requires direct assessment of drug pharmacokinetics from concentration measurements of the drug in serum or plasma of the patient. Two general techniques have been employed in computer programs that use patient drug concentrations to devise individualized dosage regimens: least-squares and Bayesian algorithms. In the "unrestricted" least-squares technique, parameters of a pharmacokinetic model are estimated from patient drug concentrations and the dosage regimen only; knowledge of disease effects on pharmacokinetics is not taken into account. Preferably four or more drug concentration measurements are required for accuracy using this technique (5). When only one or two drug levels are available, a "restricted" version of the least-squares technique has been used for estimation of a single pharmacokinetic parameter (e.g., CL), holding the other parameters fixed at the population mean value. Examples of use of the least-squares approach include the USC*PACK collection of drug programs (6) and that of Ritschel et al. (7).

In contrast to the least-squares technique, the Bayesian method, as applied to clinical pharmacokinetics of diseased individuals, incorporates knowledge of the population distribution of disease/pharmacokinetic effects as well as patient drug concentrations in estimating the individual's pharmacokinetics. Proponents of the Bayesian technique have forwarded two approaches. Sheiner et al. (8,9) described and prospectively validated (10) a Bayesian algorithm that provides optimal use of patient drug concentrations for estimation of patient-specific pharmacokinetic model parameters. This technique can work with only one drug concentration. Katz and associates recently proposed a Bayesian technique for estimating drug dosage regimens to optimally achieve target drug concentrations (11,12). Whereas the approach of Sheiner et al. concentrates on estimation of individual pharmacokinetic parameters for subsequent dosage calculation, Katz's technique focuses directly on optimal dosage regimens. Katz's technique, however, requires formidable and costly computer resources to perform the required calculations. Full evaluation of Katz's approach must await the development of an easier access to these computational requirements.

The least-squares technique for utilizing patient drug concentrations in fine-tuning dosage regimens is appealing because the essential computational algorithms, linear or nonlinear regression, are widely available. However, the requirement for four or more drug concentrations for accuracy is a severe limiting factor in actual patient application. The more desirable Bayesian technique of Sheiner et al. (8,9), although it requires fewer patient drug concentrations, may not have gained wide acceptance because of perceived computational difficulties. However, Peck and associates have shown that the nonlinear parameter estimation necessary for implementation of this Bayesian technique can be performed on inexpensive microcomputers (13,14).

EXAMPLE COMPUTER PROGRAM

In order to illustrate in detail some features of the current state-of-the-art in computer-assisted clinical pharmacokinetics, the characteristics of a program for

theophylline dosing will be described. The theophylline dosing program is implemented in BASIC on an inexpensive microcomputer (HP-85, 32K RAM) and uses
the Bayesian algorithm of Sheiner et al. (8,9) for optimal forecasting of individual
patient pharmacokinetics. Provision is made for pharmacokinetic parameter estimation and dosing recommendations with and without patient drug concentrations.
The program addresses the relative uncertainties in outpatient versus inpatient dosing
histories, as well as the relative information content of recent and remote drug
concentrations with respect to the current pharmacokinetic "state" of the patient.
The cathode-ray tube (CRT) and hard-copy high-resolution graphic outputs of the
HP-85 provide a visual summary of the time course of the drug concentration that
has clinical and educational value. Although the program is specified for the bronchodilator drug theophylline, the algorithms are general; they have been adapted
to other drugs for which the target concentration range is an appropriate strategy
for optimal therapy (26,27; and J. G. Harter, *personal communication*).

Program Organization

The program consists of two segments linked by a CHAIN command. Segment
one (TH.DOS) contains routines for patient data input and output and estimation
of subpopulation-based pharmacokinetic parameters; segment two (TH.NLR) includes routines for Bayesian nonlinear parameter estimation and graphic simulation.
The user is prompted to enter data by full-text questions flashed on the CRT display.
All times are referenced to the time of the first inpatient dosing event ($t = 0$).
General details of the program segments follow in outline form:

TH.DOS (see Appendixes A and B)

Input
Patient name
Sex
Age
Body weight
Height
Smoking history
Ethanol use/liver dysfunction degree
Heart failure degree
Benzodiazepine use
Barbiturate use
Marijuana use
Obesity degree
Oral contraceptive use
Outpatient dosing history (p.o. only)
Inpatient dosing history (p.o., i.v.)
Target theophylline concentration ([TH])
Measured [TH], times (if any)

(Optional) User-supplied theophylline clearance and distribution volume estimates
($\pm SD_0$)

Output

Abbreviations table
Patient input data
Initial estimates of patient pharmacokinetic estimates ($\pm SD_0$), elimination half-life
($T_{1/2}$)
Outpatient/inpatient dosing histories
Measured [TH] (if no measured [TH] available: (a) calculated [TH] at $t = 0$; (b)
recommended i.v. dosing regimen to achieve target [TH])

Note 1. Provision is made for tape storage of patient input data so that in a future
program run, following data retrieval by tape, the user may expeditiously proceed
with the addition of new information.

TH.NLR

Note 2. The program automatically proceeds from TH.DOS to TH.NLR. If one
or more measured [TH] is entered, the Bayesian nonlinear parameter estimates are
printed out, followed by graphic simulation output, etc. If no measured [TH] is
entered, a simulation of the time course of theophylline concentration is plotted
and followed by the dosage modification routine (see Note 3, below) (see also
Chapter 22, Figures 2 and 3).

Output

Revised estimates of patient-specific pharmacokinetic estimates ($\pm \sim SD$), $T_{1/2}$
Measured and estimated [TH] (~ 95 confidence region), time, standardized residual
Graph of measured [TH] ($\pm 10\%$ error bar) and simulated curve of [TH] versus
time
Dosage modification table and optional graphic simulation

Note 3. The dosage-modification simulation routine allows the user to experiment
with new, future dosing regimens (oral or intravenous). Input requirements include
route of administration, dose, absorption half-time, infusion rate or dosing interval,
etc. Tabular output includes the dosage regimen and simulated maximum, minimum,
average [TH] at steady state. A graphic simulation of the last entered modified
dosage regimen may be optionally printed out.

Special Algorithms

Ideal Body Weight

The subpopulation identification routine *(vide infra)* requires an estimate of ideal
body weight for calculation of the theophylline clearance and distribution volume

(16). Regression equations have been devised that relate the ideal body weight to patient height and body weight (17). These equations are based on desirable body weight tables for adults (18) and average body weight tables for infants and children (19).

Subpopulation Identification

The scheme of Jusko et al. (16) is used as a basis to obtain subpopulation mean estimates of theophylline clearance (CL, ml/hr/kg). Patient input data determine the subpopulation to which the patient belongs, which in turn determines the initial CL estimate. The subpopulation standard deviation (SD_0) of CL is arbitrarily set at 50% of CL. The population distribution volume *(Vd)* estimate is set at 0.5 liter/ kg (20) ($SD_0 = 20\%$ of *Vd*) for all patients.

Pharmacokinetic Model

The pharmacokinetic model employed in all subroutines requiring simulated theophylline concentrations is the one-compartment open linear model with first-order absorption (oral dosing) or zero-order intravenous infusion (21). When measured [TH] is entered, the program distinguishes the uncertainty in the outpatient dosing history (due to variable noncompliance) from the relative certainty of the inpatient dosing history. The initial estimated [TH] at $t = 0$, $[TH_0]$, is calculated on the basis of all available dosing information assuming 100% compliance and the subpopulation pharmacokinetic parameter estimates. Then $[TH_0]$ is considered by the TH.NLR segment as a pharmacokinetic parameter to be estimated and is refined to be patient-specific, along with CL and *Vd*. The population standard deviation of $[TH_0]$ is set at 70% of $[TH_0]$ in order to reflect the uncertainties introduced by possible outpatient noncompliance.

Weighting of Measured [TH]

The standard deviation of the most recently measured [TH] is arbitrarily set at 15% of the predicted [TH] in order to reflect analytical error (~5% of [TH]), to which is added its double in order to allow for pharmacokinetic model misspecification. However, the standard deviation of measured [TH] is inflated as the times when it is drawn, relative to the most recent [TH], become more remote. The time-dependent weighting of measured [TH] has the effect that the revised, patient-specific pharmacokinetic parameter estimates derive most heavily from recent measured [TH]. This approach is based on the notion that the current pharmacokinetic "state" of the patient is reflected most precisely in the current [TH] and progressively less so in more remote ones. These adjustments should be efficacious when the patient's physiologic/metabolic processes affecting theophylline disposition are changing during the period of observation. If the drug disposition state of the patient is stable, the effect of the weighting algorithm should be minimal. The [TH]-weighting algorithm is

$$SD_{\widehat{[TH]}} = (Q)^{t^*} \times (0.15) \times (\widehat{[TH]})$$

where $SD_{\widehat{[TH]}}$ is the SD of measured [TH], $Q = 1.01$ for theophylline, t^* is time in hours before most recent [TH], and $\widehat{[TH]}$ is predicted [TH]. The effect of the [TH]-weighting algorithm on $SD_{[TH]}$ and its relative weighting in the Bayesian pharmacokinetic parameter estimation procedure can be seen here:

Time of sample	$SD_{[TH]}$	Relative weight in objective function
Most recent	15% of [TH]	1.00
12 hr earlier	17% of [TH]	0.89
24 hr earlier	19% of [TH]	0.79
48 hr earlier	24% of [TH]	0.62
72 hr earlier	31% of [TH]	0.49
96 hr earlier	39% of [TH]	0.38

Bayesian Pharmacokinetic Parameter Estimation

The method proposed by Sheiner et al. (8,9) for obtaining pharmacokinetic parameter estimates that are refined from initial subpopulation-based estimates requires in this case the minimization of the following objective function with respect to the parameters P_i:

$$\sum_{d=1}^{q=2,3} \frac{(\bar{P}_d - P_d)^2}{SD_{0P_d}^2} + \sum_{i=1}^{m} \frac{([TH]_i - \widehat{[TH]}_i)^2}{(SD_{\widehat{[TH]}_i})^2}$$

where P_1 is the estimate of CL, P_2 is the estimate of Vd, P_3 is the estimate of $[TH_0]$, $\bar{P}_1$ is population average (disease-adjusted) of CL, $\bar{P}_2$ is population average (disease-adjusted) of Vd, $\bar{P}_3$ is population average (disease-adjusted) of $[TH_0]$, $SD_{0CL} = 0.5*\overline{CL}$, $SD_{0Vd} = 0.2*\overline{Vd}$, $SD_{0[TH0]} = 0.7*[\overline{TH_0}]$, m is number of [TH]'s input in TH.DOS, $[TH]_i$ is ith predicted [TH], $\widehat{[TH]}_i$ is ith predicted [TH] using $P_d = 1,q$, $SD_{\widehat{[TH]}_i} = (1.01)^{t'*}*(0.15)*[TH]$, $q = 2$ if no outpatient dosing, $q = 3$ if outpatient dosing occurred. The objective function is minimized within TH.NLR with a Marquardt-Levenberg routine that we adapted (13) from Horowitz and Homer (22).

Performance/Validation

A full printout of an example case that illustrates the consultative and educational value of the program is reprinted elsewhere (14). The accuracy and precision of the program's Bayesian algorithm for forecasting measured steady-state theophylline concentrations from estimates of individual pharmacokinetics were assessed (23) by retrospective analysis of 15 cases reported by Vozeh et al. (24). The mean ($\pm$ SD) prediction error of the steady state theophylline concentration, -0.3 ± 2.3 μg/ml, represents clinically acceptable accuracy and precision when the target theophylline concentrations range between 10 and 20 μg/ml.

DISCUSSION

Although the validity of computer-assisted drug therapy has been demonstrated in certain settings (10,25), it has not attained widespread use. Inaccessibility to an inexpensive user-oriented system that makes optimal use of the few precious patient drug levels usually available may be among the many possible reasons for this situation. The drug dosing program described above was devised in order to remove these obstacles by implementing an effective algorithm for pharmacokinetic forecasting on an inexpensive desk-top microcomputer. For this purpose, the HP-85 microcomputer + 32K RAM combines a number of desirable user features (e.g., ease of operation, full capability and reasonable speed in performing the necessary tasks, high-resolution graphics, hospital-chart-size printed output, tape storage) with economy of cost. The prototypical features of the program as outlined earlier have been extended to the drugs aminoglycosides (amikacin, tobramycin, and gentamicin) (26), lidocaine (27), and digoxin (J. G. Harter, *personal communication*, 1982). Program segment two, TH.NLR, is a general program that may be easily adapted to any drug that can be described pharmacokinetically by a one-compartment open linear model. The value of Q in the drug concentration weighting algorithm may be altered to reflect the rapidity with which changes in pathophysiology affect drug dispositional processes and hence drug concentrations. Other pharmacokinetic models may also be used with appropriate program changes [e.g., two-compartment open linear models (27), nonlinear models, models that take advantage of additional patient information, such as renal function tests or pharmacologic responses]. The general features of program segment one, TH.DOS, include the dosage and drug level input routines. However, the particular patient characteristics that determine subpopulation identity as well as the algorithm for the latter are unique for each drug and must be devised accordingly.

It is now feasible to employ state-of-the-art techniques in computer-assisted clinical pharmacokinetics on inexpensive desk-top microcomputers. No doubt these same capabilities will soon be available in vest-pocket microcomputers. Although the performance of these prototype Bayesian drug dosing programs has been validated on retrospective data (23,27), rigorous prospective evaluation of their clinical utility is needed before their proper place in the care of patients can be ascertained.

REFERENCES

1. Jelliffe, R. W., Buell, J., Kalaba, R., Shidhar, R., and Rockwell, R. (1970): A computer program for digitalis dosage regimens. *Math. Biosci.*, 9:179–193.
2. Mawer, G. E., Knowles, B. R., Lucas, S. B., Stirland, R. M., and Tooth, J. A. (1972): Computer-assisted prescribing of kanamycin for patients with renal insufficiency. *Lancet*, 1:12–15.
3. Peck, C. C., Sheiner, L. B., Martin, C. M., Combs, P. T., and Melmon, K. L. (1973): Computer-assisted digoxin therapy. *N. Engl. J. Med.*, 289:441–446.
4. Goicoechea, F. J., and Jelliffe, R. W. (1974): Computerized dosage regimens for highly toxic drugs. *Am. J. Hosp. Pharm.*, 31:67–71.
5. Jelliffe, R. W., Schumitzky, A., Rodman, J. H., Forrest, A., D'Argenio, D. Z., and Gilman, T. M. (1979): *Adaptive Control of Drug Dosage Regimens for Patient Care.* Syllabus, 2nd Annual Retreat on Computers and Clinical Therapeutics, University of Southern California, School of Pharmacy, Los Angeles.

6. Jelliffe, R. W., Schumitzky, A., Rodman, J., and Crone, J. (1977): A package of time-shared computer programs for patient care. In: *Proceedings of the First Annual Symposium on Computer Applications in Medical Care*, pp. 154–162. IEEE Computer Society Publications Office.

7. Ritschel, W. A., Banarer, M., and Lau Chang, E. F. (1977): Computer-calculated kanamycin dosage regimen and monitoring. *Int. J. Clin. Pharmacol.*, 15:121–125.

8. Sheiner, L. B., Rosenberg, B., and Melmon, K. L. (1972): Modeling individual pharmacokinetics for computer drug dosage. *Comp. Biomed. Res.*, 5:441.

9. Sheiner, L. B., Beal, S., Rosenberg, B., and Marathe, V. V. (1979): Forecasting individual pharmacokinetics. *Clin. Pharmacol. Ther.*, 26:294–305.

10. Sheiner, L. B., Halkin, H. H., Peck, C. C., Rosenberg, B., and Melmon, K. L. (1975): Improved computer-assisted digoxin therapy. *Ann. Intern. Med.*, 82:619–627.

11. Katz, D. (1980): A Bayesian approach to the analysis of nonlinear models with applications in pharmacokinetics. Ph.D. dissertation, University of Southern California, Los Angeles.

12. Katz, D., and Schumitzky, A. S. (1980): Bayesian analysis of pharmacokinetic models with applications to dosing regimen determination. In: *Proceedings of the 4th Annual Symposium on Computer Applications in Medical Care*, pp. 970–974. IEEE Computer Society Publications Office.

13. Peck, C. C., and Barrett, B. B. (1979): Nonlinear least-squares regression for microcomputers. *J. Pharmacokinet. Biopharm.*, 7:537–541.

14. Peck, C. C., Brown, W. D., Sheiner, L. B., and Schuster, C. G. (1980): A microcomputer drug (theophylline) dosing program which assists and teaches physicians. In: *Proceedings of the 4th Annual Symposium on Computer Applications in Medical Care*, pp. 988–994. IEEE Computer Society Publications Office.

15. Brown, W. D., and Peck, C. C. (1980): Theophylline dosing program (USUHS version 80.07.01). Technical report No. 2, Division of Clinical Pharmacology, Uniformed Services University, 4301 Jones Bridge Road, Bethesda, Md. 20814.

16. Jusko, W. J., Gardener, M. J., Mangione, A., Schentag, J., Koup, J. R., and Vance, J. W. (1979): Factors affecting theophylline clearance. *J. Pharm. Sci.*, 68:1358–1366.

17. Brown, W. D., and Peck, C. C. (1980): Simple formulas for calculating desirable body weight in adults and average body weight in children. Technical report No. 3, Division of Clinical Pharmacology, Uniformed Services University, 4301 Jones Bridge Road, Bethesda, Md. 20814.

18. Diem, K., and Lenter, C. (editors) (1970): *Documenta Geigy, Scientific Tables*, ed. 7, p. 712. Ciba-Geigy, Basle.

19. Diem, K., and Lenter, C. (editors) (1970): *Documenta Geigy, Scientific Tables*, ed. 7, p. 693. Ciba-Geigy, Basle.

20. Ogilvie, R. I. (1978): Clinical pharmacokinetics of theophylline. *Clin. Pharmacokinet.*, 3:267.

21. Gibaldi, M., and Perrier, D. (1975): *Pharmacokinetics*. Marcel Dekker, New York.

22. Horowitz, D. L., and Homer, L. D. (1970): Analysis of biomedical data by time-sharing computers. I. Non-linear regression analysis. Project No. MR 005:20–0287, *Report No. 25*, Naval Medical Research Institute, National Naval Medical Center, Bethesda, Md. 20014.

23. Peck, C. C., Brown, W. D., Sheiner, L. B., Vozeh, S., and Nichols, A. I. (1981): A prototype Bayesian drug dosing program which assists and teaches physicians. *Clin. Pharmacol. Ther.*, 29:272.

24. Vozeh, S., Kewitz, G., and Follath, F. (1980): Accurate prediction of theophylline serum concentrations using a rapid estimation of theophylline clearance (CL). *Clin. Pharmacol. Ther.*, 27:67.

25. Jelliffe, R. W., Buell, J., and Kalaba, R. (1972): Reduction of digitalis toxicity by computer-assisted glycoside dosage regimens. *Ann. Intern. Med.*, 77:891–906.

26. Perlin, E., Peck, C. C., and Nichols, A. I. (1981): An aminoglycoside dosing program using a Bayesian algorithm. In: *Proceedings of the 5th Annual Symposium on Computer Applications in Medical Care*, pp. 610–613. IEEE Computer Society Publications, New York.

27. Lenert, L., Peck, C. C., Vozeh, S., and Follath, F. (1982): Lidocaine forecaster: A two-compartment Bayesian patient pharmacokinetic computer program. *Clin. Pharmacol. Ther.*, 31:243.

Pharmacokinetic Basis for Drug Treatment,
edited by L. Z. Benet et al., Raven Press,
New York © 1984

Chapter 20

Estimation of Altered Kinetics in Populations

Lewis B. Sheiner and Stuart L. Beal

*Department of Laboratory Medicine and Department of Medicine, Division of
Clinical Pharmacology, University of California, San Franscisco,
San Francisco, California 94143*

Many of the important questions regarding the effects of disease states on pharmacokinetics are answered by investigating population pharmacokinetics: the pharmacokinetic characteristics of typical individuals with and without disease. For example, whether or not cirrhosis influences drug metabolism is determined by knowledge of population pharmacokinetics in normals and cirrhotics (see Chapters 3 and 4). To answer such questions, it may be desirable to combine data from many sources. However, the different sources may be characterized by varying amounts of data per subject and by varying data quality, and the data may have arisen from various experimental designs (including no design at all). Standard methods of data analysis may be inadequate to deal with such data, or with combining it. In this chapter we describe why this is so, and we suggest an alternative approach (1,2) with which we have had some success (3–8).

ESTIMATING POPULATION KINETICS

What We Wish to Know

Consider the following questions: Does drug clearance vary with variation in renal function? If so, what is the quantitative relationship between the two? Does protein binding of a drug vary with serum albumin concentration? If so, again, what is the quantitative relationship? These questions concern the average relationships of pathophysiology to pharmacokinetics, or the average value of a pharmacokinetic characteristic in a specific population.

Estimates of certain kinds of population pharmacokinetic parameters help answer such questions. These are the quantitative values of the proportionality between renal function (see Chapters 8 and 9) (as measured, perhaps, by creatinine clearance) and drug clearance, or serum albumin and protein binding (see Chapter 10). Population pharmacokinetic parameters of this type are called fixed-effect parameters because they quantify the relationship between certain fixed (measurable) effects (renal function, albumin level) and pharmacokinetics.

Consider some other questions: Assuming drug clearance does vary with renal function, how well do we know an individual's clearance if we know his renal function? Does variation in albumin affect clearance via its effect on protein binding? Answers to these questions are important when deciding how confident one is in one's initial dosage for the renal patient or the patient with hypoalbuminemia. Estimates of population pharmacokinetic parameters of a different type are needed here. We need to know something about the (probability) distributions of deviations of individual values of fixed-effect parameters from their population values, and how these deviations correlate with one another. The variances and covariances of the distributions provide the required information. They are population pharmacokinetic parameters of a different type: random interindividual-effect parameters (random, because individual deviations are regarded as occurring according to the probability distribution).

Finally, we may ask how much drug clearance varies from day-to-day within an individual, or how much a steady state drug level varies from day-to-day due to all causes. We might want to answer these questions in order to set reasonable thresholds for responding to changes in measured drug levels (see Chapters 21 and 22). To answer these questions, yet another random-effect population parameter (another variance) is needed: the variance of combined random intraindividual and measurement error (or just "error" variance) (random, because day-to-day fluctuation and measurement errors are also regarded as occurring according to probability distributions).

The Standard Approach

The traditional or standard approach employs an experimental paradigm. The subjects are a group of patients selected to represent a spectrum of severity of some condition (e.g., renal insufficiency) the effects of which are to be studied. Usually only 10 to 30 subjects are studied. The dosage pattern administered to the subjects is usually of simple design, perhaps a single bolus dose, or a single infusion, often to be repeated under other conditions at another time, in a balanced design. The sampling schedule (over time) for the biological fluids of interest (blood, urine, perhaps others) is usually fixed, and the same for each subject. It is designed to reveal maximum information about individual kinetics, and it consists of many samples (often more than 20) per subject.

Data analysis, applied to the standard study, proceeds in two stages. First, the data from each individual are analyzed to yield estimates of the individual pharmacokinetic parameters, such as drug clearance. This step is usually accomplished using (weighted or unweighted) nonlinear regression with the least-squares criterion (most pharmacokinetic models are statistically nonlinear). The individual parameter estimates obtained in the first step are then subjected to a second step of analysis to obtain population parameter estimates. For the fixed-effect parameters relating pharmacokinetics to physiology, least-squares regression is used, but here it is most often statistically linear (that is, the relation of drug clearance, for example, to

creatinine clearance is usually modeled as a linear one). When estimating population parameters unrelated to other factors, simple averages of the individual parameter estimates are usually taken. For estimates of the random interindividual-effect parameters, the standard deviations (or variances) of the individual parameters about the regression lines (or the average value) are used.

When random-error variance is estimated, which is rarely, the sum of the pooled squared residuals of the initial nonlinear fits divided by the (pooled) residual degrees of freedom is usually used.

Standard errors of the fixed-effect parameter estimates when the latter are estimated as averages of individual parameter estimates are usually taken to be the standard deviations of the individual parameter estimates divided by the square root of the number of sampled individuals. Standard errors of the random interindividual-effect parameter estimates are not usually computed, nor is a natural way to do so apparent.

Despite the directness, simplicity, and familiarity of the standard method, it has certain problems. First, the source of data can present problems for the standard approach. Ethical issues are encountered in planning a study of patients. It may be difficult to justify temporarily witholding a drug for study purposes or causing added risk and annoyance to an already precarious and uncomfortable patient. Consequently, traditional studies are undertaken in patient groups with lesser degrees of illness, or else adequacy of study design is sacrificed. This, in turn, leads to problems with representativeness of information obtained.

Second, because the number of study subjects is usually relatively small, the vagaries of sampling may lead to population parameter estimates that deviate substantially from true population values. This is especially so of the random interindividual-effect parameters.

Third, traditional study is quite costly. Although data analysis is not, compensation of volunteers, temporary hospitalization on a clinical research ward, assay of numerous samples, and so forth, often make the cost of a traditional study in excess of several thousands of dollars per subject.

Fourth, serendipity is often not possible. Careful control of diet, study conditions, etc., all undertaken in the interest of obtaining data with low variability, can actually prevent the discovery of unexpected but important influences on kinetics.

Finally, although problems with the standard approach's data analysis per se tend not to be major because of certain features of the experimental data, we discuss them here in order to provide background for later discussion of the analysis of routine patient data. There, the problems become acute, and they necessitate an alternative approach to data analysis.

When the method of ordinary least squares is used for the initial (individual-fitting) step in the data analysis, implicit assumptions are that all errors intervening between the "true" level and the observed level are (a) independent of each other (as one goes from concentration to concentration), (b) additive, and (c) of the same typical magnitude. All of these assumptions are open to question. Consider, in particular, the third. Absolute measurement error is often not of constant magnitude.

It can begin at a "lower limit of detectability" and then rise, often in proportion to the drug concentration itself. Measurement errors of different magnitudes are also seen when data are of more than one type (for example, when both urine concentrations and plasma concentrations of drug are available). Finally, errors of different magnitudes can be due to differences among subjects: Some may have kinetics more variable across time than others.

When using the usual method of least squares, one must use known weights to adjust for possible inhomogeneities in error magnitude. But where do the weights come from? Study of the measurement process by replication, which might offer some basis for assigning relative-error magnitudes, usually is not done. Even if it were, it might not suffice, because a considerable part of the total "error" is due not to assay measurement but to inadequacies of the pharmacokinetic model, or to transient variation in the subjects' kinetics. These "errors" must be incorporated into the weights if the latter are to be correct; yet they are not readily measurable.

Analysts often resort to weighting their data by the reciprocal of the datum itself, or the datum squared (9). Such weighting is meant to adjust for the increase in error magnitude associated with higher true values. The approach may help, but if concentrations near the minimum detectable concentration are present in the data, such weighting will tend to markedly overweight these points.

These problems may have little importance when analyzing experimental data. This is because (a) even the largest errors are often small compared with the total concentration range covered by the data, so that neither nonadditive error nor variable error magnitude nor correlated errors are important, and (b) the traditional weighting schemes *(vide supra)*, when used for data from various sources, often provide a reasonable balance.

The second step of the standard data analysis, the estimation of population parameters from individual parameter estimates, also has problems. If one were fitting a pharmacokinetic model involving four or five parameters to data for subjects with fewer concentration/time points than parameters, one might be unable to estimate all of the individual parameters. These subjects' data might then have to be discarded, even though they undoubtedly contain information about the population parameters.

Even with individual parameter estimates from all subjects, the average and variance of these estimates may be poor estimates of the population parameter and interindividual variance. This is because each individual estimate is "contaminated" to varying degrees by an irrelevant error: the error made in estimating the parameter itself. Although individual parameter estimates might be as likely to be too high as too low, so that the estimated population parameter might not be biased, still, for a precise estimate of it, less attention should be paid to the poorer individual estimates. The estimate of the population interindividual variance will have the same problems, but it *will* be biased upward. It will contain variability both from interindividual biological sources and from estimation. Independent variabilities add, rather than cancel each other.

It is the strength of the experimental design that makes the standard method acceptable: Sufficient data are gathered from everyone so that individual estimates are always possible; the amount of individual data is sufficiently large and covers a sufficiently wide range so that parameter estimates have small error relative to interindividual variability. Therefore, the fixed-effect population parameter estimates are likely to be quite good, and although undoubtedly somewhat biased, the estimates of the interindividual standard deviations may not be greatly biased.

An Alternative Approach

Because of the limitations imposed by the data source of the standard approach, the possibility of using data gathered directly from patients receiving drugs of interest is attractive. In the limit, one might attempt to extract population parameter estimates from only those data gathered by clinicians in the process of rendering care to their patients. This is "pure" routine data. One might also consider supplementing such information with a few extra samples, samples not necessary for patient care.

Such data avoid the ethical problems of experimental data. They are also representative and inexpensive.

Data analysis, however, now presents major problems. Consider the two data-analysis problems previously discussed—the assumption of homogeneous error magnitude and the estimation of population parameters from individual parameter estimates. We may no longer be confident that errors are small and error magnitude relatively (if not absolutely) homogenous. Now data are gathered in varying circumstances and have variable reliability.

Moreover, individual parameter estimates are now suspect as a means to population values. There is no experimental design; so drug concentration samples will not usually be taken at those times most likely to allow accurate parameter estimates. Varying amounts of data will be gathered from patients. None will contribute very much, and some will surely have too little data to permit accurate individual parameter estimates. When this variability is combined with that in the quality of the data, individual parameter estimates, even when they are available, will certainly have variable, and possibly often poor, accuracy. Population parameters estimated from these will be significantly "contaminated" with estimation error, and the random interindividual-effect parameter estimates may be seriously biased. Clearly, an alternative approach to data analysis is required.

Such an approach exists. It involves shifting one's point of view, and regarding the population itself as the unit of analysis. Just as when fitting an individual's data to an individual model, the goal is not the estimation of the "true" drug concentration for each time point, but rather the individual's model parameters; so, when modeling the population, the goal is the population parameter estimates, not the individual parameters. When one makes this shift, however, an essential assumption of the usual (weighted or unweighted) least-squares approach is no longer tenable. When modeling only one individual's data, each drug concentration can be approximated as being statistically independent of any other. Now, one must explicitly recognize

that only concentrations from different individuals are statistically independent of each other. The concentrations from one individual all display a systematic deviation from the expected population values because of the individual parameter shifts (from the population values) that are associated with the particular individual.

In this context, neither ordinary nor weighted simple least squares can be used. An approach that can be used, and that we do use, involves the method of extended least-squares, as applied to a nonlinear mixed-effect statistical model. The notion of extended least-squares was introduced by Beal (10). Application of the approach to pharmacokinetic models has been described by us in some detail previously (2) as an approximate maximum-likelihood procedure, which is an apt description when all random effects are assumed to be normally distributed.

The method yields direct estimates of all three types of population parameters and approximate standard errors for all parameter estimates, including the random-effect ones.

We can do no more than sketch the method here and indicate its relationship to ordinary or weighted least-squares.

In ordinary least-squares, as applied to an individual's data, one seeks the parameter values, θ, that minimize the sum of squared deviations; i.e., the values of θ minimizing

$$\sum_{i=1}^{n} [y_i - f(\theta, X_i)]^2 \tag{1}$$

where y_i is the observed response at the ith instant, and $f(\theta, X_i)$ is the predicted value of that response under the model, f, given the individual's pharmacokinetic parameters, θ, and the collection of independent variables evaluated at the ith instant, X_i, which includes time.

If there were differing error magnitudes, and one knew the (different) variances of the individual observations, one would estimate θ using weighted least-squares; i.e., one would seek θ minimizing

$$\sum_{i=1}^{n} [y_i - f(\theta, X_i)]^2 / v_i \tag{2}$$

where v_i is the variance of the ith observation. Note that usually weighted least-squares is appropriately used when it is assumed only that v_i is known up to a proportionality factor.

If, in Eq. 2, the v_i were unknown, they could perhaps be modeled as a function of θ, X_i, and some random-effect parameters, ξ. Designate the value of this function as $v(\theta, \xi, X_i)$ ($= v_i$). One usually cannot estimate θ and ξ by minimizing Eq. 2 with respect to θ and ξ because for many types of functions, v, a trivial and uninteresting solution would always result. The parameters would be chosen so as to render all v_i infinite. This choice would always minimize the expression, no matter what values were assigned to θ. It is therefore clear that one needs to add some penalty

to Eq. 2 that increases in value as ξ takes values leading to larger values of v_i. Such an expression arises in the maximum-likelihood approach to estimation when observations are normally distributed. In this case, the maximum-likelihood estimates of θ and ξ are those minimizing

$$\sum_{i=1}^{n} \left(\frac{[y_i - f(\theta, X_i)]^2}{v(\theta, \xi, X_i)} + \ln [v(\theta, \xi, X_i)] \right) \tag{3}$$

where $\ln(z)$ is the natural logarithm of z. Note here that as the value of v_i increases, so does the logarithm term. This penalty counteracts the decrease in the left-hand sum-of-squares term. Reasonable bounded estimates of all parameters are obtained from this approach. In the case that $v(\theta, \xi, X_i) = \xi$ for all i, minimizing Eq. 3 gives the exact same estimate of θ as results from minimizing Eq. 1. Also, in the case $v(\theta, \xi, X_i) = \xi \mu(X_i)$ for all i and known function μ, minimizing Eq. 3 gives the same estimate of θ as results from using weighted least-squares with weights $1/\mu(X_i)$. Even when distributions are not normal, the extended least-squares estimates provided by minimizing Eq. 3 have certain desirable statistical properties and are reasonable choices as estimates of the underlying parameters (10).

Now let us step back one level and contemplate estimating population parameters rather than individual ones. We must now regard the symbol y_i as referring to a vector of numbers, and the symbols X_i and v_i as referring to matrices, one set of y_i, X_i, and v_i for each individual studied. The vector y_i consists of all observed responses from the ith individual; the jth row of X_i consists of the collection of the values of the independent variables occurring concomitantly with y_{ij}; and v_i is the variance-covariance matrix of y_i. The length of y_i, the row dimension of X_i, and both row and column dimensions of v_i are the number of observations taken from the corresponding individual. The parameters θ and ξ are now population parameters; θ are fixed-effect parameters; ξ contains both types of random-effect parameters (i.e., random interindividual- and intraindividual-effect parameters). Some adjustments need to be made to Eq. 3 so that it deals with vectors rather than scalars, and the summation is across N individuals, not n observations; matrix notation must be used, but the spirit is the same as before.

One important difference, however, is present. Now the individual observations in each y_i vector will all correlate with each other through the common set of differences of the individual parameters from the population mean values. Thus, off-diagonal elements (the covariances of the observations) of the matrix v_i will involve the interindividual random-effect parameters, and the diagonal elements (variances of observations) will involve both the random intraindividual-effect parameters and the random interindividual-effect parameters. This is because the variances must express the typical magnitude of the deviations of the observations from their population expectation, not just from the individual expectation.

In order to make the computation of the vector f and the matrices v_i possible, one needs to approximate the population pharmacokinetic model by linearizing it in the individual parameters about the population parameters. This computation is

somewhat complicated, and it need not concern the user of the computer program we mention later. Note, too, that in Eq. 3 the "reciprocal" and the "logarithm" of the matrix v_i need to be computed; appropriate matrix analogues of these operations exist. This, too, need not concern the user of the program.

We have implemented, tested, and are distributing a computer program, NONMEM (NONlinear Mixed-Effect Model) (11) that can be used to analyze data according to the approach outlined here. The program has certain desirable features. For example, it has a convenient form for input; it provides for constraints on the parameter estimates; it provides an estimate of the asymptotic covariance matrix (from which standard errors are computed) of all the estimators; it performs "derivative-free" estimation; it produces flexible and informative tables and graphs. A tape of the program and detailed didactic documentation may be obtained by writing to the authors.

The method and program (NONMEM) have been used for several problems, as mentioned earlier. Accumulated experience indicates that it works as well as was expected. It is not, however, without some problems. The models that must be specified are more complex than in the standard approach: The entire individual and population model must be specified at once. Although this task may be seen as an advantage in that all assumptions are thereby made explicit, careful attention must be paid to it; otherwise, unfortunate errors can result. In addition, because many parameters and all data must be dealt with simultaneously, the data analysis requires a large general-purpose computer, and this is costly. This cost may be more than offset, however, by the cost savings realized in data gathering.

CONCLUSIONS

Population pharmacokinetic parameters are of three types. Fixed-effect parameters describe the relationship of physiology to kinetics. Random interindividual-effect parameters measure the magnitude of the random individual variability in the relations of the first type. Other random-effect parameters measure the magnitude of the random residual variation in observations of drug concentrations about their expected value.

The effects of disease states on pharmacokinetics can be expressed as knowledge of population pharmacokinetic parameters; their investigation is therefore a matter of some interest. The standard approach to obtaining information on them involves an experimental paradigm. In this approach, although reasonably good estimates of the pharmacokinetic parameters of some (or even all) individuals can be obtained, the population parameter estimates resulting from these may not be representative of the population of interest, or if they are representative, they may be very imprecise due to the relatively small number of individuals studied.

To analyze routine data generated in the course of patient care, or to combine data from various sources, one is faced with certain data analysis problems. These are also present when analyzing experimental data, but are probably of less import then. When the standard techniques are applied to routine data, or data from various

sources, however, the problems become acute. An alternative data analysis approach that regards the population as the unit of analysis is available. It is implemented as the exportable computer program NONMEM. The approach allows meaningful analysis of routine data, but it is costly and requires greater sophistication on the part of its users. A reasonable compromise is to use the standard approach wherever it seems applicable, and to use the alternative approach when the standard one will not suffice, as in the analysis of routine data. In this manner, the approaches need not be seen as competitive, but rather as complementary. Together, they may allow fuller use of the varied types of data available to pharmacokinetic investigators, so permitting an orderly progression from first suspecting, to detecting, to estimating, and finally to confirming the important effects of disease states on pharmacokinetics.

ACKNOWLEDGMENTS

This work was supported in part by Grants GM-26676 and GM-26691 from the United States Public Health Service.

REFERENCES

1. Sheiner, L. B., Beal, S., Rosenberg, B., and Marathe, V. V. (1979): Forecasting individual pharmacokinetics. *Clin. Pharmacol. Ther.*, 26:294–305.
2. Sheiner, L. B., Rosenberg, B., and Marathe, V. V. (1977): Estimation of population characteristics of pharmacokinetic parameters from routine clinical data. *J. Pharmacokinet. Biopharm.*, 5:445–479.
3. Holford, N., and Sheiner, L. B. (1981): The effect of quinidine and its metabolites on the electrocardiogram and systolic time intervals—concentration-response relationships. *Br. J. Clin. Pharmacol.*, 11:187–195.
4. Powell, J. R., Vozeh, S., Hopewell, P., Costello, J., Sheiner, L. B., and Riegelman, S. (1978): Theophylline disposition in acutely ill hospitalized patients. *Am. Rev. Respir. Dis.*, 118:229–238.
5. Ravenscroft, P., Vozeh, S., Weinstein, M., and Sheiner, L. B. (1978): Saliva lithium concentrations in the management of lithium therapy. *Arch. Gen. Psychiatry*, 35:1123–1127.
6. Sheiner, L. B., and Beal, S. (1981): Evaluation of methods for estimating population pharmacokinetic parameters. I. Michaelis-Menten model; routine clinical pharmacokinetic data. *J. Pharmacokinet. Biopharm.*, 9:635–651.
7. Sheiner, L. B., Vozeh, S., Stanski, D. R., Miller, R. D., and Ham, J. (1979): Simultaneous modelling of pharmacokinetics and dynamics: Application to *d*-tubocurarine. *Clin. Pharmacol. Ther.*, 25:358–371.
8. Sheiner, L. B., and Beal, S. L. (1981): Evaluation of methods for estimating population pharmacokinetic parameters. II. Biexponential model: Experimental pharmacokinetic data. *J. Pharmacokinet. Biopharm.*, 9:635–651.
9. Boxenbaum, H. C., Riegelman, S., and Elashoff, R. M. (1974): Statistical estimation in pharmacokinetics. *J. Pharmacokinet. Biopharm.*, 2:123–148.
10. Beal, S. L. (1974): Adaptive M estimation with independent nonidentically distributed data. Unpublished Ph.D. dissertation. University of California, Los Angeles.
11. Beal, S., and Sheiner, L. (1980): The NONMEM system. *American Statistician*, 34:118–119.

Pharmacokinetic Basis for Drug Treatment,
edited by L. Z. Benet et al., Raven Press,
New York © 1984

Chapter 21

Therapeutic Drug Monitoring

C. E. Pippenger and *Neil Massoud

*Departments of Biochemistry and Clinical Pathology, Cleveland Clinic Foundation,
Cleveland, Ohio 44106 and *Division of Clinical Pharmacology, Departments of
Medicine and Pharmacy, University of California, San Francisco, California 94143*

Clinicians have a continuing interest in ascertaining why a fixed drug dosage is therapeutically effective in some individuals but not in others. For centuries, appropriate drug dosage regimens were established clinically by trial and error. Modern analyticial technology has provided new insights and approaches to therapy. The ability to correlate serum drug concentrations (and, by inference, tissue concentrations) with the clinical effect observed following drug administration provides new approaches to all aspects of therapeutics. Investigations have established that the desired effect occurs only above a specific plasma concentration and that there is an optimal plasma concentration range over which drug therapy is most often successful. Above this optimal range, most patients can be expected to experience an increasing incidence of undesirable drug side effects.

The value of therapeutic drug monitoring (TDM) as an aid to rational drug therapy in patients with various disease states and genetic constitutions is firmly established. Serum drug concentrations of numerous compounds, including antiepileptic, antibiotic, antiarrhythmic, antiasthmatic, antineoplastic, and antidepressant drugs, are now measured routinely in order to establish an optimal therapeutic regimen for an individual patient at a given point in time (see Appendixes A–C). For the first time, the clinician who monitors a patient's plasma drug concentration is able to distinguish a true therapeutic failure from poor drug availability or poor compliance. With compliance rates reported to be approximately 55% for antitubercular therapy, 48% for insulin use in diabetics, 46% for patients with chronic obstructive pulmonary disease, 42% for glaucoma patients taking eyedrops, less than 60% for hypertensive patients, and 50% and 40% for neurotics and schizophrenics, respectively, this is highly relevant (1–7).

Without question, TDM has significantly improved patient care. Sherwin and his colleagues (8) have clearly demonstrated that it is possible to significantly improve seizure control in epileptic children with absence seizures through routine monitoring. Monitoring of ethosuximide concentrations and appropriate dosage adjustments resulted in a significant improvement in seizure control of absenceseizures in a population of epileptic children. Complete seizure control was achieved

in 74% of the population, as compared with 47% control prior to the availability of drug monitoring services.

Drug therapy is usually aimed at abolishing an acute or chronic pathologic state (e.g., seizures). Much more difficult to evaluate and treat, however, are diseases with only occasional clinical symptoms (e.g., certain cardiac arrhythmias, asthma, and the epilepsies). For centuries it was common for a patient to be given a fixed quantity of drug, and if the desired effect did not result, the dosage was increased until signs of toxicity appeared, at which point the dosage was reduced. If the expected response still did not occur, a second drug was prescribed. If a response to the second drug was not forthcoming, the process was repeated until the desired effect was achieved or until all possible drugs and drug combinations had been explored and exhausted. Trial-and-error therapy places both the patient and clinician at the mercy of an unknown factor—the kinetics of the prescribed drug in that particular patient.

Today, TDM allows more accurate titration of dosage to assure optimal serum concentrations and thus greater individualization of drug therapy. Only within the last three decades has a clearer understanding of the relationship between a drug's concentration within a biologic system and its therapeutic effectiveness become possible. Our current ability to monitor a wide variety of drug doses and to correlate their plasma concentrations (and, by inference, their tissue concentrations) with their therapeutic effects had to await the development of highly specific, repro-ducible, analytical technologies (see Chapter 22). Using these analytical techniques and making clinical correlations, investigators established that a minimum effective concentration (MEC) of a given drug in plasma was necessary to elicit that particular drug's therapeutic effect. Furthermore, it is now accepted that there are optimum plasma concentration ranges (see Appendixes A–C) within which therapeutic effects can be expected to occur in most patients receiving a particular drug (5–9). Still further, should plasma concentrations exceed the optimum plasma concentration range, undesirable side effects or toxicity (which may or may not be clinically demonstrable) can be expected to occur. It is essential that the clinician using drug concentrations reported by the analytical laboratory, as well as the clinical pathol-ogist, clinical pharmacist, or clinical chemist providing routine monitoring services, understand the fundamental principles and techniques of clinical pharmacology as they are applied to patient care. Such an understanding will enable a more effective interpretation of TDM data that are encountered in various clinical situations (see Chapter 22).

SITE AND MECHANISM OF DRUG ACTION

The biologic effect achieved following a given drug dose is a direct consequence of the formation of reversible bonds between the drug and tissue receptors controlling a particular response (10). For most drugs, the intensity and duration of a given pharmacologic effect are proportional to the drug concentration at the receptor site (10,11).

In order for a drug to exert the desired biologic effect, it must reach and interact with the receptors regulating that specific response. In addition, disease, age, sex, bioavailability, compliance, drug interactions, and individual differences in drug metabolism and excretion contribute to differences in interpatient drug responses (5–7,12,13). Figure 1 schematically depicts the factors that can alter the concentrations of drugs ultimately achieved and maintained at a given receptor site. Titration of drug dosage using TDM is in many cases the most precise method for achieving therapeutic plasma concentrations and compensating for these interindividual variations in responses (1,2).

For most drugs, the intensity of a pharmacologic effect is proportional to the drug concentration in extracellular fluid, which can enter tissues and interact with specific receptors to elicit a biologic effect (1,2,10). For example, antiepileptic drugs are believed to prevent seizures by binding to neural membranes or altering

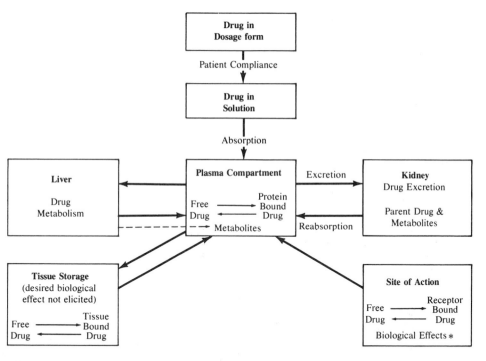

Absorption

Drug must be formulated in a manner which assures bioavailability for absorption.

Metabolism

Drug converted to a more soluble compound which may be biologically active or inactive. Metabolism can also occur in other tissues.

Excretion

Usually more water soluble drug metabolites are excreted in urine. Also drug excretion can occur via bile, feces, saliva and expired air.

Tissue Storage

Distribution of drug to sites where the desired biological effect is not elicited.

Undesirable effects may be elicited by drug interaction with a specific physiological system.

Site of Action

Free drug binds to receptor to elicit a biological effect (response). Number & type of receptors to which drug is bound determines the intensity and duration of the desired and undesired effects.

FIG. 1. Factors that regulate tissue drug concentrations. (From *Syva Monitor*, with permission.)

neurotransmitter release (14). Alteration of these functions is thought to stabilize neuronal membranes against the excessive electrical activity that is responsible for precipitating a clinical seizure.

Figure 2 is a schematic representation of drug distribution following absorption between the plasma and the various tissue compartments. Drug concentration in extracellular water is in equilibrium with the drug concentration in plasma water. The latter, representing free-drug concentration, is an indirect measure of drug concentration at the site of action. Because many drugs are partially bound to plasma proteins, an equilibrium exists between the concentration of protein-bound drug and the free-drug concentration in plasma water (15,16) (see Chapter 10). Only free drug is capable of crossing the various lipoprotein membranes that surround the receptor sites. It is impossible to directly monitor receptor-site drug concentrations *in vivo*; therefore, monitoring the total plasma drug concentrations is a reflection of the equilibrium that exists between tissue, extracellular fluid, and plasma water drug concentrations.

The site at which a given drug acts to initiate the events that lead to a specific biologic effect is arbitrarily defined as that drug's *site of action*. A drug's biologic effect may be elicited by direct interaction with a receptor that controls a specific function or by alteration of the physiologic process that regulates that specific function (5–7,9–11,14).

The *mechanism of action* of a drug refers to the actual biochemical or physical process that initiates a biologic response at a given site. The mechanism of action for most drugs depends on the drug's chemical interaction with a functionally viable component of some physiologic system. However, because the exact molecular mechanisms of action for most drugs remain obscure, theoretical models have been developed to explain these mechanisms of action. The fundamental concept on which these models are based is that there are intracellular macromolecular receptors that, when stimulated, elicit a specific biologic response. More specifically, drugs are believed to combine reversibly with receptors by means of ionic bonds, hydrogen bonds, and van der Waals forces. Such a reversible combination is thought to form a drug-receptor complex of sufficient stability to alter the physiologic response of

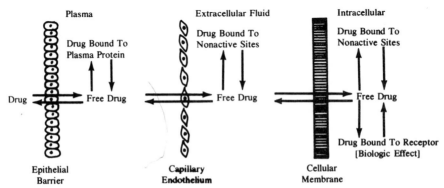

FIG. 2. Distribution of drugs between plasma and tissue. (From *Syva Monitor*, with permission.)

the target system, consequently producing the observed pharmacologic effect. Both clinical and molecular studies of the pharmacologic profiles of a wide variety of drugs have demonstrated that a much better correlation exists between the observed clinical effects of a drug and its plasma concentration than that observed between clinical effect and total daily drug dosage.

The simplest model that adequately describes this effect over a whole range of plasma concentrations is based on the hyperbolic relationship that is called the E_{max} model (19):

$$E = \frac{E_{max} \cdot C}{EC_{50} + C} \tag{1}$$

where E is effect, C is plasma concentration, E_{max} is the maximum effect attributable to the drug, and EC_{50} is the concentration producing 50% of E_{max}. This model has been extensively used in other areas, such as in enzyme kinetics (Michaelis-Menten) and protein binding. It is useful because it has three important properties: (a) it predicts the maximum effect a drug can achieve; (b) it predicts no effect when no drug is present; (c) at concentrations greater than the EC_{50}, E is not directly proportional to plasma concentration.

When the drug effect is measured as inhibition of some biologic phenomenon (e.g., hypertension), Eq. 1 can be rewritten (17) as

$$E = NODRUG - \frac{E_{max} \cdot C}{IC_{50} + C} \tag{2}$$

where NODRUG is the effect when no drug is present and IC_{50} is the concentration producing 50% of the maximum inhibition of effect (E_{max}).

Numerous factors, including individual differences in drug metabolism and excretion, age, sex, patient compliance, disease, and drug interactions (particularly during multiple-drug therapy), regulate this effect and disposition pattern within an individual patient (1,2). The rate of drug disposition regulates the amount of drug available to interact with a receptor; thus, the therapeutic response observed in a given patient is dependent on the sum of all these processes. The observed clinical effect of a given drug in a specific patient is related to the drug concentration in that patient. Interactions between all the potential factors influencing drug disposition account for the broad interpatient variability in plasma drug concentrations following either single or multiple drug doses. Individual patient response to a given drug dose, however, remains constant, because the factors that can alter drug utilization within the individual are relatively fixed (1–3,5–7,9).

Generally, interindividual variations in response, as demonstrated by the clinical response of a large population to a fixed drug dose, are more a reflection on the relationship between total daily dose and plasma concentration than a reflection of the relationship between plasma concentration and intensity of response. In other words, the probability of achieving a given plasma concentration from a given drug dose is much less than the probability of obtaining a specific biologic effect from

a given plasma concentration. This is why drugs administered at fixed doses produce marked variations within a population in observed therapeutic responses: When an average or standard drug dosage is administered to a large patient population, the desired therapeutic effect will be achieved in some patients; no therapeutic effect will occur in others; toxicity, usually associated with drug overdose, will be evident in still others (11). Titration of drug dosage to obtain an optimal therapeutic plasma concentration in the individual patient can successfully reduce undesirable responses, which are a direct consequence of interindividual variations in drug disposition. TDM can aid clinicians in achieving optimal plasma concentrations of a drug and thus assure prompt establishment and maintenance of the desired therapeutic response. This is especially true with drugs having a narrow therapeutic index (e.g., digoxin, quinidine, theophylline, phenytoin).

For most drugs, there is a direct linear relationship between the administered drug dosage and the plasma concentration achieved at steady state (6,7); that is, as the total drug dose is increased, there will be a directly proportional, concomitant linear increase in that drug's plasma concentration. Unfortunately, this is not always the case. Certain drugs, such as phenytoin, amitriptyline, salicylate, propranolol, acetaminophen, chlorpromazine, disopyramide, ethanol, mezlocillin, prednisone, valproic acid, diflunisal, and possibly theophylline (see Chapter 17), demonstrate an apparent linear dose/concentration relationship only over a given range (1–3); beyond that point, a marked elevation in plasma concentration disproportionate to the dose administered can follow what would be clinically considered a negligible dosage increase (Fig. 3). The phenomenon responsible for nonlinear increases in drug concentration is termed *saturation* or *zero-order* kinetics. Saturation kinetics is a direct reflection of the limited capacity of some drug-metabolizing enzyme mechanisms (see Chapter 17). Clinically, saturation kinetics should be suspected when a patient unexpectedly develops an adverse drug reaction associated with drug accumulation following a small dosage increment.

One of the major advantages of TDM is that it can be used to "predict" most pharmacologic responses. It functions either by assuring the clinician that the plasma concentration is within an optimal range for a given patient population or by signaling the presence of a subtherapeutic or toxic concentration in a specific patient. TDM is not a panacea, and drug concentration data must always be interpreted in conjunction with the patient's clinical status (1–3,6,7,9) (i.e., albumin, serum creatinine, bilirubin, FEV_1, α_1-acid glycoprotein). TDM, as part of routine patient care, provides clinicians with a valuable, more precise tool for assessing the pharmacologic status of the individual patient and helps them establish a regimen to achieve the desired therapeutic response.

PATIENT NONCOMPLIANCE

As noted at the beginning of this chapter, over 50% of all patients do not take their medications in the manner prescribed by their physicians (4). The most common cause of suboptimal drug concentrations, and consequent failure to achieve

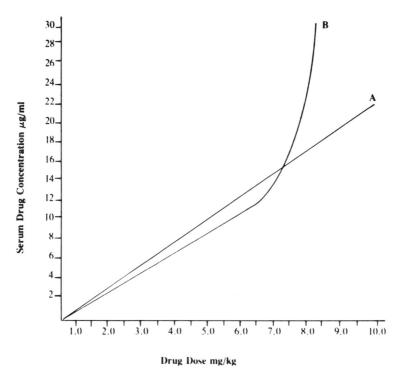

FIG. 3. Relationship between drug dose and plasma concentration: Dose–response curve for drug obeying *(A)* first-order kinetics (linear) and *(B)* zero-order kinetics (nonlinear or saturation). (From *Syva Monitor*, with permission.)

the desired therapeutic response, is patient noncompliance (Fig. 4) (17). Whenever a patient presents with consistently low plasma drug concentrations, noncompliance should be considered the possible cause. Noncompliance can usually be demonstrated by careful supervision of the patient's daily drug intake over a specified time interval (usually five half-life periods of the drug), with routine monitoring of serum drug concentrations at appropriate intervals. If there is a progressive increase in serum drug concentration over the time interval selected, the patient has been noncompliant. If the serum concentration remains low during supervised drug intake, other altered physiologic functions, such as rapid drug metabolism or altered absorption, should be considered (1–3).

If a good working relationship does not exist between the clinician and the patient, a simple yes-or-no approach based on a biochemical drug assay should be used with caution in the community setting. Here it would be difficult to distinguish the erratic user from the underuser. Methods to evaluate compliance should avoid simplistic dichotomies and should provide a continuous record to identify actual patterns of drug use (4).

Administration of the "recommended" or "average" total daily dose of a given drug without taking into account the numerous factors that alter drug disposition

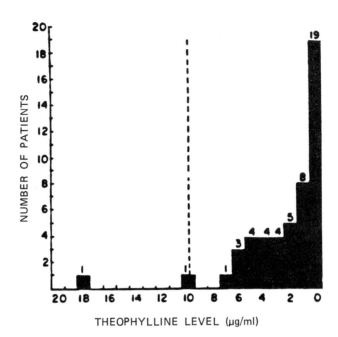

FIG. 4. Theophylline levels found in 49 of 50 pediatric patients sampled, of which all were given the standard 5-mg/kg dose every 6 hr to maintain therapeutic theophylline concentrations of 10 to 20 μg/ml. (From Sublett et al., ref. 17, with permission.)

(Fig. 5) in each patient can also lead to consistently low or high serum drug concentrations (18). Failure to individualize drug therapy (clinician noncompliance) is often responsible for suboptimal drug concentrations (1–3,5–7,9).

DRUG ABSORPTION

Entrance of drugs into the general circulation following either intravenous or intramuscular administration is generally rapid and circumvents the problems associated with drug absorption following oral administration (5,7,9,11). However, most drugs are administered orally. Following oral drug administration, a number of factors can alter the amount of drug absorbed from the gastrointestinal tract into the circulatory system. The type of drug preparation, drug solubility, concomitant administration of other drugs, whether or not the drug is taken with meals, diarrhea, or constipation can all alter the amount or rate of drug that will be absorbed following a single oral dose (see Chapter 2).

Some patients receiving appropriate drug doses will have consistently low plasma drug concentrations. Generally, these patients are classified as either noncompliant or fast drug metabolizers. However, before classifying someone as a fast metabolizer, the patient's ability to absorb the administered drug should be considered (see Chapters 2 and 4).

Because there are a significant number of factors which can alter both the extent or rate of drug absorption, the maximal concentration, after oral dosing, is rarely

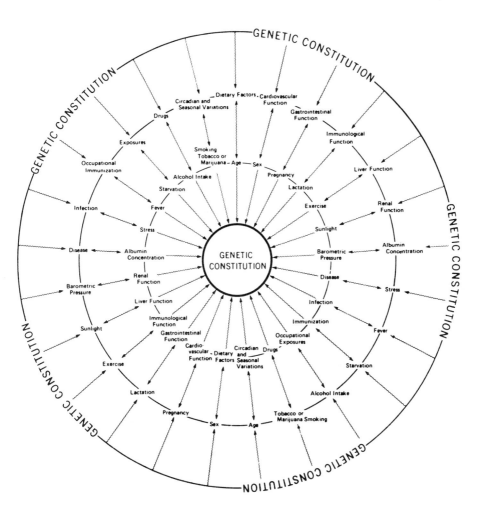

FIG. 5. The concept of concentric outer circles was developed to emphasize the multiple possibilities that exist for interaction among host factors and to suggest that the magnitude of the impact of host factors on drug response may be modulated by genetic constitution. Because in most cases these specific interactions and modulations have not yet been investigated, much less firmly established, this design is largely speculative and intended to stimulate future research rather than to depict the current state of knowledge in the field. (From Vesell, ref. 18, with permission.)

measured. For most drugs, absorption occurs within the first 60 to 90 min. For samples prior to this time, one would be uncertain of the validity of the measurement.

For those drugs with very slow absorption, the plasma concentration and half-life may be very different than when given intravenously, because it is the rate of absorption that is now the determining factor allowing the drug to be available for elimination and metabolism. This is often referred to as a "flip-flop" model.

TABLE 1. Saliva/plasma (S/P) concentration ratios of drugs

Drug	Mean S/P ratio	S/P ratio range	Conditions	No. subjects	Reference
Acebutolol	2.63 ± 1.19 (SD)	0.56–3.04	Single dose	12	Zoman et al. (1981): Br. J. Clin. Pharmacol., 12:427–429.
metabolite	0.72 ± 0.43 (SD)	0.17–1.82			
Acetaminophen	1.14 ± 0.05	0.45–3.09	Single dose	10	Glynn et al. (1973): J. Pharm. Pharmacol., 25:420–421.
Acetazolamide	0.009 ± 0.001 (SD)	0.008–0.011	Single dose	5	Wallace et al. (1977): J. Pharm. Sci., 66:527–530.
Amobarbital	0.35 ± 0.03 (SD)	0.32–0.40	Single dose	5	Inaba et al. (1975): Clin Pharmacol. Ther., 18:558–562.
Antipyrine[a]	0.92 ± 0.02		Single dose	10	Mucklow et al. (1978): Clin. Pharmacol. Ther., 24: 563–570.
	0.92 ± 0.02 (SE)		Single dose	10	Fraser et al. (1976): Br. J. Clin. Pharmacol., 3:321–325.
	1.00 ± 0.05 (SD)	0.95–1.09	Single dose	9	Welch et al. (1975): Clin. Pharmacol. Ther., 18:249–258.
	0.92 ± 0.04 (SD)	0.87–1.00	Single dose	12	Vesell et al. (1975): Clin. Pharmacol. Ther., 18:259–272.
Carbamazepine[a]	0.30	0.21–0.37	Steady state	1	Rylance (1979): Arch. Dis. Child., 54:459–467.
	0.37		Steady state	7	Troupin et al. (1975): Epilepsia, 16:223–227.
	0.26 ± 0.01 (SD)	0.25–0.28	Steady state	17	Westenberg et al. (1977): Clin. Chim. Acta, 79:155–161.
	0.42 ± 0.05 (SD)	0.34–0.51	Steady state	24	Dartels et al. (1977): Eur. J. Ped., 126: 37–44.
	0.27 ± 0.04 (SD)	0.207–0.349	Steady state		MacKichan et al. (1981): Br. J. Clin. Pharmacol., 12:31–37.
Carbamazepine epoxide	0.427 ± 0.127(SD)	0.135–0.714	Steady state	23	MacKichan et al. (1981): Br. J. Clin Pharmacol., 12:31–37.
Carbamazepine[a]	Salivary conc. correlated with dose		Steady state	11	Day et al (1981): Br. J. Clin. Prac., pp. 25–29.
Caffeine[a]	0.55		Single dose	1	Horning et al. (1977): Clin. Chem., 23:157–164.
	0.74 ± 0.08		Single dose	6	Newton et al. (1981): Eur. J. Clin. Pharmacol., 21:45–52.
Chlorpropamide		0.009–0.026	Steady state	12	Mucklow et al. (1978): Clin. Pharmacol. Ther., 24:563–570.
Cyclophosphamide	0.62	0.59–0.65	Single dose	3	Ritschel et al. (1981): J. Clin. Pharmacol., 21:461–462.
	0.77 (indicates unbound drug)		Steady state	7	Juma et al. (1979): Br. J. Clin. Pharmacol., 8:455–457.
Diazepam[a]	Salivary conc. correlated with dose		Steady state	25	Giles et al. (1980): J. Pharmacol., 71–76.
	0.029 (good correlation with free-plasma conc.)		Single dose	9	DiGregorio et al. (1978): Clin. Pharmacol. Ther., 24:720–724.
	0.016 (correlation coefficient 0.89)		Steady state	6	Hallstrom et al. (1980): Br. J. Clin. Pharmacol., 9:333–335.
	1:1 Unbound relationship between plasma and saliva, 3 hr post oral dose		Steady state	19	de Gier et al. (1980): Br. J. Clin. Pharmacol., 10:151.

Digoxin	0.66		Single dose	14	Allonen et al. (1978): Int. J. Clin. Pharmacol., 16:420.
	1.14 ± 0.48 (SD)		Steady state	34	Jusko et al. (1975): Chem. Path. Pharmacol., 10:189–192.
	0.78 ± 0.07 (SD)		Steady state	18	Huffman (1975): Clin. Pharmacol. Ther., 17:310–312.
	1.34 ± 0.44 (SD)	0.77–1.85	Steady state	4	Joubert et al. (1976): Br. J. Clin. Pharmacol., 3:1053–1056.
Ethosuximide[a]	1.68		Steady state	20	Van der Vijgh (1975): Neth. J. Med., 18:269–272.
	0.66 ± 0.20 (SD)		Steady state	12	Krivay et al. (1980): J. Pediatr., 99:810–811.
	0.88		Steady state	4	Horning et al. (1977):Clin. Chem., 23:157–164.
	1.04 ± 0.07 (SD)	0.92–1.14	Steady state	9	Horning et al. (1977): Clin. Chem., 23:157–164.
Isoniazid	0.78 ± 0.74		Steady state	19	Piredda et al. (1981): Ther. Drug Monitor., 3:321–323.
	1.02	0.90–1.17	Single dose	2	Boxenbaum et al. (1975): J. Pharmacokinet. Biopharm., 3:443–456.
Lidocaine	1.78 ± 0.39 (SD)	1.45–2.21	Single dose	3	De Boer et al. (1977): unpublished investigation.
	1.37 ± 0.79		Single dose	8	Kanto et al. (1982): Br. J. Clin. Pharmacol., 13:736–737.
Lincomycin		0.07–0.09	Single dose	15	Smith et al. (1981): J. Clin. Pharmacol., 21:411–417.
Lithium	3.1	1.6–4.5	Steady state	23	Vlaar et al. (1979): Acta Psychiatr. Scand., 60:423.
	2.85 ± 0.59 (SD)	2.13–3.47	Single dose	3	Groth et al. (1974): Clin. Pharmacol. Ther., 16:490–498.
	3.43		Single dose	2	Shimizu et al. (1977): Clin. Pharmacol. Ther., 21:212–215.
	About 2		Steady state	12	Shopsin et al. (1969): Intern. Pharmacopsych., 2:148–169.
Meperidine (pethidine)	2–5	1.37–2.60	Steady state	5	Spring et al. (1969): J. Dental Research, 48:546–549.
Methotrexate	0.04		Single dose	1	Mucklow et al. (1978): Clin. Pharmacol. Ther., 24:563–570.
			Single dose	2	Patterson et al. (1981): Int. J. Clin. Pharmacol., 19:381–385.
Norttriptyline	Highly variable and pH-dependent		Single dose	7	Virtanen (1981): Int. J. Clin. Pharmacol., 19:78–82.
Phenacetin	0.60 ± 0.19	0.41–1	Single dose	13	Vesell et al. (1975): Clin. Pharmacol. Ther., 18:259–272.
Phenobarbital[a]	0.41 ± 0.03	0.06–0.19	Steady state	11	Mucklow et al. (1978): Clin. Pharmacol. Ther., 24:563–570.
Phenytoin[a]	0.30 ± 0.03 (SE)		Steady state	8	Troupin et al. (1975): Epilepsia, 16:223–227.
	0.31 ± 0.06 (SD)		Steady state	50	Goldsmith et al. (1981): Ther. Drug Monitor., 3:151–157.
	0.13 ± 0.01 (SE)		Steady state	11	Mucklow et al. (1978): Clin. Pharmacol. Ther., 24:563–570.
	0.11		Steady state	17	Mucklow et al. (1981): Ther. Drug Monitor., 3:275–277.
	Salivary conc. correlated with dose		Steady state	15	Rylance et al. (1981): Arch. Dis. Child., 56:637–652.
	0.10 ± 0.013 (SD)		Steady state	36	Modeer et al. (1981): Acta Paediatr. Scand., 20:373–378.
	0.11 ± 0.04 (SE)		Steady state	35	Schmidt et al. (1975): Epilepsia, 16:735–741.
	0.101 ± 0.003 (SD)		Steady state	38	Cook et al. (1976): Clin. Pharmacol. Ther., 18:742–747.
	0.091 ± 0.017 (SE)		Steady state	6	Troupin et al. (1975): Epilepsia, 16:223–227.

(continued)

TABLE 1. (continued)

Drug	Mean S/P ratio	S/P ratio range	Conditions	No. subjects	Reference
Phenytoin (cont.)	0.103 ± 0.015 (SD)	0.087–0.129	Single dose	9	Paxton et al. (1977): Br. J. Clin. Pharmacol., 4:185–191.
	0.105 ± 0.004 (SD)		Steady state	17	Reynolds et al. (1976): Lancet, 2:384–386.
	0.24 ± 0.24 (SD)	0.06–1.00	Steady state	32	Bochner et al. (1974): Arch. Neurol., 31:57–59.
	0.108 ± 0.05 (SD)	0.021–0.316	Steady state	33	Barth et al. (1976): Clin. Pharmacokinet, 1:444–452.
Phenytoin + valproate	Therapeutic for phenytoin similar to when phenytoin given alone: 1–2 µg/ml		Steady state	42	Knott et al. (1982): Br. Med. J., 2:13.
Prednisolone	No correlation between saliva and plasma-free prednisolone		Single dose	6	Chakroborty et al. (1981): Eur. J. Clin. Pharmacol., 19:79–81.
Primidone	0.97 ± 0.05 (SE)	0.5–1.4	Steady state	31	Schmidt et al. (1975): Epilepsia, 16:735–741.
	1.08 ± 0.08 (SE)		Steady state	3	Troupin et al. (1975): Epilepsia, 16:223–227.
	0.95			17	Goldsmith et al. (1981): Ther. Drug Monitor., 3:151–157.
Procainamide	3.50 ± 2.34 (SD)	0.27–8.93	Steady state	12	Koup et al. (1975): J. Pharm. Sci., 64:2008–2010.
	1.62 ± 0.61 (SD)	1.35–2.12	Single dose	4	Galeazzi et al. (1976): Clin. Pharmacol. Ther., 20:278–289.
	Correlation found between QT interval and salivary concentration				
Propranolol	0.18–2.63		Steady state	19	Mucklow et al. (1978): Clin. Pharmacol. Ther., 24: 563–570.
Quinidine	0.51 ± 0.12 (SD)	0.42–0.65	Single dose	3	Jaffe et al. (1975): J. Pharm. Sci., 64:2028–2029.
Salicylate	0.033 ± 0.005 (SD)	0.029–0.039	Single dose	3	Graham et al. (1972): J. Pharm. Sci., 61:1219–1222.
Sodium valproate	0.06		Steady state	22	Schmidt (1976): Lancet, 2:639.
Streptomycin	0.15 ± 0.08 (SD)	0.06–0.27	Single dose	11	Bender et al. (1953): J. Am. Dental Assoc., 46:164–170.

Drug	Mean	Range		n	Reference
Theophylline	0.67	56–112 μmole/liter	Steady state	28	Boobis et al. (1978): Br. J. Clin. Pharmacol., 6:456p.
	0.52 ± 0.03 (SD)	0.46–0.58	Single dose	7	Koysooko et al. (1974): Clin. Pharmacol. Ther.,15:454–460.
	0.58		Steady state	16	Levy et al. (1974): Pediatrics, 53:873–876.
	0.77 ± 0.07 (SD)	0.64–0.86	Steady state	6	Knop et al. (1975): Pharmaceutisch Weekblad, 110:1297–1299.
	0.85	0.77–0.92	Single dose	2	Knop et al. (1975): Pharmaceutisch Weekblad, 110: 1297–1299.
	0.65		Steady state	22	Johnson et al. (1975): Clin. Chem., 21:144–147.
	0.49 ± 0.04 (SD)	0.44–0.52	Single dose	4	Shah et al. (1974): J. Pharm. Sci., 63:1283–1285.
	0.75		Single dose	5	De Blaey et al. (1976): Pharmaceutisch Weekblad, 111:1216–1221.
	1.52 ± 0.64 (SD) interpatient 1.52 ± 0.35 (SD) intrapatient		Steady state	19	Kelly et al. (1981): Am. J. Dis. Child.,135:137–139.
	0.45	0.3–1	Steady state	65	Goldsworthy et al. (1981): Br. J. Pharmacol., 11:434p.
	0.53	0.31–0.70	Steady state	18	Uden et al. (1981): Ther. Drug Monitor., 3:143–150.
		0.006–0.012	Single dose	1	Mucklow et al. (1978): Clin. Pharmacol. Ther., 24:563–570.
Tolbutamide	0.012 ± 0.001	0.012–0.013	Single dose	3	Matin et al. (1974): Clin. Pharmacol. Ther., 16: 1052–1058.

[a]Good correlation between plasma and salivary concentrations; salivary levels acceptable for therapeutic monitoring.

Recommendations for salivary collections (26): (a) Salivary samples should be collected immediately after oral administration. A significant amount of drug at this time indicates contaminations. (b) pH should be measured after sample collection. (c) Saliva should be collected in glass containers. (d) Saliva flow should be increased by chewing a piece of Teflon, not parafilm. (e) Timing should be consistent from dose to dose. (f) Citric acid should not be added to the tongue to increase flow.

For a recent review of the subject, see Mucklow, J. C. (1982): Ther. Drug. Monitor., 4:229–247.

Adapted from Danhof, M., and Briemer, D. D. (1978): Therapeutic drug monitoring in saliva. Clin. Pharmacokinet., 3:39–57.

DRUG-PLASMA-PROTEIN BINDING

On entering the systemic circulation, any protein-bound drug will bind to plasma proteins, and an equilibrium between free drug and bound drug will be established. By definition, bound drug is that portion of a drug bound to plasma proteins. Bound drug is unable to cross cell membranes and consequently exerts no biologic effect. Unbound or free drug is dissolved in the plasma water and can be transported across cell membranes. Only free drug can cross biologic membranes and interact with specific receptors to elicit a biologic response.

Each drug has its own characteristic protein binding pattern that is dependent on its physical and chemical properties (16–19). As a general rule, acidic drugs are bound to albumin and basic drugs to globulins, particularly α_1-acid glycoprotein (see Chapter 10). A drug may be either tightly bound or loosely bound, as determined by its affinity for plasma proteins. A weakly bound drug can be displaced from its protein sites by a drug with a greater affinity or concentration for the same binding site (see Chapter 10 for binding considerations and for a listing of drugs that are more than 90% bound).

Protein binding of a drug is also dependent on the physical characteristics of the plasma proteins and on the presence or absence of fatty acids, disease states, changes in physiology (see Chapters 9–13 and 15), or other drugs in the blood.

Certain disease states can significantly alter protein binding. For example, uremic patients have a decreased ability to bind drugs to plasma proteins. In the case of phenytoin, this lack of binding capacity ranges from uremic patients who can bind little phenytoin to those who can bind 60 to 70% of the phenytoin present in plasma. Clinically, this means that in a patient with a decreased capacity to bind phenytoin, a concentration of 3 to 7 μg/ml may be therapeutic and plasma concentrations above 15 μg/ml might precipitate phenytoin toxicity. Altered drug binding requires careful monitoring of all drugs administered in patients with abnormal renal function (20) (see Chapters 8 and 9).

If a patient presents with either clinical toxicity or a nontherapeutic response when total plasma concentration is known to be optimal, altered protein binding should be considered. Until recently, determination of protein binding was a time-consuming and tedious procedure. However, among the three methods used (equilibrium dialysis, ultrafiltration, and ultracentrifugation), new developments in ultrafiltration may be the most promising for more rapid determination of unbound drug (21,22). Because only free drug crosses into the saliva, the protein binding status of a patient can be assessed indirectly by measuring salivary drug concentrations (23,24) (Table 1). Nevertheless, caution is indicated. Salivary levels are a good indicator of free drug levels for any drug that has an ionization constant (pK_a) significantly different from the pH of plasma (i.e., very weak acidic or basic drugs). However, for acidic drugs with a pK_a under 8.2 or basic drugs with a pK_a over 6.0, salivary concentration of a drug will not consistently reflect the true free-drug concentration (25). In an attempt to provide consistent results with saliva, stimulation of saliva is suggested. Its advantages are the following: (a) Stimulation

provides large volumes of saliva. (b) Stimulated saliva has a narrower pH value (6.5–7.0), which may be of value when collecting weakly acidic or basic drugs. (c) Intersubject variability may be decreased (25,26). If the saliva/plasma ratio is used for drug monitoring, it should be consistent over a wide range of therapeutic plasma concentrations (see a recent review by Graham, ref. 26).

DRUG METABOLISM

Any foreign compound that enters the body must be eliminated. Phylogenetically from fish to humans, drug elimination mechanisms become more complex (24). As one proceeds up the phylogenetic scale, there is a progressive increase in the ability of the body to alter foreign compounds into compounds that are more water-soluble and thus more readily excreted. It is generally believed that the ability of the liver to metabolize drugs evolved as a mechanism for detoxifying ingested poisonous substances.

The drug-metabolizing enzymes of the liver are nonspecific and interact with a wide variety of chemical structures (see Chapters 3 and 4). The primary purpose of the hepatic drug-metabolizing systems is to make compounds more water-soluble; therefore, degradation of organic compounds leads to compounds that are less fat-soluble and more water-soluble (27). Metabolites of many drugs are conjugated within the liver to glucuronic acid, amino acids, or sulfates, thus further increasing water solubility and consequently the rate of renal excretion. (Renal function and drug metabolites are discussed in Chapter 9.) For example, parahydroxyphenytoin, the major metabolite of phenytoin, is conjugated with glucuronic acid. This conjugation increases its water solubility almost 100-fold.

Most drug metabolism takes place within the microsomal fraction of the hepatocyte. The microsomal enzyme systems are also responsible for the metabolism of endogenous steroids (9–12). The enzymatic systems responsible for drug metabolism are not designed to recognize specific drugs; rather, they act on classes of compounds with similar structures. The same enzyme that is responsible for the hydroxylation of phenytoin is also responsible for the hydroxylation of many other drugs containing an appropriate phenyl ring. Therefore, when phenytoin is administered simultaneously with one of these drugs, there may be some clinically significant alterations of drug concentrations that are a direct consequence as competition for metabolic sites on the enzyme increases (see Chapter 11). Clinically, one would expect to see higher serum concentrations of the drug with least affinity for the enzyme. Phenytoin has a very low affinity for microsomal enzymes. Thus, administration of a drug with a greater affinity for the enzyme than phenytoin will decrease phenytoin's rate of metabolism, and plasma phenytoin concentrations will become elevated (2,3).

One characteristic of the hepatic microsomal system is that it can be induced to metabolize drugs at a faster rate. As increasing doses of drug are administered, the body, in its attempt to eliminate the drug, synthesizes new protein in the form of enzymes capable of metabolizing that agent. But increased activity of drug-metab-

olizing enzymatic systems is not necessarily induced with every dosage increment or with the addition of another drug to the patient's regimen. There is a maximum rate at which protein synthesis can occur (2,3,28). Thus, if a patient has been regularly receiving a drug with known enzyme-induction properties, it does not follow that a second drug of similar structure added to the patient's therapeutic regimen will cause a marked increase in the rate of metabolism of both the first drug and second drug.

Genetic factors play a major role in determining the ability of a patient to metabolize drugs (29). Individuals of different ethnic origins (20–25% of Mediterranean origin, 50% of blacks, 80–90% of Asians, and 40% of Caucasians are fast-acetylator types), as well as individuals in certain families, metabolize drugs (e.g., phenytoin, dapsone, procainamide, hydralazine, sulfasalazine, or isoniazid) at a faster or slower rate than the general population (11,30). The importance of identifying fast or slow drug metabolizers is not generally appreciated. Those considered to be rapid acetylators will have a plasma isoniazid (INH) concentration of less than 2.5 µg/ml 6 hr after an oral dose of 10 mg/kg. Fast drug metabolizers of INH are not good candidates for twice-weekly therapy for the treatment of tuberculosis. Slow drug metabolizers, given standard drug dosages, will exhibit a greater incidence of drug toxicity. Absolute identification of fast and slow drug metabolizers depends on the quantitative identification of urinary drug metabolite excretion profiles as well as on serial determination of plasma drug concentrations.

The use of plasma drug concentrations alone to identify fast and slow metabolizers can be misleading. Generally, plasma drug concentrations of slow metabolizers will be significantly higher than would be observed in the general population receiving the same milligram per kilogram a day dosage. Consistently high plasma concentrations on normal or low drug doses is suggestive of slow (genetic) drug metabolism if this decrease in metabolism is not thought to be the result of a transient disease process. On the other hand, fast drug metabolizers usually exhibit consistently low plasma concentrations on standard dosage regimens. Because plasma drug levels in noncompliant patients often mimic those observed in fast metabolizers, there is a tendency to identify noncompliant patients as fast metabolizers.

Generally, a drug is metabolized from a pharmacologically active agent to an inactive product incapable of eliciting a given therapeutic response (5–7,9–11). There are exceptions to this rule (Table 2). Some organic compounds, when metabolized, have greater biologic activity than their parent compounds. For example, diazepam is rapidly metabolized to desmethyldiazepam, which is the most active antianxiety agent of all the diazepam metabolites.

As a general rule, when a compound has a less polar active metabolite, the half-life of the active metabolite is significantly longer than that of the parent compound. Such is the case with procainamide and N-acetylprocainamide (NAPA). The half-life of procainamide is 3 to 4 hr, whereas NAPA has a half-life of 6 to 9 hr in patients with normal creatinine clearance.

TABLE 2. *Active metabolites of selected drugs*[a]

Drug	Metabolite
Acetohexamide	Hydroxyhexamide
Alprenolol	4-OH-Alprenolol
Amitriptyline	Nortriptyline
Aprindine	Desethylaprindine
Carbamazepine	10,11-Epoxycarbamazepine
Cephapirin	Desacetylcephapirin
Chloral hydrate	Trichloroethanol
Chlordiazepoxide	Desmethylchlordiazepoxide
Chlorpromazine	N-Desmethylchlorpromazine
	7-Hydroxychlorpromazine
Clobazam	Desmethylclobazam
Codeine	Morphine
Diazepam	Desmethyldiazepam
Diphenoxylate	Difenoxine
Disopyramide	*N*-Dealkylated metabolite
Doxepin	Desmethyldoxepin
Encainide	*O*-Demethylencainide
	3-Methyl-*O*-demethylencainide
Ethynodiol	Norethindrone
Fenfluramine	Norfenfluramine
Flurazepam	Desmethylflurazepam
Imipramine	Desipramine
Lidocaine	Monoethylglycinexylidide (MEGX)
Loxapine	Amoxapine
Maprotiline	Desmethylmaprotiline
Meperidine	Normeperidine
Methamphetamine	Amphetamine
Methotrimeprazine	*N*-Monodesmethylmethotrimeprazine
Nomifensine	4-Hydroxyphenyl metabolite
Phenacetin	Acetaminophen
Phenylbutazone	Oxyphenbutazone
Pivampicillin	Ampicillin
Prazepam	Desmethyldiazepam
Prednisone	Prednisolone
Primidone	Phenobarbital
Procainamide	*N*-Acetylprocainamide
Propranolol	4-Hydroxypropranolol
Quinidine	3-Hydroxyquinidine
Temazepam	Oxazepam
Thioridazine	Thioridazine side-chain sulfoxide
	Thioridazine side-chain sulfone
Tolazamide	Three weakly active metabolites
Trimethadione	*N*-Desmethyl metabolite
Verapamil	Norverapamil
Zimelidine	Norzimelidine

[a]See Chapter 9 for drugs with active metabolites that are excreted renally.

RENAL EXCRETION

Urinary excretion is the major pathway for the elimination of many drugs and their metabolites (see Chapters 8 and 9). If a drug is extensively eliminated by the kidney (i.e., ≥ 25–30%) and is not extensively metabolized, changes in renal function will alter the drug's plasma concentrations to a significant degree. Uremic

patients, the elderly, and those with congestive heart failure have decreased renal drug clearance (see Chapters 6, 9, and 15).

PHARMACOKINETICS

Anyone using routine TDM must constantly keep in mind that the plasma concentration achieved and maintained following the administration of a fixed drug dosage is a direct consequence of the interactions of a wide variety of processes. These include drug absorption, distribution, metabolism, and excretion, in addition to the physiologic status of the patient. All these factors are interrelated, each playing a role in determining the steady state drug concentration that will be achieved on a fixed dosage regimen. The study of these interrelationships forms the basis of pharmacokinetics. In the practical sense, pharmacokinetics as a discipline represents an attempt to use mathematical models to predict the distribution and excretion patterns of drugs, usually at steady state concentrations, following a given dosage regimen. Applied clinical pharmacokinetics has been developed to the point where it is applicable to the study of patients receiving a given drug, provided the theoretical limitations of the model are recognized. However, in most texts, one of the unfortunate limitations of pharmacokinetics is that many models or clinical applications do not take into account multiple-drug therapy, the clinical status of the patient, or the kinetic parameters in the ill patient. Interactions between drugs can alter the kinetics of each and affect plasma drug concentrations as well (see Chapter 11). Therefore, unless specific clinical data from a given patient are available, these models should serve only as general guidelines. The availability of drug-monitoring techniques in biologic fluids resulted in attempts to correlate a given milligram per kilogram dosage of drug with the observed plasma concentration and clinical response in large patient populations. The fundamental assumption of these studies was that the patient was at steady state; that is, the intake of a drug was constant over a period of time, and drug elimination, as reflected in the rates of drug metabolism and excretion, was constant. Based on data derived from these studies, a number of computer programs have been developed that, given plasma concentration data with respect to time, will calculate the drug dosage necessary to achieve a given plasma drug concentration in a specific patient (see Chapter 19) (38). Unfortunately, these programs, and the information derived from them, are not yet widely available to clinical chemistry laboratories or clinical pharmacokinetic laboratories. Clinical establishment of a national therapeutic drug regimen does not require detailed knowledge of pharmacokinetics. However, an awareness of the terminology and fundamental principles is essential (see Chapter 1).

BASIC GUIDELINES FOR ROUTINE TDM

The ultimate responsibility of the laboratory engaged in routine TDM is to assure that all information relevant to a patient's pharmacologic profile be available to the clinician to use in individualizing that patient's therapeutic regimen.

Clinical pharmacokinetics is a valuable tool for understanding and interpreting the response of an individual patient to a given drug regimen. Computer programs that apply these principles to dosage calculations for individual patients have been developed (31–33) (see Chapter 19). These programs can be used for many drugs to calculate the expected plasma concentration that will be achieved over a fixed time interval following a given dose. Unfortunately, these programs and the information derived from them are not widely available to the clinical chemistry laboratory or to the practicing clinician. There is a series of simple guidelines that will generate approximately the same information as the computer programs without the necessity of complex mathematical formulas or computer programs (1,5,34).

There is wide individual variability in patient plasma concentration of drugs, as a direct consequence of genetic factors, multiple drug therapy, age, and so on (Fig. 5). It is extremely difficult and dangerous to generalize about the relationship between plasma concentrations and drug dose. Rather, it is necessary to apply the principles of both clinical pharmacology and pharmacokinetics to achieve the desired effect without introducing unwanted side effects in each individual patient.

The importance of individualized drug therapy is particularly significant when administering drugs to the young and the old (see Chapters 14 and 15).

In order to derive as much information as possible about the pharmacologic status of the patient, each laboratory engaged in TDM should have the following information available at the time any drug is monitored:

Patient's age. It is clearly established that there are marked age-dependent differences in drug disposition, particularly for the transition ages from neonate to infant, child to adolescent, and adult to elderly.

Patient's weight and height. The weight of the patient is essential for mathematical calculation of the relationships among drug dose, plasma concentration, and drug clearance.

Patient's other drugs. One must have knowledge of all the drugs a patient is receiving (frequency, doses, amounts, the actual times taken versus the times ordered), in addition to the agent being monitored. This is essential for identification of potential drug interactions that have been reported to alter plasma concentrations, as well as for identification of compounds that may interfere in a given analytical technique. This should include any change in brands.

Total daily doses of drugs. Knowledge of the total daily dose for each drug administered is necessary to correlate the patient's actual plasma concentrations with expected drug concentrations. Predicted drug concentrations can then be correlated with the observed (measured) drug concentrations to provide an indication of the patient's pharmacologic status.

Critical time intervals. Accuracy of dose administration should be confirmed. All doses should be timed exactly from starting time through duration of administration. They should also be consistent from nursing unit to nursing unit (see Chapter 22). Without this information, it is difficult to assess whether the actual plasma concentration represents a peak, trough, or Cp_{ss} level. Knowledge of actual sampling time and dosage interval is extremely important for accurate interpretation

of plasma concentrations of drugs with short half-life periods, such as aminoglycosides (see Appendix B). Drug administration sets that have been noted to result in loss of active drug (e.g., diazepam and nitroglycerin through plastic tubing, unprotected nitroprusside) should be recorded in the request and laboratory result form.

Clinical status of the patient. It is well established that acute or chronic disease can dramatically alter drug-utilization patterns. Awareness of the patient's current clinical status is particularly important for regulation of drug therapy in patients with hepatic or renal failure. Without knowledge of the clinical status of the patient is is impossible for those interpreting drug concentrations to distinguish an altered drug-utilization pattern that is associated with a given disease state from other factors (noncompliance, drug interactions, etc.) that can be present with a similar pattern.

If information on all the foregoing components is available, measurements of drug concentrations can provide a great deal of insight into the pharmacologic status of the patient. Clinical application of the information derived from TDM will allow individualization of drug therapy.

When long-term oral therapy is initiated, drug will continue to accumulate within the body until such time as the rate of drug clearance (elimination) is in equilibrium with the total daily drug intake. Drug clearance encompasses all distribution, metabolic, and renal processes involved in drug disposition. Over a period of time, body and plasma drug concentrations will increase exponentially until they reach a steady state or plateau.

We again emphasize that the time required to reach a stablized steady state is seven half-life periods following institution of drug therapy; however, steady state processes are 97% complete within five half-life periods. If the prescribed drug dosage is changed after a steady state has been achieved, the principles regulating the time required to achieve a new steady state plateau still apply (five times the drug half-life). For instance, if the maintenance dose of a drug were doubled, the new steady state drug concentration would not be doubled (assuming linear kinetics) until the completion of five to six half-life periods.

If a plasma drug concentration is determined before achievement of a steady state (for example, after only one or two half-lives), it will not reflect the true steady state concentration of the drug. However, the following formula may provide a general guideline to predict steady state after a given sample is taken before C_{ss} is achieved:

$$Cp_{\min(ss)} (1 - e^{-N\lambda_z\tau}) = Cp_{\min(N)}$$

where $Cp_{\min(N)}$ is the measured trough after the Nth dose that is used to approximate the $Cp_{\min(ss)}$ (minimum Cp at steady state); λ_z is the terminal disposition rate constant; and τ is the dosage interval. Measurement of plasma concentrations before steady state is achieved does not yield as much clinically useful information with respect to the patient as levels measured at steady state.

Recently however, the "single-point single-dose" method has been used to estimate the individual maintenance dose needed to achieve a desired steady state

plasma concentration for a limited number of drugs. Experimental observations have shown an excellent correlation between a single dose drug concentration determination and steady state concentrations (35). The method suggests that the maintenance dosage rate (D_M/τ) required to achieve the desired average plasma concentration (C_{av}) can be calculated from a measured plasma concentration (C^*) at an appropriate time (t^*) after a single test dose (D) knowing the disposition rate constant (λ_z). The most appropriate time to measure C^* is at $1/\lambda_z$ or approximately 1.5 times the half-life of the drug (35,36).

$$\frac{D_M}{\tau} = \frac{C_{av}}{C^*} \, D\lambda_z \, e^{-\lambda_z t^*} \approx \frac{C_{av}}{C^*} \, \frac{0.25 \, D}{t_{1/2}}$$

Using patient population half-lives (see Appendix B), reasonable estimates of D_M may be found for selected drugs that meet certain criteria. This method appears to be applicable to intravenous or oral administration and especially when the pharmacokinetic parameters (e.g., age, sex, weight/height, renal, and/or hepatic function) for that particular individual are within the normal population. This method is most appropriate for drugs where absorption is rapid (i.e., $Ka >> \lambda_z$) and where disposition follows a linear one-compartmental model. Therefore, it is not useful for drugs like phenytoin and aspirin (Chapter 17), or drugs like carbamazepine that exhibit time-dependent kinetics or drugs that have half-life periods greater than 24 to 36 hr (36). For drugs with long half-life periods, such as perhexiline $(T_{1/2} = 72{-}288 \text{ hr})$ or digitoxin $(T_{1/2} = 168{-}192 \text{ hr})$, taking a single dose and measuring a single plasma concentration 3 to 6 days later ($1\frac{1}{2}$ times $T_{1/2}$) is not any more efficient than routine monitoring of plasma concentrations following empirical maintenance doses. If this method should eventually prove to be useful for a wide variety of drugs, the ability to quickly predict maintenance dose for a desired steady state concentration should benefit patient care.

EFFECTS OF MULTIPLE-DRUG THERAPY ON DRUG DISPOSITION

Most clinically significant drug interactions are readily identifiable in the presence of elevated plasma concentrations of a given drug. Generally, it will be observed that the interfering drug has a metabolic pathway that is similar to that of the drug being monitored. In addition, multiple drug therapy can also alter absorption, protein binding, or renal clearance of a given agent. Change in any of these factors can result in altered steady state concentrations (see Chapter 11).

Any factor that alters drug clearance will alter the drug's steady state concentration:

$$Cp_{ss} = \frac{F \, \text{dose}/\tau}{\text{clearance}}$$

During multiple drug therapy, two drugs may compete for the same metabolic site. This competition will both decrease the rate of metabolism of the drug that is excluded from the site and prolong its half-life. Because the clearance is decreased, a new, higher steady state drug concentration will be achieved and maintained as

long as the multiple drug therapy is continued. For this reason it is necessary to be able to identify (a) all drugs a patient is receiving and (b) those agents that are potentially capable of altering a given drug's half-life (1,5–7,9,31,32) (see Chapters 1 and 11).

EFFECTS OF DISEASE STATES ON DRUG DISPOSITION

Drug clearance can be dramatically altered during renal disease and liver disease because the elimination rates of drugs are changed. Consequently, new steady state levels will be achieved that may differ significantly from those observed in healthy individuals. One must always consider the clinical status of the patient when interpreting plasma drug concentrations.

GENETIC CONTROL OF DRUG DISPOSITION

Drug clearance is significantly regulated by genetic factors. In a large population of patients, one can predict that if the entire population is given the same milligram per kilogram dosage of a drug, there will be marked differences in the ability of individuals within the population to utilize the drug. These genetic differences will be reflected in marked variability in the steady state plasma concentrations observed in this population. For example, in a population of patients receiving phenytoin at a standard therapeutic dosage of 5 mg/kg/day, one would theoretically expect all patients to have a therapeutic drug level of 15 μg/ml (29,31,32). In reality, plasma concentrations will range from 0 μg/ml, which suggests drug malabsorption, patient noncompliance, or rapid drug metabolism, to levels of 40 to 50 μg/ml, which may indicate the presence of hepatic disease, drug interactions, or genetically slow drug metabolizers.

The importance of genetic regulation of drug metabolism as a determinant of each individual patient's drug utilization pattern cannot be neglected. As an example, consider the incidence of fast and slow metabolizers among patients receiving isoniazid, a drug commonly used in the treatment of tuberculosis. Approximately 40% of all Caucasians are rapid acetylators of isoniazid. In contrast, over 90% of Japanese and Eskimos are rapid acetylators (7,29). This genetic variability requires individualization of therapeutic regimens to assure the maintenance of optimal isoniazid concentrations in the different populations and individuals within the population (1,5–7,9,18,29).

MINIMUM EFFECTIVE DRUG CONCENTRATIONS

Following the administration of any drug there is always a peak level, which represents the point of maximum absorption, and a trough (valley) level, which represents the lowest point achieved following a given dose of drug. The trough level occurs after the absorption process is complete. It is the lowest point achieved as a consequence of the process of drug elimination (drug metabolism and excretion) that occurs during each dosage interval.

The object of most drug therapy is to assure that a minimum effective concentration (MEC) of drug is present without reaching a potential minimum toxic concentration (MTC). One may calculate the maximum maintenance dose ($D_{M,max}$) and the maximum dosage internal (τ_{max}) to assure that the plasma concentrations at steady state will remain between MTC and MEC.

$$D_{M,max} = \frac{MTC - MEC}{FV}$$

$$\tau_{max} = 1.44 \, t_{1/2} \, \ln(MTC/MEC)$$

Therefore, the blood specimens for routine therapeutic monitoring should, for most drugs, be drawn immediately prior to the next drug dose at steady state. The actual plasma concentration observed at that time should be within the optimal therapeutic range. It is imperative to recognize that the MEC of a given drug necessary to achieve the desired therapeutic effect can vary from patient to patient. The severity of the disease process plays a major role in determining MEC for many drugs. Therefore, it is possible to achieve a therapeutic response at suboptimal concentrations in some patients, whereas others will require toxic concentrations to achieve control. Plasma concentrations must always be interpreted in conjunction with the clinical status of the patient and the desired therapeutic endpoint (1,2,5,7,12).

INTERPRETATION OF PLASMA DRUG CONCENTRATIONS

There are a number of advantages to TDM that provide the clinician with clinically useful information. Plasma drug concentrations in conjunction with a thorough assessment of the patient's clinical status and the therapeutic goals to be achieved provide a means of successfully and rapidly individualizing a patient's therapeutic regimen to assure optimal benefits with minimal risk:

1. Noncompliance can be identified (37). Many patients, in particular those who have chronic disease requiring therapy over a prolonged period of time, do not take their medications as prescribed. Moreover, patients with chronic diseases that do not necessarily cause pain or other unusual discomfort (for example, the epilepsies, asthma, hypertension) may easily neglect to take their medicine. The end result of such noncompliance is an exacerbation of the existing disorder some time in the future. Studies have clearly demonstrated that noncompliance is a major factor in treatment failures (5–7,9).

2. Individual variations in drug utilization patterns can be dealt with appropriately. In any population of individuals, a drug dosage based solely on body weight results in a fixed steady state serum concentration. If the plasma concentrations following a specific dosage are analyzed in a large patient population, however, the distribution of drug levels will be Gaussian (a bell-shaped curve). The vast majority of patients will show levels within the range expected for a given milligram per kilogram dosage. Patients who are genetically either fast or slow drug metabolizers will have levels at extreme ends of the curve. The fast drug metabolizers

require significantly higher doses to achieve the same plasma concentrations and consequently the desired therapeutic effect. Patients who are slow drug metabolizers become intoxicated and experience side effects from standard therapeutic doses of the drugs; therefore, optimal drug levels can be maintained in these patients with dosages well below the standard regimen.

TDM allows identification of individuals who are fast or slow metabolizers and ensures that their medication regimens can be appropriately adjusted to fit their own metabolic patterns. Without TDM, a prolonged period (sometimes lasting months) of trial-and-error therapy is required to achieve the appropriate dosage regimen, thus unnecessarily subjecting the patient to a time interval when the disease process is uncontrolled (1,28,29).

A common factor (characteristic of a few drugs, including acetaminophen, propranolol, diflunisal, phenytoin, and aspirin) associated with abnormal drug elevations is the phenomenon of saturation (zero-order) kinetics. In TDM, this is often reflected by a rapid rise in serum drug concentrations following a small increment of drug dosage. Thus, a small dosage increment will cause a large increase in serum concentration. The therapeutic index, that is, the margin of safety between therapeutic and toxic drug concentrations, is extremely small for many drugs. If the enzymes responsible for the metabolism of these drugs become saturated, drug intoxication can develop quickly (see Chapter 17).

3. Altered drug utilization as a consequence of disease can be readily identified. Patients on long-term drug therapy may become acutely ill (see Chapter 6) and require the administration of additional therapeutic agents. Drug interactions (see Chapter 11) may then cause these patients to respond in an unexpected manner to a fixed dosage of some adjunctive therapy. Acute or chronic uremia (see Chapters 8 and 9) can dramatically decrease the elimination of a drug that is primarily dependent on urinary excretion, and renal failure can alter the protein binding characteristics for many drugs that are bound to albumin. In both situations the ratio of free drug to total drug may increase to the point where free-drug concentrations are high enough to produce a clinically evident toxic drug response, although the total serum drug concentrations are well within optimal therapeutic range. Hepatic disease (see Chapters 3 and 4) can extensively alter a given therapeutic response by impairing a patient's ability to metabolize drugs. Most drugs depend on liver detoxification for conversion to water-soluble products, which are easily eliminated from the body. Thus, a precipitous rise in parent drug concentrations can occur as the unmetabolized drug, which normally would have been eliminated from the system, accumulates (9–11,27).

TDM provides a means of accurately calculating and correcting dosage regimens to coincide with the disease status of the patient.

4. An altered physiologic state can be compensated for. Normal alterations in physiologic state also change drug utilization patterns. Three areas in which TDM is crucial to successful dosage regimen adjustments should be emphasized.

Most important, the normal process of maturation involves a large number of physiologic changes that can dramatically alter drug utilization. Children (see Chap-

ter 14) utilize drugs at a faster rate than adults and therefore, as a rule of thumb, require almost twice as much drug on a body-weight basis as an adult to achieve the same therapeutic drug concentration. As a child enters puberty, drug utilization patterns rapidly change to those of adulthood, to the extent that by early pubescence the conversion to adult patterns is complete. These changes usually occur between the ages of 10 and 13, appearing earlier in girls than in boys. It is imperative that TDM be carried out carefully for any drug administered chronically to early pubescent and pubescent children. Failure to adjust the child's therapeutic regimen to compensate for the associated physiologic changes may result in exposure to unnecessary and prolonged drug toxicity, with its attendant sequelae (12,34).

As the maturation process continues, however, the efficiency of normal physiologic functions decreases, as does the ability to bind drugs to plasma protein. Geriatric patients (see Chapter 15) often exhibit reduced rates of drug elimination, thereby requiring reduced drug dosages. It is possible for geriatric patients to have total plasma drug concentrations within the optimal therapeutic range and, at the same time, elevated free-drug concentrations that can produce adverse side effects. The clinical signs of drug intoxication in the elderly often present clinically as lethargy and confusion, and TDM provides a means of distinguishing drug-induced confusion from organic deterioration (9).

Anyone involved in the utilization of information derived from TDM must always bear in mind that the interpretation of plasma drug concentrations must always be carried out in conjunction with an assessment of the clinical status of the patient. Therapeutic ranges should more correctly be described as optimal concentrations. The optimal concentration (therapeutic range) of a drug is defined as that concentration of drug present in plasma or some other biologic fluid or tissue that provides the desired therapeutic response in most patients. The severity of the disease process determines the amount of drug necessary to achieve a given therapeutic effect. Thus, it is quite possible that a patient may achieve the desired therapeutic effect at a plasma concentration well below the optimal range. Conversely, some patients will not achieve the desired therapeutic effect even when plasma concentrations are elevated into the toxic range. If the desired therapeutic effect is achieved at suboptimal plasma concentrations, every attempt should be made to avoid the prescription of additional drugs simply to increase the plasma concentration into what is commonly referred to as the therapeutic range. Obviously, the interpretation of plasma drug concentration must take into account the various factors that can alter the steady state plasma concentration achieved on a given dosage regimen.

REFERENCES

1. Pippenger, C. E. (1979): Therapeutic drug monitoring: An overview. *Ther. Drug Monitor.*, 1: 3–9.
2. Koch-Weser, J. (1981): Serum drug concentrations in clinical perspective. *Ther. Drug Monitor.*, 3:3–16.
3. Baer, D. M., and Dito, W. R. (eds.) (1981): *Interpretations in Therapeutic Drug Monitoring.* American Society of Clinical Pathologists, Chicago.
4. Dirks, J. F., and Kinsman, R. A. (1982): Nondichotomous patterns of medication usage: The yes-no fallacy. *Clin. Pharmacol. Ther.*, 31:413–417.

5. Melmon, K. L., and Morelli, H. I. (eds.) (1978): *Clinical Pharmacology: Basic Principles in Therapeutics*, 2nd Ed. Macmillian, New York.
6. Gilman, A. G., Goodman, L. S., and Gilman, A. (eds.) (1980): *The Pharmacological Basis of Therapeutics*, 6th Ed. Macmillian, New York.
7. Avery, G. S. (ed.) (1980): *Drug Treatment: Principles and Practice of Clinical Pharmacology and Therapeutics*, 2nd Ed. Adis Press, Sydney.
8. Sherwin, A. L. (1978): Clinical pharmacology of ethosuximide. In: *Antiepileptic Drugs: Quantitative Analysis and Interpretation*, edited by C. E. Pippenger, J. K. Penry, and H. Kutt, pp. 283–295. Raven Press, New York.
9. O'Malley, K., Judge, T. G., and Crooks, J. (1980): *Geriatric Clinical Pharmacology and Therapeutics in Drug Treatment*, 2nd Ed., edited by G. S. Avery, pp. 158–181. Adis Press, Sydney.
10. Goldstein, A., Aronow, L., and Kalman, S. M. (1974): *Principles of Drug Action: The Basis of Pharmacology*, 2nd Ed., John Wiley & Sons, New York.
11. Mayer, S. E., Melmon, K. L., and Gilman, A. G. (1980): Introduction: The dynamics of drug absorption, distribution, and elimination. In: *The Pharmacological Basis of Therapeutics*, 6th Ed., edited by A. G. Gilman, L. S. Goodman, and A. Gilman, pp. 1–27. Macmillian, New York.
12. Morselli, P. L. (1977): Antiepileptic drugs. In: *Drug Disposition During Development*, edited by P. L. Morselli, pp. 311–360. Spectrum Publications, New York.
13. Mirkin, B. L. (ed.) (1976): *Perinatal Pharmacology and Therapeutics*. Academic Press, New York.
14. Glaser, G. H., Penry, J. K., and Woodbury, D. M. (eds.) (1980): *Antiepileptic Drugs: Mechanisms of Action*. Raven Press, New York.
15. Koch-Weser, J., and Sellers, E. M. (1976): Binding of drugs to serum albumin. *N. Engl. J. Med.*, 294:311–316, 526–531.
16. Levy, R. H. (1980): Monitoring of free valproic acid levels. *Ther. Drug. Monitor.*, 2:199–201.
17. Sublett, J. L., Pollard, S. J., Kadlec, G. J., and Karibo, J. M. (1979): Non-compliance in asthmatic children. *Ann. Allergy*, 43:95–97.
18. Vesell, E. S. (1982): On the significance of host factors that affect drug disposition. *Clin. Pharmacol. Ther.*, 31:1–7.
19. Holford, N. H. G., and Sheiner, L. B. (1981): Understanding the dose-effect relationship. *Clin. Pharmacokinet.*, 6:429–453.
20. Benet, L. Z. (ed.) (1976): *The Effect of Disease States on Drug Pharmacokinetics*. American Pharmaceutical Association, Washington, D.C.
21. Pippenger, C. E. (1980): Rationale and clinical application of therapeutic drug monitoring. *Pediatr. Clin. North Am.*, 27:891–925.
22. Garlock, C. M., Pippenger, C. E., Desaulniers, C. W., and Sternberg, S. (1979): A rapid ultrafiltration technique for the determination of free drug concentrations. I and II. *Clin. Chem.*, 25:1117.
23. McAuliffe, J. J., Sherwin, A. L., Leppick, I. E., Fayle, S. A., and Pippenger, C. E. (1977): Salivary levels of anticonvulsants: A practical approach to drug monitoring. *Neurology (Minneap.)*, 27:409–413.
24. Danhof, M., and Breimer, D. D. (1978): Therapeutic drug monitoring in saliva. *Clin. Pharmacokinet.*, 3:39–57.
25. Mucklow, J. C., Bending, M. R., Kahn, G. C., and Dollery, C. T. (1978): Drug concentration in saliva. *Clin. Pharmacol. Ther.*, 24:563–570.
26. Graham, G. G. (1982): Noninvasive chemical methods of estimating pharmacokinetic parameters. *Pharmacol. Ther.*, 18:333–349.
27. Conney, A. H. (1967): Pharmacological implications of microsomal enzyme induction. *Pharmacol. Rev.*, 19:317–366.
28. Kutt, H. (1978): Evaluation of unusual antiepileptic drug concentrations. In: *Antiepileptic Drugs: Quantitative Analysis and Interpretation*, edited by C. E. Pippenger, J. K. Penry, and H. Kutt, pp. 307–314. Raven Press, New York.
29. Kromann, N., Christiansen, J., Flachs, H., Dom, M., and Huidberg, E. F. (1981): Differences in single dose kinetics between Greenland Eskimos and Danes. *Ther. Drug Monitor.*, 3:239–246.
30. Winter, M. E. (1980): *Basic Clinical Pharmacokinetics*. Applied Therapeutics, San Francisco.
31. Kaka, J. S., and Buchanan, E. C. (1983): Aminoglycoside pharmacokinetics on a microcomputer. *Drug Intell. Clin. Pharm.*, 17:33–38.
32. Koup, J. R., and Benjamin, D. R. (1980): Numerical integration simulation programs for the microcomputer. *Ther. Drug Monitor.*, 2:243–247.

33. Lafrate, P. R., Gotz, V. P., Robinson, J. D., and Lupkiewicz, S. M. (1982): Computer-simulated conversion of theophylline dosage forms. *Drug Intell. Clin. Pharm.*, 16:19–25.
34. Pippenger, C. E. (1978): Pediatric clinical pharmacology of antiepileptic drugs: A special consideration. In: *Antiepileptic Drugs: Quantitative Analysis and Interpretation*, edited by C. E. Pippenger, J. K. Penry, and H. Kutt, pp. 315–319. Raven Press, New York.
35. Slattery, J. T. (1981): Single point maintenance dose prediction: Role of interindividual differences in clearance and volume of distribution in choice of sampling time. *J. Pharm. Sci.*, 70:1174–1175.
36. Unadkat, J. D., and Rowland, M. (1982): Further considerations of the "Single-point single-dose" method to estimate individual maintenance dosage requirements. *Ther. Drug Monitor.*, 4:201–208.
37. Evans, L., and Spelman, M. (1983): The problem of noncompliance with drug therapy. *Drugs*, 25:63–67.
38. Bowman, J. D., and Mungell, D. (1983): The use of programmable calculations in clinical pharmacokinetics. In: *Applied Clinical Pharmacokinetics*, edited by D. Mungell, pp. 389–434. Raven Press, New York.

Pharmacokinetic Basis for Drug Treatment,
edited by L. Z. Benet et al., Raven Press,
New York © 1984

Chapter 22

Establishing a Clinical Pharmacokinetics Laboratory

Robert M. Elenbaas and *Neil Massoud

*Schools of Pharmacy and Medicine, University of Missouri–Kansas City, and Department of Emergency Health Services, Truman Medical Center, Kansas City, Missouri 64108 and *Division of Clinical Pharmacology, Departments of Medicine and Pharmacy, University of California, San Francisco, San Francisco, California 94143*

In 1981, 12% of North America's health-care costs were due to laboratory testing procedures. Unfortunately, training in the interpretation of test results has not kept pace with advances in laboratory analytical procedures. Hence, the clinican may be confronted with laboratory data contributing little to the patient's care. One area of major growth within recent years has been the development of readily available analytical procedures for measuring serum drug concentrations. Whereas the majority of hospital laboratories can provide the physician with this service for a fairly wide variety of drugs, very few provide any assistance in correct interpretation of such data. The difficult task of correlating the test results to the patient's condition (e.g., hypoalbuminemia, genetic makeup, decreased renal function, pregnancy, social habits, etc.) (see Chapter 21, Fig. 5), and subsequently tailoring the drug dosage regimen to fit the needs of the individual patient, is left to the clinician. Unfortunately, again, a general lack of training in pharmacokinetics may impair appropriate interpretation, such that the laboratory test may actually impede more than aid achievement of optimal patient care (1–3).

Effective application of pharmacokinetics to the clinical setting is dependent on two principal factors: (a) accurate, timely measurement of drug concentrations in serum or other biologic fluids (see Chapter 21) and (b) an interpretive consultation from a practitioner knowledgeable in clinical pharmacokinetics, allowing the design of a patient-specific drug dosage regimen (4). It is our belief that development of a specialized clinical pharmacokinetics laboratory (CPL) is the most effective means to achieve an acceptable level of performance within both of these areas.

The following discussion deals with the practical aspects of developing and maintaining a pharmacokinetics *service* laboratory. A number of administrative, financial, and political questions must be answered, and decisions must be made by the individual considering the development of such a specialty laboratory. A

prospective review of the matter should ease the development and growth of pharmacokinetics service laboratories in other settings.

SCOPE OF CPL SERVICES

Drug Assay

Many hospitals internally assay three or four commonly ordered drugs and refer the balance to an outside reference laboratory. However, these reference laboratories may not individually provide a broad scope of service, and therefore the hospital or clinic must deal with two or more laboratories. By consolidating these activities within a specialty CPL, it may be possible to provide a broader range of analyses at lesser cost. For example, a hospital laboratory asked to assay only one or two aminoglycoside blood levels per week may not be able to provide this service internally or may find it necessary to hold samples for a weekly "batch run." The clinical utility of the test, of course, declines as the length of time between sampling and return of results increases. However, a laboratory receiving specimens from several hospitals could find it economically feasible to provide the service on a daily basis.

Other benefits may result from the construction of a specialty pharmacokinetics laboratory. The analytical chemistry expertise and alternative drug assay methods that may exist here can serve as a major advantage in quality control and assay development for specialty needs. Whereas this latter point is possibly of decreasing importance with improved commercial technology in the drug assay field, problems encountered in the clinical setting will probably continue to demand this expertise. For example, HPPH (the parahydroxyphenyl derivative of phenytoin) may accumulate in patients with decreased renal function (see Chapter 9) and interfere with the homogenous enzyme immunoassay (e.g., EMIT®) for phenytoin, falsely elevating the result by 1.7 to 2.1-fold (5). If an alternative assay method, like high-performance liquid chromatography (HPLC), were available, it could be used in settings such as this to avoid possible confusion in complicated cases.

The need for an effective system of quality control in determining of serum drug concentrations is pivotal to effective application of this information to patient care. Some skepticism has been voiced in questioning if the benefits achieved through drug concentration determination (DCD) outweigh the costs. Although many factors may prohibit consistent correlation (2,6) of the drug blood concentration to the clinical state of the patient (Table 1), problems with assay methods warrant special mention (2,3,7).

It has been found that considerable variability may exist among and within laboratories in the analysis of drug blood concentrations. McCormick et al. (8) submitted samples containing identical amounts of either digoxin, phenytoin, or phenobarbital to three hospital laboratories. In each case, one sample was labeled as a quality-control specimen, and its twin was made to simulate a clinical specimen. All hospital laboratories performed well in the analysis of the quality-control spec-

TABLE 1. *Cautions in the interpretation of drug concentrations*

Patient variability
1. Patient compliance
2. Individual capacity to absorb or distribute drugs
3. Individual capacity to metabolize or excrete drugs
4. Acute severe pathologic condition vs treated improved pathologic condition
5. Body weight/height ratio, body surface area
6. Concomitant drugs and nutritional status
7. First-pass effect
8. Tissue responsiveness (e.g., geriatrics vs neonates; low serum albumin vs normal)

Nursing, assay, and medication variability
1. Quality of pharmaceutical formulations (generic vs brand)
2. Medication errors
3. Route, technique, and timing of administration (highly variable between wards and between hospitals)
4. Time course of treatment [steady state? acute dose(s)?]
5. Reproducibility of the assay method
6. Time of sampling
7. Interferences in laboratory determinations: drug-drug or drug-laboratory values (e.g., cefoxitin interfering with serum creatinine values)
8. False measurement of active drug via degradation of the inactive glucuronide to the active form of the drug during assay procedure
9. Metabolite interference of drug assay

---

imen; however, performance on the clinical specimen was variable and generally poor, often falling outside the 90% confidence interval for the mean of the corresponding quality-control sample. In another study, Pippenger and associates (4) found that almost half of identical samples distributed to 112 American and Canadian laboratories gave results outside 1 standard deviation of the mean for five reference laboratories. This indicates laboratory and/or technician laxity in the analysis of clinical specimens. Although not evaluated, one could speculate that this laxity would be less likely to exist within a specialty pharmacokinetics laboratory in which its personnel are oriented toward a primary mission of accurate quantitative drug analysis and in which the clinical importance of the test results are understood. Laboratory biological procedures with a 10% to 20% margin of error (e.g., Hgb, sodium, white blood cell count) are acceptable in most cases. However, such a level of measurement error for drugs with a narrow therapeutic window (see Appendixes A–C, which include most of these drugs) could result in an unwarranted dosage modification.

Consultation

Several surveys of selected drug blood levels have indicated that tests are ordered, specimens sampled, or data interpreted inappropriately as much as 25% to 65% of the time (9–13). Even in situations where the test is indicated, failure to sample at the correct time within the dosage regimen may (a) markedly diminish or negate

the test's worth and (b) result in inappropriate dosage adjustments. Hospital phlebotomists or ward nurses often cannot obtain samples at the exact time needed, even though a very specific order may be written to do so. A DCD should therefore be regarded as a component of a pharmacokinetic consultation, and the CPL should be involved in the sampling, data reporting, and test interpretation processes.

Elenbaas et al. (9) have shown that a policy of prerequisite consultation with a clinical pharmacist prior to sampling or specimen analysis can have a significant influence on the use of DCDs, and they noted a 40% reduction in the frequency of these analyses after its initiation. This policy states that a physician may request a DCD in consultation with a clinical pharmacist who advises on the true need and timing of the sample; all samples must be approved by an appropriately trained clinical pharmacist associated with the CPL before they will be assayed. Further, assay results are communicated to this clinical pharmacist, who enters the data into the patient's record along with an appropriate interpretive consultation and recommendations. It is estimated that this policy saves patients and third-party payers in excess of $20,000 annually in expenditures for drug blood concentrations within a 250-bed acute-care institution.

In addition to the time of sampling, consideration should be given to the actual method of collecting and storing the sample until time of analysis. In general, storage of whole blood should be discouraged, because the erythrocyte/plasma concentration ratio varies between drugs, and sample hemolysis may variably influence assay results and interpretation (2). The plasma sample should be adequately stored to prevent decomposition (refrigeration, freezing). It has been found, for example, that plasma specimens containing both carbenicillin and either of the aminoglycosides gentamicin or tobramycin may demonstrate a progressive loss of aminoglycoside when stored for a period of time prior to assay; the rate of loss is dependent in part on temperature (2,7). Lastly, care should be taken in certain circumstances when using vacutainer tubes or "butterfly" needles for specimen collection of basic drugs. Plasticizers within certain devices are believed to displace basic drugs from α_1-acid glycoprotein, thus decreasing the fraction bound (as with propranolol) (see Table 2) (14).

In many institutions it will not be possible for a representative of the CPL to review every drug concentration determination prior to its analysis. In such situations it is especially important that the form used by hospital personnel to order the test be designed with input from the CPL and be structured so as to record patient information pertinent to the test's interpretation (e.g., body weight, height, drugs to be analyzed, relevant diet restrictions, admitting disease state, other diseases, concurrent drugs, renal and/or hepatic function). When these data are not available, it has been found that plasma analyses are of little or no value except to confirm that the patient has been receiving the drug. Evaluation of a DCD and clinical interpretation by an appropriately trained professional, either directly or through a form more elaborate than that used by most clinical chemistry departments, is a must (2). This same form can be used for reporting results and providing an

TABLE 2. *Effects of vacutainers on binding*

Drug	Effect	Reference
Propranolol	Decreased plasma concentration, decreased protein binding	Cotham et al. (1975): *Clin. Pharmacol. Ther.*, 18:535–538.
Alprenolol	Decreased binding	Piafsky et al. (1976): *Lancet*, 2:963.
Quinidine	Decreased protein binding, decreased plasma concentration	Fremstad et al. (1976): *Acta Pharmacol. Toxicol.*, 39:570–572. Kessler et al. (1979): *Clin. Pharmacol. Ther.*, 25:204–210.
Meperidine (pethidine)	Increased blood-to-plasma ratio (? secondary to decreased protein binding)	Wilkinson et al. (1976): *Clin. Pharmacol. Ther.*, 19:46–48.
Chlorimipramine	Decreased plasma concentration	Mellstrom et al. (1977): *J. Chrom.*, 143:597–605.
Demethylchlorimipramine		
Lidocaine	Decreased plasma concentration, decreased binding	Stargel et al. (1979): *Clin. Chem.*, 25:617–619.
Amitriptyline	Small decrease in plasma concentration	Cochran et al. (1979): *Commun. Psychopharmacol.*, 2:495–503.
Imipramine		
Desmethylimpramine		
Nortriptyline		
Imipramine	Decreased plasma protein binding	Borga et al. (1977): *Clin. Pharmacol. Ther.*, 22:539–544.
Amitriptyline	Decreased plasma concentration	Veith et al. (1978): *Commun. Psychopharmacol.*, 2:491–494.
Doxepin		
Desmethylimipramine		
Nortriptyline		
Neuroleptics	Increase in free fraction (10- to 80-fold)	Freedberg et al. (1979): *Life Sci.*, 24:2467–2474.
Methadone	Decreased protein binding	Romach et al. (1979): *Clin. Pharmacol. Ther.*, 25:246.

From Piafsky (14), with permission.

interpretive consultation. Figures 1–3 provide examples of individualized drug monitoring forms, and Fig. 4 provides one for multi-use drug monitoring.

CONSIDERATIONS IN DEVELOPING AND MAINTAINING A CPL

Service Versus Research

A conscious commitment to patient care services must be made and balanced against whatever research activities may be planned for the laboratory. A tendency often exists in the university-based program to place an emphasis on research and allow service to assume a secondary role. It is difficult to use the same equipment

SUGGESTED SAMPLING TIMES

(   ) how many doses given _____
(   ) suggested sampling time _____
(   ) sample not indicated at this time

DATE	DRUG/DOSE/ROUTE	BUN/CR	PREDICTED CRCL ML/MIN	PEAK MCG/ML	TROUGH MCG/ML

RECOMMENDED PEAK ANTIBIOTIC CONCENTRATIONS

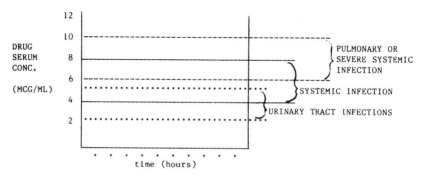

a) Peak concentrations should be within the appropriate areas for the type of infection for which the drug is ordered.

b) Corresponding troughs should fall below 2 mcg/ml PRIOR to each dose. If this does not occur there may be an associated increase of nephro-/ototoxicity.

COMMENTS/RECOMMENDATIONS

_____
_____
_____
_____
_____
_____
_____
_____
_____
_____

Clinician _____ Date _____

PATIENT FACTORS CONSIDERED
IN CALCULATIONS

AGE _____ SEX _____
HEIGHT _____ CM
ACTUAL BODY WEIGHT _____ KG
IDEAL BODY WEIGHT _____ KG
SERUM CREATININE _____ MG/DL
BUN _____ MG/DL
PREDICTED CRCL _____ ML/MIN
HGB _____
TEMP _____
AREA OF INFECTION _____
CULTURE _____

FIG. 1. Gentamicin/tobramycin drug predictions form. *Note:* The use of serum creatinine values may not be accurate for determining creatinine clearance in the following conditions or when the patient is on the following drugs: (a) patients with nephrotic syndrome, renal transplants, dialysis, pregnancy (second or third trimester), acute burns ($\geq$ 25% of body surface), diabetes mellitus (with ketoacidosis), gross ascites, muscular dystrophy, or amputated limbs (38); (b) patients on $\geq$ 2 g methyldopa/day, $\geq$ 3 g L-DOPA/day, $\geq$ 4 g ASA/day, $\geq$ 4 g vitamin C/day, or Cefoxitin (39–44).

LOADING DOSE
Has the patient received theophylline or related compounds within the past 12 hours???

NO (Group A)   YES (Group B)

1) obtain or estimate patient's total body weight   1) if in emergency, draw 2-5ml blood
2) select loading dose according to nomogram   for drug concentration determination
                                                          2) give half the dose according to
                                                              nomogram

AMINOPHYLLINE LOADING DOSE NOMOGRAM

Total Body Weight (Kg)							(Kg)
	50	60	70	80	90	100	

Normal Loading Dose (mg)
250   300   350   400   450   500   550

Reduced Loading Dose (mg)
(for patients with CHF,   200   250   300   350   400   425
liver disease, acute
pulmonary edema or over 65 years)

(Draw a perpendicular line down from the patient's
total body weight to find the loading dose of Aminophylline in milligram's: this can be given in 250-
500 ml D5W, to run in over 30 minutes)

MAINTENANCE DOSE

Use patient's lean body weight (LBW):

Females: LBW(Kg) = 45Kg + 2.3Kg for every inch over 5ft
Males: LBW(Kg) = 50Kg + 2.3Kg for every inch over 5ft

PATIENT CATEGORY	IV AMINOPHYLLINE INFUSION RATE (mg/Kg LBW/Hr)	ORAL DOSE (mg/Kg LBW)
1) No CHF or liver disease & over 65 years	0.6	A. multiply by 8 for q8hr oral AMINOPHYLLINE
2) mild to moderate CHF	0.5	B. multiply by 10.0 for q8hr oral CHOLEDYL[R]
3) severe CHF	0.4	C. multiply by 10 for q12hr THEO-DUR[R]
4) cirrhosis, bili<2	0.4	
5) cirrhosis, bili>2	0.3	
6) cirrhosis, bili>2 and albumin<2.5	0.15	
7) no CHF or liver disease		A. multiply by 6 for q6hr oral AMINOPHYLLINE
a) light or non-smoker	0.7	B. multiply by 8 for q6hr oral CHOLEDYL[R]
b) heavy smoker	0.9	C. multiply by 10 for q12hr oral THEO-DUR[R]
c) heavy marijuana smoker	0.9	

CAUTION: The maintenance dose cannot be safely recommended in severe pulmonary edema due to
the variability (20 fold) in theophylline clearance in this group of patients.
The risk of toxicity & the fact that frequently the patient with acute LVF
is improved clinically within a few hours of initiating treatment may
justify only administering a loading dose & monitoring closely for response.

(Piafsky K.M., Sitar D.S., Rangno R.E., Ogilivie R.I., Theophylline kinetics in
acute pulmonary edema, Clin Pharmacol Ther, 31:310-316, 1977)

FACTORS THAT AFFECT THEOPHYLLINE SERUM CONCENTRATION:

Pneumonia(↔↑), Acute Fever(↔↑), Erythromycin(↔↑), Cimetidine(↑)
Pnenobarbital(↔↓), High CHO diet(↔↑), High Protein Diet(↔↓)
Chronic Allopurinol Therapy(↔↑), Metoprolol(↔↑), Oral Contraceptives(↔↑)
(McElnay J.C., Smith G.D., Helling D.K., Apractical guide to interactions in-
volving theophylline kinetics, Drug Intell Clin Pharm, 16:533-542, 1982)

SUGGESTED SAMPLING TIME: Draw 2-5ml of blood

1) continous IV infusion: draw sample 24-36 hours after infusion started
2) oral dosing: after 2 days of therapy, draw sample 2 hours after midday dose
    For Theo-Dur[R] or slow release preparation of theophylline, after
    3 days of therapy, draw sample 4-6 hours after morning dose.

FIG. 2. Suggested guidelines for adults in maintaining aminophylline steady state serum concentrations between 8 to 20 mg/liter, with a target of 12 to 14 mg/liter. Recommendations for
oral Theo-Dur have been slightly underdosed to allow for a certain degree of variability in the
rate of oral absorption sometimes seen with any zero order oral medication.

THEOPHYLLINE PHARMACOKINETICS

Suggested sampling times.
( ) how many doses given_____
( ) suggested sampling time_____
( ) sample not indicated at this time.

IV AMINOPHYLLINE   YES   NO   ORAL_____
LOADING DOSE:_____   DOSE:_____
MAINTENANCE DOSE:_____   DATE STARTED:_____TIME STARTED_____
DATE STARTED:_____TIME STARTED:_____ DOSING SCHEDULE:_____

          LABORATORY SERUM CONCENTRATIONS:
IV ROUTE: SERUM CONCENTRATION_____DATE DRAWN_____TIME DRAWN_____STEADY STATE: YES NO
ORAL ROUTE: SERUM CONCENTRATION_____DATE DRAWN_____TIME DRAWN_____STEADY STATE: YES NO

PHARMACOKINETIC PROFILE

ACUTE HALF LIFE($t\frac{1}{2}$):_____hours   NON-ACUTE HALF LIFE:_____hours

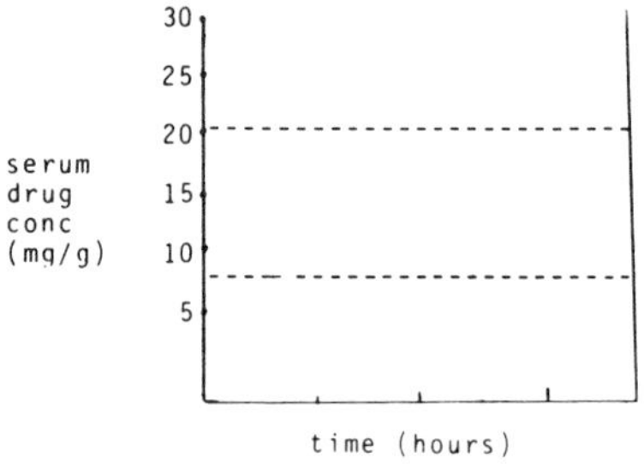

serum
drug
conc
(mq/g)

time (hours)

FACTORS CONSIDERED IN CALCULATIONS:
ACTUAL BODY WEIGHT:_____LEAN BODY WEIGHT:_____HEIGHT:_____AGE:___SEX:___
TEMP.:_____HGB:_____BLOOD pH:_____
CURRENT DIAGNOSIS:_____

PULM. EDEMA:	YES	NO	N/R	EXTENT:_____
CHF:	YES	NO	N/R	EXTENT:_____
HEPATITIS	YES	NO	N/R	EXTENT:_____
CIRRHOSIS	YES	NO	N/R	EXTENT:_____
PNEUMONIA	YES	NO	N/R	EXTENT:_____
OBESITY	YES	NO	N/R	EXTENT:_____
SMOKING	YES	NO	CIGS/DAY:_____	HX OF SMOKING: YES NO
ALCOHOL	YES	NO	QUANTITY:_____	

THEOPHYLLINE PRODUCT USED AT HOME:_____

FIG. 3. Theophylline prediction and recommendation form. Usual therapeutic serum concentrations are between 8 and 20 mcg/ml, but certain patients respond to lower concentrations (e.g., 5–8 mcg/ml).

DATE TIME COLLECTED	LOG NUMBER	DATE AND TIME SPECIMEN RECEIVED IN LAB	
		SUGGESTED SAMPLE TIME:	
RESULTS	NORMAL VALUES		
		TEST	HOUSE STAFF
ug/ml		PHENOBARBITAL	
ug/ml		PHENYTOIN (DILANTIN)[R]	ATTENDING
ug/ml		PRIMIDONE (MYSOLINE)[R]	
ug/ml		CARBAMAZEPINE (TEGRETOL)[R]	MEDICAL STUDENT
ug/ml		ETHOSUXIMIDE (ZARONTIN)[R]	
ug/ml		THEOPHYLLINE	DIAGNOSIS
ug/ml		QUINIDINE	
ug/ml		PROCAINAMIDE (PRONESTYL)[R]	
ug/ml		NAPA	
ug/ml		THIOCYANATE	
ug/ml		GENTAMICIN	
ug/ml		PROPRANOLOL	
	MISC TESTS		
			LAB COMMENT ☐ STAT

AGE   WEIGHT   HEIGHT

INPATIENT ?   OUTPATIENT ?

LAST DOSE

DRUG   DATE/TIME   DOSE

MEDICATION HISTORY

PERTINENT LAB DATA

COMMENTS

REFER ALL QUESTIONS TO 474-4100 x251

called by _____, date _____ tech_____

received by _____, date completed _____

FIG. 4. Multiple drug prediction and recommendation form.

or laboratory technicians in both research and service activities, unless the volume of work in each area is quite small. Attempting to do so will generally put the two activities in competition at any given time and tend to decrease the responsiveness of the laboratory to the clinical situation. However, it is certainly possible to conduct both service and research activities once defined personnel and equipment commitments to each of these areas have been made.

Independent or Hospital-Shared Facilities

It must be decided whether the pharmacokinetics laboratory is to be physically and/or fiscally separate from the hospital and is to provide its services on a contractual basis (independent) or is to be developed as a part of the pathology, clinical chemistry, or some other hospital department (shared). Advantages and disadvantages exist in both arrangements, and the optimal choice in a given situation will depend on the interplay of several factors. Advantages of independent facilities include the following:

1. Control and direction of the laboratory can more easily rest with an individual specifically trained in pharmacokinetics and/or analytical chemistry. It may, therefore, be easier to develop laboratory policies and procedures sensitive to the unique needs of the clinicans incorporating pharmacokinetics into their practice.

2. There may be concrete financial incentives to see that the laboratory performs acceptably and provides a real service. If it is fiscally independent of the hospital, monies gained from contracted patient services can probably be more easily fed back into the laboratory to facilitate its growth and increase its spectrum of activities.

3. If appropriate, the activities of the laboratory can probably be more easily incorporated into the teaching programs of the university.

Disadvantages of independent facilities include the following:

1. Start-up costs in developing a specialty drug-assay laboratory are considerable. At least $30,000 to $75,000 will have to be spent before even the simplest laboratory can initiate activity, an amount of money that may be difficult for the average clinical pharmacy, clinical pharmacology, or clinical chemistry program to raise initially.

2. Overhead costs may be higher in that rent and utilities may have to be paid and accounts receivable and payable must be managed.

3. A liability for financial losses exists if the laboratory does not generate enough income to balance expenditures.

4. A laboratory physically separated from the institution it serves may be less responsive to clinical needs.

5. The laboratory must be able to stand alone and will not have the strength of a pathology department to draw on: (a) It will not have any major financial "loss leaders." (b) Many state regulations require that clinical laboratories be directed by a pathologist. (However, changes in New York State law allow a doctor with a Pharm.D. or Ph.D. to be the acting laboratory director of a special therapeutic substances monitoring service within a hospital or institution. California allows an

individual with a doctorate in toxicology or related science to become a director of a clinical laboratory. These two changes may set the pace for further direction of CPLs.) (c) It will have to independently assume medico-legal liability and be insured accordingly.

Conversely, the advantages of hospital-shared facilities include potentially reduced overhead costs, possibly a lesser need to financially break even, and the collective strengths of the department of pathology. The disadvantages include a potential loss of control in the laboratory's direction and thrust, loss of financial incentives, and possibly more complex affiliation agreements between university and institution if joint college-hospital ventures are planned.

Level of Service

Presumably, a specialty pharmacokinetics laboratory will be developed in order to provide a higher level of service than already exists in the community. Decisions must be made regarding the drugs to be assayed, the hours the laboratory is to be open, the availability of stat services, and turnaround time.

A formal and informal "marketing survey" can be used to identify those drug assays that should be provided. Although specialty needs must exist within a particular institution or locale, the drugs phenytoin, phenobarbital, theophylline, digoxin, and the aminoglycosides (Table 3) provide the core of commonly ordered tests on which the financial solvency of the laboratory will usually be based (7). Although the numbers of Table 3 represent a major teaching institution, the percentages of specific drugs assayed are very similar to those in the average 200- to 300-bed hospital.

Routine hours of operation of the laboratory must be determined. Is the laboratory to be opened the basic 5-day 40-hr week, or are night and/or weekend services to be available? If these latter services are to be provided, can it be effectively done with a technician on call, or must someone be constantly present in the laboratory? If the technician is on call, what system will exist to prevent abuse and unnecessary "stat" specimens? Will the laboratory close on holidays? An effective clinical laboratory must be able to provide its services on a stat basis on those occasions when an immediate need truly exists. In actuality, however, this need is not common, and not all assays need to be available on a stat basis (i.e., theophylline, for which there may be an immediate need to know, versus gentamicin, for which a stat level is probably never indicated). In general, a stat level may be warranted when immediate therapy is dictated by the drug level when clinical assessment of the patient cannot allow one to estimate the drug concentration and when the drug has a narrow therapeutic index.

Turnaround time, that is, elapsed time from specimen arrival to availability of results, must be in line with the clinical need for information. Test results for routine analyses should be available on the same day that the specimen is obtained. Although special circumstances may exist in individual settings, a basic 40-hr week for laboratory operations will serve almost all clinical needs quite adequately.

TABLE 3. *Drugs for which routine plasma level determinations were available at UCSF during 1981*

Drug	Number of assays requested in 1981	Assay method[a]	Clinically significant metabolites	Percentage of drug excreted unchanged in urine	Usual therapeutic serum levels
Acetaminophen	45	HPLC	S-Conjugates (overdose)	<5	NA[b]
Carbamazepine	260	HPLC	10,11-Epoxide	<5	4–12 μg/ml
Digoxin	1,668	RIA		60–80	0.8–2.4 ng/ml
Ethosuximide	25	HPLC		10–20	40–100 μg/ml
Gentamicin	221	RIA, HPLC		>96	4–12 μg/ml
Isoniazid	58	COL	N-Acetylisoniazid		NA
Lidocaine	49	GC	N-Desethyllidocaine	<5	1.5–6 μg/ml
Lithium	1,013	AA		>95	0.6–1.2 mEq/liter
Methotrexate	236	PBA, HPLC	7-Hydroxymethotrexate	90	NA
Phenobarbital	626	HPLC		20–50	10–40 μg/ml
Phenytoin	1,464	HPLC	4'-OH-Phenytoin	<5	10-20 μg/ml
Primidone	15	HPLC	Phenobarbital, phenylethyl-malondiamide	20–50	5–10 μg/ml (10–40 μg/ml phenobarbital)
Procainamide	465	HPLC	N-Acetylprocainamide	40–55	4–10 μg/ml
Propranolol	48	HPLC	4-OH-Propranolol	<5	20–80 ng/ml
Quinidine	288	HPLC	3-OH-Quinidine; further metabolites (?)	<20	1–5 μg/ml
Salicylate	255	COL		3–20	15–30 mg/dl
Sulfonamides	18	COL			
Theophylline	2,664	HPLC		<15	5–20 μg/ml
Tobramycin	1,027	HPLC		>96	4–12 μg/ml

[a]HPLC, high-performance liquid chromatography; RIA, radioimmunoassay; COL, colorimetry; AA, atomic absorbance; PBA, protein binding assay; GC, gas chromatography.
[b]NA, not applicable.
Adapted from Sadee and Beelen (7).

Assay Methods, Equipment, and Space

Once the level of service to be provided has been determined, appropriate assay methods may be chosen. Numerous drug assay methods are available; Table 4 provides examples available as of 1980 (7). The decision to use a particular method should consider the number of specimens anticipated, the possible interference in method, the time required per specimen, and its cost, reproducibility, and reliability. The ability to hold specimens and provide a single daily (or occasionally weekly or semiweekly) run of the assay is an important way to reduce costs and time spent per individual test. One should also consider the degree to which the method is technician-dependent; results are likely to vary from one operator to another or from day-to-day because of subtle technician variability. Obviously, such a method should be avoided. For internal quality control, it is advisable to provide technicians with a known drug of known concentration on a twice-monthly basis and have them measure it with their routine daily samples. It is also a good idea to unexpectedly provide spiked samples as if they were patient samples from the wards. Lastly, the shelf-life of the method's reagents should be contrasted with their expected rate of utilization to minimize wastage. An assay method that is inexpensive on an individual-run basis may become very expensive if it uses a reagent with a short shelf-life, most of which must be discarded because of a low rate of utilization.

Equipment and methods already at hand often dictate the procedures to be used. As a general rule, however, if a low assay volume is anticipated within the laboratory, HPLC methods are probably preferred, whereas a high volume tends to make methods like enzyme immunoassay more desirable, assuming a reasonable choice exists. Considered on a single-assay basis, HPLC is relatively inexpensive in reagent costs, although time-consuming, whereas enzyme immunoassay (e.g., EMIT®) is usually more time-efficient but requires more expensive reagents. However the EMIT system does not allow one to see where any potential problems may occur (i.e., peak overlaps). Obviously, the method chosen must be reliable, and the laboratory director and clinicians must be confident in the validity of its results; selections should not be made simply because a particular method is inexpensive or easy to perform. At present, for the drugs listed in Table 4, approximately 90% to 95% can be assayed by HPLC, 70% by gas chromatography (GC), 45% by radioimmunoassay (RIA), 50% by mass spectrometry (MS), and 25% by enzyme immunoassay (EIA). For most drugs routinely monitored, EIA, HPLC, or RIA generally provides the optimal balance of efficiency, reliability, and reasonable cost for a relatively busy CPL. However, one must remember that the method of choice for a particular laboratory varies with personnel and laboratory focus. One should anticipate requiring about 600 to 900 sq ft of space to provide the CPL services described in this chapter. A good microprocessor would be an exceptional added asset.

Developing a Fee Schedule

There will be a recurring question: "Can we do it cheaper than they can?" Hospital pathology departments generally do not like to refer tests to other laboratories, and

TABLE 4. Survey of analytical techniques

Drug	Analytical technique[a]														
	HPLC	GC	MS	TLC	UV	Fluor	Col	Pol	RIA	EIA	IA	PBA	EA	Micro	Various assays
Acetaminophen	+	+	+		+		+	+							
Acetazolamide	+	+	+				+	+					+		
ε-Aminocaproic acid	+	+													
Aminopyrine		+	+	+	+										
Amphetamine		+	+	+	+	+	+		+	+			+		
Anticonvulsants	+	+	+	+	+	+	+		+	+					
Atropine			+			+	+		+						+
BCNU			+												
Barbiturates	+	+	+	+	+		+		+	+					
Carbamazepine	+	+	+	+	+		+		+	+					
Chloramphenicol	+	+	+	+		+	+	+	+				+	+	
Chlordiazepoxide	+	+		+		+	+	+	+						
Chloroquine	+	+	+	+		+	+	+	+						
Chlorpromazine	+	+	+	+	+	+	+	+	+						
Clofibrate	+	+			+										
Clonazepam	+	+	+	+				+	+						
Clonidine		+	+												
Cocaine	+	+	+	+	+				+	+					+
Cyclophosphamide	+					+	+								
Dexamethasone	+	+					+		+						
Diatrizoate sodium				+	+		+		+						
Diazepam	+	+	+	+	+				+						
Diazoxide	+	+	+		+										
Digoxin		+	+	+	+		+		+	+		+	+		
Diphenhydramine	+	+	+	+	+				+						
Doxorubicin	+	+		+		+			+						
Ethambutol			+	+			+								
Ethosuximide		+	+	+					+	+				+	
Ethynylestradiol	+	+	+						+			+			

Drug															
5-Fluorouracil	+	+	+						+	+	+		+	+	
Gentamicin	+								+					+	
Haloperidol	+	+							+						+
Hydralazine	+	+							+						
Hydrochlorothiazine	+	+							+	+	+	+	+		
Hydrocortisone	+	+							+						
Imipramine	+	+	+						+						
Indomethacin	+	+													
Isoniazid	+													+	
Isosorbide dinitrate															
Lidocaine	+									+					+
Lithium	+														
Lysergide									+						
Melphalan	+								+						
Meperidine	+								+	+					
6-Mercaptopurine	+								+	+	+				
Methadone	+								+	+					
Methaqualone	+									+	+	+	+	+	
Methotrexate	+								+	+					
Methyldopa	+	+							+	+	+				
Metronidazole	+								+	+	+			+	+
Morphine	+	+							+	+				+	
Nicotine								+							
Nitrofurantoin	+							+	+						
Oxazepam	+							+							
Penicillin	+								+						
Phencyclidine	+								+	+	+				
Phenylbutazone	+	+							+	+					
Phenytoin	+	+							+	+					
Primidone	+								+						
Procainamide	+	+							+						
Procarbazine	+														
Propoxyphene	+						+		+	+					
Propranolol	+	+					+		+						
Quinidine							+		+						
Reserpine							+								
Salicylic acid	+						+		+						

(continued)

TABLE 4. (continued)

Drug	Analytical technique[a]														
	HPLC	GC	MS	TLC	UV	Fluor	Col	Pol	RIA	EIA	IA	PBA	EA	Micro	Various assays
Spironolactone	+					+									
Succinylcholine	+	+	+												
Sulfonamides	+	+		+		+	+								
Tetracyclines	+					+	+							+	+
Tetrahydrocannabinol	+	+	+	+					+						
Theophylline	+	+	+		+					+					
Tolbutamide		+								+	+				
Valproic acid		+					+								
Warfarin	+	+			+	+									+
Total number of assays	52	58	40	24	22	26	26	10	29	17	5	4	6	8	5
Percent of listed drugs	70	77	53	32	29	35	35	13	39	23	7	5	8	11	7

[a]High-performance liquid chromatography (HPLC); gas chromatography (GC); mass spectrometry (MS); thin-layer chromatography (TLC); ultraviolet spectrophotometry (UV); fluorescence (Fluor); colorimetry (Col); polarography (Pol); radioimmunoassay (RIA); enzyme immunoassay (EIA); other immunoassays (IA); protein binding assays (PBA) (excluding immunoassays); enzymatic assays (EA); microbiological assays (Micro).
From Sadee and Beelen (7), with permission.

if they believe the test can be performed internally for almost the same cost, they would prefer to do so. As commercial technology advances and hospital laboratories begin to perform these tests for reasonable cost at relative ease, it may become increasingly difficult for the low- or moderate-volume independent pharmacokinetics laboratory to survive. Unfortunately, considerations of turnaround time or pharmacokinetic expertise may take on secondary importance for the laboratory director or hospital administrator who must balance the budget.

Simplistically put, the cost of performing an individual test is determined by summing equipment, personnel, supply, and overhead expenditures for a given period of time and dividing that amount by the number of assays performed in the same time interval. The fee charged, then, is determined by the test's cost and some predetermined amount of desired profit (which could be zero if private enterprise is not the goal).

Calculation of equipment costs should not only include their initial purchase price but also allow for replacement and purchase of backup items. Vulnerable pieces (i.e., lamps, printers, columns, etc.) should be kept on hand so that down-time is obviated or minimized. In circumstances where this is not economically feasible, it is wise to be in contact with places where equipment may be borrowed or shared if breakdowns occur. Also, one should locate a reliable manufacturer's representative who can guarantee 1- to 2-day delivery. Whereas it may be frustrating to have a research project halted for a few days because of inoperable equipment, such a delay is devastating to the activities and reputation of a service laboratory and cannot be tolerated.

Personnel costs should include technicians, secretarial support, and the laboratory's director, although the latter two need not be included in the service budget if they can be supported by other sources (i.e., university or hospital department). Importantly, technician needs will exceed 1.0 full time equivalent (FTE), even if the laboratory is open only 40 hr per week, because allowance must be made for vacations, sick leave, and holidays. The service laboratory obviously cannot suspend operation just because its technician is ill or is on vacation; an alternative is to have the laboratory's director act as the second backup to provide these technical services. This allows the laboratory director to be occasionally involved in these services, the better to appreciate current needs, level of service, etc. This may be of greater importance in setting up the CPL, as contrasted to the situation once it is running smoothly. At least 1.2 technician FTEs should be committed to service activities, with all technicians equally familiar with the CPL's procedures and assay methods.

Supply costs include assay kits, reagents, glassware, etc., but one should also consider reagent or kit shelf-life, anticipated rate of use, and expected wastage. The costs of discarded unused materials should be incorporated into calculation of operating expenses. Overhead includes not only such items as rent, utilities, and employee fringe benefits but also expenditures necessitated in maintaining the laboratory's quality-control procedures. Annual inflationary adjustments should be considered in these calculations.

The foregoing calculations may produce an unreasonably expensive fee (although a high fee for unique tests requiring special methods may not be unreasonable). If this occurs, there are three possibilities: costs must be reduced, or the number of assays must be increased, or additional sources of income must be found. For example, can equally reliable but less expensive assay methods be used? Can overhead costs be reduced by sharing facilities? Can personnel costs be reduced? Has too high a goal been set for the level of service of the laboratory? Are the hours of operation needlessly extensive? Are too many "low-volume assays" with high attendant costs being proposed and consuming the laboratory's resources? Can samples be held for batch analysis and still be sensitive to the needs of the clinician? Can the volume of assays be increased by dealing with a greater number of institutions? Can the laboratory generate income by providing analysis services to clinical investigators? Can fees for pharmacokinetic consultations be used to support the laboratory? And, lastly, is the university willing to support the service activities of the laboartory (e.g., salary of director, secretarial support, overhead) because it benefits their teaching programs?

Quality Control

Quality control in this setting refers not only to evaluation of assay methods but also to the entire sampling, data reporting, and interpretation processes (see Chapter 21). Within individual states, a bureau of laboratories will specify certain quality-control procedures for assay methods. Contractual quality-control services are available through such organizations as the College of American Pathologists, but it must be the responsibility of drug assay laboratories to develop their own internal programs. It is control over the sampling and data interpretation process that provides the real challenge, but this should be a major thrust of a specialty CPL.

Potential Problems

From the foregoing comments it can be seen that administrative, political, and financial problems may arise when developing and maintaining a pharmacokinetics service laboratory, especially if it is independent of the hospital's pathology department. Who is to direct the laboratory? Some states have very specific regulations in this area and require that a pathologist serve in this capacity. In laboratories housed within schools of pharmacy, a pharmacokineticist/pharmaceutical chemist is most commonly the director. We have found real value in having the kineticist/chemist serve as director and a clinical pharmacist act as associate director. This arrangement appears to offer an appropriate balance in the laboratory's direction, and it facilitates effective communication and problem solving between the laboratory, clinical environment, and institutions served by the CPL.

Political problems stem largely from the competition for provision of service likely to exist between hospitals, reference laboratories, and a specialty pharmacokinetics laboratory housed elsewhere than in the pathology department. Additionally, therapeutic drug monitoring (TDM) is a topic now actively discussed within pathology and clinical chemistry circles; it represents a real service that these

individuals, located in almost every hospital in the United States, would like to offer the practicing physician and his patients. Exactly how TDM differs from "clinical pharmacokinetics" and clinical pharmacy is not exactly clear. Early, effective communication with the hospital pathology department is needed if these problems are to be minimized. If the pharmacokinetics laboratory is administratively located within the school of pharmacy, the school's affiliation agreement with the institution should make specific reference to the level of service provided by the laboratory and the understanding it has with the pathology department.

Developing a pharmacokinetics service laboratory is a relatively expensive proposition requiring considerable expenditure before any income is expected. Also, as with most specialty laboratory services, its volume is relatively low and ongoing costs relatively high. Therefore, reliance on a single health care institution to maintain financial stability is often impossible, and the service must be sold to the community. Also a very real potential for conflict of interest exists when clinical pharmacy practitioners have a stimulus to generate specimens to maintain the activities of the laboratory or support a pharmacokinetic consultation program.

CONCLUSIONS AND RECOMMENDATIONS

Although a specialty pharmacokinetics laboratory can be constructed and directed by an individual competent in the discipline, such a laboratory can probably be most easily constructed by working with the hospital pathology or clinical chemistry department and developing it as a joint service of that department and the clinical pharmacy/pharmacology department. The CPL should also be available for clinical toxicology consultation. Other tasks the CPL can become involved in include (a) prospective and retrospective monitoring of therapeutics, (b) development of criteria for the choice of drugs to be admitted to the hospital formulary, (c) design and testing of therapeutic guidelines and instructions, and (d) pharmacokinetic research, e.g., metabolite identification and kinetics in health and disease states, qualitative and quantitative drug-interaction studies, placental transfer, pharmacokinetics in children, qualitative and quantitative adverse-effects evaluation, drug formulation, and bioavailability and product testing (2). Importantly, however, control of the sampling, analysis, and data interpretation processes must be under the supervision of individuals well educated and experienced in clinical pharmacokinetics.

REFERENCES

1. Young, D. S., Pestaner, L. C., and Gibberman, V. (1975): Effects of drugs on clinical laboratory tests. *Clin. Chem.*, 21:922.
2. van der Kleijn, E., Baars, A. M., Damsma, J. E., Guelen, P. J. M., Schobben, A. F. A. M., Termond, E., and Vree, T. B. (1980): Pharmacokinetic interpretation of the fate of drugs in body fluid. In: *The Serum Concentration of Drugs*, edited by F. W. H. M. Merkus, pp. 18–47. International Congress Series 501. Excerpta Medica, Amsterdam.
3. Koch-Weser, J. (1981): Serum drug concentrations in clinical perspective. *Ther. Drug. Monitor.*, 3:3–16.
4. Koch-Weser, J. (1980): Serum concentration of drugs as guides to pharmacotherapy. In: *The Serum Concentration of Drugs*, edited by F. W. H. M. Merkus, pp. 3–17. International Congress Series 501. Excerpta Medica, Amsterdam.
5. McDonald, D. M. (1980): Renal disease may increase apparent phenytoin in serum as measured by enzyme multiplied immunoassay. *Clin. Chem.*, 26:361–362.

6. Ayers, G., Burnett, D., Griffiths, A., and Richens, A. (1981): Quality control of drug assays. *Clin. Pharmacokinet.*, 6:106–117.
7. Sadee, W., and Beelen, G. C. M. (1980): *Drug Level Monitoring: Analytical Techniques, Metabolism, and Pharmacokinetics*, pp. 28–48. Wiley Interscience, New York.
8. McCormick, W., Ingelfinger, J. H., Isakson, G., and Goldman, P. (1978): Errors in measuring drug concentrations. *N. Engl. J. Med.*, 299:1118–1121.
9. Elenbaas, R. M., Payne, V. W., and Bauman, J. L. (1980): Influence of clinical pharmacist consultation on the use of drug blood level tests. *Am. J. Hosp. Pharm.*, 37:61–64.
10. Anderson, A. C., Hodges, G. R., and Barnes, W. G. (1976): Determination of serum gentamicin sulfate levels. Ordering patterns and use as a guide to therapy. *Arch. Intern. Med.*, 136:785–787.
11. Flynn, T. W., Pevonka, M. P., Yost, R. L., Weber, C. E., and Stewart, R. B. (1978): Use of serum gentamicin levels in hospitalized patients. *Am. J. Hosp. Pharm.*, 35:806–808.
12. Slaughter, R. L., Schneider, P. J., and Visconti, J. A. (1978): Appropriateness of the use of serum digoxin and digitoxin assays. *Am. J. Hosp. Pharm.*, 35:1376–1379.
13. Floyd, R. A., and Taketomo, R. (1979): Serum drug level usage review. A clinical pharmacy service. *Drug Intell. Clin. Pharmacol.*, 13:44–45.
14. Piafsky, K. M. (1980): Disease-induced changes in the plasma binding of basic drugs. *Clin. Pharmacokinet*, 5:246–262.
15. McCracken, G. H., Threlheld, N., and Thomas, M. L. (1977): Intravenous administration of kanamycin and gentamicin in newborn infants. *Pediatrics*, 60:463–466.
16. Gill, M. A., and Kern, J. W. (1979): Altered gentamicin distribution in ascitic patients. *Am. J. Hosp. Pharm.*, 36:1704–1706.
17. Sketris, I., Lesar, T., Zaske, D., and Cipolle, R. J. (1981): Effect of obesity on gentamicin pharmacokinetics. *J. Clin. Pharmacol.*, 21:288–293.
18. Mombelli, G. (1981): Anti-pseudomonas activity: Bronchial secretions of patients receiving amikacin or tobramycin as a continuous infusion. *Antimicrob. Agents Chemother.*, 19:72–75.
19. Bauer, L. A., and Blowin, R. A. (1981): Influence of age on theophylline clearance in patients with chronic obstructive pulmonary disease. *Clin. Pharmacokinet.*, 6:469–474.
20. Barclay, J., Whiting, B., Meredith, P. A., and Addis, G. J. (1981): Theophylline-salbutamol interaction: Bronchodilator response to salbutamol at maximally effective plasma theophylline concentrations. *Br. J. Clin. Pharmacol.*, 11:203–208.
21. Antal, E. J., Kramer, P. A., Mercik, S. A., Chapron, D. J., and Lawson, I. R. (1981): Theophylline pharmacokinetics in advanced age. *Br. J. Clin. Pharmacol.*, 12:637–645.
22. Vicuna, N., McNay, J. L., Ludden, T. M., and Schwertner, H. (1979): Impaired theophylline clearance in patients with cor pulmonale. *Br. J. Clin. Pharmacol.*, 7:33–37.
23. Piafsky, K. M., Sitar, D. S., Rangno, R. E., and Ogilvie, R. I. (1977): Theophylline kinetics in acute pulmonary edema. *Clin. Pharmacol. Ther.*, 21:310–316.
24. Piafsky, K. M., Sitar, D., Rangno, R. E., and Ogilvie, R. I. (1977): Disposition of theophylline in patients with hepatic cirrhosis. *N. Engl. J. Med.*, 296:1495–1497.
25. Scott, P. H., Tabachneck, E., MacLeod, S., and Correia, J. (1981): Sustained-release theophylline for childhood asthma: Evidence for circadian variation of theophylline pharmacokinetics. *J. Pediatr.*, 99:476.
26. Resar, R. K., Walson, P. D., Fritz, W. L., Perry, D. F., and Barbee, R. A. (1970): Kinetics of theophylline; variability and effect of arterial pH in chronic obstructive lung disease. *Chest*, 76:11–16.
27. Jenne, J., Nagasawa, R., McHugh, R., MacDonald, F., and Wyse, E. (1975): Decreased theophylline half-life in cigarette smokers. *Life Sci.*, 17:195–198.
28. Kappas, A., Alvares, A. P., Anderson, K. E., Pantuck, E. J., Pantuck, C. B., Change, M. S., and Conney, A. H. (1978): Effect of charcoal-broiled beef on antipyrine and theophylline metabolism. *Clin. Pharmacol. Ther.*, 23:445–450.
29. Vozeh, S., Powell, J. R., Riegelman, S., Costello, J. F., Sheiner, L. B., and Hopewell, P. C. (1978): Changes in theophylline clearance during acute illness. *J.A.M.A.*, 240:1882–1884.
30. Lawey, C. H. (1977): Theophylline in liver disease. *N. Engl. J. Med.*, 297:1122–1124.
31. Noone, P., Beale, D. F., Pollach, S. S., Perera, M. R., Amirak, I. D., Fernando, O. N., and Moorhead, J. F. (1978): Monitoring aminoglycosides use in patients with severely impaired renal function. *Br. Med. J.*, 2:470–474.
32. Burkle, W. S. (1981): Comparative evaluation of the aminoglycoside antibiotics for systemic use. *Drug. Intell. Clin. Pharmacol.*, 15:847–862.

33. Barza, M., and Scheife, R. T. (1977): Drug therapy reviews. Part 4. Aminoglycosides. *Am. J. Hosp. Pharm.*, 34:723–737.
34. Pechere, J. C., and Dugal, R. (1979): Clinical pharmacokinetics of aminoglycoside antibiotics. *Clin. Pharmacokinet.*, 4:170–199.
35. Benet, L. Z., and Sheiner, L. B. (1980): Appendix II. Design and optimization of dosage regimens; pharmacokinetic data. In: *The Pharmacological Basis of Therapeutics*, 6th ed., edited by A. G. Gilman, L. S. Goodman, and A. Gilman, pp. 1675–1737. Macmillan, New York.
36. Massoud, N. (1981): Update on the treatment of bacterial urinary tract infection. *Drug. Intell. Clin. Pharmacol.*, 15:738–750.
37. Chung, M., Schrogie, J. J., and Symchowicz, S. (1981): Pharmacokinetic study of sisomicin in human. *J. Pharmacokinet. Biopharm.*, 9:535–551.
38. Friedman, R. B., Anderson, R. E., Entine, S. M., and Hirshberg, S. B. (1980): Effects of diseases on clinical laboratory tests. *Clin. Chem.*, 26:86–87D.
39. Yosselson-Superstine, S. (1982): Drug interference with clinical tests performed by a 20-channel computerized autoanalyzer. *Am. J. Hosp. Pharm.*, 39:848–849.
40. Saah, A. J., Koch, T. R., and Drusano, G. L. (1982): Cefoxitin falsely elevates creatinine levels. *J.A.M.A.*, 247:205–206.
41. Krupp, M. A., and Chatton, M. J. (1982): *Current Medical Diagnosis and Treatment*, p. 1053. Lange Medical Publications, Los Altos, CA.
42. Kampmann, J. P., and Hanson, J. M. (1981): Glomerular filtration rate and creatinine clearance. *Br. J. Clin. Pharmacol.*, 12:7–14.
43. Burry, H. C., and Dieppe, P. A. (1976): Apparent reduction of endogenous creatinine by salicylate treatment. *Br. Med. J.*, 2:16–17.
44. Kijima, Y., Sasaoka, T., Kanayama, M., and Kubota, S. (1977): L-dopa effects on renal function. *N. Engl. J. Med.*, 297:112–113.

APPENDIXES

In the appendixes to follow pharmacokinetic values are provided from a number of original and review articles. The values in the tables have been obtained from healthy adult subjects. In many instances specific disease or physiological alterations are provided in the previous chapters. However, even in healthy volunteers the mean values (± the standard deviation) may not always account for a particular patient, as depicted in the figure below. One must remember:

1. The pharmacokinetic values provided are the best we have to date and may therefore change with time as we gain knowledge.
2. If the observed patient's pharmacokinetic parameters are not consistent with the literature, perhaps one should then further evaluate the possible mechanisms for the differences.

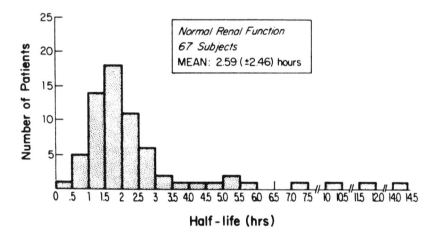

The half-life of amikacin is illustrated for 67 patients who had a normal serum creatinine. (From Zaske, D. E. (1980): Aminoglycosides. In: *Applied Pharmacokinetics, Principles of Therapeutic Drug Monitoring*, edited by W. E. Evans, J. J. Schentag, and W. J. Jusko. Applied Therapeutics. San Francisco, with permission.)

Appendix A: Theophylline Pharmacokinetics

TABLE 1. *Theophylline pharmacokinetics (therapeutic concentration 5–20 µg/ml)**

Factors	Age (mean ± SD) (years)	No. of patients	V_d (liter/kg)	Clearance (mean ± SD) (ml/min/kg)	Half-life (mean ± SD) (hr)	Ref.
Age						
Premature neonates with apnea[a]	7.5 ± 4.4 days	6	0.72–2.82	0.29 ± 0.10	30 ± 6.5	1
Infants under 6 months	41 ± 12 days	8		0.64 ± 0.30	20 ± 5.3	2
	12 ± 4 weeks	8		Incomplete data	14 ± 4	3
	18 ± 2 weeks	3		0.8 ± 0.1	6.9 ± 1.0	4
Infants 6–11 months	34 ± 10 weeks	4		2.0 ± 0.5	4.6 ± 1.2	4
	34 ± 7 weeks	5		Incomplete data	3.7 ± 1.0	5
Young children 1–4 years	2.5 ± 0.9	10		1.7 ± 0.6	3.4 ± 1.1	6
Older children						
4–12 years	9.4 ± 3	17		1.5 ± 0.4	Not measured	7
13–15 years	14 ± 0.8	6		0.8 ± 0.2	Not measured	7
16–17 years	10.7 ± 2.6	30		1.4 ± 0.6	3.7 ± 1.1	8
Adults						
Otherwise healthy nonsmoking asthmatics	31 ± 10	16		0.65 ± 0.19	8.7 ± 2.2	9
Healthy nonsmoking volunteers	22–35	19		0.82 ± 0.35	8.1 ± 2.4	10
Healthy nonsmoking volunteers	20–32	15	0.47 ± 0.08	0.67 ± 0.13	8.2 ± 1.2	11
Young students	19–31 (23)	14	V_d unbound (1.38 ± 0.23)	35 ± 12 ml/min 113 ± 40 ml/min (unbound)	8.5 ± 2.5	15 15
Elderly						
Ambulatory	70–85 (76)	14	V_d unbound (0.86 ± 0.14)	30 ± 10 ml/min 80 ± 30 ml/min (unbound)	9.8 ± 4.0	15
COPD smokers	64–79 (70.5)	6		1.04 ± 0.26		12
COPD smokers with CHF	64–81 (70.1)	10		0.47 ± 0.22		12
Nonsmokers with normal cardiac, liver, and renal function	67.0 ± 5.7	9		0.59 ± 0.07	7.4 ± 1.1	13
Single dose study	53–72 (64)	12	0.53 ± 0.12	0.69 ± 0.24	9.5 ± 1.0	14
Abnormal physiology[b]						
Fever associated with acute viral upper respiratory tract illness	9–15	6 (during illness) (1 month later)		Not measured Not measured	7.0 ± 3.0 4.1 ± 2.4	16

Cor pulmonale	64	8			Not measured	17
Acute pulmonary edema	71 ± 10	9	0.56 (0.40–0.80)	0.48 ± 0.20	22.9 (3.1–82)	18
Hepatic cirrhosis[c]	52.0 ± 8.2	9	0.785	0.041 (liters/hr/kg)	14.1 (7.1–59.1)	19
				0.43 (0.13–3.3)	32 (10.4–56)	20
				0.21 (0.1–0.6)	8.6 (5.7–12.4)	21
Obesity: overweight > 30% of IBW	23–58	14	0.38 ± 0.07 TBW; 0.77 ± 0.19 IBW	0.54 ± 0.19 TBW; 1.1 ± 0.34 IBW		
Congestive heart failure with COPD	63.0 ± 8.3	3 (acute); 3 (nonacute)	0.43 ± 0.17; 0.52 ± 0.12	0.44 ± 0.22; 1.1 ± 0.41		22
Circadian rhythm?	6–13	40			Time to peak longer when given at bedtime	23
Circadian rhythm?	50–82	12			Time to peak longer when given at bedtime	24
Acidosis	No data	12	→ pH increases Vd??			25
Smoking history						
Marijuana alone	20–25	7		1.2 ± 0.5	4.3 ± 1.2	10
Marijuana and cigarettes	19–27	7		1.5 ± 0.4	4.3 ± 1.0	10
Cigarettes	33	10		Not measured	4.1 ± 1.0	26
Cigarettes (heavy smokers)	22–31 (27)	7		1.05 ± 0.32	5.4 ± 1.0	11
Ex-cigarette-smokers (for at least 2 years)	22–39 (28)	6		0.85 ± 0.20	6.4 ± 1.0	11
Concurrent drugs						
Allopurinol (300 mg b.i.d.)	21–30	12 (day 0); 12 (day 28)	0.43 ± 0.02; 0.43 ± 0.02	0.59 ± 0.03; 0.44 ± 0.02	8.5 ± 0.4; 11 ± 0.4	27
Erythromycin	No data	5 (controls); 5 (erythromycin)	0.55 ± 0.05; 0.66 ± 0.03	0.99 ± 0.14; 0.77 ± 0.09	6.8 ± 0.6; 10.8 ± 2.2	28
Triacetyloleandomycin (TAO)	39 ± 15	8 (before); 8 (during)		0.70 ± 0.14; 0.34 ± 0.05	Not measured; Not measured	29
Erythromycin base	23 ± 2.2	8 (before); 8 (after)		0.82 ± 0.17; 0.60 ± 0.11	6.7 ± 1.9; 8.3 ± 1.8	30
Erythromycin (250 mg q.i.d.)	26–32 (29)	8 (before); 8 (after 1 wk)	0.42 ± 0.09; 0.53 ± 0.15		7.8 ± 1.7; 9.5 ± 1.4	31
Cimetidine (smoker—1 pkg/day)	71	1	↓ by 30–65%		↑ by 50–97%	32

(continued)

TABLE 1. *(Continued)*

Factors	Age (mean ± SD) (years)	No. of patients	Vd (liter/kg)	Clearance (mean ± SD) (ml/min/kg)	Half-life (mean ± SD) (hr)	Ref.
Phenobarbital	23–32 (27)	6 (before)		0.75 ± 0.35	Not measured	33
		(after 1 mo)		1.0 ± 0.5	Not measured	
Phenobarbital (6 smokers < 10 cig./day)	23–35	4 (placebo)	0.57 ± 0.06	1.3 ± 0.1	5.11 ± 0.71	34
		8 (after 2 wk)	0.54 ± 0.02	1.4 ± 0.2	5.68 ± 1.02	
Erythromycin						
Bronchial asthma	49 ± 3	15	24.3 ± 1.2 liters	2.1 ± 0.2	8.7 ± 0.6	43
Chronic airflow obstruction	65 ± 5	8	26.3 ± 1.7 liters	2.4 ± 0.3	8.2 ± 0.9	43
Metoprolol						
Smoker	24–31	6	0.39 ± 0.05	0.05 ± 0.02	5.6 ± 1.1	42
Nonsmoker	22–28	3	0.40 ± 0.03	0.03 ± 0.01	9.9 ± 1.6	42
Propranolol (smoker)	24–31	6	0.41 ± 0.04	0.03 ± 0.02	9.3 ± 2.7	42
Nonsmoker		3	0.44 ± 0.04	0.02 ± 0.01	14 ± 3.2	42
Aberrant diets						
Low carbohydrate/high protein	22–29	6 (before)			8.1 ± 2.4	35
		(after 2 wk)			5.2 ± 1.0	
Charcoal-broiled beef	22–32	8 (before)			6.0 ± 1.0	36
		(after 7 days)			4.7 ± 0.4	
Caffeine, theobromine, cabbage, or brussels sprouts					increased	37
					decreased	37

[a]Maintenance theophylline dosage of 2 mg/kg/day results in caffeine concentration of 1.0 ± 1.0 (0–3.37) (38,39).

[b]Hypoxemia may partially account for noted decreases in theophylline clearance (40).

[c]Patients with a serum albumin of <3 g/dl and a bilirubin of >1.5 mg/dl have associated longer half-lives and lower clearances. In the presence of cirrhosis, patients may have higher free theophylline as a result of lower serum albumin (41).

Abbreviations: COPD, chronic obstructive lung disease; AVH, acute viral hepatitis; CHF, congestive heart failure.

*Adapted from Hendeles, L.: First North American Conference on the Effects of Disease States on Clinical Pharmacokinetics, Vancouver, B.C., Canada, October, 1980.

REFERENCES

1. Aranda, J. V., Sitar, D. S., Parsons, W. E., Loughnan, P. M., and Neims, A. H. (1976): Pharmacokinetic aspects of theophylline in premature newborns. *N. Engl. J. Med.*, 295:413–416.
2. Giacoia, G., Jusko, W. J., Menke, J., and Koup, J. R., (1976): Theophylline pharmacokinetics in premature infants with apnea. *J. Pediatr.*, 89:829–832.
3. Nassif, E. G., Weinberger, M., Guiang, S. F., and Jimenez, D. (1979): Theophylline disposition in infancy. Presented at American Academy of Pediatrics Annual Meeting, San Francisco.
4. Rosen, J. P., Danish, M., Ragni, M. C., Saccar, C. L., Yaffe, S. J., and Lecks, H. I., (1979): Theophylline pharmacokinetics in the young infant. *Pediatrics*, 64:248–251.
5. Simons, F. E. R., and Simons, K. J. (1978): Pharmacokinetics of theophylline in infancy. *J. Clin. Pharmacol.*, 18:472–476.
6. Loughnan, P. M., Sitar, D. S., Ogilvie, R. I., Eisen, A., Fox, Z., and Neims, A. H. (1976): Pharmacokinetic analysis of the disposition of intravenous theophylline in young children. *J. Pediatr.*, 88:874–879.
7. Ginchansky, E., and Weinberger, M. (1977): Relationship of theophylline clearance to oral dosage in children with chronic asthma. *J. Pediatr.*, 91:655–660.
8. Ellis, E. F., Koysooko, R., and Levy, G. (1976): Pharmacokinetics of theophylline in children with asthma. *Pediatrics*, 58:542–547.
9. Hendeles, L., Weinberger, M., and Bighley, L. (1978): Disposition of theophylline following a single intravenous aminophylline infusion. *Am. Rev. Respir. Dis.*, 118:97–103.
10. Jusko, W. J., Schentag, J. J., Clark, J. H., Gardner, M., and Yurchak, A. M. (1978): Enhanced biotransformation of theophylline in marijuana and tobacco smokers. *Clin. Pharmacol. Ther.*, 24:406–410.
11. Powell, J. R., Thiercelin, J., Vozeh, S., Sansom, L. and Riegelman, S. (1977): The influence of cigarette smoking and sex on theophylline disposition. *Am. Rev. Respir. Dis.*, 116:17–23.
12. Bauer, L. A., Blouin, R. A., (1981): Influence of age on theophylline clearance in patients with chronic obstructive pulmonary disease. *Clin. Pharmacokinet.*, 6:469–474.
13. Nielsen-Kudsk, F., Magnussen, I., and Jakobsen, P. (1978): Pharmacokinetics of theophylline in ten elderly patients. *Acta Pharmacol. Toxicol.*, 42:226–234.
14. Barclay, J., Whiting, B., Meredith, P. A., and Addis, G. J. (1981): Theophylline-salbutamol interaction: Bronchodilator response to salbutamol at maximally effective plasma theophylline concentrations. *Br. J. Clin. Pharmacol.*, 11:203–208.
15. Antal, E. J., Kramer, P. A., Mercik, S. A., Chapron, D. J., and Lawson, I. R. (1981): Theophylline pharmacokinetics in advanced age. *Br. J. Clin. Pharmacol.*, 12:637–645.
16. Chang, K. C., Bell, T. D., Lauer, B. A., and Chai, H. (1978): Altered theophylline pharmacokinetics during acute respiratory viral illness. *Lancet*, 1:1132–1134.
17. Vicuna, N., McNay, J. L., Ludden, T. M., and Schwertner, H. (1979): Impaired theophylline clearance in patients with cor pulmonale. *Br. J. Clin. Pharmacol.*, 7:33–37.
18. Piafsky, K. M., Sitar, D. S., Rangno, R. E., and Ogilvie, R. I. (1977): Theophylline kinetics in acute pulmonary edema. *Clin. Pharmacol. Ther.*, 21:310–316.
19. Piafsky, K. M., Sitar, D., Rangno, R. E., and Ogilvie, R. I., (1977): Disposition of theophylline in patients with hepatic cirrhosis. *N. Engl. J. Med.*, 296:1495–1497.
20. Mangione, A., Imhoff, T. E., Lee, R. V., Shum, L. Y., and Jusko, W. (1978): Pharmacokinetics of theophylline in hepatic disease. *Chest*, 73:616–622.
21. Gal, P., Jusko, W. J., Yurchak, A. M., and Franklin, B. A. (1978): Theophylline disposition in obesity. *Clin. Pharmacol. Ther.*, 23:438–444.
22. Powell, J. R., Vozeh, S., Hopewell, P., Costello, J., Sheiner, L. B., and Riegelman, S. (1978): Theophylline disposition in acutely ill hospitalized patients. *Am. Rev. Respir. Dis.*, 118:229–238.
23. Scott, P. H., Tabachnik, E., MacLeod, S., Correia, J., Newth, C., and Levison, H. (1981): Sustained-release theophylline for childhood asthma: Evidence for circadian variation of theophylline pharmacokinetics. *J. Pediatr.*, 99:476.
24. Thompson, P. J., Butcher, M. A., Frazer, L. A., and Marlin, G. E. (1981): Pharmacokinetics of a single evening dose of slow-release theophylline in patients with chronic lung disease. *Br. J. Clin. Pharmacol.*, 12:443–444.
25. Resar, R. K., Walson, P. D., Fritz, W. L., Perry, D. F., and Barbee, R. A. (1979): Kinetics of theophylline: Variability and effect of arterial pH in chronic obstructive lung disease. *Chest*, 76:11–16.

26. Jenne, J., Nagasawa, R., McHugh, R., MacDonald, F., and Wyse, E. (1975): Decreased theophylline half-life in cigarette smokers. *Life Sci.*, 17:195–198.
27. Manfredi, R. L., and Vesell, E. S. (1981): Inhibition of theophylline metabolism by long-term allopurinol administration. *Clin. Pharmacol. Ther.*, 29:224–229.
28. Pfeifer, H. J., Greenblatt, D. J., and Friedman, P. (1978): Effect of antibiotics on theophylline kinetics in humans. *Clin. Pharmacol. Ther.*, 23:124–125.
29. Weinberger, M., Hudgel, D., Spector, S., and Chidsey, C. (1977): Inhibition of theophylline clearance by troleandomycin. *J. Allergy Clin. Immunol.*, 59:228–231.
30. Wing, D., Prince, R., Weinberger, M., and Hendeles, L. (1981): The effect of erythromycin on theophylline kinetics. *J. Allergy Clin. Immunol.*, 68:427–431.
31. Branigan, T. A., Robbins, R. A., Cady, W. J., Nickols, J. G., and Ueda, C. T. (1981): The effects of erythromycin on the absorption and disposition kinetics of theophylline. *Eur. J. Clin. Pharmacol.*, 21:115–120.
32. Campbell, M. A., Plachetka, J. R., Jackson, E. J., Moon, J. F., and Finley, P. R. (1981): Cimetidine decreases theophylline clearance. *Ann. Intern. Med.*, 95:68–69.
33. Landay, R. A., Gonzalez, M. A., and Taylor, J. C. (1978): Effect of phenobarbital on theophylline disposition. *J. Allergy Clin. Immunol.*, 62:27–29.
34. Piafsky, K. M., Sitar, D. S., and Ogilvie, R. I. (1977): Effect of phenobarbital on the disposition of intravenous theophylline. *Clin. Pharmacol. Ther.*, 22:336–339.
35. Kappas, A., Anderson, K. E., Conney, A. H., and Alvares, A. P. (1976): Influence of dietary protein and carbohydrate on antipyrine and theophylline metabolism in man. *Clin. Pharmacol. Ther.*, 20:643–653.
36. Kappas, A., Alvares, A. P., Anderson, K. E., Pantuck, E. J., Pantuck, C. B., Chang, R., and Conney, A. H. (1978): Effect of charcoal-broiled beef on antipyrine and theophylline metabolism. *Clin. Pharmacol. Ther.*, 23:445–450.
37. Monks, T. J., Caldwell, J., and Smith, R. L. (1979): Influence of methylxanthine-containing foods on theophylline metabolism and kinetics. *Clin. Pharmacol. Ther.*, 26:513.
38. Weinberger, M., Hendeles, L. and Bighley, L. (1978); The relation of product formulation to absorption of oral theophylline. *N. Engl. J. Med.*, 299:852–857.
39. Boda, H. S., Khanna, N. N., Somani, S. M., and Tin, A. A. (1979): Interconversion of theophylline and caffeine in newborn infants. *J. Pediatr.*, 94:993–995.
40. Vozeh, S., Powell, J. R., Riegelman, S., Costello, J. F., Sheiner, L. B., and Hopewell, P. C. (1978): Changes in theophylline clearance during acute illness. *J.A.M.A.*, 240: 1882–1884.
41. Lawey, C. H., (1977): Theophylline in liver disease. *N. Engl. J. Med.*, 297:1122–1124.
42. Conrad, K. A., and Nyman, D. W. (1982): Effects of metoprolol and propranolol on theophylline elimination. *Clin. Pharmacol. Ther.*, 28:463–467, 1980.
43. Christine, R., Mathiew, M., Bah, H., Thuillez, C., Duroux, P., and Guidicelli, J. F. (1982): Kinetics and ventilatory flow in bronchial asthma and chronic airflow obstruction: Influence of erythromycin. *Clin. Pharmacol. Ther.*, 31:579–586.

Appendix B: Pharmacokinetics and Therapeutic Concentrations

1. Beta-blocking agents
2. Antiarrhythmics
3. Anticonvulsants
4. Psychiatric and antianxiety agents
5. Aminoglycosides
6. Anti-infective agents

TABLE 1. Pharmacokinetic parameters of beta-blocking agents (1–11)

Drug	Extent of absorption: % dose/time to peak (p.o.)	Extent of bioavailability (% dose)	Nature (acid or base)/pK_a	Beta-blocking plasma concentration	Half-life (hr)/Vd (liter/kg)	Clearance (ml/min/kg)/plasma protein binding (%)[d]	Urinary recovery unchanged drug (% dose)/total urinary recovery (% dose)
Acebutolol[c,e]	/1–4 hr	37 ± 12	Base/9.4	0.2–2 µg/ml	2.7 ± 0.4/1.2 ± 0.3	7/26 ± 3	40 ± 11/
Alprenolol[a,e,f,h]	≥90/1–2 hr	8.6 ± 5.5	Base/9.7	30–100 ng/ml	2–3/3.4 ± 1.2	15 ± 9/85 ± 3	≤1/≥90
Atenolol[c,e,g]	/2–4 hr	50–60	Base/9.6	0.2–1.3 µg/ml	6.3 ± 1.8/0.7	1.3 (liter/min)/≤ 5	80/
Labetalol	/1–2 hr	≈40			4.0 ± 0.5/	/50	
Metoprolol[c,g,h]	≥95/1–2 hr	40–50	Base/9.7	25–100 ng/ml	3.2 ± 0.2/4.2 ± 0.7	15 ± 3/13	10 ± 3/≥95
Nadolol[g]	/1–4 hr	34 ± 5	Base/	25–275 ng/ml	14–24/2.1 ± 1.0	2.9 ± 0.6/20 ± 4	73 ± 4/≥90
Oxprenolol[b,e,g,h]	70–95/0.5–1.5 hr	24–60	Base/9.5	40–100 ng/ml	2/1.5	0.6 (liter/min)/75	/70–95
Penbutolol[e]	/1.5 hr	≈90					
Pindolol[b,g,h]	≥90/1–3 hr	86 ± 21	Base/8.8	50–150 ng/ml	3.4 ± 0.2/2.0 ± 0.3	6.2 ± 2.4/51 ± 3	≈41/≥90
Practolol[b,c,g]	≥95/1–3 hr	≥95	Base/9.5	1.5–5 µg/ml	6–8/1.6	0.14 (liter/min)/≤10	≥90/≥90
Propranolol[a,e,f,h]	≥90/1–3 hr	36 ± 10	Base/9.45	20–80 ng/ml	2.9–0.3/3.9 ± 0.6	12 ± 3/93 ± 2	≤0.5/≥90
Sotalol[h]	/2–3 hr	≥60	Base/9.8	0.5–4 µg/ml	5–13/0.7	/54	≈60/
Talindolol	/1 hr	≈60			1.7/		
Timolol	≥90/1–2 hr	75	Base/	5–10 ng/ml	2.7 ± 0.5/1.3	6.3 ± 1.2/10	≈20/
Tolamolol[e]	/2 hr	≈30	Base/9.2		2.5/3.2	/91	
Toliprolol[e]	/2 hr	≈90	Base/		2–3/		

[a]Highly lipophilic.
[b]Weakly lipophilic.
[c]Cardioselective.
[d]A recent review of binding considerations is given by Schneider et al. (11).
[e]Active metabolites of clinical importance.
[f]Dose-dependent bioavailability.
[g]Non-dose-dependent bioavailability.
[h]Variation in plasma level greater than threefold, from oral dosing.

REFERENCES

1. Benet, L. Z. and Sheiner, L. B. (1980): Design and optimization of dosage regimens, pharmacokinetic data. In: *The Pharmacological Basis of Therapeutics*, 6th Ed., edited by A. G. Gilman, L. S. Goodman, and A. Gilman, pp. 1675–1737. Macmillan, New York.
2. Ritschel, W. A. (1980): Pharmacokinetic parameters of beta-adrenergic blocking agents. *Drug Intell. Clin. Pharmacol.*, 14:746–756.
3. Frishman, W. (1979): Clinical pharmacology of the new beta-adrenergic blocking drugs. Part I. *Am. Heart J.*, 97:663–670.
4. Heel, R. C., Brogden, R. N., Pakes, G. E., Speight, T. M., and Avery, G. S. (1980): Nadolol: A review. *Drugs*, 20:1–23.
5. Frishman, W., and Silverman, R. (1979): Clinical pharmacology of the new beta-adrenergic blocking drugs. Part 2. *Am. Heart J.*, 97:797–807.
6. Avery, G. S. (editor) (1980): *Drug Treatment*, 2nd Ed., pp. 1211–1223. Adis Press, New York.
7. Duchin, K. L., Vukovich, R. A., Dennick, L. G., Groel, J. T., and Willard, D. A. (1980): Effects of nadolol β-blockade on blood pressure in hypertension. *Clin. Pharmacol. Ther.*, 27:57–63.
8. Silke, B., John, V. A., Calvert, R. T., and Taylor, S. H. (1983): Initiation and maintenance of beta-blockade with intravenous oxprenolol. *Eur. J. Clin. Pharmacol.*, 24:7–14.
9. Wilson, T. W., Firor, W. B., Johnson, G. E., Holmes, G. I., Tsianco, M. C., Huber, P. B., and Davies, R. O. (1982): Timolol and propranolol; bioavailability, plasma concentrations, and beta blockade. *Clin. Pharmacol. Ther.*, 32:676–685.
10. Mullane, J. F., Kaufman, J., Dvornik, D., and Coelho, J. (1982): Propranolol dosage, plasma concentrations, and beta-blockade. *Clin. Pharmacol. Ther.*, 32:692–699.
11. Schneider, R. E., and Bishop, H. (1982): Beta-blocker plasma concentrations and inflammatory disease: Clinical implications. *Clin. Pharmacokinet.*, 7:281–284.

TABLE 2. Cardiac antiarrhythmics (1–18)

Drug	Extent of absorption (% dose)	Bioavailability (% dose)	Therapeutic plasma level (μg/ml)	Half-life (hr)	Vd (liter/kg)	Clearance (ml/min/kg)	Plasma protein binding (%)	Urinary recovery (% dose unchanged)
Quinidine	≥95	76	1–5 (80%) 6–8 (20%)	6.2 ± 1.8 (3–16)[a]	V_c = 0.9[f] V_d = 3.0	4.7 ± 1.8	71 ± 11	18 ± 5 (varies with urine pH)
Procainamide[e]	≥90	75–90	3.5–8 (90%) 8–12 (10%)	α 5 min[g] β 2.5–7.4[b,d]	V_c = 0.1 V_d = 2.2	11.8	16 ± 5	67 ± 8
Lidocaine	90–100	35 ± 11	1.5–6	α 9.5 min β 1.8	V_c = 0.5 V_d = 1.8 ± 0.4	12.3 ± 5.8 (↓CHF, cirrhosis, ↔ uremia, AVH)[h]	51 ± 8	<5
Phenytoin	≥95	98	8–18	6–60 (dose-depend.) (mean 22 ± 9 hr)	V_d = 0.5–0.8	0.3 at linear kinetics	88–96	<5
Disopyramide[e]	≥90	83 ± 11	2–7.5	α 2 min β 7.8 ± 1.6[c,d]	V_c = 0.13 V_d = 0.78 ± 0.26	1.3 ± 0.7	28 (4 μg/ml) 68 (0.4 μg/ml)	55 ± 6
Propranolol[e]	≥90	30	0.02–0.10	3.5–6	V_d = 3–4	6–14	90–96	<1
Mexiletine	90–100	90–100	0.5–2	10–20[d]	V_d = 5.3 ± 0.2	5	70	10
Tocainide	≥95	≥95	4–10 (90%) 10–15 (10%)	12–15	V_c = 1.0 V_d = 1.6	2.2	50	40 (20–70)
Aprinidine	≥95	85–95	1–3	α 1.7 β 13–30	V_c = 1.7 V_d = 3.7	2.6	85–95	<1

Drug								
Verapamil	≥95	22 ± 5.6	100–400 ng/ml	6.7 ± 4.3[a]	$Vc = 2.1$ $Vd = 4.0–6.5$	≈15	90	70
Digoxin[j,k]	≥80	75 ± 11	0.8–2.4 ng/ml	42 ± 19[b,d]	0.5 ± 0.18	0.046 ± 0.023	25 ± 5	72 ± 9
Digitoxin	≥90	>90	10–30 ng/ml	6.9 ± 2.7 days			90 ± 2	33 ± 15
Bretylium	Low	?[i]	0.5–1	9.8				High
N-acetylprocainamide	85	83 ± 12	9.4–19.5	(4–17)[d] 9.5 ± 3[d]	$Vc = 0.7$ $Vd = 1.4 ± 0.2$	3.1 ± 0.4	11	85
Amiodarone	High	?	0.6–3.0	18–40 days				
Encainide[e]	High	High	10–150 ng/ml	3.4 ± 2				
Ethmozin	High	High		5–13				
Lorcainide	High	Low	100–500 ng/ml	7.8 ± 2.2	6.33 ± 2.23	14.4 ± 3.3	83 ± 4	80
Nifedipine	High	65–70	25–100 ng/ml	8–12			92–98	
Pirmenol	83 ± 24		0.7–2.0	6–12				
Diltiazem	High	20	30–130 ng/ml	0.4	$Vc = 14.2$ liters	900–1015 ml/min	77–86	35

[a]Increased in liver disease.
[b]Increased in cardiac failure.
[c]Increased following myocardial infarction.
[d]Increased in renal failure.
[e]Clinically important metabolite.
[f]Vd = volume of distribution, steady state; Vc = volume distribution of central compartment.
[g]α = half-life for fast disposition phase; β = half-life for terminal phase.
[h]AVH = acute viral hepatitis.

[i]? = not known.
[j]For a recent review of the effects of disease states on cardiac glycosides, see Ochs et al. (9).
[k]Plasma clearance in ml/min/kg: with no congestive heart failure, 1.0 × creatinine clearance (ml/min/kg) + 0.8; with congestive heart failure, 0.9 × creatinine clearance (ml/min/kg) + 0.33. Volume of distribution is equal to 3.8 + [3.1 × creatinine clearance (ml/min/kg)]. (Vd in liter/kg.)

Note: Monitoring of antiarrythmic drugs has been recently reviewed by Follath, et al. (11).

REFERENCES

1. Benet, L. Z., and Sheiner, L. B. (1980): Design and optimization of dosage regimens, pharmacokinetic data. In: *The Pharmacological Basis of Therapeutics*, 6th Ed., edited by A. G. Gilman, L. S. Goodman and A. Gilman, pp. 1675–1737. Macmillan, New York.
2. Nademanee, K., and Singh, B. N. (1982): Advances in antiarrhythmic therapy. *J.A.M.A.*, 247: 217–222.
3. Opie, L. H. (1980): IV antiarrhythmic drugs. *Lancet*, 1:861–867.
4. Keefe, D. L. D., Kates, R. E., and Harrison, D. C. (1981): New antiarrhythmic drugs. *Drugs*, 22:363–400.
5. Anderson, J. L., Harrison, D. C., Meffin, P. J., and Winkle, R. A. (1978): Antiarrhythmic drugs. *Drugs*, 15:271–309.
6. Singh, B. N., Cho, Y. W., and Kuemmerle, H. P. (1981): Clinical pharmacology of antiarrhythmic drugs: A review and overview. Part I. *Int. J. Clin. Pharmacol.*, 19:139–151.
7. Tartaglione, T. A., Pepine, C. J., and Pieper, J. A. (1982): Diltiazem: A review of its clinical efficacy and use. *Drug Intell. Clin. Pharmacol.*, 16:371–379.
8. Connolly, S. J., and Kates, R. E. (1982): Clinical pharmacokinetics of *N*-acetylprocainamide. *Clin. Pharmacokinet.*, 7:206–220.
9. Ochs, H. R., Greenblatt, D. J., Bodem, G., and Dengler, H. J. (1982): Disease-related alterations in cardiac glycoside disposition. *Clin. Pharmacokinet.*, 7:434–451.
10. Vozeh, S., Katz, G., Steiner, V., and Follath, F. (1982): Population pharmacokinetic parameters in patients treated with oral mexiletine. *Eur. J. Clin. Pharmacol.*, 23:445–451.
11. Follath, F., Ganzinger, U., and Schuetz, E. (1983): Reliability of antiarrythmic drug plasma concentration monitoring. *Clin. Pharmacokinet.*, 8:63–82.
12. Bennett, P. N., Aarons, L. J., Bending, M. R., Steiner, J. A., and Rowland, M. (1982): Pharmacokinetics of lidocaine and its deethylated metabolite. *J. Pharmacokinet. Biopharm.*, 10:265–281.
13. Hammill, S. C., Shand, D. G., Harrell, F. E., Zimmerman, J., Reiter, M. J., Verghese, C., and Pritchett, E. L. C. (1982): Pirmenol kinetics and effective oral dose. *Clin. Pharmacol. Ther.*, 32:686–691.
14. Kates, R. E., Harrison, D. C., and Winkle, R. A. (1982): Metabolite cumulation during long-term oral encainide administration. *Clin. Pharmacol. Ther.*, 31:427–431.
15. Canada, A. J., Lesko, L. J., Haffajee, G. I., Johnson, B., and Asdourian, G. K. (1983): Amiodarone for tachyarrhythmias: Pharamacology, kinetics, and efficacy. *Drug. Intell. Clin. Pharm.*, 17:100–104.
16. Karim, A., Nissen, C., and Azarnoff, D. L. (1982): Clinical pharmacokinetics of disopyramide. *J. Pharmacokinet. Biopharm.*, 10:465–493.
17. Karlsson, E. (1975): Procainamide and phenytoin: Comparative study of their antiarrhythmic effects at apparent therapeutic plasma levels. *Br. Heart J.*, 37:731–740.
18. Kates, R. E. (1983): Calcium antagonists: Pharmacokinetic properties. *Drugs*, 25:113–124.

TABLE 3. Pharmacokinetics of anticonvulsants (1-6)

Drug	Extent of bioavailability (% of dose)	Time to peak (hr)	Therapeutic plasma range (μg/ml)	Half-life (hr)	V_d (liters/kg)	Clearance (liter/hr/kg)	Plasma protein binding (%)
Ethosuximide	100 ± 10	t_{max} 3–7[a]	40–100	56–60 (adult) 30 (child)	0.72 ± 0.07	1.013	<5
Phensuximide	?			5–12			<10
Methsuximide* ↓	?		10–40	2.6			<10
N-desmethylmethsuximide			10–40	36–45			
Troxidone (trimethadione*) ↓	?		>700	16			<5
Dimethadione				240			
Valproic acid	100 ± 10	t_{max} ≤ 1.5	50–150	16 ± 3	0.15–0.4 (0.13 ± 0.04 mean)	0.006	93 ± 4[b]
Diazepam* ↓	100 ± 14	t_{max} ≤ 1.5	>600 ng/ml	20–90 18 (child)	1–2 (1.1 ± 0.3 mean)	0.03	98.7 ± 0.2[b]
Desmethyldiazepam				50–99			
Nitrazepam	78 ± 16	t_{max} 1–3	30–180 (114 mean)	21–25	2.4 ± 0.8	1.0 ± 0.5 (ml/min/kg)	83–86
Clonazepam	98 ± 31	t_{max} 2–4	15–70	20–60 (39 ± 12 mean)	2–6 (3.2 ± 1.1 mean)	0.05	47–82
Phenobarbitone* ↓		t_{max} 6–18	10–40	72–120 (adult) 37–73 (child)	0.7–1.0 (0.88 ± 0.33 mean)	0.004	50–60
Methylphenobarbitone* Primidone* ↓	92 ± 18	t_{max} 0.5–8 (mean 3)	5–12	24–45 8 ± 4.8	0.59 ± 0.47	0.06	0–20
Phenylethylmalonamide							
Carbamazepine* ↓	>70	t_{max} 6–18	4–12	29–36 36 ± 15	0.8–1.4	0.2	82 ± 5
10, 11-epoxy							
Phenytoin	98 ± 7	t_{max} 3–12	10–20	17 ± 5 V_{max} = 8.4 ± 4.6 mg/kg/day K_m = 4.4 ± 1.2 mg/liter	0.5–0.8 (0.64 ± 0.04 mean)	0.02[c]	87–93[b]

[a] t_{max} = time to peak after oral administration.
[b] Decreased protein binding in uremia.
[c] At low doses when exhibiting linear kinetics.
*Has active metabolite, which is shown directly below indicated drug; ↓ indicates active metabolite formed.

REFERENCES

1. Benet, L. Z., and Sheiner, L. B. (1980): Design and optimization of dosage regimens, pharmaco-kinetic data. In: *The Pharmacological Basis of Therapeutics*, 6th Ed., edited by A. G. Gilman, L. S. Goodman, and A. Gilman. pp. 1675–1737. Macmillan, New York.
2. Hvidberg, E. F., and Dam, M. (1976): Clinical pharmacokinetics of anticonvulsants. *Clin. Pharmacokinet.*, 1:161–188.
3. Eadie, M. J. (1976): Plasma level monitoring of anticonvulsants. *Clin. Pharmacokinet.*, 1:52–66.
4. Kutt, H., and McDowell, F. H. (1980): Neurological diseases. In: *Drug Treatment*, 2nd Ed., edited by G. S. Avery, pp. 1010–1056. Adis Press, New York.
5. Merkus, F. W. (1980): *The Serum Concentration of Drugs*, pp. 65–105. International Congress Series 501. Excerpta Medica, Amsterdam.
6. Kangas, L., and Breimer, D. D. (1981): Clinical pharmacokinetics of nitrazepam. *Clin. Pharmacokinet.*, 6:346–366.

TABLE 4. *Psychiatric and antianxiety medications (1–18)*

Drug	Extent of bioavailability (% of dose)	Therapeutic level (ng/ml)[a] (9,10)	Half-life (hr)	Vd (liters/kg)	Plasma protein binding (%)
Imipramine[b]	29–68	≥45 ⎱ 120–240	13 ± 3	15 ± 6	89–94
Desipramine	33–68	≥75 ⎰	18 ± 5	34 ± 8	92 ± 1
Amoxapine		?			
Amitriptyline[b]	31–61	≥70 ⎱ 160–250	17–46	6.4–36	82–96
Nortriptyline	51 ± 5	50–150 ⎰	31 ± 13	18 ± 4	93–95
Protriptyline	77–93	70–220	78 ± 11	22 ± 1	92
Clomipramine[b]		80–100	12–84	7–20	
Maprotiline	36–67	200–300 (80–180)	21–58	15–28	88
Doxepin[b]	13–45	>40 ⎱ 110–150	8–24	20 ± 8	
Desmethyldoxepin		⎰	33–81		
Bupropion	60–80	?	10.7–13.8	19–24	85
Viloxazine	90	1–3 μg/ml	2–5	1.5	85–90
Mianserin[b]	30	15–72	14–33	35–48	90
Nomifensine[b]		25–75?	2–4	5.4–14	60–75
Trazodone	85	?	8		89–95
Zimelidine[b]	30–60		5–15		
Chlorpromazine[c]	32 ± 19	40–300 (lower for child)	23–37	12–30	95–98
Lithium	95 ± 5	0.7–1.5 mEq/liter	22 ± 8	0.8 ± 0.3	0
Haloperidol		1–15[d]	13–40	18–30	92
Clovamine		60?	6–14		
Diazepam	100	>600	20–90	1.1 ± 0.3	98.7 ± 0.2
Chlordiazepoxide	100	>700	9.9 ± 2.5	0.3 ± 0.03	96.5 ± 1.8
Clonidine[e]	75 ± 4	?		2.1 ± 0.4	

[a] For antidepressants, a response to dexamethasone test may also provide a measure of therapeutic efficacy (9).
[b] Has active metabolite.
[c] The plasma concentrations can be diminished by concomitant use of anticholinergics (14).
[d] For Gilles de la Tourette (1–3 ng/ml), for psychotic syndromes (10–15 ng/ml), for mania (2.5–4.5 ng/ml). In general, children require lower plasma levels for the same therapeutic effects (13).
[e] Has been shown to be of some benefit in acute mania (15), Tourette syndrome (16), and possible schizophrenia (17).
? = questionable therapeutic concentrations.

REFERENCES

1. Hollister, L. E. (1981): Current antidepressant drugs. *Drugs*, 22:129–152.
2. Borga, O., Azarnoff, D. L., Forshell, G. P., and Sjoqvist, F. (1969): Plasma protein binding of tricyclic antidepressants in man. *Biochem. Pharmacol.*, 18:2135–2143.
3. Asberg, M. (1976): Treatment of depression with tricyclic drugs. *Pharmakopsychiatr.*, 9:18–26.
4. Brogden, R. N., Heel, R. C., Speight, T. M., and Avery, G. S. (1978): Mianserin: A review of its pharmacological properties and therapeutic efficacy. *Drugs*, 16:273–301.
5. Brogden, R. N., Heel, R. C., Speight, T. M., and Avery, G. S. (1979): Nomifensine: A review of its pharmacological properties and therapeutic efficacy. *Drugs*, 18:1–24.
6. Brogden, R. N., Heel, R. C., Speight, T. M., and Avery, G. S. (1981): Trazodone: A review of its pharmacological properties and therapeutic use in depression and anxiety. *Drugs*, 21:401–429.
7. Findlay, J. W. A., Van Wyck Fleet, J., Smith, P. G., Butz, R. F., Hinton, M. L., Blum, M. R., and Schroeder, D. H. (1981): Pharmacokinetics of bupropion, a novel antidepressant agent, following oral administration to healthy subjects. *Eur. J. Clin. Pharmacol.*, 21:127–135.
8. Burrows, G. D., Norman, T. R., Maguire, K. P., Rubinstein, G., Scoggins, B. A., and Davies, B. (1977): A new antidepressant butriptyline: Plasma levels and clinical response. *Med. J. Aust.*, 2:604–606.
9. Carroll, B. J. (1981): Clinical applications of the dexamethasone suppression test. *Intern. Drug. Ther. Newsletter*, 16:1–4.
10. Davis, K. L. (1981): Neuroendocrine and neurochemical measurements in depression. *Am. J. Psychiatry*, 138:1555–1561.
11. Scoggins, B. A. (1982): Pharmacokinetic study of mianserin. *Eur. J. Clin. Pharmacol.*, 21:517–520.
12. Rawls, W. N. (1982): Trazodone. *Drug. Intell. Clin. Pharm.*, 16:7–13.
13. Morselli, P. L., Bianchetti, G., and Dugas, M. (1982): Haloperidol plasma level monitoring in Neuropsychiatric patients. *Ther. Drug Monitor*, 4:51–58.
14. Calimlim, L. R. (1982): Problems in therapeutic blood monitoring of chlorapromazine. *Ther. Drug Monitor*, 4:41–49.
15. Jouvent, R., Lecrubier, Y., Puech, A. J., Simon, P., and Widlocker, D. (1980): Antimaniac effect of clonidine. *Am. J. Psych.*, 137:1275–1276.
16. McKeith, I. G., Williams, A., and Nicol, A. R. (1981): Clonidine in Tourette syndrome. *Lancet*, 1:270–271.
17. Freedom, R., Kirch, D., Bell, J., Adler, L. E., Pecevich, M., and Denver, P. (1982): Clonidine treatment in schizophrenia. *Acta Psychiat. Scand.*, 65:35–45.
18. Pinder, R. M., Van Delft, A. M. L. (1983): The potential therapeutic role of the enantiomers and metabolites of mianserin. *Br. J. Clin. Pharmacol.*, 15:2695–2765.

TABLE 5. Clinical pharmacokinetics of aminoglycosides (1–7)

Drug	Desired serum conc (mcg/ml) Peak	Trough	Toxic serum conc. (mcg/ml) Peak	Trough	Serum $T_{1/2}$ (hr) Adult	Neonate	Anephric	V_d (liters/kg)	Ke determination	Plasma protein binding (%)	24-hr urinary recovery (%) (in normals, Clcr >80 ml/min)	Dialysis clearance (ml/min) H	P
Streptomycin	25–30	<4	≥10	?	2–3	7	100–110	0.26		30–35	30–90	17	
Kanamycin	15–25	<7.5	≥30	≥8	2.1 ± 0.2 or [$T_{1/2}$ = 3.1 (Cr) + 0.2]	18	27–36	0.26 ± 0.05	Ke = 0.0025 (Clcr) + 0.01	0–3	52–90	30–40	5–8
Gentamicin[a]	4–10	<2	?≥12	≥2	2–3 or log $T_{1/2}$ = −0.838 (Clcr) +2	5–11	24–48	0.25 ± 0.08	%Ke = 0.249 (Clcr) + 0.21 Ke = 0.5 (Clcr)/V_d	<10	≥90	26–48	5–10
Tobramycin[a]	4–10	<2	?≥12	≥2	2–3 or log $T_{1/2}$ = 0.1303 (Cr) + 0.649	5–9	24–48	0.31	%Ke = 0.6 (Clcr) + 4.2 Ke = 0.00293 (Clcr) + 0.0186	<10	80–90	50–60	15
Amikacin[a]	15–30	<7.5	?≥30	≥8	2.3 ± 0.4 [$T_{1/2}$ = 2.3 (Cr)$^{1.37}$] [$T_{1/2}$ = 3.3 (Cr) − 1.4]	5–8	36–48	0.21 ± 0.08	%Ke = 0.331 (Clcr) − 0.42)	<10	94	22	6.4
Netilmicin[a]	4–8	<2	?≥15	?≥2–4	2.2 [$T_{1/2}$ = 2.275 (Cr) + 2.865]	3.4–4.7	40–50	0.25	Ke = 0.002 (Clcr) + 0.017 %Ke = 0.31 (Clcr) − 0.56	<10	45	20–40	
Sisomicin	4–8	<2	?≥12	2.34 ± 0.47	2.5–3.5 [$T_{1/2}$ = 2.13 (Cr)]		45–60	0.19 ± 0.04	Ke = 0.0024 (Clcr) + 0.0034 %Ke = 0.312 (Clcr) + 3.16	0–20	40–50		
Neomycin	—	—	Less than 3% absorbed orally		2–3		12–24			?		30–50	10

[a]In adults, clearance is often considered to be equal to creatinine clearance, in ml/min. Time for peak serum concentrations after intramuscular injection is ~0.5–1 hr.

Abbreviations: Clcr, creatinine clearance in ml/min; Cr, serum creatinine in mg%; H, hemodialysis; %Ke, elimination rate constant expressed as percent hourly loss. Ke, elimination rate constant (hr^{-1}) best fit for different degrees of renal dysfunction; P, peritoneal dialysis; V_d, volume of distribution.

REFERENCES

1. Pechere, J. C., and Dugal, R. (1979): Clinical pharmacokinetics of aminoglycoside antibiotics. *Clin. Pharmacokinet.*, 4:170–199.
2. Chung, M., Schrogie, J. J., and Symchowicz, S. (1981): Pharmacokinetic study of sisomicin in humans. *J. Pharmacokinet Biopharm.*, 9:535–551.
3. Counts, G. W., Blair, A. D., Wagner, K. F., and Turck, M. (1982): Gentamicin and tobramycin kinetics. *Clin. Pharmacol. Ther.*, 31:662–668.
4. Sanders, C. (1980): The aminoglycosides: An overview. *Syva Monitor.*, 6:1–8.
5. Barza, M., and Scheife, R. T. (1977): Drug Therapy reviews: Antimicrobial spectrum, pharmacology and therapeutic use of antibiotics—Part 4: Aminoglycosides. *Am. J. Hosp. Pharm.*, 34:723–737.
6. Appel, G. B., Neu, H. C. (1978): Gentamicin in 1978. *Ann. Intern. Med.*, 89:528–538.
7. Guay, D. R. P. (1983): Netilmicin. *Drug. Intell. Clin. Pharm.*, 17:83–91.

TABLE 6. *Anti-infective agents*

Drug	Oral availability (%)	Half-life (hr)	Volume of distribution (liters)	Clearance (ml/min)	Plasma protein binding (%)	Urinary excretion (%)	Plasma conc. (mcg/ml) after: 250 mg	500 mg	1 g
Amantadine	95 (5)	9–37				90	0.5[a]		
Amoxicillin	93 (10)	1 (0.1)	29 (13)	370 (90)	18	52 (15)	3.2[a]	7–8[a]	
Amphotericin B	<10	15 (2) days	260 (30)	28 (5)	>90	<5	35 mg[b] gave 1 mcg/ml		
Ampicillin	25–70	1.3 (0.2)	26 (5)	270 (50)	18	90 (8)		2–6[e]	
Azlocillin		1.0				60–70		400[b]	
Aztreonam		1.6	12.6	25		67 (2)			
Bacampicillin		1–2.2	24.5						
Carbenicillin	<10	1.0 (0.2)	12.6		50	80 (10)			140[b]
Cefaclor	90	0.6–1.0	17 (2)	82	25	54–68	6[a]	13[a]	25[a]
Cefadroxil		1.3	10.5		<10	90–95		15[a]	
Cefamandole	96 (3)	0.8	11.2 (0.4)	218 (70)	74	68–75	1 g im 20–30; 1 g iv 70–80; 1 g iv 90–150		
Cefazolin		1.8 (0.4)	8.8 (0.2)	65 (12)	73–84	80–90			50–60[c]
Cefmenoxime		1.3				75–80			45[b]
Cefoperazone	<10	1.6–2.1	658–770	80 (20)	90	15–36			70–140[b]
Ceforanide		2.8	13.1	49	80	90		30[c]	85[b]
Cefotaxime		0.9–1.5	27	250	40	50–78			85[b]
Cefoxitin	78	0.7	11 (3)	390	65–80	80–90		40[b]	40–85[b]
Ceftazidime		1.8	16–19	138 (10)	17	88			22[c], 60[b]
Ceftizoxime	<10	0.9–1.4	18	160 (10)	48 (10)	70			67[b]
Ceftriaxone		8.0	10.7	14.2	83–96	60			41[c], 62[b]
Cefuroxime		1.4	19–20	75–96	35	80	50		150
Cephalexin	90 (10)	0.9 (0.2)	18	300 (80)	14 (3)	96			40[c]
Cephalothin		0.6 (0.3)	18 (8)	470 (120)	71 (3)	52			
Cephapirin		0.4	16		54	68	1 G im 15–20		
Chloramphenicol	80–90	2.7 (0.8)	64	250 (120)	53 (5)	5 (1)	4–8[a]	10–20[b]	40–100[b]
Cinoxacin		1–4.2			60–80	50–65		3–28[a]	70[b]
Clindamycin	85	2.7 (0.4)	46 (7)	245 (56)	94	9–14	2–3[a]	10[b]	
Cloxacillin	49	0.6	24.5		93	35–45	5–8[a]	7–14[a]	

(continued)

TABLE 6. (continued)

Drug	Oral availability (%)	Half-life (hr)	Volume of distribution (liters)	Clearance (ml/min)	Plasma protein binding (%)	Urinary excretion (%)	Plasma conc. (mcg/ml) after: 250 mg	500 mg	1 g
Dicloxacillin	50–85	0.8	6.0 (0.2)	112 (21)	94 (2)	60 (7)		15–18[a]	
Doxycycline	60–93	20 (4)	105		86 (4)	40 (4)	2.5–3[a]		
Econazole		8.5 & 81				30–40	1–20[b]		
Erythromycin (base)	18–45	1.1–3.0	50 (14)	420 (170)	72 (3)	10–15	0.18–15[a]	10[b]	
Ethambutol	77 (8)	3.1 (0.4)	105 (14)	600 (60)	20–30	79 (3)	0.4–2[a]		
Griseofulvin	95	9–24				<5			
Flucloxacillin	44–54	0.8	8.0		96	41	11–20[a]		
Flucytosine	>80	5.3 (0.7)	40		<5	74 (10)	1 g iv 15–25 1.5 g po 45–50		
Inosiplex		0.5			as uric acid?				
Interferon		2–9							
Isoniazid	5	1.2–3.0 6.5–9.0	42 (7)	135–490	0	7–29	3–5[a]		
Ketoconazole		0.9 (0.2)			99	<5			
Methicillin			30 (7)	427	28–49	88			
Metronidazole	80	6–11.5	48–56		10	8	5[a]	9–20[a,b,d]	19[a]
Mezlocillin		1.0				45–70			50[b]
Miconazole	25–30	20–25	1474		90–93	<10	oral 500 mg 0.4 iv 500 mg 2–9		
Minocycline	100	18 (4)	28 (7)	21 (8)	76	11	2.5–3.5[a]		

Moxalactam	30	2.4	90		50	40–70		1 g iv 40–100
Nafcillin		0.6–1.0	77 (21)	41	86 (2)	25	5–6[a]	20–30[b]
Nitrofurantoin		0.5			60	30–45	0.2–2[a]	
Penicillin G	15–30	0.6	14		60	15–30	1–3[a]	
Penicillin V	60				80	26	3–5[a]	
Piperacillin		1.0				70–90		
Pivmecillinam (mecillinam)		1.0					2.5[a]	
Rifampin		2.1 (0.3)	112 (14)	600 (63)	89	16 (4)	9[a]	
Ribavirin		24 hr?						
Streptomycin		2.5	17.5		30	30–80	15–20[c]	
Sulfamethoxazole	100	8.6 (0.3)	15 (1)	22 (3)	62 (5)	30 (1)		
Sulfisoxazole	100	5.9 (0.9)	10.5 (1.4)	23 (3.5)	88–92	53 (9)	60–90[a]	
Tetracycline	77	9.9 (1.5)	91–105	130	65 (3)	48	4[a]	
Ticarcillin		1.2	15	132	55–65	86	6–8[b]	
Tinidazole		12.3	44	147			110[b]	10–25[b]
Trimethoprim	100	11.0 (1.4)	130 (15)	150 (40)	70 (5)	53 (2)	2.5–4[a]	9–18[b]
Vancomycin		5–6	29	35	<10	>90		20–30[b]
Vidarabine		1.5			50		3.5–5.5[b]	

SDs given in parentheses.
[a]Peak concentration after oral dosing.
[b]Peak concentration after intravenous dosing.
[c]Intramuscular dosing.
[d]Ten to 14 for oral and i.v. dosing; 9–20 for suppositories.

REFERENCES

1. Nightingale, C H., Greene, D. S., and Quintiliani, R. (1975): Pharmacokinetics and clinical use of cephalosporin antibiotics, *J. Pharm. Sci.,* 64:1899–1927.
2. Wise, R., (1982): Penicillins and cephalosporins: Antimicrobial and pharmacological properties. *Lancet,* 2:140–144.
3. Eliopoulos, G. M., and Moellering, R. C. (1982): Azlocillin, mezlocillin, and piperacillin: New broad-spectrum penicillins, *Ann. Intern. Med.,* 97:755–760
4. Barza, M. and Weinstein, L (1976): Pharmacokinetics of the penicillins in man. *Clin. Pharmacokinet.,* 1:297–308.
5. Neu, H. C. (1982): The new beta-lactamase-stable cephalosporins. *Ann. Intern. Med.,* 97:408–419.
6. Thompson, R. L. (1977): The cephalosporins. *Mayo Clin. Proc.,* 52:625–630.
7. Polk, R. E. (1982): Moxalactam. *Drug Intell. Clin. Pharm.,* 16:104–112.
8. Guay, R. P. (1982): Cinoxacin. *Drug Intell. Clin. Pharm.,* 16:916–921.
9. Benet, L. Z. (1982): Pharmacokinetics: 1. Absorption, distribution, and excretion. In: *Basic and Clinical Pharmacology,* edited by B. G. Katzung, Chapter 3, pp. 22–34. Lange Medical Publications, Los Altos, California.
10. Chang, W. Te., and Heel, R. C. (1981): Ribavirin and inosiplex: A review of their present status in viral diseases. *Drugs,* 22:111–128.
11. Lyon, J. A. (1983): Cefoperazone. *Drug Intell. Clin. Pharm.,* 17:7–10.
12. Brogden, R. N., Heel, R. C., Speight, T. M., and Avery, G. S. (1978): Metronidazole in anaerobic infections: A review of its activity. *Pharmacokinet. Ther. Use,* 16:387–417.
13. Heel, R. C., Brogden, R. N., Pakes, G. E., Speight, T. M., and Avery, G. S. (1980): Miconazole: A preliminary review of its therapeutic efficacy in systemic fungal infections. *Drugs.,* 19:7–30.
14. Daneshmend, T. K., and Warnock, D. W. (1983): Clinical pharmacokinetics of systemic antifungal drugs. *Clin. Pharmacokinet.,* 8:17–42.
15. Ralph, E. D. (1983): Clinical pharmacokinetics of metronidazole. *Clin. Pharmacokinet.,* 8:43–62.
16. Brogden, R. N., Carmine, A., Heel, R. C., Morley, P. A., Speight, T. M., and Avery, G. S. (1981): Cefoperazone: A review of its *in vitro* antimicrobial activity, pharmacological properties and therapeutic efficacy. *Drugs,* 22:423–460.
17. Garzone, P., Lyon, J., and Yu, V. L. (1983): Third-generation and investigational cephalosporins: 1. Structure-activity relationships and pharmacokinetic review. *Drug Intell. Clin. Pharm.,* 17:507–515.
18. Aronoff, G. R., Sloan, R. S., Stanish, R. A., and Fineberg, N. S. (1982): Mezlocillin dose-dependent elimination kinetics in renal impairment. *Eur. J. Clin. Pharmacol.,* 21:505–509.
19. Bergan, T., and Arnold, E. (1980): Pharmacokinetics of metronidazole in healthy adult volunteers after tablets and suppositories. *Chemotherapy,* 26:231–241.

Appendix C: Information Pertinent in Monitoring Plasma Drug Concentrations

TABLE 1. *Information pertinent in monitoring plasma drug concentrations*

Drug (reference)	Concurrent disease states, altered physiologic conditions, or drugs altering serum drug concentrations/interpretation[a]	Comments[b]		Assay method[i]
Acetaminophen (1–4)	GI (2); geriatrics (15); Stanbio kit false concentrations with high bilirubin	Therapeutic conc. (N.A.) ↓ prealbumin levels parallel liver damage		COL, HPLC Spectrophotometric
Carbamazepine (5,6)	GI (2); interactions (11); cimetidine (↑ C_{ss}); isoniazid (↑ C_{ss})	Therapeutic conc. 4–12 μg/ml		HPLC
Digoxin (7–18,36)	GI (2); CHF (6); renal disease (8,9); geriatrics (15); thyroid abnormalities, verapamil (↓ CL, ↓ V); amiloride (↓ CL and inotropic effect); nifedipine (↓ CL); quinidine (↓ CL, ↓ Vd); quinine (↓ CL, ↓ Vd); tetracycline or erythromycin (↑ C_{ss}—change in metabolism in about 10% of patients); amiodarone (C_{ss} ↔ ↑); spironolactone (↓ CL, may result in up to 200% error in assay)	Therapeutic conc. 0.8–2.4 ng/ml Cross-reactivity with (RIA) Spironolactone (e.g., 25 mg q.i.d.) Amiloride 50 ng/ml Triamterene 0.5 μg/ml	1.4 ng/ml[c] 0.6 ng/ml[c] 0.3 ng/ml[c]	EMIT RIA
Ethosuximide (19)	Valproic acid (↑ C_{ss})	Therapeutic conc. 40–100 μg/ml		HPLC
Gentamicin[e] (20–22,37,40)	Renal disease (8,9); burns (19); Laboratory (22) caution with heparinized tubes when sampling for bioassay; incompatible with many drugs when mixed directly within same i.v. (↓ $T_{1/2}$), fever (↔ C_{ss}), third trimester (↔ ↑ $T_{1/2}$), a serum bilirubin of ≥4 mg% altered EMIT results when compared to biological assay	Nephrotoxicity associated with troughs > 2 μg/ml, polyuria, urine osmolarity, ↓ GFR, or ↑ urinary β₂-microglobulin		RIA HPLC Bioassay EMIT

Drug	Factors/Interactions	Comments	Method
Isoniazid	GI (2); interactions (11); renal (9)	If hepatitis occurs—usually within first 3–5 months of therapy (↑ bili., ↑ LDH_5, ↑ SGOT)	GC
Lidocaine[f]	Liver (4); CHF (6); renal (9); interactions (11); pregnancy (13); geriatrics (15); smoking (16)	Therapeutic conc. 1.4–6 µg/ml	GC
Lithium[g] (23–25)	Renal (8,9); pregnancy (13); geriatrics (15); chrono (12); diuretics (↑ C_{ss}); marijuana (↑ C_{ss})	Therapeutic conc. 0.7–1.5 mEq/liter[d]; renal toxicity associated with ↓ concentrating ability, nephrogenic diabetes insipidus	AA
Methotrexate (26)	Salicylates and phenylbutazone (↑ C_{ss} and free conc.); PABA (↑ free conc.); probenecid (↑ C_{ss}); trimethoprim interferes with PBA	Therapeutic conc. (N.A.)	PBA HPLC RIA HPLC
Phenobarbital (27)	Renal (8,9); interactions (11); valproic acid (↓ CL); poor solubility in i.v. solutions containing acidic medium	Therapeutic conc. 10–40 µg/ml	HPLC
Phenytoin (28)	GI (2); renal (8,9); binding (10); interactions (11); chrono (12); pregnancy (13); geriatrics (15); thioridazine (↑ C_{ss}, → CL); phenylbutazone (↑ C_{ss}); chloramphenicol (↑ C_{ss}); isoniazid (↑ C_{ss}); disulfiram (↑ C_{ss}); valproic acid, sulfonamides, salicylates (↑ free conc.) should not be mixed in i.v.s other than sodium chloride 0.9% or Ringer's lactate, with EMIT higher reported values in renal-failure patients (Chapter 22)	Therapeutic conc. 10–20 µg/ml	EMIT
Procainamide (29)	Cardiac (6); renal (9); propranolol (↑ $T_{1/2}$, ↓ CL)	Therapeutic conc. 3–8 µg/ml	HPLC
Propranolol	GI (2); liver (4); cardiac (6); renal (9); chrono (12); geriatrics (15); smoking (16); interactions (11); pregnancy (13); chlorpromazine (↔ ↑ C_{ss})	Therapeutic conc. 20–100 ng/ml	HPLC
Quinidine (32)	Liver (4); cardiac (6); renal (8,9); geriatrics (15); interactions (11); food—with slow-release form	Therapeutic conc. 1–4 µg/ml	HPLC
Salicylates	Renal (9); interactions (11); chrono (12); pregnancy (13); geriatrics (15); probenecid (↑ C_{ss})	Therapeutic conc. 15–30 mg/liter (antiinflammatory concentrations)	COL

(continued)

TABLE 1. *Information pertinent in monitoring plasma drug concentrations*

Drug (reference)	Concurrent disease states, altered physiologic conditions, or drugs altering serum drug concentrations/interpretation[a]	Comments[b]	Assay method[i]
Theophylline[h] (30,38)	GI (2); liver (4); cardiac (6); interactions (11); chrono (12); pregnancy (13); nonlinear (17); Appendix A—caution, interpretation of results by HPLC if patient on ampicillin, cephalothin, chloramphenicol, sulfamethoxazole, sulfisoxazole; many i.v. incompatibilities	Therapeutic conc. 5–20 μg/ml	HPLC EMIT
Valproic acid (32)	GI (2); renal (9); binding (10); caution with Teflon screw caps in GLC extraction step	Therapeutic conc. 50–150 μg/ml	GLC EMIT

Abbreviations: N.A., not applicable; PBA, protein binding assay; COL, colorimetric; HPLC, high-pressure liquid chromatography; EMIT, enzyme-multiplied immunoassay; RIA, radioimmunoassay; GC, gas chromatography; AA, atomic absorption; PABA, para-aminobenzoic acid; GLC, gas-liquid chromatography.

[a] Suggested chapters in parentheses for further reading.

[b] Suggested therapeutic concentrations for which 85% of patients respond with minimal side effects (see preceding tables).

[c] Measured digoxin concentrations by RIA when digoxin was not given.

[d] Ayd, F. J., (1982): Lithium mania and lithium responders. *Intern. Drug Ther. News*, 17:17–20. Ayd, F. J. (1982): Monitoring plasma concentrations of psychoactive drugs. *Intern. Drug Ther. News*, 17:13–16.

[e] In uremic patients on concomitant carbenicillin, the gentamicin half-life may decrease. Also, if the samples taken are not assayed within a given time frame, carbenicillin may begin to inactivate gentamicin within the sample tube.

[f] For two recent reviews concerning lidocaine plasma concentrations, see Routledge et al. (33) and Lopez et al. (39).

[g] For a recent review of serum lithium levels and clinical response, see Sashidharan (34).

[h] See also Slaughter et al. (35).

[i] See also Chapter 22.

REFERENCES

1. Hutchinson, D. R., Smith, M. G., and Parke, D. V. (1980): Prealbumin as an index of liver function after acute paracetamol poisoning. *Lancet*, 2:121–123.
2. Swanson, M. B., and Walters, M. I., (1981): Elimination of interference by salicylate in spectrophotometric analysis of serum acetaminophen. *Clin. Chem.*, 27:1104.
3. Bailey, D. N. (1982): Colorimetry of serum acetaminophen (paracetamol) in uremia. *Clin. Chem.*, 28:187–189.
4. Kellmeyer, K., Yates, C., Parker, S., and Hilligoso, D., (1982): Bilirubin interference with kit determination of acetaminophen. *Clin. Chem.*, 28:554–555.
5. Telerman-Toppet, N., Duret, M. E., and Coers, C. (1981): Cimetidine interaction with carbamazepine. *Ann. Intern. Med.*, 94:544.
6. Block, S. H. (1982): Carbamazepine-isoniazid interaction. *Pediatrics*, 64:494–495.
7. Shenfield, G. M. (1981): Influence of thyroid dysfunction on drug pharmacokinetics. *Clin. Pharmacokinet.*, 6:275–297.
8. Pedersen, K. E., Pedersen, A. D., Hvidt, S., Klitgaard, N. A., and Nielsen-Kudsk, F. (1981): Digoxin-verapamil interaction. *Clin. Pharmacol. Ther.*, 30:311–316.
9. Waldorff, S., Hansen, P. B., Kjaergard, H., Buch, J., Egebald, H., and Steiness, E. (1981): Amiloride-induced changes in digoxin dynamics and kinetics: Abolition of digoxin-induced inotropism with amiloride. *Clin. Pharmacol. Ther.*, 30:172–176.
10. Belz, G. G., Aust, P. E., and Munkes, R. (1981): Digoxin plasma concentrations and nifedipine. *Lancet*, 1:844–845.
11. Gustafsson, K. S., Jogestrand, T., Norlander, R., and Dahlqvist, R. (1981): Effect of quinidine on digoxin concentration in skeletal muscle and serum in patients with atrial fibrillation. *N. Engl. J. Med.*, 305:209–301.
12. Aronson, J. K., and Carver, J. G. (1981): Interaction of digoxin with quinine. *Lancet*, 1:1418.
13. Thomas, R. W., and Maddox, R. R.. (1981): Spironolactone-digoxin interaction. *Ther. Drug Monitor.*, 3:117–120.
14. Lindenbaum, J., Rudd, D. G., Butler, V. P., Tse-Eng, D., and Saha, J. R. (1981): Inactivation of digoxin by the gut flora: Reversal by antibiotic therapy. *N. Engl. J. Med.*, 305:789–794.
15. Moysey, J. D., Jaggarao, N. S. V., Grundy, E. N., and Chamberlin, D. A., (1981): Amiodarone increases plasma digoxin concentrations. *Br. Med. J.*, 1:272.
16. Achilli, A., and Serra, N. (1981): Amiodarone-digoxin interaction. *Br. Med. J.*, 1:1630.
17. George, C. F., (1982): Interactions with digoxin: More problems. *Br. Med. J.*, 1:291–292.
18. Zeegers, J. J. W., Maas, A. H. J., Willebrands, A. F., Kruyswijk, H. H., and Jambroes, G. J. (1973): The radioimmunoassay of plasma-digoxin. *Clin. Chem. Acta*, 44:109–117.
19. Mattson, R. H., and Cramer, J. A. (1980): Valproic acid and ethosuximide interaction. *Ann. Neurol.*, 7:583–584.
20. Di Piro, J. T., Rush, D. S., Record, K. E., and Bivins, B. A. (1980): Gentamicin nephrotoxicity during dosing controlled by gentamicin serum levels. *Drug Intell. Clin. Pharm.*, 14:53–55.
21. Trissel, L. A. (1980): *Handbook on Injectable Drugs*, 2nd Ed., pp. 231–233. American Society of Hospital Pharmacists, Washington, D.C.
22. Yourassowsky, E. Broe, M. E., and Wieme, R. J. (1972): Effect of heparin on gentamicin concentration in blood. *Clin. Chem. Acta*, 42:189–191.
23. Hwang, S., and Tuason, V. B. (1980): Long-term maintenance lithium therapy and possible irreversible renal damage. *J. Clin. Psychiatry*, 41:11–19.
24. Kerry, R. J., Ludlow, J. M., and Owen, G. (1980): Diuretics are dangerous with lithium. *Br. Med. J.*, 2:371.
25. Ratey, J. J. (1981): Lithium-marijuana interaction. *J. Clin. Psychopharmacol.*, 1:32–35.
26. Hande, K., Gober, J., and Fletcher, R. (1980): Trimethoprim interferes with serum methotrexate assay by the competitive protein binding technique. *Clin. Chem.*, 26:1617–1619.
27. Kapetanovic, I. M., Kuperferberg, H. J., Porter, R. J., Theodore, W., Schulman, E., and Perry, J. K. (1982): Mechanism of valproate-phenobarbital interaction in epileptic patients. *Clin. Pharmacol. Ther.*, 29:480–486.
28. Vincent, F. M. (1980): Phenothiazine-induced phenytoin intoxication. *Ann. Intern. Med.*, 93:56–57.
29. Weidler, D. J., Garg, D. C., Jallad, N. S., and McFarland, M. A. (1981): The effect of long-term propranolol administration on the pharmacokinetics of procainamide in humans. *Clin. Pharmacol. Ther.*, 29:289.

30. Weider, N., McDonald, J. M., Tieber, V. L., Smith, C. H., Kessler, G., Ladenson, J. H. and Dietzler, D. N. (1979): Assay of theophylline: Comparison of EMIT on the ABA-100 to HPLC, GLC, and UV procedures with detailed evaluation of interferences. *Clin. Chem. Acta*, 97:9–17.
31. Leroux, M., Budnik, K., Hall, J., Irvine-Meek, J., Otten, N., and Seslva, S. (1981): Comparison of gas liquid chromatograph (GLC) and EMIT assay for serum valproic acid (VPA). *Clin. Chem.*, 27:1093.
32. Spenard, J., Sirois, G., and Gagnon, M. A. (1982): The second peak in the serum levels curve after oral administration of a slow-release quinidine dosage form: Effect of food. *Br. J. Clin. Pharmacol.*, 13:752–754.
33. Routledge, P. A., Stargel, W. W., Barchowsky, A., Wagner, G. S., and Shand, D. G. (1982): Control of lidocaine therapy: New perspectives. *Ther. Drug Monitor.*, 4:264–270.
34. Sashidharan, S. P. (1982): The relationship between serum lithium levels and clinical response. *Ther. Drug Monitor.*, 4:249–264.
35. Slaughter, R. L., Green, L., and Kohli, R. (1982): Hemodialysis clearance of theophylline. *Ther. Drug Monitor.*, 4:191–193.
36. Jodestrand, T., and Norlander, R. (1983): Serum digoxin determination in outpatients: Need for standardization. *Br. J. Clin. Pharmacol.*, 15:55–58.
37. Giordano, D., Breslin, D., Kampa, I. S., and Veentra, A. (1982): Comparison of three assay procedures for gentamicin determination. *Ther. Drug Monitor.*, 4:405–408.
38. Robinson, J. D., and Steeves, R. A. (1982): EMIT: Theophylline assay at reduced cost. *Ther. Drug Monitor.*, 4:427–431.
39. Lopez, L. M., Mehta, J. L., Robinson, J. D., and Roberts R. J. (1982) : Optimal lidocaine dosing in patients with myocardial infarction. *Ther. Drug Monitor.*, 4:271–276.
40. Wagner, J. C., Misinski, J. and Slama, T. G. (1983): Falsely elevated aminoglycoside serum levels in jaundice patients. *Drug Intell. Clin. Pharm.*, 17:544–546.

Appendix D: Additional Disease States Altering Drug Pharmacokinetics

1. Obesity
2. Thyroid Dysfunction

TABLE 1. *Drug pharmacokinetics in the obese (>20–25% of ideal body weight)[a]*

Drug	Weight (kg)	Half-life (hr)	Volume[b] (liter/kg)	Clearance[b] (ml/min/kg)	Reference
Acetaminophen	>120% IBW	2.5 (2.6)			Lee et al. (2)
Acetaminophen	135 (71)	2.55 (2.76)	0.81 (1.09)	3.74 (4.55)	Abernethy et al. (3)
N-Acetyl procainamide	>60 ± 19% IBW	5.5 ± 1.0 (6.5 ± 1.0)		6.13 ± 1.84 (liters/hr/m²)[d] (9.15 ± 1.94)	Christoff et al. (10)
Amikacin	>90% IBW	2.0 ± 0.4 (2.2 ± 0.3)	0.18 ± 0.02 (0.26 ± 0.03)	1.07 ± 0.26 (1.37 ± 0.30)	Bauer et al. (11)
Antipyrine	100.3 (62.5)	15.0 (10.7)	0.46 (0.63)	0.41 (0.76)	Abernethy et al. (4)
Diazepam	101.1 (60.4)	95 (40)	2.81 (1.53)		Abernethy et al. (4)
Digoxin	100 (65)	35.6 (41.2)	10.7 (14.3)	3.28 (4.27)	Abernethy et al. (5)
Fentanyl		4.8 (3.8)	398 (L) (390)	964 (ml/min) (1116)	Bentley et al. (6)
Gentamicin[c]		1.8 (2)	0.19 (0.24)	1.22 (1.39)	Abernethy et al. (1)
Procainamide	>60 ± 19% IBW	2.5 ± 0.4 (3.1 ± 1.0)	1.64 ± 0.75 (2.22 ± 0.34)	24.7 ± 3.6 (liters/hr/m²) (22.9 ± 6.9)	Christoff et al. (10)
Theophylline		8.6 (6)	0.38 (0.48)	0.547 (1.05)	Gal et al. (7)
Thiopental	138	31.9 (6.6)	4.7 (1.4)	3 (3.5)	Mayersohn et al. (8)
Tobramycin[c]		1.8 (1.85)	0.23 (0.3)	1.48 (1.87)	Abernethy and Greenblatt (1)
Tobramycin	>90% IBW	1.9 ± 0.4 (2.1 ± 0.5)	0.19 ± 0.03 (0.26 ± 0.02)	1.11 ± 0.22 (1.43 ± 0.34)	Bauer et al. (11)
Vancomycin	111–226 (66–89)	3.2 (4.8)	43 (L) (28.9)	187.5 (ml/min) (80.8)	Blouin et al. (9)

[a]Data in parentheses indicate normal values (i.e., non-obese).
[b]Data based on total body weight.
[c]It is suggested that with aminoglycosides the volume term should be calculated using ideal body weight (IBW) + 0.4 of excess body weight.
[d]Renal clearance.

REFERENCES

1. Abernethy, D. R., and Greenblatt, D. J. (1982): Pharmacokinetics of drugs in obesity. *Clin. Pharmacokinet.*, 7:108–124.
2. Lee, W. H., Kramer, W. G., and Granville, G. E. (1981): The effects of obesity on acetaminophen pharmacokinetics in man. *J. Clin. Pharmacol.*, 21:284–287.
3. Abernethy, D. R., Divoll, M., Greenblatt, D. J., and Ameer, B. (1982): Obesity, sex, and acetaminophen disposition. *Clin. Pharmacol. Ther.*, 31:783–790.
4. Abernethy, D. R., Greenblatt, D. J., Divoll, M., Harmatz, J. S., and Shader, R. I. (1981): Alteration in drug distribution and clearance due to obesity. *J. Pharmacol. Exp. Ther.*, 217:681–685.
5. Abernethy, D. R., Greenblatt, D. J., and Smith, T. W. (1981): Digoxin disposition in obesity, clinical pharmacokinetic investigation. *Am. Heart J.*, 102:740–744.
6. Bentley, J. B., Borel, J. D., Gillespie, T. J., Vaughen, R. W., and Gandolfi A. J. (1981): Fentanyl pharmacokinetics in obese and nonobese patients. Anesthiology, 55A (Suppl):177.
7. Gal, P., Jusko, W. J. Yurchak, A. M., and Franklin, B. A. (1978): Theophylline disposition in obesity. *Clin. Pharmacol. Ther.*, 23:438–444.
8. Mayersohn, M., Calkins, J. M., Perrier, D. G., Jung, D. and Saunders, R. J. (1981): Thiopental kinetics in obese surgical patients. Anesthiology, 55A (Suppl):178.
9. Blouin, R. A., Bauer, L. A., Miller, D. D., Record, K. E., and Griffen, W. O. (1982): Vancomycin pharmacokinetics in normal and morbidly obese subjects. *Antimicrob. Agents Chemother.*, 21:575–580.
10. Christoff, P. B., Conti, D. R., Naylor, C., and Jusko, W. J. (1983): Procainamide disposition in obesity. *Drug Intell. Clin. Pharm.*, 17:516–522.
11. Bauer, L. A., Edwards, W. A. D., Dellinger, E. P., and Simonowitz, D. A. (1983): Influence of weight on aminoglycoside pharmacokinetics in normal weight and morbidly obese patients. *Eur. J. Clin. Pharmacol.*, 24:643–647.

TABLE 2. Drug pharmacokinetics with altered thyroid function[a]

Drug	"Absorption"	Half-life (hr)	Volume (liter/kg)	Clearance (ml/min/kg)	Reference
Acetaminophen	34.9 (mg/liter)[b] (36.6) '28.3'	2.38 (2.77) '2.03'	0.83 (0.81) '0.94'	4.1 (3.6) '5.4'	Forfar et al. (2)
Anticoagulants (warfarin[c], dicoumarol)	↓ sensitivity in hypothyroidism ↑ sensitivity in hyperthyroidism				Self et al. (3)
Atenolol	2.98 (μmol/liter)[b] '2.21'	4.6 '4.3'			Hallengren et al. (4)
Antipyrine		10.95 (23.6) '7.4'			Shenfield (1)
Digoxin[d]			420–1026 (liter) (492 ± 10.2) '1399 ± 88.7'		Shenfield (1)
Methimazole (via carbimazole)		3.7 '3.2'			Kampmann et al. (5) Skellern et al. (6)
Methimazole[e]	618.7 (nmol/liter)[b] '568.6'	2.96' '2.9'			Skellern et al. (6)
Metoprolol		3.9	'19.8'[f]	'92' (ml/min)	Hallengren et al. (4)
Phenytoin		14 (13.1) '17.2'	45.1 (46.6) '49.8'	33.8–42.8 (43.4) '38.3'	Hansen et al. (7)

Drug					Reference
Prolactin	45 (ml/min/m²)g (38) '52'				Cooper et al. (8)
Propranololc	43–285 (ng/ml)b '38–194' Cp_{ss} 74 ± 15 (ng/ml) Cp_{ss} '60 ± 15' (ng/ml)	4.4 ± 0.6 '3.8 ± 1.0' '2.9'	3.8 ± 0.5 '5.5 ± 0.4' '3.8 ± 1.0'	725 ± 114 (ml/min) '1193 ± 274'	Hallengren et al. (4) Shenfield (1) Wells et al. (11)
Propylthiouracil		1.14 '0.9'			Shenfield (1) Kampmann et al. (5)
Sotalol	1.57–2.61 (mg/liter)b '1.11–3.63'		'53' (liter)	'204' (ml/min)	Aro et al. (9)
Thyroid (T_3)		36 '20'	15.6 (liter/m²) (17.8) '22.6'	15.3 (liter/day/m²) (11.4) '33.4'	Shenfield (1) Woeber et al. (12)

aWhere possible the control values are given first, parentheses indicate hypothyroid and single quotes indicate hyperthyroid.

bCp_{max}.

cPlasma protein binding for propranolol: hyperthyroid '84.9%', euthyroid 87.9%, hypothyroid (89.3%), for warfarin: '99.33%', 99.46%, (99.45%), respectively (10).

dThe degree of cardiac tissue uptake and required digoxin plasma concentrations in thyroid dysfunction is still in question.

eStudy involved female patients only.

fApparent V area.

gA recent review of the clinical pharmacokinetics of beta-blocking drugs in thyroid disease is provided by Feely, J. (1983): Clin. Pharmacokinet., 8:1–16.

REFERENCES

1. Shenfield, G. M. (1981): Influence of thyroid dysfunction on drug pharmacokinetics. *Clin. Pharmacokinet.*, 6:275–297.
2. Forfar, J. C., Pottage, A., Toft, A. D., Irvine, W. J., Clements, J. A., and Prescott, L. F. (1980): Paracetamol pharmacokinetics in thyroid disease. *Eur. J. Clin. Pharmacol.*, 18:269–273.
3. Self, T., Weisburst, M., Wooten, E., Straughn, A., and Oliver, J. (1975): Warfarin induced hypoprothrombinaemia potentiation by hyperthyroidism, *J.A.M.A.*, 231:1165–1166.
4. Hallengren, B., Nilson, O. R., Karlberg, B. E., Melander, A., Tegler, L., and Wahlin-Boll, E. (1982): Influence of hyperthyroidism on the kinetics of methimazole, propranolol, metoprolol, and atenolol. *Eur. J. Clin. Pharmacol.*, 21:379–384.
5. Kampmann, J. P., and Hansen, J. M. (1981): Clinical pharmacokinetics of antithyroid drugs. *Clin. Pharmacokinet.*, 6:401–428.
6. Skellern, G. G., Knight, B. I., Low, C. K. L., Alexander, W. D., McLarty, D. G., and Kalk, W. J. (1980): The pharmacokinetics of methimazole after oral administration of carbimazole and methimazole in hyperthyroid patients. *Br. J. Clin. Pharmacol.*, 9:137–143.
7. Hansen, J. M., Skovsted, L., Kampmann, J. P., Lumholtz, B. I., and Sierback-Nielson, K. (1978): Unaltered metabolism of phenytoin in thyroid disorders. *Acta Pharmacol. Tox.*, 42:343–346.
8. Cooper, D. S., Ridgway, E. C., Kliman, B., Kjellberg, R. N., and Maloof, F. (1979): Metabolic clearance and production rates of prolactin in man. *J. Clin. Invest.*, 64:1669–1680.
9. Aro, A., Anttila, M., Korhonen, T., and Sundquist, H. (1982): Pharmacokinetics of propranolol and sotalol in hyperthyroidism. *Eur. J. Clin. Pharmacol.*, 21:373–377.
10. Feely, J., Stevenson, H. I., and Crooks, J. (1981): Altered plasma protein binding of drugs in thyroid disease. *Clin. Pharmacokinet.*, 6:298–305.
11. Wells, P.G., Feely, J., Nadeau, J., Wilkinson, G. R., and Wood, A. J. J. (1981): Propranolol disposition in thyrotoxicosis. *Clin. Res.*, 29:279A.
12. Woeber, K. A., Sobel, R. J., Ingbar, S. H., and Sterling, K. S. (1970): The peripheral metabolism of triiodothyronine in normal subjects and in patients with hyperthyroidism. *J. Clin. Invest.*, 49:643–649.

SUBJECT INDEX

Subject Index